HARRISON'S

Principles of INTERNAL MEDICINE

SELF-ASSESSMENT AND BOARD REVIEW

Editorial Board

17th Edition

HARRISON'S

Principles of

INTERNAL MEDICINE

SELF-ASSESSMENT AND BOARD REVIEW

For use with the 17th edition of HARRISON'S PRINCIPLES OF INTERNAL MEDICINE

EDITED BY

CHARLES WIENER, MD
Professor of Medicine and Physiology
Vice Chair, Department of Medicine
Director, Osler Medical Training Program
The Johns Hopkins University School of Medicine
Baltimore

Contributing Editors

Gerald Bloomfield, MD, MPH

Cynthia D. Brown, MD

Joshua Schiffer, MD

Adam Spivak, MD

Department of Internal Medicine
The Johns Hopkins University School of Medicine
Baltimore

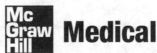 **Medical**

New York   Chicago   San Francisco   Lisbon   London   Madrid   Mexico City
New Delhi   San Juan   Seoul   Singapore   Sydney   Toronto

Harrison's
PRINCIPLES OF INTERNAL MEDICINE, 17e
Self-Assessment and Board Review

3 4 5 6 7 8 9 0   QPD/QPD   0 9

ISBN   978-0-07-149619-3
MHID   0-07-149619-X

Notice

Medicine is an ever-changing science. As new research and clinical experience broaden our knowledge, changes in treatment and drug therapy are required. The authors and the publisher of this work have checked with sources believed to be reliable in their efforts to provide information that is complete and generally in accord with the standards accepted at the time of publication. However, in view of the possibility of human error or changes in medical sciences, neither the authors nor the publisher nor any other party who has been involved in the preparation or publication of this work warrants that the information contained herein is in every respect accurate or complete, and they disclaim all responsibility for any errors or omissions or for the results obtained from use of the information contained in this work. Readers are encouraged to confirm the information contained herein with other sources. For example and in particular, readers are advised to check the product information sheet included in the package of each drug they plan to administer to be certain that the information contained in this work is accurate and that changes have not been made in the recommended dose or in the contraindications for administration. This recommendation is of particular importance in connection with new or infrequently used drugs.

This book was set in Minion by Silverchair Science + Communications, Inc.
The editors were James Shanahan and Mariapaz Ramos Englis.
The production supervisor was Catherine H. Saggese.
Quebecor World was printer and binder.

This book is printed on acid-free paper.

Library of Congress Cataloging-in-Publication Data

Harrison's principles of internal medicine: self assessment and board review / edited by Charles M. Wiener ; contributing editors, Gerald Bloomfield ... [et al.]. -- 17th ed.
    p. cm.
  "For use with the 17th edition of Harrison's principles of internal medicine."
  Includes bibliographical references.
  ISBN 978-0-07-149619-3 (hardcover)
    1. Internal medicine--Examinations, questions, etc. I. Wiener, Charles M. II. Title: Principles of internal medicine.
RC46.H333 2008 Suppl.
616.0076--dc22

                                                                        2008008340

CONTENTS

PREFACE

People who pursue careers in Internal Medicine are drawn to the specialty by a love of patients, mechanisms, discovery, education, and therapeutics. We love hearing the stories told to us by our patients, linking signs and symptoms to pathophysiology, solving the diagnostic dilemmas, and proposing strategies to prevent and treat illness. It is not surprising given these tendencies that internists prefer to continue their life-long learning through problem solving.

This book is offered as a companion to the remarkable 17th edition of *Harrison's Principles of Internal Medicine.* It is designed for the student of medicine to reinforce the knowledge contained in the parent book in an active, rather than passive, format. This book contains over 1000 questions, most centered on a patient presentation. Answering the questions requires understanding pathophysiology, epidemiology, differential diagnosis, clinical decision making, and therapeutics. We have tried to make the questions and the discussions timely and relevant to clinicians. All answer discussions are referenced to the relevant chapter(s) in the par-

ent book and often contain useful figures or algorithms appropriate to the question. We recommend this book to students and clinicians looking for an active method of life-long learning and as a resource for preparing for the Internal Medicine board examination.

We appreciate the confidence of the editors of *Harrison's,*17th edition, to allow us to do this book. We thank our families and loved ones who had to watch us pore over page proofs to come up with original questions and answers. All of the authors are (or were) affiliated with Osler Medical Training Program at the The Johns Hopkins School of Medicine. The dedicated physicians of the Osler Medical Service inspire us daily to constantly learn and improve. We thank them for their constant appreciation of high standards and their dedication to outstanding patient care. Many of the case presentations derive from actual patients we've cared for, and we thank the patients of Johns Hopkins Hospital for their nobility and their willingness to participate in our clinical and educational missions.

I. INTRODUCTION TO CLINICAL MEDICINE

QUESTIONS

DIRECTIONS: Choose the **one best** response to each question.

I-1. A physician is deciding whether to use a new test to screen for disease X in his practice. The prevalence of disease X is 5%. The sensitivity of the test is 85%, and the specificity is 75%. In a population of 1000, how many patients will have the diagnosis of disease X missed by this test?

- A. 50
- B. 42
- C. 8
- D. 4

I-2. How many patients will be erroneously told they have diagnosis X on the basis of the results of this test?

- A. 713
- B. 505
- C. 237
- D. 42

I-3. Which type of health care delivery system encourages physicians to see more patients but to provide fewer services?

- A. Capitation
- B. Fee-for-service
- C. Fixed salary compensation
- D. Out-of-pocket

I-4. The curve that graphically represents the family of cut-off points for a positive vs. negative test is a receiver operating characteristic (ROC) curve. The area under this curve is a quantitative measure of the information content of a test. The ROC axes are

- A. negative predictive value vs. (1 – positive predictive value)
- B. positive predictive value vs. (1 – negative predictive value)
- C. sensitivity vs. (1 – specificity)
- D. specificity vs. (1 – sensitivity)

I-5. A patient is seen in the clinic for evaluation of chest pain. The patient is 35 years old and has no medical ill-

I-5. *(Continued)*

nesses. She reports occasional intermittent chest pain that is unrelated to exercise but is related to eating spicy food. The physician's pretest probability for coronary artery disease causing these symptoms is low; however, the patient is referred for an exercise treadmill test, which shows ST depression after moderate exercise. Using Bayes' theorem, how does one interpret these test results?

- A. The pretest probability is low, and the sensitivity and specificity of exercise treadmill testing in females are poor; therefore, the exercise treadmill test is not helpful in clinical decision making in this case.
- B. Regardless of the pretest probability, the abnormal result of this exercise treadmill testing requires further evaluation.
- C. Because the pretest probability for coronary artery disease is low, the patient should be referred for further testing to rule out this diagnosis.
- D. Because the pretest probability was low in this case, a diagnostic test with a low sensitivity and specificity is sufficient to rule out the diagnosis of coronary artery disease.
- E. The testing results suggest that the patient has a very high likelihood of having coronary artery disease and should undergo cardiac catheterization.

I-6. An effective way to measure the accuracy of a diagnostic test is a positive likelihood ratio [sensitivity/(1 – specificity)], which is also defined as the ratio of the probability of a positive test result in a patient with disease to the probability of a positive test result in a patient without disease. What other piece of information is needed along with a positive likelihood ratio to estimate the possibility of a given disease in a certain patient with a positive test result?

- A. Disease prevalence in the patient's geographic region
- B. Negative predictive value of the test
- C. Positive predictive value of the test
- D. Pretest probability of the disease in a patient

I-7. Drug X is investigated in a meta-analysis for its effect on mortality after a myocardial infarction. It is found that mortality drops from 10 to 2% when this drug is administered. What is the absolute risk reduction conferred by drug X?

   A.   2%
   B.   8%
   C.   20%
   D.   200%
   E.   None of the above

I-8. How many patients will have to be treated with drug X to prevent one death?

   A.   2
   B.   8
   C.   12.5
   D.   50
   E.   93

I-9. A healthy 23-year-old female is referred to your clinic after being seen in the emergency department for intermittent severe chest pain. During her visit, she is ruled out for cardiac ischemia, with negative biomarkers for cardiac ischemia and unremarkable electrocardiograms. An exercise single photon emission CT (SPECT) myocardial perfusion test was performed, and a reversible exercise-induced perfusion defect was noted. The test was read as positive. The patient was placed on aspirin. She is quite concerned that she continues to have chest pain intermittently on a daily basis without any consistency in regards to time or antecedent activity. She is otherwise active and feeling well. She smokes socially on weekends. She has no family history of early coronary disease. What would be the best next course of action?

   A.   Cardiac catheterization
   B.   CT of her coronary arteries
   C.   Dobutamine stress echocardiogram
   D.   Evaluation for non-cardiac source of her chest pain
   E.   Repeat exercise SPECT test

I-10. Which of the following statements regarding gender health is true?

   A.   Alzheimer's disease affects men and women at equal rates.
   B.   Alzheimer's disease affects men two times more commonly than women.
   C.   In a recent placebo-controlled trial, postmenopausal hormone therapy did not show improvement in disease progression in women with Alzheimer's disease.
   D.   Women with Alzheimer's disease have higher levels of circulating estrogen than women without Alzheimer's disease.

I-11. All of the following statements regarding women's health are true *except*

   A.   Coronary heart disease mortality rates have been falling in men over the past 30 years, while increasing in women.

I-11. *(Continued)*

   B.   Women have longer QT intervals on resting ECG, predisposing them to higher rates of ventricular arrhythmia.
   C.   Women are more likely than men to have atypical symptoms of angina such as nausea, vomiting, and upper back pain.
   D.   Women with myocardial infarction (MI) are more likely to present with ventricular tachycardia, whereas men are more likely to present with cardiogenic shock.
   E.   Women under the age of 50 experience twice the mortality rate compared to men after MI.

I-12. When ordering an evaluation of coronary artery disease in a female patient, all of the following are true *except*

   A.   Exercise stress testing has more false positives in women than in men.
   B.   Exercise stress testing has more false negatives in women than in men.
   C.   Women are less likely than men to undergo angioplasty and coronary artery bypass grafting (CABG).
   D.   Women undergoing coronary artery bypass surgery have lower 5- and 10-year survival rates than men.
   E.   Women undergoing coronary artery bypass surgery have less relief of angina and less graft patency than men.

I-13. Which of the following statements regarding cardiovascular risk is true?

   A.   Aspirin is effective as a means of primary prevention in women for coronary heart disease.
   B.   Cholesterol-lowering drugs are less effective in women than in men for primary and secondary prevention of coronary heart disease.
   C.   Low high-density lipoprotein (HDL) and diabetes mellitus are more important risk factors for men than for women for coronary heart disease.
   D.   Total triglyceride levels are an independent risk factor for coronary heart disease in women but not in men.

I-14. Which of the following alternative medicines has shown proven benefit compared to placebo in a large randomized clinical trial?

   A.   Echinacea root for respiratory infection
   B.   *Ginkgo biloba* for improving cognition in the elderly
   C.   Glucosamine/chondroitin sulfate for improving performance and slowing narrowing of the joint space in patients with moderate to severe osteoarthritis
   D.   Saw palmetto for men with symptomatic benign prostatic hyperplasia (BPH)
   E.   St.-John's-wort for major depression of moderate severity

I-15. You prescribe an extended-release antihypertensive agent for your patient at a dosing interval of 24 h. The

I-15. *(Continued)* *See explanation*

half-life of the agent is 48 h. Three days later the patient's blood pressure is not controlled. At this point you should

A. add a second agent
B. double the dose of the current agent
C. increase the frequency of the current dose to twice/day
D. recheck the blood pressure in 1 week
E. switch to an agent from a different class

I-16. A 56-year-old patient arrives in your clinic with worsening somnolence, per his wife. You have followed him for several years for his long-standing liver disease related to heavy alcohol use in the past and hepatitis C infection, as well as chronic low back pain related to trauma. He has recently developed ascites but has had a good response to diuretic therapy. He has no history of gastrointestinal bleeding, he denies fever, chills, abdominal pain, tremor, or any recent change in his medicines, which include furosemide, 40 mg daily; spironolactone, 80 mg daily; and extended-release morphine, 30 mg twice a day. He is afebrile with normal vital signs. His weight is down 5 kg since initiating diuretic therapy. Physical examination is notable for a somnolent but conversant man with mild jaundice, pinpoint pupils, palmar erythema, spider hemangiomas on his chest, a palpable nodular liver edge at the costal margin, and bilateral 1+ lower extremity edema. He does not have asterixis, abdominal tenderness, or an abdominal fluid wave. Laboratory results compared to 3 months previously reveal an increased INR, from 1.4 to 2.1; elevated total bilirubin, from 1.8 to 3.6 mg/dL; and decreased albumin from 3.4 to 2.9 g/L; as well as baseline elevations of his aspartate and alanine aminotransferases (54 U/L and 78 U/L, respectively). Serum NH_4 is 16. What would be a sensible next step for this patient?

A. Decrease his morphine dose by 50% and reevaluate him in a few days
B. Initiate antibiotic therapy
C. Initiate haloperidol therapy
D. Initiate lactulose therapy
E. Perform a paracentesis

See expl. frostbite

I-17. A homeless male is evaluated in the emergency department. He has noted that after he slept outside during a particularly cold night his left foot has become clumsy and feels "dead." On examination, the foot has hemorrhagic vesicles distributed throughout the foot distal to the ankle. The foot is cool and has no sensation to pain or temperature. The right foot is hyperemic but does not have vesicles and has normal sensation. The remainder of the physical examination is normal. Which of the following statements regarding the management of this disorder is true?

A. Active foot rewarming should not be attempted.
B. During the period of rewarming, intense pain can be anticipated.
C. Heparin has been shown to improve outcomes in this disorder.

I-17. *(Continued)*
D. Immediate amputation is indicated.
E. Normal sensation is likely to return with rewarming.

I-18. A 78-year-old female is seen in the clinic with complaints of urinary incontinence for several months. She finds that she is unable to hold her urine at random times throughout the day; this is not related to coughing or sneezing. The leakage is preceded by an intense need to empty the bladder. She has no pain associated with these episodes, though she finds them very distressing. The patient is otherwise independent in the activities of daily living, with continued ability to cook and clean for herself. Which of the following statements is true?

A. The abrupt onset of similar symptoms should prompt cystoscopy.
B. First-line therapy for this condition consists of desmopressin.
C. Indwelling catheters are rarely indicated for this disorder.
D. Referral to a genitourinary surgeon is indicated for surgical correction.
E. Urodynamic testing must be performed before the prescription of antispasmodic medications.

I-19. All of the following statements regarding medications in the geriatric population are true *except*

A. Falling albumin levels in the elderly lead to increased free (active) levels of some medications, including warfarin.
B. Fat-soluble drugs have a shorter half-life in geriatric patients.
C. Hepatic clearance decreases with age.
D. The elderly have a decreased volume of distribution for many medications because of a decrease in total body water.
E. Older patients are two to three times more likely to have an adverse drug reaction.

I-20. Which of the following class of medicines has been linked to the occurrence of hip fractures in the elderly?

A. Benzodiazepines
B. Opiates
C. Angiotensin-converting enzyme inhibitors
D. Beta blockers
E. Atypical antipsychotics

I-21. Patients taking which of the following drugs should be advised to avoid drinking grapefruit juice?

A. Amoxicillin
B. Aspirin
C. Atorvastatin
D. Prevacid
E. Sildenafil

enzyme inhibit.

I-22. A recent 18-year-old immigrant from Kenya presents to a university clinic with fever, nasal congestion, severe

I-22. *(Continued)*

fatigue, and a rash. The rash started with discrete lesions at the hairline that coalesced as the rash spread caudally. There is sparing of the palms and soles. Small white spots with a surrounding red halo are noted on examination of the palate. The patient is at risk for developing which of the following in the future?

A. Encephalitis
B. Epiglottitis
C. Opportunistic infections
D. Postherpetic neuralgia
E. Splenic rupture

Koplik spots

I-23. You are a physician working in an urban emergency department when several patients are brought in after the release of an unknown gas at the performance of a symphony. You are evaluating a 52-year-old female who is not able to talk clearly because of excessive salivation and rhinorrhea, although she is able to tell you that she feels as if she lost her sight immediately upon exposure. At present, she also has nausea, vomiting, diarrhea, and muscle twitching. On physical examination the patient has a blood pressure of 156/92, a heart rate of 92, a respiratory rate of 30, and a temperature of 37.4°C (99.3°F). She has pinpoint pupils with profuse rhinorrhea and salivation. She also is coughing profusely, with production of copious amounts of clear secretions. A lung examination reveals wheezing on expiration in bilateral lung fields. The patient has a regular rate and rhythm with normal heart sounds. Bowel sounds are hyperactive, but the abdomen is not tender. She is having diffuse fasciculations. At the end of your examination, the patient abruptly develops tonic-clonic seizures. Which of the following agents is most likely to cause this patient's symptoms?

A. Arsine
B. Cyanogen chloride
C. Nitrogen mustard
D. Sarin
E. VX

I-24. All the following should be used in the treatment of this patient *except*

A. atropine
B. decontamination
C. diazepam
D. phenytoin
E. 2-pralidoxime chloride

I-25. A 24-year-old male is brought to the emergency department after taking cyanide in a suicide attempt. He is unconscious on presentation. What drug should be used as an antidote?

A. Atropine
B. Methylene blue
C. 2-Pralidoxime
D. Sodium nitrite alone
E. Sodium nitrite with sodium thiosulfate

I-26. A 40-year-old female is exposed to mustard gas during a terrorist bombing of her office building. She presents to the emergency department immediately after exposure without complaint. The physical examination is normal. What is the next step?

A. Admit the patient for observation because symptoms are delayed 2 h to 2 days after exposure and treat supportively as needed.
B. Administer 2-pralidoxime as an antidote and observe for symptoms.
C. Irrigate the patient's eyes and apply ocular glucocorticoids to prevent symptoms from developing.
D. Discharge the patient to home as she is unlikely to develop symptoms later.
E. Discharge the patient to home but ask that she return in 7 days for monitoring of the white blood cell count.

I-27. A 24-year-old healthy man who has just returned from a 1-week summer camping trip to the Ozarks presents to the emergency room with fever, a severe headache, mild abdominal pain, and severe myalgias. He is discharged home but 1 day later feels even worse and therefore returns. Temperature is 38.4°C, heart rate is 113 beats/min; blood pressure is 120/70. Physical examination is notable for a well-developed, well-nourished, but diaphoretic and distressed man. He is alert and oriented to time and place. His lungs are clear to auscultation. He has no heart murmur. His abdomen is mildly tender with normal bowel sounds. Neurologic examination is nonfocal. There is no evidence of a rash. Laboratory evaluation is notable for a platelet count of 84,000/μL. A lumbar puncture is notable for 5 monocytes, no red blood cells, normal protein levels, and normal glucose levels. What should be the next step in this patient's management?

A. Atovaquone
B. Blood cultures and observation
C. Doxycycline
D. Rimantadine
E. Vancomycin, ceftriaxone, and ampicillin

I-28. A 23-year-old woman with a chronic lower extremity ulcer related to prior trauma presents with rash, hypotension, and fever. She has had no recent travel or outdoor exposure and is up to date on all of her vaccinations. She does not use IV drugs. On examination, the ulcer looks clean with a well-granulated base and no erythema, warmth, or pustular discharge. However, the patient does have diffuse erythema that is most prominent on her palms, conjunctiva, and oral mucosa. Other than profound hypotension and tachycardia, the remainder of the examination is nonfocal. Laboratory results are notable for a creatinine of 2.8 mg/dL, aspartate aminotransferase of 250 U/L, alanine aminotransferase of 328 U/L, total bilirubin of 3.2 mg/dL, direct bilirubin of 0.5 mg/dL, INR of 1.5, activated partial thromboplastin time of 1.6 × control, and platelets at 94,000/μL. Ferritin is 1300 μg/mL. The patient is started on broad-spectrum antibiotics after

I-28. *(Continued)*
appropriate blood cultures are drawn and is resuscitated with IV fluid and vasopressors. Her blood cultures are negative at 72 h: at this point her fingertips start to desquamate. What is the most likely diagnosis?

A. Juvenile rheumatoid arthritis (JRA)
B. Leptospirosis
C. Staphylococcal toxic shock syndrome
D. Streptococcal toxic shock syndrome
E. Typhoid fever

I-29. The Centers for Disease Control and Prevention (CDC) has designated several biologic agents as category A in their ability to be used as bioweapons. Category A agents include agents that can be easily disseminated or transmitted, result in high mortality, can cause public panic, and require special action for public health preparedness. All the following agents are considered category A *except*

A. *Bacillus anthracis*
B. *Francisella tularensis*
C. ricin toxin from *Ricinus communis*
D. smallpox
E. *Yersinia pestis*

I-30. A 50-year-old alcoholic woman with well-controlled cirrhosis eats raw oysters from the Chesapeake Bay at a cookout. Twelve hours later she presents to the emergency department with fever, hypotension, and altered sensorium. Her extremity examination is notable for diffuse erythema with areas of hemorrhagic bullae on her shins. What is the most likely diagnosis?

A. *Escherichia coli* sepsis
B. Hemolytic uremic syndrome
C. Meningococcemia
D. Staphylococcal toxic shock syndrome
E. *Vibrio vulnificus* infection

I-31. Hyperthermia is defined as

A. a core temperature >40.0°C
B. a core temperature >41.5°C
C. an uncontrolled increase in body temperature despite a normal hypothalamic temperature setting
D. an elevated temperature that normalizes with antipyretic therapy
E. temperature >40.0°C, rigidity, and autonomic dysregulation

I-32. A patient in the intensive care unit develops a temperature of 40.8°C, profoundly rigid tone, and hemodynamic shock 2 min after a succinylcholine infusion is started. Immediate therapy should include

A. intravenous dantrolene sodium
B. acetaminophen
C. external cooling devices
D. A and C
E. A, B, and C

I-33. Which of the following conditions is associated with increased susceptibility to heat stroke in the elderly?

A. A heat wave
B. Antiparkinsonian therapy
C. Bedridden status
D. Diuretic therapy
E. All of the above

I-34. A 68-year-old alcoholic arrives in the emergency department after being found in the snow on a cold winter night in Chicago. His core temperature based on rectal and esophageal probe is 27°C. Pulse is 30 beats/min and blood pressure is 75/40 mmHg. He is immobile and lacks corneal, oculocephalic, and peripheral reflexes. He is immediately intubated and placed on a cardiac monitor. He then converts to ventricular fibrillation: a defibrillation attempt at 2 J/kg is not successful. What should be the next immediate step in management?

A. Active rewarming with forced-air heating blankets, heated humidified oxygen, heated crystalloid infusion
B. Amiodarone infusion
C. Insertion of a transvenous pacemaker
D. Passive rewarming with numerous blankets for insulation
E. Repeat defibrillation

I-35. In the evaluation of malnutrition, which of the following proteins has the shortest half-life and thus is most predictive of recent nutritional status?

A. Albumin
B. Fibronectin
C. Retinol-binding protein complex
D. Prealbumin
E. Transferrin

I-36. A 45-year-old man is stranded overnight in the cold after an avalanche. He is airlifted to your medical center and found to have anesthesia and a clumsy sensation in the distal extent of the fingers on his left hand (see Color Atlas, Figure I-36). What is the best initial management of his hand?

A. Intravenous nitroglycerine
B. Oral nifedipine
C. Rapid rewarming
D. Surgical debridement
E. Topical nitroglycerine paste

I-37. Fecal occult blood testing (FOBT) was shown to decrease colon cancer–related mortality from 8.8/1000 persons to 5.9/1000 persons over a 13-year period. What is the approximate absolute risk reduction (ARR) of this intervention in the studied population?

A. 50%
B. 30%
C. 3%
D. 0.3%
E. 0%

I-38. Which preventative intervention leads to the largest average increase in life expectancy for a target population?

A. A regular exercise program for a 40-year-old man
B. Getting a 35-year-old smoker to quit smoking
C. Mammography in women aged 50–70
D. Pap smears in women aged 18–65
E. Prostate specific antigen (PSA) and digital rectal examination for a man >50 years old

I-39. All of the following patients should receive a lipid screening profile *except*

A. a 16-year-old male with type 1 diabetes
B. a17-year-old female teen who recently began smoking
C. a 23-year-old healthy male who is starting his first job
D. a 48-year-old woman beginning menopause
E. a 62-year-old man with no past medical history

I-40. A 46-year-old female presents to her primary care doctor complaining of a feeling of anxiety. She notes that she always had been what she describes as a "worrier," even in grade school. The patient has always avoided speaking in public and recently is becoming anxious to the extent where she is having difficulty functioning at work and in social situations. She has difficulty falling asleep at night and finds that she is always "fidgety" and has a compulsive urge to move. The patient owns a real estate company that has been in decline since a downturn in the local economy. She recently has been avoiding showing homes for sale. Instead, she defers to her partners because she finds that she is nervous to the point of being unable to speak to her clients. She has two children, ages 16 and 12, who are very active in sports. She feels overwhelmed with worry over the possibility of injury to her children and will not attend their sports events. You suspect that the patient has a generalized anxiety disorder. All of the following statements regarding this diagnosis are true *except*

A. The age at onset of symptoms is usually before 20 years, although the diagnosis usually occurs much later in life.
B. Over 80% of these patients will have concomitant mood disorders such as major depression, dysthymia, or social phobia.
C. As in panic disorder, shortness of breath, tachycardia, and palpitations are common.
D. Experimental work suggests that the pathophysiology of generalized anxiety disorder involves impaired binding of benzodiazepines at the γ-aminobutyric acid (GABA) receptor.
E. The therapeutic approach to patients with generalized anxiety disorder should include both pharmacologic agents and psychotherapy, although complete relief of symptoms is rare.

I-41. For which of the following herbal remedies is there the best evidence for efficacy in treating the symptoms of benign prostatic hypertrophy?

I-41. *(Continued)*

A. Saint John's wort
B. Gingko
C. Kava
D. Saw palmetto
E. No herbal therapy is effective

I-42. Which of the following personality traits is most likely to describe a young female with anorexia nervosa?

A. Depressive
B. Borderline
C. Anxious
D. Perfectionist
E. Impulsive

I-43. Why is it necessary to coadminister vitamin B_6 (pyridoxine) with isoniazid?

A. Vitamin B_6 requirements are higher in tuberculosis patients.
B. Isoniazid causes decarboxylation of γ-carboxyl groups in vitamin K–dependent enzymes.
C. Isoniazid interacts with pyridoxal phosphate.
D. Isoniazid causes malabsorption of vitamin B_6.
E. Isoniazid causes a conversion of homocysteine to cystathionine.

I-44. The prevalence of hypertension in American persons aged >65 years old is

A. 10–35%
B. 35–60%
C. 60–85%
D. >85%

I-45. Diabetes is associated with all of the following in the elderly *except*

A. cerebrovascular accident
B. cognitive decline
C. fall risk
D. myocardial infarction
E. urinary incontinence

I-46. Which of the following is the best indicator of prognosis and longevity in a geriatric patient?

A. Functional status
B. Life span of first-degree relatives
C. Marital status
D. Number of medical comorbidities
E. Socioeconomic status

I-47. Diagnostic criteria for delirium as a cause of a confused state in a hospitalized patient include all of the following *except*

A. agitation
B. altered level of consciousness
C. disorganized thinking

I-47. *(Continued)*

    D.   fluctuating mental status

    E.   poor attention

I-48. Fall risks in the elderly include all of the following *except*

    A.   creatinine clearance <65 mL/min

    B.   diabetes mellitus

    C.   fear of falling

    D.   history of falls

    E.   hypertension

    F.   psychotropic medications

I-49. A stage 1 decubitus ulcer (nonblanchable erythema of intact skin or edema and induration over a bony pressure point) can progress to a stage 4 decubitus ulcer (full-thickness skin loss with tissue necrosis as well as damage to bone, muscle and tendons) over what period of time?

    A.   Several hours

    B.   1–2 days

    C.   1–2 weeks

    D.   1–2 months

I-50. A 74-year-old woman complains of leaking urine when she coughs, laughs, or lifts her groceries. She denies polydipsia and polyuria. She delivered four children vaginally and underwent total abdominal hysterectomy for fibroids 20 years earlier. She has mild fasting hyperglycemia that is controlled with diet. What is likely to be the best management for her problem?

    A.   Bladder retraining exercises (planned urinations every 2 h)

    B.   Doxazosin plus finasteride

    C.   Metformin

    D.   Oxybutynin

    E.   Surgery

I-51. A 38-year-old man with multiple sclerosis develops acute flaccid weakness in his left arm and left leg. Physical examination reveals normal sensorium, normal cranial nerve function, 1/5 strength in his left upper extremity, 0/5 strength in his left lower extremity, impaired proprioception in his left leg, intact proprioception in his right leg, decreased pain and temperature sensation in his right arm and leg, and normal light touch/pain and temperature sensation in his right leg. Where is his causative lesion most likely to be?

    A.   Cervical nerve roots

    B.   High cervical spinal cord

    C.   Medulla

    D.   Pons

    E.   Right cortical hemisphere

I-52. A 32-year-old man with a history of HIV infection presents to the hospital with nausea, abdominal disten-

I-52. *(Continued)*

tion and projectile vomiting that developed over the previous 8–12 h. He denies fevers, chills, diaphoresis, melena, or diarrhea. Over the past 3 months, he has lost 30 lb in the context of advanced HIV infection. He has never had abdominal surgery. On examination, his abdomen is distended, with high-pitched intermittent bowel sounds and guarding but no rebound. A periumbilical bruit is also detected. Abdominal x-ray reveals a small-bowel obstruction with a probable cut-off point in the mid duodenum. What is the diagnostic test of choice for diagnosing the cause of the underlying obstruction?

    A.   Abdominal CT with abdominal angiogram

    B.   Enteroscopy

    C.   Laparoscopy

    D.   Serum carcinoembryonic antigen (CEA) level

    E.   Stool acid-fast bacillus culture

    F.   Upper gastrointestinal (GI) series with small bowel follow through

I-53. A 64-year-old man with primary light chain amyloidosis develops orthostatic symptoms despite maintaining adequate oral intake. He also notes early satiety, with bloating and vomiting if he eats too rapidly. To combat this, he has decreased the size of his meals but eats twice as frequently during the day, with some positive effect. What is the most likely explanation for his gastrointestinal symptoms?

    A.   Diverticulosis

    B.   Gastric cancer

    C.   Gastroparesis

    D.   Irritable bowel syndrome

    E.   Small-bowel obstruction

I-54. A 42-year-old man with a history of end-stage renal disease is on hemodialysis and has been taking a medication chronically for nausea and vomiting. Over the past week he has developed new-onset involuntary lip smacking, grimacing, and tongue protrusion. This side effect is most likely due to which of the following antiemetics?

    A.   Erythromycin

    B.   Methylprednisolone

    C.   Ondansetron

    D.   Prochlorperazine

    E.   Scopolamine

I-55. Which of the following is *not* a common cause of persistent cough lasting more than 3 months in a nonsmoker?

    A.   Asthma

    B.   Gastroesophageal reflux disease

    C.   Lisinopril

    D.   *Mycoplasma* infection

    E.   Postnasal drip

I-56. A 64-year-old alcoholic presents to the emergency department with occasional hemoptysis, productive cough, and low-grade fever over the past several weeks. His CT scan shows an abnormality in the right lower lobe. He reports several contacts with tuberculosis-infected patients while in prison several years ago. Sputum examination reveals putrid-smelling thick green sputum streaked with blood. The Gram stain shows many polymorphonuclear leukocytes and a mix of gram-positive and -negative organisms. What is the most likely diagnosis?

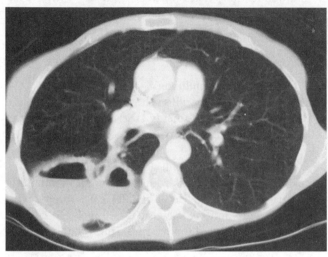

FIGURE I-56

A. Bronchogenic carcinoma
B. Polymicrobial lung abscess
C. Pulmonary tuberculosis
D. Tricuspid valve endocarditis
E. Wegener's granulomatosis

I-57. A 74-year-old man with known endobronchial carcinoma of his left mainstem bronchus develops massive hemoptysis (1 L of frank hemoptysis productive of bright red blood) while hospitalized. All of the following should be considered in his initial management *except*

A. bronchial artery embolization
B. cough suppressants
C. direct bronchoscopic electrocautery
D. placing the patient in the lateral decubitus position with his right side down
E. selective intubation of the right main stem bronchus under bronchoscopy

I-58. A patient with proteinuria has a renal biopsy that reveals segmental collapse of the glomerular capillary loops and overlying podocyte hyperplasia. The patient most likely has

A. diabetes
B. HIV infection
C. multiple myeloma
D. systemic lupus erythematosus
E. Wegener's granulomatosis

I-59. A 35-year-old woman comes to your clinic complaining of shortness of breath. It is immediately apparent that she has a bluish tinge of her face, trunk, extremities, and mucus membranes. Which of the following diagnoses is most likely?

A. Atrial septal defect
B. Myocarditis
C. Raynaud's phenomenon
D. Sepsis
E. Vasospasm due to cold temperature

I-60. A 43-year-old man with alcoholic liver disease complains of dyspnea upon sitting up. Physical examination is notable for chest spider angiomas and palmar erythema. His arterial oxygen saturations fall from 96% to 88% upon transition from lying to sitting. His lung fields are clear and heart sounds are crisp. Abdominal examination is notable for a palpable nodular liver edge but no fluid wave or shifting dullness. He has 1+ lower extremity edema. What is the most likely cause of his dyspnea?

A. Chronic thromboembolic disease
B. Congestive heart failure
C. Pulmonary arteriovenous fistula
D. Portal hypertension
E. Ventricular septal defect

I-61. A 30-year-old woman complains of lower extremity swelling and abdominal distention. It is particularly troublesome after her daily shift as a toll booth operator and is at its worst during hot weather. She denies shortness of breath, orthopnea, dyspnea on exertion, jaundice, foamy urine, or diarrhea. Her symptoms occur independently of her menstrual cycle. Physical examination is notable for 2+ lower extremity edema, flat jugular venous pulsation, no hepatojugular reflex, normal S_1 and S_2 with no extra heart sounds, clear lung fields, a benign slightly distended abdomen with no organomegaly, and normal skin. A complete metabolic panel is within normal limits, and a urinalysis shows no proteinuria. What is the most likely diagnosis?

A. Cirrhosis
B. Congestive heart failure
C. Cyclical edema
D. Idiopathic edema
E. Gastrointestinal malabsorption
F. Nephrotic syndrome

I-62. All of the following factors are associated with a greater risk of ventricular arrhythmia versus anxiety/panic attack in a patient complaining of palpitations *except*

A. history of congestive heart failure
B. history of coronary artery disease
C. history of diabetes mellitus
D. palpitations lasting >15 min
E. palpitations provoked by ethanol

I-63. A 25-year-old healthy woman visits your office during the fifth month of pregnancy. Her blood pressure is 142/86 mmHg. What should be your next step in management?

A. Have her return to your clinic in 2 weeks for a blood pressure check
B. Initiate an angiotensin-converting enzyme inhibitor
C. Initiate a beta blocker
D. Recheck her blood pressure in the seated position in 6 h
E. Recheck her blood pressure in the lateral recumbent position in 6 h

I-64. A 33-year-old woman with diabetes mellitus and hypertension presents to the hospital with seizures during week 37 of her pregnancy. Her blood pressure is 156/92 mmHg. She has 4+ proteinuria. Management should include all of the following *except*

A. emergent delivery
B. intravenous labetalol
C. intravenous magnesium sulfate
D. intravenous phenytoin

I-65. Which cardiac valvular disorder is the most likely to cause death during pregnancy?

A. Aortic regurgitation
B. Aortic stenosis
C. Mitral regurgitation
D. Mitral stenosis
E. Tricuspid regurgitation

I-66. A 27-year-old woman develops left leg swelling during week 20 of her pregnancy. Left lower extremity ultrasonogram reveals a left iliac vein deep vein thrombosis (DVT). Proper management includes

A. bedrest
B. catheter-directed thrombolysis
C. enoxaparin
D. inferior vena cava filter placement
E. Coumadin

I-67. In which of the following categories should women undergo routine screening for gestational diabetes?

A. Age >25 years
B. Body mass index >25 kg/m^2
C. Family history of diabetes mellitus in a first-degree relative
D. African American
E. All of the above

I-68. All of the following should be components of the routine evaluation of any patient undergoing medium- or high-risk non-cardiac surgery *except*

A. 12-lead resting electrocardiogram
B. chest radiograph
C. detailed history

I-68. (*Continued*)
D. physical examination
E. treadmill stress test

I-69. Noninvasive cardiac imaging/stress testing should be considered in patients with how many of the following six proven risk factors (high-risk surgery, ischemic heart disease, congestive heart failure, cerebrovascular disease, diabetes mellitus, and renal insufficiency) for perioperative cardiac events (including pulmonary edema, myocardial infarction, and heart block)?

A. 1
B. 2
C. 3
D. 4
E. 5

I-70. A 72-year-old white man with New York Heart Association II ischemic cardiomyopathy, diabetes mellitus, and chronic renal insufficiency (creatinine clearance = 42 mL/min) undergoes dobutamine echocardiography prior to carotid endarterectomy. He is found to have 7-mm ST depressions in his lateral leads during the test and develops dyspnea at 70% maximal expected dosage, requiring early cessation of the stress test. His current medicines include an angiotensin-converting enzyme inhibitor, a beta blocker, and aspirin. What would be your advice to the patient?

A. Cancel the carotid endarterectomy
B. Proceed to cardiac catheterization
C. Maximize medical management
D. Proceed directly to carotid endarterectomy
E. Proceed directly to carotid endarterectomy and coronary artery bypass surgery

I-71. Parkinson's disease can often be differentiated from the atypical Parkinsonian syndromes (multiple system atrophy, progressive supranuclear palsy) by the presence of which of the following?

A. Axial stiffness
B. Pill-rolling tremor
C. Shuffling gait
D. Stooped posture
E. Turning en bloc

I-72. A wide-based gait with irregular lurching and erratic foot placement but no subjective dizziness characterizes which type of gait ataxia?

A. Cerebellar dysfunction
B. Frontal gait abnormality
C. Inner ear dysfunction
D. Parkinsonian syndromes
E. Sensory ataxia

I-73. A patient with a narrow-based gait instability complains that he needs to look at his feet while he walks to prevent falling. He feels wobbly standing with his eyes

I-73. *(Continued)*
closed and notes frequent falls. On examination, he has no difficulty initiating gait, his stride is regular, strength is normal, and there is no tremor. Review of routine blood work drawn 3 months prior reveals a hematocrit of 29% with an elevated mean corpuscular volume. Which of the following is the most likely diagnosis?

A. Amyotrophic lateral sclerosis
B. Cerebellar tumor
C. Cerebrovascular disease
D. Parkinson's disease
E. Pernicious anemia

I-74. Which of the following is an effective method to evaluate for cortical sensory deficits?

A. Graphesthesia (the capacity to recognize letters drawn by the examiner on the patient's hand)
B. Stereognosis (the ability to recognize common objects, such as coins, by palpation)
C. Touch localization
D. Two-point discrimination testing
E. All of the above

I-75. A 23-year-old female patient complains of visual blurriness. On examination, her pupils are equally round. Shining a flashlight into her right eye causes equal, strong constriction in both of her eyes. When the light is flashed into her left eye, both pupils dilate slightly though not to their previous size prior to light confrontation. Where is there most likely to be anatomic damage?

A. Left cornea
B. Left optic nerve or retina
C. Optic chiasm
D. Right cornea
E. Right optic nerve or retina

I-76. A patient complains of blurred vision in both eyes particularly in the periphery with the right being worse than the left. Visual field examination with finger confrontation reveals a decreased vision in the left periphery in the left eye and right periphery in the right eye. Where is there most likely to be a lesion?

A. Bilateral optic nerves
B. Left lateral geniculate body
C. Left occipital cortex
D. Post-chiasmic optic tract
E. Suprasellar space

I-77. Which of the following methods is most effective for the diagnosis of corneal abrasions?

A. Fluorescein and cobalt-blue light examination
B. Intraocular pressure measurement
C. Lid eversion for foreign body examination
D. Oculoplegia and dilation
E. Viral culture of the cornea

I-78. Which of the following criteria best differentiates episcleritis from conjunctivitis?

A. Concurrent connective tissue disease such as lupus
B. Lack of discharge
C. More diffuse ocular involvement
D. Reduced eye motility
E. Severe pain

I-79. Which diagnosis can be easily confused with adenoviral conjunctivitis and is a major cause of blindness in the United States?

A. Endophthalmitis
B. Herpes simplex virus keratitis
C. Angle-closure glaucoma
D. Uveitis
E. Trachoma

I-80. A 34-year-old male patient is referred to your clinic after a new diagnosis of anterior uveitis. All of the following diseases should be screened for by history and physical and/or laboratory examination because they may cause anterior uveitis *except*

A. ankylosing spondylitis
B. Lyme disease
C. sarcoidosis
D. syphilis
E. toxoplasmosis

I-81. A 22-year-old female is referred to your clinic after being started on glucocorticoids for a new diagnosis of left optic neuritis seen on examination with disc pallor, and it is confirmed with quantitative visual field mapping. What further evaluation is indicated?

A. Antinuclear antibodies
B. Brain MRI
C. Erythrocyte sedimentation rate
D. No further evaluation unless symptoms recur
E. Temporal artery biopsy

I-82. A 69-year-old male dialysis patient with poorly controlled diabetes, heart failure and chronic indwelling catheters presents with fever and loss of vision in the left eye developing over the past 6 h. Vital signs are notable for a temperature of 101.3°F, heart rate of 105/min, and blood pressure of 125/85. Which test is most likely to confirm the diagnosis?

A. Blood cultures
B. Blood smear
C. Brain MRI
D. Rheumatic panel
E. Rapid plasma reagin

I-83. Exposure to which of the following types of radiation would result in thermal injury and burns but would not cause damage to internal organs because the particle size is too large to cause internal penetration?

I-83. *(Continued)*
- A. Alpha radiation
- B. Beta radiation
- C. Gamma radiation
- D. Neutron particles
- E. X-rays

I-84. A "dirty" bomb is detonated in downtown Boston. The bomb was composed of cesium-137 with trinitrotoluene. In the immediate aftermath, an estimated 30 people were killed due to the power of the blast. The fallout area was about 0.5 mile, with radiation exposure of ~1.8 gray (Gy). An estimated 5000 people have been potentially exposed to beta and gamma radiation. Most of these individuals show no sign of any injury, but about 60 people have evidence of thermal injury. What is the most appropriate approach to treating the injured victims?

- A. All individuals who have been exposed should be treated with potassium iodide.
- B. All individuals who have been exposed should be treated with Prussian blue.
- C. All individuals should be decontaminated prior to transportation to the nearest medical center for emergency care to prevent exposure of health care workers.
- D. Severely injured individuals should be transported to the hospital for emergency care after removing the victims' clothes, as the risk of exposure to health care workers is low.
- E. With this degree of radiation exposure, no further testing and treatment are needed.

I-85. A 54-year-old man is admitted to the hospital with severe nausea, vomiting, and diarrhea. These symptoms began 36 h ago. He briefly improved for a few hours yesterday, but today has progressively worsened. He states he is concerned about possible poisoning because of his role in espionage and counterterrorism for the U.S. government. He met with an informant 2 days previously at a hotel bar, where he drank three cups of coffee but did not eat. He does state that he left the table to place a phone call during the meeting and is concerned that his coffee may have been contaminated. He otherwise is quite healthy and takes no medications. On physical examination, he appears ill. The vital signs are: blood pressure 98/60 mmHg, heart rate 112 beats/min, respiratory rate 24 breaths/min, Sa_{O_2} 94%, and temperature 37.4°C. Head, ears, eyes, nose, and throat examination shows pale mucous membranes. Cardiovascular examination is tachycardic, but regular. His lungs are clear. The abdomen is slightly distended with hyperactive bowel sounds. There is no tenderness or rebound. Extremities show no edema, but a few scattered petechiae are present. Neurologic examination is normal. A complete blood count is performed. The results are: white blood cell (WBC) count 150/µL, red blood cell count 1.5/µL, hemoglobin 4.5 g/dL,

I-85. *(Continued)*
hematocrit 15%, platelet count 11,000/µL. The differential on the WBC count is 98% PMNs, 2% monocytes, and 0% lymphocytes. A blood sample is held for HLA testing. A urine sample is positive for the presence of radioactive isotopes, which are determined to be polonium-210, a strong emitter of alpha radiation. The mode of exposure is presumed to be ingestion. What is the best approach to the treatment of this patient?

- A. Bone marrow transplantation
- B. Gastric lavage
- C. Potassium iodide
- D. Supportive care only
- E. Supportive care and dimercaprol

I-86. Several victims are brought to the emergency room after a terrorist attack in the train station. An explosive was detonated that dispersed an unknown substance throughout the station, but several people reported a smell like that of horseradish or burned garlic. Prior to transport to the emergency room, exposed individuals had their clothing removed and underwent showering and decontamination. On initial presentation, there was no apparent injury except eye irritation. Over the next few hours, most of those exposed complain of nasal congestion, sinus pain, and burning in the nares. Beginning about 2 h after exposure, many of the exposed individuals began to notice diffuse redness of the skin, particularly in the neck, axillae, antecubital fossae, and external genitalia. In addition, a few people also developed blistering of the skin. Hoarseness, cough, and dyspnea are noted as well. What is the most likely chemical agent that was released in the terrorist attack?

- A. Chlorine
- B. Cyanide
- C. Mustard gas
- D. Phosgene oxime
- E. Soman

I-87. An unknown chemical agent was released in a terrorist attack in the food court of a shopping mall. Several victims who were close to the site of the release of the gas died prior to arrival of the emergency medical teams. Upon arrival, the survivors were complaining of difficulty with vision and stated that they felt the world was "going black." The victims were also noted to be drooling and have increased nasal secretions. A few individuals were dyspneic with wheezing. The most severely affected victims fell unconscious and soon thereafter developed seizures. What medication(s) should be administered immediately to the survivors?

- A. Atropine, 6 mg IM
- B. 2-Pralidoxime chloride, 1800 mg IM
- C. Diazepam, 5 mg IV
- D. A and B
- E. B and C
- F. All of the above

I-88. A 7-month-old child is brought to clinic by his parents. He was the product of a healthy pregnancy, and there were no perinatal complications. The parents are concerned that there is something wrong; he is very hyperactive and is noted to have a 'mousy' odor. On examination the child is found to have mild microcephaly, hypopigmentation and eczema. Laboratory studies are sent and a diagnosis is made. How could this clinical scenario have been prevented?

A. Screening at 6 months of age for urine ketones
B. Screening at birth for phenylalanine in blood
C. Screening at birth for chromosomal abnormalities
D. Genetic screening of parents prior to delivery
E. Cord blood sampling at 2 months' pregnancy for glutamine synthase

I-89. A 35-year-old woman with a history of degenerative joint disease comes to clinic complaining of dark urine over the past several weeks. She has had arthritis in her hips, knees, and shoulders for about 2 years. On examination, she is noted to have gray-brown pigmentation of the helices of both ears. Which of the following disorders is most likely?

A. Alkaptonuria
B. Hawkinsinuria
C. Homocystinuria
D. Hyperprolinemia type I
E. Tryptophanuria

I-90. A 22-year-old man presents to a local emergency room with severe muscle cramps and exercise intolerance. His symptoms have been worsening over a period of months. He has noticed that his urine is frequently dark. Examination reveals tenderness over all major muscle groups. A creatine phosphokinase (CK) is markedly elevated. He reports a normal childhood but since age 18 has noticed worsening exercise intolerance. He no longer plays basketball and recently noticed leg fatigue at two flights of stairs. After intense exercise, he occasionally has red-colored urine. Which of the following is the most likely diagnosis?

A. Glucose-6-phosphatase deficiency
B. Lactate dehydrogenase deficiency
C. McArdle disease (type V glycogen storage disease)
D. Pyruvate kinase deficiency
E. von Gierke's disease (type I glycogen storage disease)

I-91. An enzymatic assay of muscle tissue is sent and a diagnosis is made. Which of the following represents a major source of morbidity in this disease which should be explained thoroughly to the patient?

A. Fulminant liver failure
B. Myocarditis and subsequent heart failure
C. Progressive proximal muscle weakness
D. Rhabdomyolysis leading to renal failure
E. This is a benign disorder without major clinical risks

I-92. A 21-year-old woman comes to clinic to establish new primary care. She has a history of type III glycogen storage disease (debranching deficiency), for which she takes a high-protein, high-carbohydrate diet. She has a normal physical examination except for short stature, mild weakness, and a slightly enlarged liver. She works as an administrative assistant and is planning to be married in the next 6 months. She is concerned about her long-term prognosis and the chances of the disease developing in a child. All of the following statements about her prognosis are true *except*

A. Cardiomyopathy is a possible complication.
B. Chronic liver disease is a possible complication.
C. Dementia is a possible complication.
D. Her child will not have the disease unless her fiancé is a carrier.
E. Prenatal testing is available for the disease.

I-93. A 36-year-old man comes to your office asking for genetic testing for Alzheimer's disease. He has no cognitive complaints but notes that all four of his grandparents have had Alzheimer's and his father has mild cognitive impairment at the age of 62. His Mini-Mental Status Examination is 29/30, losing one point on the serial-7's examination. He requests testing for the apolipoprotein E allele (ε4). This request is an example of which of the following?

A. Early-onset dementia
B. Genetic discrimination
C. Predisposition testing
D. Presymptomatic testing

I-94. A recently married couple comes to see you in clinic for prenatal counseling. They are both in their mid-thirties and have read extensively on the internet about pregnancy and increasing maternal age. They want to know the risk of miscarriage as well as the risk of having a child with Down syndrome. Which of the following is true regarding chromosome disorders and increasing maternal age?

A. About half of trisomy conceptions will survive to term.
B. In women under the age of 25, trisomy occurs in <1% of all pregnancies.
C. Lower socioeconomic status is a recognized risk factor in trisomic conceptions.
D. The risk of Down syndrome increases 1% per year of maternal age.
E. Women over the age of 42 have a 33% chance of a trisomic conception.

I-95. In what percentage of pregnancies do chromosomal disorders occur?

A. 0.01%
B. 0.1–0.5%
C. 1–2%
D. 2–5%
E. 10–25%

I-96. All the following disorders can cause ambiguous sexual differentiation *except*

- A. 21-hydroxylase deficiency
- B. androgen insensitivity syndrome
- C. Klinefelter syndrome
- D. mixed gonadal dysgenesis
- E. testicular dysgenesis

I-97. An 18-year-old female is evaluated in an outpatient clinic for a complaint of amenorrhea. She reports that she feels as if she never developed normally compared with other girls her age. She has never had a menstrual period and complains that she has had only minimal breast growth. Past medical history is significant for a diagnosis of borderline hypertension. In childhood the patient frequently had otitis media and varicella infections. She received the standard vaccinations. She recently graduated from high school and has no learning difficulties. She is on no medications. On physical examination, the patient is of short stature with a height of 56 in. Blood pressure is 142/88. The posterior hairline is low. The nipples appear widely spaced, with only breast buds present. The patient has minimal escutcheon consistent with Tanner stage 2 development. Her external genitalia appear normal. Bimanual vaginal examination reveals an anteverted, anteflexed uterus. The ovaries are not palpable. What is the most likely diagnosis?

- A. Hypothyroidism
- B. Hyperthyroidism
- C. Malnutrition
- D. Testicular feminization
- E. Turner syndrome (gonadal dysgenesis)

I-98. A 30-year-old male is seen for a physical examination when obtaining life insurance. The last time he saw a physician was 15 years ago. He has no complaints. Past medical history is notable for scoliosis that was surgically corrected when the patient was a teenager and a recent shoulder dislocation. He takes no medications and does not smoke, drink, or use illicit drugs. Family history is notable for a father and a brother with colon cancer at ages 45 and 50 years, respectively. Physical examination is notable for normal vital signs, a tall habitus with hypermobile joints, normal skin, and ectopia lentis. Rectal examination is normal, and stool is guaiac-negative. The remainder of the examination is normal. Appropriate recommendations for follow-up should include which of the following annual studies?

- A. Colonoscopy
- B. Echocardiography
- C. Fecal occult blood testing
- D. Serum periodic acid–Schiff (PSA) measurement
- E. Serum thyroid-stimulating hormone (TSH)

I-99. All the following diseases are caused by errors in DNA repair *except*

I-99. *(Continued)*
- A. ataxia-telangiectasia (AT)
- B. Fanconi's anemia (FA)
- C. fragile X (FX) syndrome
- D. hereditary nonpolyposis colorectal cancer (HNPCC)
- E. xeroderma pigmentosum (XP)

I-100. A 45-year-old male is evaluated for weakness and a progressive change in mental status. After extensive evaluation, he is diagnosed with a mitochondrial disorder. All of the following statements about mitochondrial disorders are true *except*

- A. The mitochondrial genome does not recombine.
- B. Inheritance is maternal.
- C. The proportion of wild-type and mutant mitochondria in different tissues is identical.
- D. Cardiomyopathy is a feature of many mitochondrial disorders.
- E. Acquired somatic mitochondrial mutations may play a role in age-related degenerative disorders.

I-101. Prader-Willi syndrome (PWS) is a rare disorder that is characterized by diminished fetal activity, obesity, mental retardation, and short stature. A deletion on the paternal copy of chromosome 15 is the cause. A deletion on the same site on chromosome 15, but on the maternal copy, results in a different syndrome: Angelman's syndrome. This syndrome is characterized by mental retardation, seizures, ataxia, and hypotonia. What is the name of the genetic mechanism that results in this phenomenon?

- A. Genetic anticipation
- B. Genetic imprinting
- C. Lyonization
- D. Somatic mosaicism
- E. Uniparental disomy

I-102. All the following are inherited disorders of connective tissue *except*

- A. Alport syndrome
- B. Ehlers-Danlos syndrome
- C. Marfan syndrome
- D. McArdle's disease
- E. osteogenesis imperfecta

I-103. A 30-year-old male comes to your office for genetic counseling. His brother died at age 13 years with Tay-Sachs disease. His sister is unaffected. The patient and his wife wish to have children. Which of the following statements concerning Tay Sachs disease is true?

- A. It is seen most commonly in Scandinavian populations.
- B. It is caused by mutations in the galactosidase gene.
- C. Most patients die in the third or fourth decade of life.
- D. Death occurs as a result of progressive neurologic decline.
- E. Splenomegaly is common in these patients.

I-104. All of the following statements about Gaucher disease are true *except*

   A.   Bone pain is common.
   B.   Disease frequency is highest in Ashkenazi Jews.
   C.   Inheritance is autosomal recessive.
   D.   Splenomegaly is rare.
   E.   The disease is caused by mutations in the gene for acid β-glucosidase.

I-105. The following pedigree is an example of what pattern of inheritance?

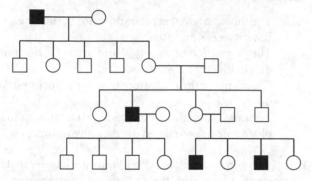

Solid figure = Affected individual
Open figure = Unaffected individuals

FIGURE I-105

   A.   X-linked recessive inheritance
   B.   X-linked dominant inheritance
   C.   Autosomal recessive inheritance
   D.   Autosomal dominant inheritance
   E.   Cannot be determined by the limited information provided in this pedigree

I-106. Diseases that are inherited in a multifactorial genetic fashion (i.e., not autosomal dominant, autosomal recessive, or X-linked) and are seen more frequently in persons bearing certain histocompatibility antigens include

   A.   gluten-sensitive enteropathy
   B.   neurofibromatosis
   C.   adult polycystic kidney disease
   D.   Wilson's disease
   E.   cystic fibrosis

I-107. A 32-year-old man seeks evaluation for ongoing fevers of uncertain cause. He first noted a feeling of malaise about 3 months ago, and for the past 6 weeks, he has been experiencing daily fevers to as high as 39.4°C (103°F). He awakens with night sweats once weekly and has lost 4.5 kg. He complains of nonspecific myalgias and arthralgias. He has no rashes and reports no ill contacts. He has seen his primary care physician on three separate occasions during this time and has had documented temperatures of 38.7°C (101.7°F) while in the physician's office. Multiple laboratory studies have been performed that have shown nonspecific findings only. A complete blood count showed a white blood cell count of 15,700/μL with 80% polymorphonu-

I-107. *(Continued)*
clear cells, 15% lymphocytes, 3% eosinophils, and 2% monocytes. The peripheral smear is normal. The hematocrit is 34.7%. His erythrocyte sedimentation rate (ESR) is elevated at 57 mm/h. Liver and kidney function are normal. HIV, Epstein-Barr virus (EBV), and cytomegalovirus (CMV) testing are negative. Routine blood cultures for bacteria, chest radiograph, and purified protein derivative (PPD) testing are negative. In large groups of patients similar to this one with fever of unknown origin, which of the following categories comprises the largest group of diagnoses if one is able to be determined?

   A.   Drug or other ingestion
   B.   Hereditary periodic fever syndromes, such as familial Mediterranean fever
   C.   Infection
   D.   Neoplasm
   E.   Noninfectious inflammatory disease

I-108. Chronic hypoxia causes biochemical changes whereby oxygen delivery to tissues is not impaired. In comparison to someone living at sea level, which of the following changes would be expected in a healthy person acclimated to living at high altitude?

   A.   Basal temperature <37°C
   B.   Serum pH >7.45
   C.   Increased red blood cell levels of 2,3-diphosphoglycerate
   D.   Hemoglobin concentration <10 mg/dL
   E.   Arterial P_{CO_2} <30 mmHg

I-109. Independent of insurance status, income, age, and comorbid conditions, African-American patients are less likely to receive equivalent levels of care when compared to white patients for the following scenarios:

   A.   Prescription of analgesic for pain control
   B.   Referral to renal transplantation
   C.   Surgical treatment for lung cancer
   D.   Utilization of cardiac diagnostic and therapeutic procedures
   E.   All of the above

I-110. Which of the following would be present in an individual who has lost nondeclarative memory?

   A.   Inability to recall a spouse's birthday
   B.   Inability to recall how to tie one's shoe
   C.   Inability to recognize a photo that was taken at one's wedding
   D.   Inability to recognize a watch as an instrument for keeping time
   E.   Inability to remember the events of one's high school graduation

I-111. A 24-year-old woman presents for a routine checkup and complains only of small masses in her groin. She states that they have been present for at least 3 years. On physical

I-111. *(Continued)*

examination, she is noted to have several palpable 1-cm inguinal lymph nodes that are mobile, nontender, and discrete. There is no other lymphadenopathy on examination. What should be the next step in management?

A. Bone marrow biopsy
B. CT scan of the chest, abdomen, and pelvis
C. Excisional biopsy
D. Fine-needle aspiration for culture and cytopathology
E. Pelvic ultrasound
F. Reassurance

I-112. Which of the following findings associated with lymphadenopathy is usually suggestive of metastatic cancer rather than a benign etiology?

A. Hard, matted texture of involved nodes
B. Splenomegaly
C. Supraclavicular lymphadenopathy
D. Tender adenopathy of the anterior cervical chain
E. A and B
F. A and C
G. A and D

I-113. All of the following diseases are associated with massive splenomegaly (spleen extends 8 cm below the costal margin or weighs >1000 g) *except*

A. autoimmune hemolytic anemia
B. chronic lymphocytic leukemia
C. cirrhosis with portal hypertension
D. myelofibrosis with myeloid metaplasia
E. none of the above

I-114. The presence of Howell-Jolly bodies, Heinz bodies, basophilic stippling, and nucleated red blood cells in a patient with hairy cell leukemia prior to any treatment intervention implies which of the following?

A. Diffuse splenic infiltration by tumor
B. Disseminated intravascular coagulation (DIC)
C. Hemolytic anemia
D. Pancytopenia
E. Transformation to acute leukemia

I-115. Which of the following is true regarding infection risk after elective splenectomy?

A. Patients are at no increased risk of viral infection after splenectomy.
B. Patients should be vaccinated 2 weeks after splenectomy.
C. Splenectomy patients over the age of 50 are at greatest risk for postsplenectomy sepsis.
D. *Staphylococcus aureus* is the most commonly implicated organism in postsplenectomy sepsis.
E. The risk of infection after splenectomy increases with time.

I-116. A 64-year-old man comes to your office complaining of erectile dysfunction. He is not able to generate an erec-

I-116. *(Continued)*

tion. His past medical history is significant for coronary artery bypass grafting many years ago, status post-carotid endarterectomy, and a mildly reduced left ventricular ejection fraction. His medications include aspirin, carvedilol, simvastatin, lisinopril and furosemide. He does not take nitrates. On physical examination, you note normal-sized testes and a normal prostate. There are no fibrotic changes along the penile corpora. His libido is intact. What is the most likely cause of this patient's erectile dysfunction?

A. Disturbance of blood flow
B. Low testosterone
C. Medication related
D. Psychogenic

I-117. You perform a nocturnal tumescence study on the patient in the preceding scenario. He does not have any erections during rapid-eye-movement sleep. Which treatment modality do you offer at this time?

A. Couple sex therapy
B. Implantation of a penile prosthesis
C. Intraurethral alprostadil
D. Vardenafil

I-118. The wife of the patient in the preceding scenario also reports to you that she has experienced a low sexual desire lately. She is not distressed by this and the couple reports no conflict as a result of her low desire. She is 61 years old and also has a history of a coronary artery bypass graft remotely. She experienced menopause at the age of 53. Her medications include an aspirin, metoprolol, simvastatin, verapamil, and a multivitamin. She asks whether an oral agent will assist with her sexual desire. What is the best answer for this patient?

A. Phosphodiesterase type 5 (PDE-5) inhibitors have been shown to improve sexual function in premenopausal women
B. PDE-5 inhibitors have been shown to improve sexual function in postmenopausal women
C. PDE-5 inhibitors have no role in the treatment of female sexual dysfunction
D. PDE-5 inhibitors treat orgasmic disorder but not sexual arousal disorder

I-119. A 54-year-old male patient of yours presents to your clinic complaining of unexplained weight loss. On review of his chart, you do notice that he has lost 8% of his total body weight in the past year. He has well-treated hypertension for which he takes a thiazide diuretic. Other than recently being widowed, he has no pertinent social history. He is a lifelong nonsmoker and worked as a hospital administrator. An extensive review of systems is unrevealing. Your physical examination reveals no masses or other pathology. A brief psychiatric examination shows no signs of depression. You perform initial testing with a complete blood count; electrolytes, renal function, liver

I-119. *(Continued)*
function, urinalysis, thyroid-stimulating hormone, and a chest x-ray, which are unrevealing. He is up to date on his routine cancer screening. What is the next step in the workup of this patient?

   A. Chest CT scan
   B. Close follow-up
   C. Positron emission tomography (PET) scan
   D. Total-body CT scan
   E. Upper endoscopy

I-120. You are conducting research on a novel nonsteroidal anti-inflammatory drug (NSAID). To ascertain the safety profile of the drug you recruit 100 volunteers who lack the ability to produce IgE. All subjects receive the drug. A minority of participants experience an anaphylactic reaction within minutes of ingesting the drug. IgE levels are undetectable in all 100 subjects. What is the most likely explanation for this phenomenon?

   A. The drug itself directly triggered the immune system in a minority of patients.
   B. The IgE receptor in the patients with anaphylaxis is constitutively activated.
   C. The patients who had anaphylaxis have received this drug before.
   D. The patients who had anaphylaxis overexpress CD8+ T cells.

I-121. Anthrax spores can remain dormant in the respiratory tract for how long?

   A. 1 week
   B. 2 weeks
   C. 3 weeks
   D. 6 weeks
   E. 12 weeks

I-122. Twenty recent attendees at a National Football League game arrive at the emergency department complaining of shortness of breath, fever, and malaise. Chest roentgenograms show mediastinal widening on several of these patients, prompting a concern for inhalational anthrax as a result of a bioterror attack. Antibiotics are initiated and the Centers for Disease Control and Prevention is notified. What form of isolation should be instituted for these patients?

   A. Airborne
   B. Contact
   C. Droplet
   D. None

I-123. Typical *Variola major* (smallpox) infection can be distinguished from *Varicella* (chicken pox) infection based on which of the following clinical characteristics?

   A. Lesions at different stages of development at any location
   B. Lesions in the same stage of development at any location

I-123. *(Continued)*
   C. Maculopapular rash that begins on the face and trunk and spreads to the extremities (centrifugal spread)
   D. Maculopapular rash that begins on the face and extremities and spreads to the trunk (centripetal spread)
   E. B and C
   F. B and D

I-124. You are working in an urban-based intensive care unit and two cases of severe pneumonia are admitted. *Francisella tularensis* is cultured from both patients' sputum samples. Neither patient recalls contact with wild or domesticated animals in the past 2 weeks. You should do all of the following *except*

   A. Alert the Centers for Disease Control and Prevention (CDC) authorities about the potential for a bioterrorist attack.
   B. Alert the microbiology laboratory director.
   C. Institute droplet precaution for the involved patients.
   D. Treat with broad-spectrum antibiotics.

I-125. All of the following are well-documented physical effects of smoking marijuana *except*

   A. decreased sperm count
   B. chronic bronchial irritation
   C. delayed gastric emptying
   D. exercise-induced angina
   E. impaired single-breath carbon monoxide diffusion capacity ($D_{L_{CO}}$)

I-126. A young man is brought to the emergency department by his parents. For the past 12 h he has barricaded himself in his room out of fear of being taken away by "the guys in black." He fears he is losing control and fears that he is going to die. His parents found him trembling and sweating in his room with various pills and plant leaves in his possession. He feels like he is choking and that he is about to die at any minute. On examination, his pupils are dilated and he has a heart rate of 143 beats/min. What substance is most likely to have caused these symptoms?

   A. Heroin
   B. Lysergic acid diethylamide (LSD)
   C. Marijuana
   D. Methamphetamine

I-127. A 37-year-old woman arrives at the emergency department after experiencing a transient state of altered mental status on route to the United States as an immigrant from Nigeria. From the reports of the other passengers and flight attendants on the plane, she was normally interactive throughout most of the flight but was difficult to arouse from sleep upon landing. Upon trying to exit the plane, she fell over and became disarticulate. Her mental status immediately improved when she received naloxone, thiamine, and IV glucose via an emergency response team. Upon arrival at the emergency department 1 h later, she appears

I-127. *(Continued)*
anxious but is alert, oriented, and appropriate. Temperature is 36.8°C, blood pressure is 162/84 mmHg, heart rate is 108 beats/min, respiratory rate is 22 breaths/min, and oxygen saturation is 99% on room air. Her pupils are equal and reactive. Cranial nerves are intact. Her oropharynx is slightly dry. There is no lymphadenopathy. Lungs are clear. She has a regular heart beat with normal S_1, S_2, and no extra heart sounds. Her abdomen has normal bowel sounds with slight epigastric tenderness. Her skin is normal without any track marks or rash. A complete metabolic panel and complete blood count are normal. A urine toxicology screen reveals heroin metabolites. Further evaluation should include:

A. arterial blood gas
B. blood cultures
C. cerebrospinal fluid (CSF) analysis
D. echocardiogram
E. orifice examination

I-128. Which of the following is a distinguishing feature of amphetamine overdose versus other causes of sympathetic overstimulation due to drug overdose or withdrawal?

A. Hallucination
B. Hot, dry, flushed skin and urinary retention
C. History of benzodiazepine abuse
D. Markedly increased blood pressure, heart rate, and end-organ damage in the absence of hallucination
E. Nystagmus

I-129. Which of the following findings suggests an opiate overdose?

A. Anion gap metabolic acidosis with a normal lactate
B. Hypotension and bradycardia in an alert patient
C. Mydriasis
D. Profuse sweating and drooling
E. Therapeutic response to naloxone

I-130. A patient with metabolic acidosis, reduced anion gap, and increased osmolal gap is most likely to have which of the following toxic ingestions?

A. Lithium
B. Methanol
C. Oxycodone
D. Propylene glycol
E. Salicylate

I-131. Which of the following is true regarding drug effects after an overdose in comparison to a reference dose?

A. Drug effects begin earlier, peak earlier, and last longer
B. Drug effects begin earlier, peak later, and last longer
C. Drug effects begin earlier, peak later, and last shorter
D. Drug effects begin later, peak earlier, and last shorter
E. Drug effects begin later, peak later, and last longer

I-132. A 28-year-old man with bipolar disorder, who is on lithium, is found in his room 2 days after not showing up to work. He is arousable but dysarthric and has a markedly abnormal gait when trying to walk. Upon arrival at the emergency department, he has a grand mal seizure. The seizure is not sustained but recurs an hour after 6 mg lorazepam is infused IV. In the postictal stage, he is not arousable to sternal rub and lacks a gag reflex. His serum sodium returns at 158 meq/L. In reference to his seizures, all of the following are next steps in his management *except*

A. barbiturates
B. benzodiazepines
C. endotracheal intubation
D. free water replacement
E. phenytoin

I-133. Which of the following statements regarding gastric decontamination for toxin ingestion is true?

A. Activated charcoal's most common side effect is aspiration.
B. Gastric lavage via nasogastric tube is preferred over the use of activated charcoal in situations where therapeutic endoscopy may also be warranted.
C. Syrup of ipecac has no role in the hospital setting.
D. There are insufficient data to support or exclude a benefit when gastric decontamination is used more than 1 h after a toxic ingestion.
E. All of the above are true.

I-134. What is the main contributor to the resting energy expenditure of an individual?

A. Adipose tissue
B. Exercise level
C. Lean body mass
D. Resting heart rate
E. None of the above

I. INTRODUCTION TO CLINICAL MEDICINE

ANSWERS

I-1 and I-2. The answers are C and C. *(Chap. 3)* In evaluating the usefulness of a test, it is imperative to understand the clinical implications of the sensitivity and specificity of that test. By obtaining information about the prevalence of the disease in the population—the specificity and sensitivity—one can generate a two-by-two table, as shown below. This table is used to generate the total number of patients in each group of the population:

	Disease Status	
Test Result	Present	Absent
Positive	True-positive	False-positive
Negative	False-negative	True-negative
	Total number of patients with disease	Total number of patients without disease

The sensitivity of the test is $TP/(TP + FN)$. The specificity is $TN/(TN + FP)$. In this case the table is filled in as follows:

	Disease Status	
Test Result	Present	Absent
Positive	42	237
Negative	8	713
	Total number of patients with disease = 50	Total number of patients without disease = 950

I-3. The answer is A. *(Chap. 3)* A capitation system provides physicians with a fixed payment per patient per year. This has the potential to encourage physicians to take on more patients but to provide patients with fewer services because the physician is liable for expenses. A fixed salary system encourages physicians to take on fewer patients. A fee-for-service system encourages physicians to provide more services. Out-of-pocket services not covered by insurers are available only to patients with adequate means to receive the service.

I-4. The answer is C. *(Chap. 3)* A receiver operating characteristic curve plots sensitivity on the *y*-axis and (1 – specificity) on the *x*-axis. Each point on the curve represents a cutoff point of sensitivity and 1 – specificity. The area under the curve can be used as a quantitative measure of the information content of a test. Values range from 0.5 (a 45° line) representing no diagnostic information to 1.0 for a perfect test. See Figure I-4.

I-5. The answer is A. *(Chap. 3)* Bayes' theorem is used in an attempt to quantify uncertainty by employing an equation that combines pretest probability with the testing characteristics of specificity and sensitivity. The pretest probability quantitatively describes the clinician's certainty of a diagnosis after doing a history and physical examination. The equation is

$$\text{Posttest probability} = \frac{\text{Pretest probability} \times \text{test sensitivity}}{\text{Pretest probability} \times \text{test sensitivity} + (1 - \text{disease prevalence}) \times \text{test false-positive rate}}$$

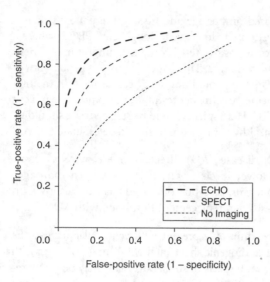

FIGURE I-4 The receiver operating characteristic (ROC) curves for three diagnostic exercise tests for detection of CAD: exercise ECG, exercise SPECT, and exercise echo. Each ROC curve illustrates the trade-off that occurs between improved test sensitivity (accurate detection of patients with disease) and improved test specificity (accurate detection of patients without disease), as the test value defining when the test turns from "negative" to "positive" is varied. A 45° line would indicate a test with no information (sensitivity = specificity at every test value). The area under each ROC curve is a measure of the information content of the test. Moving to a test with a larger ROC area (e.g., from exercise ECG to exercise echo) improves diagnostic accuracy. However, these curves are not measured in the same populations and the effect of referral biases on the results cannot easily be discerned. *(From KE Fleischmann et al: JAMA 280:913, 1998, with permission.)*

In this manner, the uncertainty one faces in clinical decision making is quantified. By inserting numbers into the equation, one can see that a low pretest probability combined with a poorly sensitive and specific test will yield a low posttest probability. However, the same test result, when combined with a high pretest probability, will yield a high posttest probability. There have been criticisms of this theorem. Unfortunately, few tests have only two outcomes: positive and negative. This theorem does not take into account the useful information that is gained from nonbinary test results. Further, it is cumbersome to calculate the posttest probability for each individual circumstance and patient. Perhaps the most useful lesson from Bayes' theorem is to take into account pretest probability when ordering tests or interpreting test results. To be clinically useful, a clinical scenario with a low pretest probability will require a test with high sensitivity and specificity. Conversely, a high pretest probability presentation can be confirmed by a test with only average sensitivity and specificity.

I-6. **The answer is D.** *(Chap. 3)* A positive likelihood ratio can only be interpreted in the context of a pretest probability of disease. Disease prevalence in a certain region contributes to the patient's pretest probability. However, other factors such as the patient's age, clinical history and risk factors for the disease in question are also important in determining pretest probability. Armed with an estimated pretest probability and a positive test with a known likelihood ratio, the clinician can estimate a posttest probability of disease. Generally, diagnostic tests are most useful in patients with a medium pretest probability (25–75%) of having a disease. For example, in a patient with a low pretest probability of disease, a positive test can be misleading in that the patient's posttest probability of disease is still low. The same applies for a patient with a high pretest probability of disease with a negative test: the negative test usually does not rule out disease. It is therefore incumbent upon the physician to have a rough estimate of the pretest probability of disease, positive likelihood ratio of the diagnostic test, and negative likelihood ratio of the diagnostic test prior to ordering the test.

I-7 and I-8. **The answers are B and C.** *(Chap. 3)* The goal of a meta-analysis is to summarize the treatment benefit conferred by an intervention. Risk reduction is frequently expressed by relative risk or odds ratios; however, clinicians also find it useful to be familiar with the absolute risk reduction (ARR). This is the difference in mortality (or another endpoint) between the treatment and the placebo arms. In this case, the absolute risk reduction is 10% − 2% = 8%. From this number, one can calculate the number needed to treat (NNT), which is 1/ARR. The NNT is the number of patients who must receive the intervention to prevent one death (or another outcome assessed in the study). In this case the NNT is 1/8% = 12.5 patients.

I-9.   **The answer is D.** *(Chaps. 3 and 219)* Based on her age and history, the patient's pretest probability of coronary artery disease is extremely low. Even though the SPECT scan is a test with good performance characteristics, a positive test is only meaningful in a patient with medium pretest probability of coronary disease. This patient's posttest probability of coronary disease is still low to medium. The test should not have been ordered in the first place and is an example of defensive medicine. Any further testing could expose the patient to undue invasive testing and further anxiety. Her aspirin should be stopped; she should be reassured; other causes of chest pain in a healthy young woman should be evaluated.

I-10. **The answer is C.** *(Chap. 6)* Alzheimer's disease (AD) affects women twice as commonly as men. Women with AD have lower levels of circulating estrogen than age-controlled women without disease. Despite this, placebo-controlled trials have shown no benefit in terms of cognitive decline for estrogen replacement in women with AD.

I-11. **The answer is D.** *(Chap. 54)* Men more commonly present with ventricular tachycardia and women more commonly present with cardiogenic shock after MI. Younger women with MI are more likely to die than their male counterparts of similar age. This may be partly related to the observation that physicians are less likely to suspect heart disease in women with chest pain and are less likely to perform diagnostic and therapeutic procedures in women.

I-12. **The answer is D.** *(Chap. 6)* Exercise electrocardiographic testing has *both* higher false positives and false negatives in women than in men. Women with myocardial infarctions less often receive angioplasty, thrombolytics, aspirin, beta blockers, or CABGs than men. While women have a greater perioperative mortality, lower graft patency rate, and less angina relief than men after CABG, their 5- and 10-year mortality rates are not different from those of men.

I-13. **The answer is D.** *(Chap. 6)* Aspirin does not provide primary prevention for myocardial infarction for women with coronary heart disease, but it does provide primary prevention for ischemic stroke and is therefore a useful drug for women at risk for atherosclerotic disease. Cholesterol-lowering drugs are as effective in women as in men for primary and secondary prevention of coronary heart disease. Low HDL and diabetes mellitus are more important risk factors in women than in men. Overall, women receive fewer risk modification interventions than men, likely because of the perception that they are at lower risk of coronary heart disease.

I-14. **The answer is C.** *(Chap. 10)* Echinacea constituents have in vitro activity to stimulate humoral and cellular immune responses. Yet clinical trials have not shown convincing efficacy for respiratory infections. *Ginkgo biloba* is being evaluated in a large trial to evaluate its efficacy in reducing the rate of onset or progression of dementia. However, there is no current evidence that it improves cognition. Saw palmetto and African plum are widely purchased by Americans to relieve symptomatic BPH, yet clinical trials of saw palmetto have not shown efficacy. While St.-John's-wort showed benefit in small and non-controlled trials, high-quality placebo-controlled trials showed no superiority compared to placebo for patients with major depression of moderate severity. Only glucosamine/chondroitin sulfate have proven benefit in a large multicenter controlled trial. It is not known if it slows cartilage degeneration.

I-15. **The answer is D.** *(Chap. 5)* Steady-state serum levels are achieved after five elimination half-lives, when the dosing interval is 50% of the half-life. Therefore, from a pharmacokinetic standpoint, the patient may not achieve full efficacy of the antihypertensive agent until 10 days into therapy. Therefore checking for effect at 3 days is premature. Doubling the dose or increasing the frequency may predispose to toxicity. There is no reason to add a second agent or switch to another agent until completing a trial of adequate duration on the current agent.

I-16. **The answer is A.** *(Chap. 5)* The patient is developing full-blown cirrhosis and as a result has impaired hepatic clearance of his morphine. This is due to impaired first-pass metabolism as a consequence of abnormal liver architecture, depressed cytochrome P450 activity, and perhaps portacaval shunting. Physical and laboratory examinations reveal evidence of worsening cirrhosis and opiate toxicity. Hepatic encephalopathy and sub-acute bacterial peritonitis are considerations in the cirrhotic patient with impaired mental status. However, the patient has no discernible ascites and no evidence of hepatic encephalopathy on examination. The focus should be on reducing centrally acting therapies such as morphine, rather than adding another medicine such as haloperidol.

I-17.   The answer is B. *(Chap. 20)* This patient presents with frostbite of the left foot. The most common presenting symptom of this disorder is sensory changes that affect pain and temperature. Physical examination can have a multitude of findings, depending on the degree of tissue damage. Mild frostbite will show erythema and anesthesia. With more extensive damage, bullae and vesicles will develop. Hemorrhagic vesicles are due to injury to the microvasculature. The prognosis is most favorable when the presenting area is warm and has a normal color. Treatment is with rapid rewarming, which usually is accomplished with a 37 to 40°C (98.6 to 104°F) water bath. The period of rewarming can be intensely painful for the patient, and often narcotic analgesia is warranted. If the pain is intolerable, the temperature of the water bath can be dropped slightly. Compartment syndrome can develop with rewarming and should be investigated if cyanosis persists after rewarming. No medications have been shown to improve outcomes, including heparin, steroids, calcium channel blockers, and hyperbaric oxygen. In the absence of wet gangrene or another emergent surgical indication, decisions about the need for amputation or debridement should be deferred until the boundaries of the tissue injury are well demarcated. After recovery from the initial insult, these patients often have neuronal injury with abnormal sympathetic tone in the extremity. Other remote complications include cutaneous carcinomas, nail deformities, and, in children, epiphyseal damage.

I-18.   The answer is C. *(Chap. 9)* Urinary incontinence occurring randomly without associated Valsalva or other stress is most likely detrusor overactivity. This disorder is the most common type of incontinence in the elderly, both males and females. In females there is no need to do further testing in a patient with long-standing incontinence; however, in males urethral obstruction is often coexistent, and urodynamic testing is indicated to investigate this possibility. An abrupt onset of symptoms or associated suprapubic pain in either sex should prompt cystoscopy and urine cytologic testing to evaluate for bladder stones, tumor, or infection. First-line therapy is behavioral therapy with or without biofeedback. Frequent timed voiding is often successful. If drugs are imperative, oxybutynin or tolterodine can be tried with close follow-up to ensure that urinary retention does not occur. Desmopressin must be used with extreme caution in this population. Indeed, patients with heart failure, chronic kidney disease, or hyponatremia should not take this medication. Indwelling catheters are rarely indicated for this disorder; instead, external collection devices or protective pads or undergarments are favored.

I-19.   The answer is B. *(Chaps. 5 and 9)* Adverse drug reactions in the geriatric population are common, occurring two to three times more frequently than they do in younger patients. This is due to several factors. Drug clearance is altered because of decreased renal plasma flow and glomerular filtration as well as decreased hepatic clearance. Furthermore, the volume of distribution of many drugs is decreased with a drop in total body water. However, in older persons there is a relative increase in fat, which will lengthen the half-life of fat-soluble medications. Serum albumin levels decline in general in the elderly, particularly in the hospitalized and sick population. As a result, drugs that are primarily protein-bound, such as warfarin and phenytoin, will have higher free or active levels at similar doses. Care must be taken in interpreting total serum levels for these drugs because a low total level may be accompanied by a normal free level and thus be appropriately therapeutic.

I-20.   The answer is A. *(Chap. 5)* In population surveys of noninstitutionalized elderly, up to 10% had at least one adverse drug reaction in the prior year. Adverse drug reactions are common in the elderly and are related to altered drug sensitivity, impaired renal or hepatic clearance, impaired homeostatic mechanisms, and drug interactions. Long half-life benzodiazepines are linked to the increased occurrence of hip fractures in the elderly. The association may be due to the increased risk of falling (related to sedation) in a population with a high prevalence of osteoporosis. This association may also be true for other drugs with sedative properties such as opioids or antipsychotics. Exaggerated responses to cardiovascular drugs such as ACE inhibitors may occur because of a blunted vasoconstrictor or chronotropic response to reduced blood pressure. Conversely, elderly patients often display decreased sensitivity to beta blockers.

I-21.   The answer is C. *(Chap. 5)* Grapefruit juice inhibits CYP3A4 in the liver, particularly at high doses. This can cause decreased drug elimination via hepatic metabolism and increase potential drug toxicities. Atorvastatin is metabolized via this pathway. Drugs that may enhance atorvastatin toxicity via this mechanism include phenytoin, ritonavir, clarithromycin, and azole antifungals. Aspirin is cleared via renal mechanisms. Prevacid can cause impaired absorption of other drugs via its effect on gastric pH. Sildenafil is a phosphodiesterase inhibitor that may enhance the effect of nitrate medications and cause hypotension.

I-22.   The answer is A. *(Chaps. 18 and 185)* Based on the characteristic rash and Koplik's spots, this patient has measles. A rare but feared complication of measles is subacute sclerosing panencephalitis. His examination does not support epiglottitis as he has no drooling or dysphagia. His rash is not characteristic of acute HIV infection, and he lacks the pharyngitis and arthralgias commonly seen with this diagnosis. The rash is not consistent with herpes zoster, and he is quite young to invoke this diagnosis. Splenic rupture occasionally occurs with infectious mononucleosis, but this patient has no pharyngitis, lymphadenopathy, or splenomegaly to suggest this diagnosis.

I-23 and I-24.   The answers are D and D. *(Chap. 215)* This patient has symptoms of an acute cholinergic crisis as seen in cases of organophosphate poisoning. Organophosphates are the "classic" nerve agents, and several different compounds may act in this manner, including sarin, tabun, soman, and cyclosarin. Except for agent VX, all the organophosphates are liquid at standard room temperature and pressure and are highly volatile, with the onset of symptoms occurring within minutes to hours after exposure. VX is an oily liquid with a low vapor pressure; therefore, it does not acutely cause symptoms. However, it is an environmental hazard because it can persist in the environment for a longer period. Organophosphates act by inhibiting tissue synaptic acetylcholinesterase. Symptoms differ between vapor exposure and liquid exposure because the organophosphate acts in the tissue upon contact. The first organ exposed with vapor exposure is the eyes, causing rapid and persistent pupillary constriction. After the sarin gas attacks in the Tokyo subway in 1994 and 1995, survivors frequently complained that their "world went black" as the first symptom of exposure. This is rapidly followed by rhinorrhea, excessive salivation, and lacrimation. In the airways, organophosphates cause bronchorrhea and bronchospasm. It is in the alveoli that organophosphates gain the greatest extent of entry into the blood. As organophosphates circulate, other symptoms appear, including nausea, vomiting, diarrhea, and muscle fasciculations. Death occurs with central nervous system penetration causing central apnea and status epilepticus. The effects on the heart rate and blood pressure are unpredictable.

Treatment requires a multifocal approach. Initially, decontamination of clothing and wounds is important for both the patient and the caregiver. Clothing should be removed before contact with the health care provider. In Tokyo, 10% of emergency personnel developed miosis related to contact with patients' clothing. Three classes of medication are important in treating organophosphate poisoning: anticholinergics, oximes, and anticonvulsant agents. Initially, atropine at doses of 2 to 6 mg should be given intravenously or intramuscularly to reverse the effects of organophosphates at muscarinic receptors; it has no effect on nicotinic receptors. Thus, atropine rapidly treats life-threatening respiratory depression but does not affect neuromuscular or sympathetic effects. This should be followed by the administration of an oxime, which is a nucleophile compound that reactivates the cholinesterase whose active site has been bound to a nerve agent. Depending on the nerve agent used, oxime may not be helpful because it is unable to bind to "aged" complexes that have undergone degradation of a side chain of the nerve agent, making it negatively charged. Soman undergoes aging within 2 min, thus rendering oxime therapy useless. The currently approved oxime in the United States is 2-pralidoxime. Finally, the only anticonvulsant class of drugs that is effective in seizures caused by organophosphate poisoning is benzodiazepines. The dose required is frequently higher than that used for epileptic seizures, requiring the equivalent of 40 mg of diazepam given in frequent doses. All other classes of anticonvulsant medications, including phenytoin, barbiturates, carbamazepine, and valproic acid, will not improve seizures related to organophosphate poisoning.

I-25. **The answer is E.** *(Chap. 215)* Cyanide is an asphyxiant that causes death by inhibiting cellular respiration. It is a colorless liquid or gas that has a typical smell of almonds. The onset of symptoms after cyanide exposure is rapid and usually begins with eye irritation. The skin is flushed. The patient rapidly develops confusion, tachypnea, and tachycardia. With severe poisoning, death results from acute respiratory distress syndrome (ARDS) and hypoxemia with lactic acidosis. The antidote for cyanide poisoning is a combination of sodium nitrite and sodium thiosulfate.

I-26. **The answer is A.** *(Chap. 215)* Sulfur mustard was the first weaponized chemical and was first used in World War I, accounting for 70% of the estimated 1.3 million chemical casualties in that war. It remains a significant terrorist threat today because of simplicity of manufacture and effectiveness. Sulfur mustard constitutes both a vapor and a liquid chemical threat. It acts as a DNA-alkylating agent and affects rapidly dividing cells. The effects of sulfur mustard are delayed 2 h to 2 days, depending on the severity of exposure. The organs most commonly affected are the skin, eyes, and airways. Late bone marrow suppression also occurs 7 to 21 days after exposure. Erythema resembling a sunburn is the mildest form of injury. This progresses to large flaccid bullae containing sterile serous fluid. Large portions of body-surface area may be affected, similar to the situation in burn victims. The primary airway lesion is necrosis of the mucosa. Clinically, this causes pseudomembrane formation and, in the most severe cases, airway obstruction. Laryngospasm may also occur. The effects on the eyes include conjunctivitis, blepharospasm, pain, and corneal damage. Death results from airway obstruction, pneumonia, secondary skin infections, or sepsis with neutropenia. There is no antidote to mustard gas or liquid exposure. Treatment is supportive, ensuring adequate analgesia and hydration. Application of topical glucocorticoids before denudation of skin may be useful. Small blisters should be left intact, but large bullae should be unroofed. The fluid is sterile and does not contain mustard derivatives. Silver sulfadiazine or other topical antibiotics should be used to prevent secondary skin infections. Conjunctival irritation should be treated with topical solutions, including antibiotics. Petroleum jelly should be applied to the eyelids to prevent them from sticking together. Intubation may be necessary for protection against airway obstruction. Repeated bronchoscopy may also be needed to remove pseudomembranes. Finally, careful follow-up for the development of marrow suppression is needed.

I-27. **The answer is C.** *(Chaps. 18 and 167)* This patient likely has Rocky Mountain spotted fever. The headache and thrombocytopenia after a recent camping trip in a rickettsial endemic region are typical findings. As this is usually a serologic diagnosis requiring significant laboratory processing time, and can be fatal, empirical therapy with doxycycline is warranted. The lack of a rash does not preclude this diagnosis because the characteristic macular rash spreading from the wrists and ankles centripetally appears 2–5 days after the first fever. Atovaquone is used for babesiosis, a disease that is defined by hemolysis and is not prevalent in the Ozarks. The patient has no evidence of bacterial meningitis to warrant empirical coverage. While fever and myalgias are typical of influenza, it is most common in winter and does not typically cause thrombocytopenia.

I-28. **The answer is C.** *(Chaps. 18 and 129)* This case is likely toxic shock syndrome, given the clinical appearance of septic shock with no positive blood cultures. The characteristic diffuse rash, as well as the lack of a primary infected site, make staphylococcus the more likely inciting agent. Streptococcal toxic shock usually has a prominent primary site of infection, but the diffuse rash is usually much more subtle than in this case. Staphylococcal toxic shock can be associated with immunosuppression, surgical wounds, or retained tampons. Mere *Staphylococcus aureus* colonization (with an appropriate toxigenic strain) can incite toxic shock. Centers for Disease Control and Prevention guidelines state that measles, Rocky Mountain spotted fever, and leptospirosis need to be ruled out serologically to confirm the diagnosis. However, this patient is at very low risk for these diagnoses based on vaccination and travel history. JRA would become a consideration only if the fevers were more prolonged and there was documented evidence of organomegaly and enlarged lymph nodes.

I-29.   The answer is C. *(Chap. 214)* Using the characteristics listed in the question, the CDC developed classifications of biologic agents that are based on their potential to be used as bioweapons. Six types of agents have been designated as category A: *Bacillus anthracis*, botulinum toxin, Yersinia pestis, smallpox, tularemia, and the many viruses that cause viral hemorrhagic fever. Those viruses include Lassa virus, Rift Valley fever virus, Ebola virus, and yellow fever virus.

I-30.   The answer is E. *(Chaps. 18 and 149)* *Vibrio vulnificus* is a marine-borne gram-negative rod that causes overwhelming sepsis in the immunocompromised host, particularly cirrhotic patients. Modes of infection are direct wound inoculation or ingestion via raw seafood. Presentation is rapid with the classic skin findings described in this case, which approximate purpura fulminans as the illness progresses. Mortality is >50%, even with appropriate and early antibiotics.

I-31.   The answer is C. *(Chap. 17)* *Hyperthermia* occurs when exogenous heat exposure or an endogenous heat-producing process, such as neuroleptic malignant syndrome or malignant hyperthermia, leads to high internal temperatures despite a *normal* hypothalamic temperature set point. *Fever* occurs when a pyrogen such as a microbial toxin, microbe particle, or cytokine resets the hypothalamus to a higher temperature. A particular temperature cutoff point does not define hyperthermia. Rigidity and autonomic dysregulation are characteristic of malignant hyperthermia, a subset of hyperthermia. Fever, not hyperthermia, responds to antipyretics.

I-32.   The answer is D. *(Chap. 17)* This patient has malignant hyperthermia, for which dantrolene and external cooling are appropriate interventions. Malignant hyperthermia occurs in individuals with a genetic predisposition that causes elevated skeletal muscle intracellular calcium concentration after exposure to some inhaled anesthetics or succinylcholine. Cardiovascular instability is common within minutes. Although malignant hyperthermia is rare, these drugs are used commonly, and without prompt recognition the condition may be fatal. There is no role for antipyretics as the thalamic set point for temperature is likely not altered in the setting of hyperthermia.

I-33.   The answer is E. *(Chap. 17)* The elderly and the very young are at highest risk of nonexertional heat stroke. Environmental stress (heat wave) is the most common precipitating factor, particularly in the bedridden or for those living in poorly ventilated or non-air-conditioned conditions. Medications such as antiparkinson treatment, diuretics, or anticholinergic therapy increase the risk of heat stroke.

I-34.   The answer is A. *(Chap. 20)* Initial focus should be aggressive rewarming. Further attempts at defibrillation are unlikely to work until core temperature is normalized. Pharmacologic strategies are also ineffective in the setting of hypothermia, though the possibility of toxicity based on accumulation of drug does exist once successful rewarming is achieved. If initial active rewarming techniques are ineffective, cardiopulmonary bypass, warmed hemodialysis, peritoneal lavage with warmed fluid, or pleural lavage with warmed fluid should be considered on an emergent basis. A pacemaker will not be effective for ventricular fibrillation and may provoke arrhythmias due to ventricular irritability.

I-35. **The answer is B.** *(Chap. 72)* Albumin has a half-life of 2 to 3 weeks and is a sensitive but nonspecic measure of protein-calorie malnutrition. Other situations in which albumin is low include sepsis, surgery, overhydration, and increased plasma volume, including congestive heart failure, renal failure, and chronic liver disease. Among the other markers of nutritional state, transferrin has a half-life of 1 week. Prealbumin and retinol-binding protein complex have the same half-life of 2 days. Fibronectin has the shortest half-life: 1 day.

I-36. **The answer is C.** *(Chap. 20)* This patient has severe frostbite vesiculations implying deep tissue injury, including the microvasculature. Medical therapy with intravenous or topical vasodilators is not effective in this setting. Decisions regarding surgical debridement and amputation are best made in the chronic stage of management rather than acutely in the absence of infection. Initially, rewarming and aggressive analgesia with opiates are the mainstay of therapy.

I-37. **The answer is D.** *(Chap. 4)* It is important to contrast the relative risk reduction of an intervention versus the absolute risk reduction. The ARR is 0.88% − 0.59% = 0.29% (note: rates are per 1000 persons). The relative risk reduction in this case is ~30%. It might be predicted, therefore, that this intervention might result in a 30% decrease in colon cancer mortality if widely implemented in a target population. However, the ARR is much smaller; 1 divided by the absolute risk reduction (1/ARR) equals the number needed to treat to prevent one colon cancer death. In this case, that number is ~330. Therefore, while the impact on a population level might be large, it takes a large number of patients to prevent one event with the intervention (FOBT).

I-38. **The answer is B.** *(Chap. 4)* Predicted increases in life expectancy are average numbers that apply to populations, not individuals. Because we often do not understand the true nature of risk of disease, screening and lifestyle interventions usually benefit a small proportion of the total population. For screening tests, false positives may also increase the risk of diagnostic tests. While Pap smears increase life expectancy overall by only 2–3 months, for the individual at risk of cervical cancer, Pap smear screening may add many years to life. The average life expectancy increases resulting from mammography (1 month), PSA (2 weeks), or exercise (1–2 years) are less than from quitting smoking (3–5 years).

I-39. **The answer is B.** *(Chaps. 4 and 235)* Current guidelines from the National Cholesterol Education Project Adult Treatment Panel III recommend screening in all adults >20 years old. The testing should include fasting total cholesterol, triglycerides, low-density lipoprotein cholesterol, and high-density lipoprotein cholesterol. The screening should be repeated every 5 years. All patients with Type 1 diabetes should have lipids followed closely to decrease cardiovascular risk by combining the results of lipid screening with other risk factors to determine risk category and intensity of recommended treatment.

I-40. **The answer is C.** *(Chap. 386)* Generalized anxiety disorder is common, with a lifetime prevalence of approximately 5% and with the onset of symptoms often occurring before age 20. These patients frequently report having feelings of anxiety and social phobia that date back to childhood. Clinically, these patients report persistent, excessive, and unrealistic worries that prevent normal functioning. In addition, there is often the complaint of feeling "on edge" with nervousness, arousal, and insomnia. However, unlike panic disorder, palpitations, tachycardia, and shortness of breath are rare. Pathophysiologically, there is likely to be impaired function of the GABA receptor with decreased binding of benzodiazepines at that receptor. Therapy should include a combination of drugs and psychotherapy. Drugs that may be used include benzodiazepines, buspirone, and anticonvulsants with GABAergic properties, such as gabapentin, tiagabine, and divalproex.

I-41. **The answer is D.** *(Chap. 10; Wilt et al.)* Because plant products are in widespread use in the well-accepted therapeutic armamentarium of Western medicine (e.g., digoxin, taxol, penicillin), it should not be surprising that several "herbal remedies" have been demonstrated in prospective clinical trials to be beneficial. For example, Saint John's wort is more effective than placebo for mild to moderate depression; the mechanism is not known, although the metabolism of several neurotransmitters is inhibited by this substance. Kava products have antianxiolytic activity. Extracts of the fruit of the saw palmetto, *Serona repens*, have been shown to decrease nocturia and improve peak urinary flow compared with placebo in males with benign prostatic hypertrophy. Saw palmetto extracts affect the metabolism of androgens, including the inhibition of dihydrotestosterone binding to androgen receptors.

I-42.   The answer is D. *(Chap. 76)* The most important feature of patients with anorexia nervosa is refusal to maintain even a low-normal body weight. The full syndrome of anorexia nervosa occurs in about 1 in 200 individuals. These patients are always markedly underweight, hardly ever menstruate, and often engage in binge eating. The mortality rate is 5% per decade. The etiology of this serious eating disorder is unknown but probably involves a combination of psychological, biologic, and cultural risk factors. This illness often begins in an obsessive or perfectionist patient who starts a diet. As weight loss progresses, the patient has increasing fears of gaining weight and engages in stricter dieting practices. This disorder essentially occurs only in cultures in which thinness is valued, suggesting a strong cultural influence. Bulimia nervosa, in which patients continue to maintain a normal body weight but typically engage in overeating with binges followed by compensatory purging or purging behavior, has a higher than expected prevalence in patients with childhood or parental obesity. It is unclear whether anorexia nervosa is hereditary in nature.

I-43.   The answer is C. *(Chap. 71)* Certain medications, including isoniazid used for tuberculosis, L-dopa used for Parkinson's disease, and penicillamine used for scleroderma, promote vitamin B_6 (pyridoxine) deficiency by reacting with a carbonyl group on 5-pyridoxal phosphate, which is a cofactor for a host of enzymes involved in amino acid metabolism. Foods that contain vitamin B_6 include legumes, nuts, wheat bran, and meat. Vitamin B_6 deficiency produces seborrheic dermatitis, glossitis, stomatitis, and cheliosis (also seen in other vitamin B deficiencies). A microcytic, hypochromic anemia may result from the fact that the first enzyme in heme synthesis (aminolevulinic synthetase) requires pyridoxal phosphate as a cofactor. However, vitamin B_6 is also necessary for the conversion of homocysteine to cystathionine. Consequently, a deficiency of this vitamin could produce an increased risk of cardiovascular disease caused by the resultant hyperhomocystinemia.

I-44.   The answer is C. *(Chap. 9)* Hypertension and diabetes are the most important chronic diseases whose prevalence increases with age. In those >65 years old, the prevalence of hypertension is estimated at 60–85%. These numbers will likely increase in the near future as the population ages and obesity is more prevalent. Recent data suggest that the frequency of uncontrolled hypertension is increasing in older adults in the United States. The presence of uncontrolled hypertension accelerates functional and cognitive decline in older adults. These data also have important implications on the frequency of cardiovascular disease and stroke in older adults.

I-45.   The answer is B. *(Chap. 4)* The prevalence of diabetes in older adults is ~18–21%. This rate will likely increase with increasing obesity in older adults. Diabetes has been linked with physical decline, while hypertension has been linked with cognitive decline. However, both disorders are commonly present in the elderly. Diabetes and stroke are most consistently associated with a diminished capacity for functional recovery in the elderly.

I-46.   The answer is A. *(Chap. 9)* Functional status, as defined by a patient's ability to provide for his or her own daily needs, is the most important indicator for prognosis. A decline in functional status should prompt a search for medical illness, dementia, change in social support, or depression. Screening for functional status should include assessment of activities of daily living, gait and balance, cognition, vision, hearing, and dental and nutritional health.

I-47.   **The answer is A.** *(Chaps. 9 and 26)* Delirium can cause prolonged hospitalization and may be life threatening. It is often underdiagnosed. The Confusion Assessment Method (CAM) is highly sensitive and specific for identifying delirium. One common misconception is that all delirious patients are agitated. In fact, delirium is often associated with a decreased level of consciousness, and patients can appear withdrawn or aloof, rather than agitated, combative, or anxious. Another crucial diagnostic criterion is that the patient's mental state represents a clear, acute deviation from their baseline status.

I-48.   **The answer is E.** *(Chap. 9)* Fall rates increase with age and have substantial effect on mortality and morbidity. Some 3–5% of falls result in fracture, and falls are an independent risk factor for nursing home placement. All older adults should have at least annual fall risk assessment and be asked about falls during clinic visits. Fall prevention necessitates a multidisciplinary approach including management of medical conditions associated with falls, limitation of psychotropic medicines (especially benzodiazepines), frequent visual examinations, interventions such as tai-chi geared towards stabilizing gait, and close examination of circumstances associated with past falls.

I-49.   **The answer is B.** *(Chap. 9)* Physical examination of all immobilized or bed-bound patients must include careful examination of common sites for pressure sores. The heels, lateral malleoli, sacrum, ischia, and greater trochanters account for 80% of pressure sores. Shear forces and moisture are predisposing factors. In older adults and nursing home residents, the development of a pressure sore increases mortality fourfold. Infectious complications include osteomyelitis and sepsis. A fairly innocuous-appearing lesion can progress to a deep, easily infected, and very difficult-to-manage stage 4 decubitus ulcer in a very short period of time without aggressive wound care and off-loading by nursing staff.

I-50.   **The answer is E.** *(Chap. 9)* This patient has stress incontinence. Stress incontinence, due to dysfunction of the urethral sphincter, is common in women and uncommon in men. It most often occurs with activities that increase abdominal pressure. The most common risks are previous childbearing, gynecologic surgery, and menopause. Kegel exercises may be useful, but surgery is considered the most effective intervention. Oxybutynin and bladder training exercises are sometimes effective for urge incontinence, which is more common in men. α-Adrenergic blockers and 5-α-reductase inhibitors are used for prostate hypertrophy in men. Close monitoring for hyperglycemia and diabetes is useful in elderly patients with incontinence, but this patient does not describe polyuria and her past vaginal deliveries and pelvic surgery put her at risk for stress incontinence.

I-51.   **The answer is B.** *(Chap. 23)* The patient has Brown-Séquard syndrome, likely because of a new multiple sclerosis plaque. The lack of cranial nerve involvement and other cortical deficits, in the presence of upper extremity and lower extremity deficits, suggests a high cord lesion. These often lead to differing ipsilateral and contralateral sensory deficits, as in this patient. The combination of left side motor deficit and right side sensory deficit makes the cortical lesion unlikely. Brainstem lesions will also not account for the localization and bilaterality. A cervical cord root lesion would not be bilateral.

I-52.   **The answer is A.** *(Chaps. 23 and 292)* The patient's weight loss predisposes him to superior mesenteric artery (SMA) syndrome. Due to loss of the omental fat pad, the SMA compresses the duodenum in this condition, leading to obstruction. Laparoscopy is less likely to be of diagnostic benefit (i.e., for adhesions) as the patient has never had abdominal surgery. An upper GI series may be useful for evaluation of an obstructing mass, though SMA syndrome is more likely in this clinical context. While patients with advanced HIV are at risk of a variety of infectious causes of diarrhea, they are unlikely to present with acute small-bowel obstruction. Serum CEA levels may be elevated in colon cancer but would not be helpful in explaining the cause of acute small-bowel obstruction.

I-53.   **The answer is C.** *(Chap. 23)* Amyloidosis predisposes to autonomic neuropathy, which in turn causes both orthostasis and gastroparesis. Gastrointestinal amyloidosis is another possibility in this patient, though his early satiety and bloating are typical for gastroparesis. Treatment can include pro-motility agents, such as metoclopramide as well as dietary changes that this patient has already instituted on his own. Small-bowel obstruction would not be relieved by smaller frequent meals. Gastric cancers may present with early satiety and vomiting as well as weight loss. Diverticulosis and irritable bowel syndrome present with lower gastrointestinal symptoms.

I-54.   The answer is D. *(Chap. 39)* This patient has developed tardive dyskinesia that may be irreversible. Prochlorperazine is an antidopaminergic agent that suppresses emesis by acting centrally at the dopamine D_2 receptors. This class of agents is most effective for the treatment of medication-, toxin-, and metabolic-induced emesis. However, these agents freely cross the blood-brain barrier and can cause anxiety, galactorrhea, sexual dysfunction, and dystonic reactions. Tardive dyskinesia is the most serious of these neurologic toxicities. Erythromycin is a prokinetic that may worsen nausea and vomiting. Ondansetron acts at the $5-HT_3$ receptor and has no antidopaminergic activity. Scopolamine is an anticholinergic that may cause delirium, stupor, and other neurologic side effects, but not tardive dyskinesia. Glucocorticoids also do not cause tardive dyskinesia.

I-55.   The answer is D. *(Chap. 34)* Chronic cough is defined as a cough present for >8 weeks. *Mycoplasma* infection can cause a cough acutely or a postinfectious cough that persists for as long as 8 weeks. Asthma, postnasal drip, and reflux disease are the three most common causes of chronic cough in a nonsmoker not taking angiotensin-converting enzyme (ACE) inhibitors. All ACE inhibitors, including lisinopril, can cause chronic cough, possibly due to altered bradykinin metabolism. Patients with ACE inhibitor cough may be switched to an angiotensin receptor blocker, which does not cause cough.

I-56.   The answer is B. *(Chaps. 34 and 252)* The putrid smell and polymicrobial gram stain suggest a polymicrobial lung abscess consisting of normal oral flora, including anaerobes and *Streptococcus viridans*. The anaerobes contribute to the putrid smell of the sputum. The patient's protracted mild clinical course is typical for this process, and his alcoholism is a clear risk factor as well. The superior segment of the right lower lobe is the most common site of aspiration and lung abscess, followed by the posterior segment of the right upper lobe and the superior segment of the left lower lobe. Tricuspid valve endocarditis may cause lung abscess due to staphylococcal (*S. aureus*) bacteremia. The patient is clearly at risk for pulmonary tuberculosis (TB) given his imprisonment; however, the sputum would not likely be putrid and purulent with this microscopic appearance. The cavitary lesions of TB are typically in the upper lobes. Wegener's granulomatosis may cause cavitary masses, but they are usually multiple and would not have putrid sputum. Squamous cell lung cancer may also cavitate by outgrowing its blood supply and may be secondarily infected, although usually not with this degree of anaerobic characteristics.

I-57.   The answer is D. *(Chap. 34)* Hemoptysis in these conditions originates from the bronchial circulation that is supplied by the aorta or intercostal arteries, not the pulmonary artery. Because of the high pressures, bleeding may be sudden and massive. Embolization of bronchial arteries feeding the suspected area may stop the bleeding. Cough suppressants may help decrease the irritating effects on the submucosa of coughing. Direct bronchoscopic cautery may be beneficial for friable tumors. Selective intubation of the right main bronchus may be supportive by protecting the non-bleeding right lung. Occlusion of the right lung bronchus by coagulating blood could lead to respiratory failure. The patient should be placed with his non-bleeding lung up, not down, as the goal is to prevent blood from entering the non-bleeding lung.

I-58.   The answer is B. *(Chaps. e9 and 277)* A collapsing variant of focal segmental glomerulosclerosis is typically diagnostic of HIV nephropathy, which presents with proteinuria and subacute loss of renal function. Diabetes typically causes thickening of glomerular basement membrane, mesangial sclerosis, and arteriosclerosis. Multiple myeloma causes proteinuria via deposition of light chains in the glomeruli and tubules and the development of renal amyloidosis. Microscopy shows amyloid proteins with Congo red staining. SLE causes membranous and proliferative nephritis due to immune complex deposition. Wegener's granulomatosis and microscopic polyangiitis cause pauci-immune necrotizing glomerulonephritis.

I-59. **The answer is A.** *(Chaps. 35 and 244)* This patient has central cyanosis, which is due to arterial desaturation. In central cyanosis, skin and mucus membranes are affected. Peripheral cyanosis is the result of peripheral hypoperfusion of various causes either due to hypotension, as with heart failure (e.g., myocardial infarction, myocarditis) or sepsis, or due to peripheral vasoconstriction, as with cold exposure or Raynaud's phenomenon. In these cases, the extremities are most affected, with the mucus membranes usually spared. This patient has Eisenmenger's physiology with right-to-left shunting of deoxygenated blood. Other causes of central cyanosis include severe lung disease, pulmonary arteriovenous malformations, alveolar hypoventilation, or hemoglobin abnormalities.

I-60. **The answer is C.** *(Chap. 35)* Cirrhotic patients are at risk of developing pulmonary arteriovenous fistulas. These, as well as portopulmonary shunts, cause platypnea and orthodeoxia (dyspnea and desaturation with sitting up). The fistulas, which are preferentially at the base of the lungs, increase the right-to-left shunting (and therefore hypoxemia) when upright. In the supine position, the apex of the lung is better perfused and the hypoxemia improves. The oxygen desaturation in the upright position causes the platypnea. Congenital pulmonary arteriovenous malformations may also cause platypnea and orthodeoxia. Ventricular septal defects will not cause hypoxemia until they develop right-to-left shunting.

I-61. **The answer is D.** *(Chap. 36)* The patient's positional edema that is worse in hot weather strongly suggests idiopathic edema. Idiopathic edema occurs mostly in women and is characterized by episodes of edema that may include abdominal distention. It is typically diurnal, with worsening after being upright for prolonged periods or in hot weather. Cyclical edema occurs with menstruation and is related to estrogen stimulation of fluid retention. Congestive heart failure, nephrotic syndrome, and cirrhosis are ruled out by history and by physical and laboratory examinations. Initially, therapy should include patient education regarding the need to lie flat for a few hours each day, as well as compression stockings put on in the mornings. Idiopathic edema may be related to abnormal activation of the renin-angiotensin system, and angiotensin-converting enzyme inhibitors may play a role if conservative interventions are not effective. Diuretics may be beneficial initially but may lose effectiveness if used continuously.

I-62. **The answer is D.** *(Chap. 37)* Palpitations are a common complaint among patients who report fluttering, pounding, or thumping sensation in the chest. Palpitations may arise from cardiac, psychiatric, miscellaneous (thyrotoxicosis, drugs, ethanol, caffeine, cocaine), or unknown causes. While most arrhythmias do not cause palpitations, patients with palpitations and known heart disease or risk factors are at risk of atrial or ventricular arrhythmias. Overall, patients complaining of palpitations >15 min are more likely to have psychiatric causes. Most patients with palpitations do not have serious arrhythmias. History, physical examination, Holter monitoring, and electrocardiography may be used to evaluate for arrhythmias.

I-63. **The answer is D.** *(Chap. 7)* Blood pressure >140/90 mmHg during the second trimester is markedly abnormal. During the second trimester, blood pressure should fall due to a decrease in systemic vascular resistance. Elevated blood pressure is associated with an increase in perinatal morbidity and mortality. Delaying diagnosis may be harmful. Blood pressure should be performed in the sitting position because in the lateral recumbent position the decrease in preload may cause a reduced blood pressure. The diagnosis of hypertension requires measurement of two elevated blood pressures at least 6 hours apart. Hypertension may be caused by preeclampsia, chronic hypertension, gestational hypertension, or renal hypertension. If hypertension is diagnosed, a safe antihypertensive should be initiated and a referral to a high-risk obstetrician should be considered.

I-64. **The answer is D.** *(Chap. 7)* This patient has severe eclampsia, and delivery should be performed as rapidly as possible. Mild eclampsia is the presence of new-onset hypertension and proteinuria in a pregnant woman after 20 weeks' gestation. Severe eclampsia is eclampsia complicated by central nervous system symptoms (including seizure), marked hypertension, severe proteinuria, renal failure, pulmonary edema, thrombocytopenia, or disseminated intravascular coagulation. Delivery in a mother with severe eclampsia before 37 weeks' gestation decreases maternal morbidity but increases fetal risks of complications of prematurity. Aggressive management of blood pressure, usually with labetalol, decreases maternal risk of stroke. Angiotensin-converting enzyme inhibitors and angiotensin-receptor blockers should not be used due to the potential of adverse effects on fetal development. Eclamptic seizures should be controlled with magnesium sulfate; it has been shown to be superior to phenytoin.

I-65.   **The answer is D.** *(Chap. 7)* Mitral stenosis is associated with flash pulmonary edema, atrial arrhythmias, and risk of maternal death. The risk is likely related to the increase in cardiac output and circulating blood volume during pregnancy. Sudden death due to arrhythmia or pulmonary hypertension may occur. During delivery, patients with mitral stenosis should be managed with careful heart rate control. Balloon valvuloplasty may be performed during pregnancy. The decrease in systemic vascular resistance during pregnancy makes mitral, tricuspid, and aortic regurgitation generally well tolerated because heart failure is not likely. If aortic stenosis is severe, balloon valvuloplasty may be necessary.

I-66.   **The answer is C.** *(Chap. 7)* Pregnancy causes a hypercoagulable state, and DVT occurs in about 1 in 2000 pregnancies. DVT occurs more commonly in the left leg than the right leg during pregnancy due to compression of the left iliac vein. Approximately 25% of pregnant women with DVT have a factor V Leiden mutation, which also predisposes to preeclampsia. Prothrombin G20210A mutation (homozygotes and heterozygotes), and methylenetetrahydrofolate reductase C677 mutation (homozygotes) are also risk factors for DVT during pregnancy. Coumadin is strictly contraindicated during the first and second trimesters due to risk of fetal abnormality. Low-molecular-weight heparin is appropriate therapy but may be switched to heparin infusion at delivery, if an epidural is likely. Ambulation, rather than bedrest, should be encouraged as with all DVTs. There is no proven role for local thrombolytics or an inferior vena cava filter in pregnancy. The latter would be considered only in scenarios where anticoagulation is not possible.

I-67.   **The answer is E.** *(Chap. 7)* Pregnancy complicated by diabetes is associated with greater maternal and perinatal morbidity and mortality rates. Women with gestational diabetes are at increased risk of preeclampsia, delivering infants large for gestational age, and birth lacerations. Their infants are at risk of hypoglycemia and birth injury. Appropriate therapy can reduce these risks. Not performing diabetes screening during pregnancy should be considered only in low-risk patients (age <25, no obesity, no history of gestational or other diabetes, no diabetes in first-degree relatives).

I-68.   **The answer is B.** *(Chap. 8)* The goal of the evaluation is to identify patients at intermediate or high risk of postoperative complications. The history and physical examination should focus on detecting symptoms or signs of occult cardiac or pulmonary disease. Preoperative laboratory testing should be carried out for specific conditions based on the clinical examination. Many questionnaires exist to identify patients at intermediate or high risk. There is no proven role for chest radiograph in this context provided that the cardiopulmonary history and physical examination are within normal limits.

I-69.   **The answer is C.** *(Chap. 8)* The six criteria listed in the question represent the Revised Cardiac Risk Index (RCRI). A patient with none of the risk factors has a <1% chance of a postoperative major cardiac event. Patients with three of the criteria have a 10% chance of having a cardiac event in the perioperative or intraoperative period. This is therefore considered an appropriate cut-off point for noninvasive cardiac imaging/stress testing to occur.

I-70. **The answer is B.** *(Chap. 8)* Pharmacologic stress tests, such as dopamine, persantine, or adenosine, are more useful than exercise testing in patients with functional limitation. While their positive predictive value is poor, they have excellent negative predictive value for identifying patients at risk for perioperative myocardial infarction or death. The patient is on adequate medical therapy for his ischemic cardiomyopathy but nevertheless had a very high-risk stress test. He should proceed to cardiac catheterization for either endovascular stenting or referral to bypass surgery.

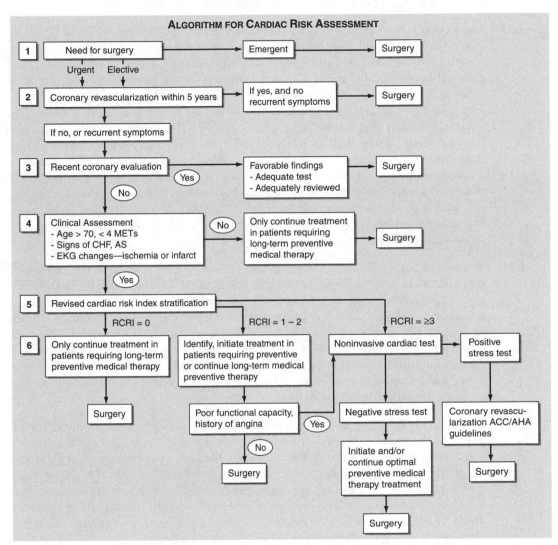

FIGURE I-70 Composite algorithm for cardiac risk assessment and stratification in patients undergoing noncardiac surgery. Stepwise clinical evaluation: [1] Emergency surgery; [2] Prior coronary revascularization; [3] Prior coronary evaluation; [4] Clinical assessment; [5] Revised cardiac risk index; [6] Risk modification strategies. Preventative medical therapy = beta blocker and statin therapy. RCRI, revised cardiac risk index. *(Adapted from KA Eagle et al and TH Lee et al.)*

I-71. **The answer is B.** *(Chaps. 24 and 366)* Parkinson's disease is common, affecting 1–2% of the population >65 years. Axial stiffness, stooped posture, shuffling gait, and pill-rolling tremor are distinctive. Other progressive neurologic disorders such as those listed above may present with Parkinsonian features. The atypical Parkinsonian syndromes can be difficult to differentiate from Parkinson's disease. However, the presence of a pill-rolling tremor is specific for Parkinson's disease.

I-72. **The answer is A.** *(Chap. 24)* The gait of cerebellar dysfunction most closely resembles a drunken gait with very poor balance, frequent lurching, and high risk of fall. However, unlike patients with inner ear dysfunction, these symptoms are usually not associated with subjective dizziness, vertigo, and nausea. Frontal gait disorder or gait apraxia is common in the elderly and has a variety of causes. Typical features include a wide base of support, short strides, shuffling, and difficulty with starts and turns. The most common cause of frontal gait is subcortical small-vessel cerebrovascular disease. Patients with Parkinsonian syndromes have a shuffling gait, with difficulty initiating and turning en bloc. Sensory ataxia may be caused by tabes dorsalis or vitamin B_{12} neuropathy. Patients have a narrow base and look down; their gait is regular with path deviation. They have no difficulty initiating gait but have postural instability and falls.

I-73.   The answer is E. *(Chap. 24)*   The inability to walk in a stable fashion without direct visual observation of the feet suggests a deficit in proprioception due to large-fiber neuropathy. The narrow-based gait with no difficulty initiating gait and normal strength is consistent with sensory ataxia. Classically this was caused by tabes dorsalis, although vitamin B_{12} deficiency is a treatable disease that may present with this form of neuropathy and gait disorder. This suspicion is even greater in the context of a macrocytic anemia, a finding that is consistent with vitamin B_{12} deficiency. Further signs of impaired proprioception, such as decreased ability to sense joint position, are even more suggestive of the diagnosis. Cerebellar ataxia will have a wide-based gait with a lurching stride. Cerebrovascular disease may present with a frontal gait disorder that is characterized by a wide-based, slow, shuffling gait. Parkinson's disease also causes a shuffling gait with difficulty initiating and turning en bloc. Amyotrophic lateral sclerosis does not cause a sensory or proprioceptive neuropathy but will alter gait due to muscle weakness.

I-74.   The answer is E. *(Chap. 25)*   Abnormalities of the tests listed with intact primary sensation in an alert cooperative patient identify lesions in the parietal cortex or the thalamocortical projection to the parietal lobe. Though two-point discrimination is a common screening technique for cortical sensory deficits, each of the above techniques is a quick and helpful alternative to evaluate for a cortical sensory deficit. Two-point discrimination is best tested with a set of calipers that simultaneously touch the skin. Normally, one can distinguish 3-mm separation of points on the pads of the fingers. Touch localization is performed by having the patient close his or her eyes and identify the site of the examiner touching the patient lightly (with finger or cotton swab).

I-75.   The answer is B. *(Chap. 29)*   This patient has a Marcus Gunn pupil, or afferent pupil defect. As the response is only abnormal when light is shone in her left eye, this implies an afferent defect in that eye mediated by retinal or optic nerve damage. The right and left efferent systems are intact, based on normal pupillary constriction bilaterally with light exposure to the right eye. A corneal defect in the left eye may impair vision but would not block light transmission to the left retina and optic disc: pupillary responses would therefore remain intact. Common causes of a Marcus Gunn pupil include retrobulbar optic neuritis and other optic nerve diseases.

I-76.   The answer is E. *(Chap. 29)*   This patient has a bitemporal hemianopia implying a lesion at the optic chiasm. Crossed fibers are more damaged than uncrossed lesions by compression. Therefore mass lesions at the chiasm may cause bilateral temporal visual field defects. Sellar lesions such as pituitary adenoma, meningioma, craniopharyngioma, and aneurysm can lead to this bitemporal hemianopia, which may be subtle to the patient and the examiner. Optic nerve lesions such as ischemic optic neuropathy, retinal vascular occlusion, advanced glaucoma, or optic neuritis will cause a horizontal scotoma. Post-chiasmic lesions, cortical lesions, or geniculate body lesions will cause homonymous hemianopia.

I-77.   The answer is A. *(Chap. 29)*   A red and painful eye is often caused by a corneal abrasion. History is very useful to determine the pretest probability of this type of lesion, because it will be increased in the context of contact lens use, recent eye trauma, or particulate exposure. Cobalt-blue examination with fluorescein is then used to confirm the presence of corneal abrasion. It is particularly important as it occasionally reveals a dendritic pattern consistent with Herpes simplex virus keratitis, a diagnosis that necessitates a very different type of treatment. Lid eversion is useful if there is suspicion that the foreign body is still present. Corneal abrasion should be treated with topical antibiotic ointment and patching. Cycloplegia may reduce pain by relaxing the ciliary body.

I-78.   The answer is B. *(Chap. 29)* Conjunctivitis is the most common cause of a red, irritated eye. Pain is minimal and visual acuity is only minimally impacted. It is usually due to adenovirus infection. Bacterial infection causes a mucopurulent discharge. Conjunctivitis invariably presents with ocular discharge, whereas episcleritis does not. Episcleritis, inflammation of the episclera, a thin layer between the sclera and the conjunctiva, is often more localized than conjunctivitis, but this cannot always be used to discriminate the two. Scleritis, a deeper, more intense inflammatory condition than episcleritis, is associated commonly with various connective tissue disorders and should always be considered in patients with these conditions.

I-79.   The answer is B. *(Chap. 29)* Herpes simplex virus (HSV) keratitis is a major cause of blindness in the developed world. Several clues to the diagnosis of HSV keratitis may be present on examination, including periocular vesicles on the skin and a dendritic pattern of cornea ulceration on fluorescein examination (which is pathognomonic). However, these findings are not always present. Viral culture and corneal examination by an experienced ophthalmologist should always be performed in cases where the diagnosis is unclear. Angle-closure glaucoma is rare but can be easily ruled out by an ophthalmologist with a measure of ocular pressure and slit-lamp examination. Uveitis is notable for "cells and flare" and occasionally hypopyon in the iris and perilimbic sparing. Endophthalmitis involves the entire globe and evokes pain with ocular movement. Internationally, keratitis due to trachoma is a common cause of blindness, but it is uncommon in the developed world.

I-80.   The answer is E. *(Chap. 29)* Uveitis involving the anterior portion of the eye is referred to as *iritis* or *iridocyclitis*. It is diagnosed by slit-lamp examination. The differential diagnosis for anterior uveitis includes sarcoidosis, ankylosing spondylitis, juvenile rheumatoid arthritis, inflammatory bowel disease, reactive arthritis, and Behçet's disease. It may also be associated with Lyme disease, syphilis, and other infections. Often no cause is found. Posterior uveitis involves the vitreous, retina, or choroid. It may also accompany autoimmune diseases, Behçet's disease, sarcoid, and inflammatory bowel disease. A wide variety of infections may cause posterior uveitis. Toxoplasmosis specifically causes a posterior uveitis rather than an anterior uveitis. The extent of screening for diseases associated with anterior uveitis should depend on a risk assessment for each disorder based on the history and physical examination.

I-81.   The answer is B. *(Chap. 29)* Optic neuritis is a common inflammatory lesion of the optic nerve. In a large clinical study, the mean age of patients was 32 years and 75% of the patients were female. Pain is common with eye movement. Vision loss usually recovers somewhat even without treatment. Steroids hasten vision gain but do not alter the final visual acuity. Multiple sclerosis (MS) is a primary concern for all newly diagnosed cases of optic neuritis. The 10-year cumulative likelihood of developing multiple sclerosis after an episode of optic neuritis is almost 40%. Patients with a first episode of optic neuritis should receive a brain MRI to evaluate for MS. It may show characteristic lesions of the disease prior to the development of CNS symptoms and is a helpful tool for monitoring progression of disease of this condition while on therapy.

I-82.   The answer is A. *(Chap. 29)* Sudden blindness in a patient with fever and high risk of endovascular infection is endocarditis until proven otherwise. Even primary bacteremia in the absence of cardiac vegetation can seed the eye, often leading to endogenous endophthalmitis or central retinal artery occlusion. Another consideration in this patient would be septic thrombophlebitis with septic emboli to the eye. Stroke, vasculitis, syphilis, and hematologic malignancy are possible causes of acute blindness, but are less likely given the acute presentation with fever.

I-83.   The answer is B. *(Chap. 216)* Beta radiation consists of small negatively charged electrons. These particles can only travel short distances in tissue and lead primarily to burns similar to thermal injury. Plastic layers and clothing can prohibit penetration of most beta particles. Beta radiation is frequently released in radiation accidents, and radioactive iodine is the best-recognized member of this group. Alpha radiation consists of heavy positively charged particles consisting of two protons and two neutrons. Because of the large size, alpha particles cannot penetrate tissue. However, if alpha particles are internalized, they will cause damage to cells within the immediate proximity. The most damaging particles emitted during a nuclear explosion are gamma rays, x-rays, and neutrons. Gamma rays and x-rays are both photons and have similar ability to penetrate through matter. They are the principal type of radiation to cause total body exposure. Neutrons are heavy, but uncharged, and possess a range of energy. These neutrons can ionize DNA directly or through generation of free radicals.

I-84.   The answer is D. *(Chap. 216)* Much of the initial damage related to a "dirty" bomb is related to the power of the blast rather than the radiation. Following a terrorist attack, it is important to identify all individuals who might have been exposed to radiation. The initial treatment of these individuals should be to stabilize and treat the most severely injured. Those with severe injuries should have contaminated clothing removed prior to transportation to the emergency room, but further care should not be withheld for additional decontamination as the risk of exposure to health care workers is low. Individuals with minor injuries who can be safely decontaminated without increasing the risk of medical complications should be transported to a centralized area for decontamination. A further consideration regarding treatment following radiation exposure is the total dose of radiation that an individual was exposed to. At a dose <2 Gy, there are usually no significant adverse outcomes, and no specific treatment is recommended unless symptoms develop. Many individuals will develop flulike symptoms. However, a complete blood count should be obtained every 6 h for the first 24 h because bone marrow suppression can develop with radiation exposure as low as 0.7 Gy. The earliest sign of this is a fall in the lymphocyte count of >50%. Potential treatments of radiation exposure include use of colony-stimulating factors and supportive transfusions. Stem cell transfusion and bone marrow transplantation can be considered in the case of severe pancytopenia that does not recover. However, this is controversial, given the lack of experience with the procedure for this indication. Following the Chernobyl nuclear reactor accident, none of the bone marrow transplants were successful.

I-85.   The answer is E. *(Chap. 216)* This patient has been exposed to radioactive polonium-210, a strong emitter of alpha radiation, which can be used as a calibration source or neutron source in nuclear reactors. The patient is presenting with acute radiation sickness after an unknown ingestion amount. However, his symptoms began early after ingestion, and there is also severe bone marrow suppression, suggesting that the dose was >2 Gy. Polonium accumulates in the spleen and kidneys. In addition to supportive care with transfusions and colony-stimulating factors, chelation with dimercaprol should be attempted as polonium has a radiologic half-life of 138.4 days and a biologic half-life of 60 days. A bone marrow transplant could be considered if his bone marrow fails to recover. The presumed ingestion occurred >36 h previously, and a gastric lavage is unlikely to be helpful. Potassium iodide is useful in radioactive iodine poisoning or overdose.

I-86.   The answer is C. *(Chap. 215)* Mustard gas (sulfur mustard) is a vesicant agent that has been used as a chemical agent of warfare and terrorism since World War I. In World War I, sulfur mustard was responsible for 70% of the 1.3 million individuals killed by chemical warfare, but overall, it had a mortality rate of only 1.9%. Sulfur mustard is composed of both vapor and liquid components that can cause damage to epithelial surfaces. However, the effects of mustard gas exposure are delayed several hours after exposure. An initial clue to which agent the individuals were exposed was the smell of horseradish or burned garlic, which is characteristic of mustard gas. The earliest effects of mustard exposure involve the nose, sinuses, and pharynx. Common symptoms include burning in the nares, epistaxis, sinus pain, and pharyngeal pain. Damage to the upper airway may cause laryngitis and nonproductive cough. Lower airway involvement results in nonproductive cough and dyspnea, but pulmonary hemorrhage is rare. Pseudomembranes may form and cause airway obstruction. The eyes are the most sensitive organ to mustard vapor injury with a shorter latency to symptoms than the skin. Ocular symptoms include irritation, conjunctivitis, photophobia, blepharospasm, pain, and corneal damage. Erythema of the skin begins 2 h to 2 days after exposure and is greatest at warm, moist locations such as the axillae, neck, antecubital fossae, perineum, and genitalia. Small vesicles may develop, which coalesce to form bullae. The bullae are usually large and flaccid and filled with a clear to straw-colored fluid. Death from mustard gas exposure is usually due to sepsis and respiratory failure, although high-dose exposure can lead to bone marrow failure 7–21 days after the initial exposure. Phosgene oxime is also a vesicant agent that may present with similar symptoms, but it can be differentiated from mustard gas by its pungent pepperish odor. Further, phosgene presents with immediate symptoms and pain. Chlorine is a gas that causes inhalant damage to the lungs with noncardiogenic pulmonary edema as the primary presentation. Cyanide is an asphyxiant with rapid onset of symptoms, including death. Soman is a nerve agent that would present with cholinergic symptoms of miosis, salivation, muscle fasciculations, and copious secretions. The symptoms have a rapid onset, with respiratory depression and death within minutes of exposure.

I-87.   **The answer is F.** *(Chap. 215)* These individuals have been exposed to organophosphorus nerve agents (soman, sarin, tabun, cyclosarin, and VX) that act by inhibition of tissue synaptic acetylcholinesterase. The symptoms of nerve agents are those of a cholinergic crisis. Symptoms manifest in the order in which organ systems are exposed. When nerve agents are released as a vapor, the first organ that is usually affected is the eyes with miosis and a feeling that the world is "going black," as was reported during the Tokyo subway terrorist attack in which sarin was released. Exposure of the nasopharynx to organophosphates causes rhinorrhea, excessive salivation, and drooling. Bronchorrhea and cough frequently occur. After inhalation of the toxin, it is rapidly absorbed into the blood across the alveolar-capillary membrane. The gastrointestinal tract is usually rapidly affected once the agents are in the bloodstream, with resultant diarrhea, cramping, nausea, and vomiting. When death occurs due to nerve agents, it is usually because of the central nervous system (CNS) effects of these agents. Acetylcholine and its receptor are widely distributed in the brain, and exposure to large amounts of organophosphate agents leads to rapid unconsciousness, seizures, and central apnea. Nerve agents have a short half-life in circulation, and thus, if intervention is made rapidly, improvement in symptoms should likewise be rapid, without subsequent recurrence of symptoms. The initial treatment for nerve agents is administration of atropine, which is widely available worldwide. Atropine acts quickly at muscarinic acetylcholine receptors to alleviate the central apnea but does not reverse the neuromuscular effects. In addition to anticholinergic therapy with atropine, use of oximes is also recommended after nerve gas exposure. Oximes such as 2-pralidoxime (2-PAM) reactivate the cholinesterase to restore normal enzyme function. In individuals with severe CNS toxicity and seizures, benzodiazepines, such as diazepam, are the treatment of choice. Typical anticonvulsant drugs, such as phenytoin, carbamazepine, phenobarbital, and valproic acid are ineffective in treating the seizures caused by nerve agents.

I-88.   **The answer is B.** *(Chap. 358)* This child has the classic clinical findings of phenylketonuria, an autosomal recessive disorder of amino acid metabolism in which phenylalanine cannot be converted to tyrosine. It is the most common inherited disorder of amino acid metabolism. Untreated or unrecognized cases will usually have a normal birth but will rapidly begin to show signs of this illness, which include microcephaly, mental retardation, and seizures. The "mousy" odor is due to phenylacetate accumulation in skin, hair, and urine. The toxicity of phenylalanine is due to its inhibition of transport of other amino acids necessary for normal protein, myelin, and neurotransmitter synthesis. Screening for phenylalanine in the blood should occur prior to 3 weeks of age (usually this is done at birth) to prevent symptoms. Treatment consists of lifelong dietary phenylalanine restriction and tyrosine supplementation. If detected at birth, affected children do not develop the aforementioned complications. Women with phenylketonuria who become pregnant must maintain strict control before and during pregnancy to avoid congenital defects, microcephaly, growth retardation, and mental retardation in the baby.

I-89.   The answer is A. *(Chap. 358)* Alkaptonuria is a rare disorder of homogentisic acid oxidase deficiency which leads to urinary excretion and tissue accumulation of oxidized homogentisic acid. Patients may present in their thirties or forties with arthritis and darkly colored urine, as well as tissue pigmentation (ochronosis) from homogentisic acid. The arthritis is typically in the large joints such as hips, knees, shoulders, and low back. The gray-brown pigmentation is characteristic and can involve the sclera and the ear. The diagnosis should be suspected in a patient whose urine darkens to blackness. Hawkinsinuria is a related disorder of amino acid metabolism, in which a 4-hydroxyphenylpyruvate dioxygenase enzyme defect leads to failure to thrive in infancy. Unlike most amino acid disorders, it is autosomal dominant. Tryptophanuria results in mental retardation, skin photosensitivity, and ataxia; however, the enzyme defect leading to this phenotype has not been identified. Hyperprolinemia type I is caused by a proline oxidase defect and is typically benign. Homocystinuria is caused by a cystathionine β-synthase defect and leads to mental retardation.

I-90 and I-91.   The answers are C and D. *(Chap. 356)* Myophosphorylase deficiency (type V glycogen storage disease), also known as McArdle disease, is the most common adult glycogen storage disease. The enzyme deficiency limits ATP production via glycogenolysis. It is characterized by exercise intolerance, muscle cramping, myoglobinuria, and elevated CKs (at rest and increased with exercise). Symptoms usually develop in adulthood as a result of either brief intense activity or sustained exertion. Rhabdomyolysis after intense activity may cause myoglobinuria and subsequent renal failure and is the major clinical risk about which patients should be warned. Heart disease does not occur. The most common childhood disorder glycogen storage disease is glucose-6-phosphatase deficiency (type I), also known as von Gierke's disease, which presents at age 3–4 months with growth retardation and hepatosplenomegaly. Lactate dehydrogenase deficiency and pyruvate kinase deficiency present similarly to McArdle disease but are very rare.

I-92.   The answer is C. *(Chap. 356; J Shen et al.)* Type III glycogen storage disease, a deficiency in debranching enzyme, causes abnormalities in glycogen degradation. Clinical manifestations include hepatomegaly, hypoglycemia, short stature, variable skeletal myopathy, and cardiomyopathy. Dementia does not occur. When liver and muscle are involved, the disease is termed type IIIa; however, in 15% of patients, liver disease predominates and these patients are characterized as having type IIIb disease. Fasting ketosis will occur if glucose/protein intake is not maintained. In most patients, hepatomegaly improves with age; however, chronic liver disease and cirrhosis may occur in adulthood, requiring liver transplantation. Hepatocellular carcinoma has also been reported. Treatment consists of dietary management with frequent high-carbohydrate meals and possible nocturnal drip feeding to avoid hypoglycemia. Linkage analysis markers can be used for screening carriers and prenatal diagnosis.

I-93.   The answer is C. *(Chap. 64)* Presymptomatic testing applies to diseases where a specific genetic alteration is associated with a near 100% likelihood of developing the disease, such as Huntington's disease. In contrast, predisposition testing predicts a risk for disease that is <100%. The presence of the apolipoprotein E allele (ε4) does not predict with 100% accuracy individuals who will develop Alzheimer's; therefore, this patient's testing is an example of predisposition testing. Not everyone with this marker will develop the disease, and individuals without this marker may develop Alzheimer's. Other examples of predisposition testing include hereditary breast cancer. The patient does not have any signs or symptoms of dementia, and he is not being discriminated against in this scenario.

I-94.   The answer is E. *(Chap. 63)* There is a very tight association between increasing maternal age and trisomy. Race, geography, and socioeconomic factors do not affect this relationship. In women under 25, 2% of all conceptions are trisomic. The vast majority of trisomic conceptions will spontaneously abort; only trisomy 13, 18, 21 (Down syndrome) and sex chromosome trisomies survive to term in measurable numbers. Women >42 years of age have a 33% chance of a trisomic conception. Despite this well-described association, little is known about the mechanism that drives it.

I-95. The answer is E. *(Chap. 63)* Human cells contain 46 chromosomes: 22 pairs of autosomal chromosomes and one pair of sex chromosomes, XX in females and XY in males. Deviation in the number or structure of these chromosomes is common and is estimated to occur in 10–25% of all pregnancies. They are the most common cause of fetal loss. In pregnancies surviving to term, they are the leading known cause of birth defects and mental retardation.

I-96. The answer is C. *(Chap. 343)* This group of genetic conditions often presents with disorders of sexual differentiation. Genetically, Klinefelter syndrome results from a meiotic nondysjunction of sex chromosomes during gametogenesis, producing a 47,XXY individual. Phenotypically, these individuals are male but have eunuchoid features, small testes, decreased virilization, and gynecomastia. The other disorders listed in the question may result in sexual ambiguity, more commonly in males. In mixed gonadal dysgenesis, there is mosaicism resulting from the genotype 46,XY/45,X. Depending on the proportion of cells with the 46,XY genotype, the phenotype can be either male or female. Testicular dysgenesis results from the absence of müllerian inhibiting substance during embryonic development and may be caused by multiple genetic mutations and may be associated with the absence of müllerian-inhibiting substance and reduced testosterone production. Feminization may also occur through androgen insensitivity and mutations in the androgen receptor. Virilization of females with resultant ambiguous sexual differentiation most commonly occurs in patients with congenital adrenal hyperplasia (CAH). The most common cause of CAH is 21-hydroxylase deficiency, which results in ambiguous female genitalia, hypotension, and salt wasting.

I-97. The answer is E. *(Chap. 343)* Turner syndrome, or gonadal dysgenesis, is a common chromosomal disorder that affects 1 in 2500 female births. The most common genetic defect is the 45,XO karyotype, which causes half of all phenotypic cases of this syndrome. Age at diagnosis is variable, based on the clinical manifestations. Most cases are diagnosed perinatally on the basis of reduced fetal growth or lymphedema at birth with nuchal folds, a low posterior hairline, or left-sided cardiac defects. Some girls may not be diagnosed in childhood and come to attention much later in life because of delayed growth and lack of sexual maturation. Limited pubertal development occurs in up to 30% of girls with Turner syndrome, with approximately 2% reaching menarche. Owing to the frequency of congenital heart and genitourinary defects, a thorough workup should be done after the diagnosis, including an echocardiogram and renal imaging. Long-term management includes growth hormone replacement during childhood and estrogen replacement to maintain bone mineralization and feminization.

I-98. The answer is B. *(Chap. 357)* This patient presents with the classic findings of an inherited disorder of connective tissue, particularly Marfan syndrome. The presentation is not consistent with the bony deformities or blue sclera seen in patients with osteogenesis imperfecta, and he is tall with long extremities, which makes chondroplasia very unlikely. However, his hypermobility and lens disorders suggest Marfan syndrome or, less commonly, Ehlers-Danlos syndrome. Given the high risk of aortic root disease in Marfan syndrome, echocardiography is indicated in this patient. The other screening tests are not specific to Marfan syndrome and are not appropriate in a 30-year-old male.

I-99. The answer is C. *(Chap. 62)* Neoplastic disorders may arise from mutations in DNA that affect oncogenes, tumor suppressor genes, apoptotic genes, and DNA repair genes. Several genetic disorders involving DNA repair enzymes underscore the importance of these mutations. Patients with xeroderma pigmentosum have defects in DNA damage recognition and in nucleotide excision and repair. These patients often have skin cancers as a result of the mutagenic effects of ultraviolet light. Ataxia-telangiectasia is characterized by large telangiectatic lesions on the face, cerebellar ataxia, immunologic defects, and hypersensitivity to ionizing radiation. Mutation in the ATM gene that causes AT gives rise to defects in meiosis and increasing damage from ionizing radiation. Fanconi's anemia is caused by mutations in multiple complementation groups that are characterized by various congenital anomalies and a marked predisposition to aplastic anemia and acute myeloid leukemia. HNPCC is caused by mutations in one of several mismatch repair genes that result in microsatellite instability and a high incidence of colon, ovarian, and uterine cancers. Fragile X syndrome is caused by unstable trinucleotide repeats that destabilize DNA. It is characterized by X-linked inheritance and typical large ears, macroorchidism, and mental retardation.

I-100. **The answer is C.** *(Chap. 62)* Mendelian inheritance patterns do not apply to mitochondrial genetics. Mitochondrial DNA (mtDNA) consists of small encoding transfer and ribosomal RNAs and various proteins that are involved in oxidative phosphorylation and adenosine triphosphate (ATP) generation. mtDNA exists as a circular chromosome within cells. The mitochondrial genome does not recombine. The genetic material that is introduced into the egg by the sperm does not contain mitochondrial DNA, therefore, inheritance is maternal. All the children of an affected mother will inherit the disorder. An affected father will not transmit the disorder. The clinical manifestations of the various disorders in mitochondrial genetics are characterized by alterations in oxidative phosphorylation that lead to reductions in the ATP supply and apoptosis. Areas of high dependence on oxidative phosphorylation include skeletal and cardiac muscle and the brain. During replication, the number of mitochondria can drift among various cells and tissues, resulting in heterogeneity, or heteroplasmy. This results in further variation in the clinical phenotype. Acquired mutations in the mitochondrial genome are thought to play a significant role in age-related degenerative disorders such as Alzheimer's disease and Parkinson's disease.

I-101. **The answer is B.** *(Chap. 62)* Genetic imprinting is gene inactivation that results in preferential expression of an allele depending on its parental origin. It has an important role in a number of diseases, including malignancies. Abnormal expression in the paternally derived copy of the insulin-like growth factor II (IGF-II) gene results in the cancer predisposing Beckwith-Wiedemann syndrome. Uniparental disomy is the inheritance of dual copies of either maternal or paternal chromosomes. This may result in similar phenotypes, as in the case of imprinting. The Prader-Willi and Angelman's syndromes may result from uniparental disomy involving inheritance of defective maternal or paternal chromosomes, respectively. Similarly, hydatidiform moles may contain normal numbers of diplid chromosomes, all of which are of paternal origin. The opposite occurs in ovarian teratomas. Lyonization is epigenetic inactivation of one of the two X chromosomes in every cell of the female. Somatic mosaicism is the presence of two or more genetically distinct cell lines in the tissue of an individual. The term *anticipation* is often used to refer to diseases caused by trinucleotide repeats that are often characterized by worsening of clinical phenotypes in successive generations. These diseases, such as Huntington's disease and fragile X syndrome, are characterized by expansion of these repeats in subsequent generations of individuals, resulting in earlier and often more severe clinical phenotypes.

I-102. **The answer is D.** *(Chap. 357)* Connective tissue is composed of macromolecules (collagen, elastin, fibrillin, proteoglycans, etc.) that are assembled into an insoluble extracellular matrix. Disorders of any of these macromolecules may result in a disorder of connective tissue. Osteogenesis imperfecta is caused by mutations in type I procollagen. Over 400 mutations have been found in patients with OI. Clinically, it is characterized by decreased bone mass, brittle bones, blue sclerae, dental abnormalities, joint laxity, and progressive hearing loss. The phenotype may range from severe disease with in utero death to milder forms with lesser severity and survival into adulthood. Ehlers-Danlos syndrome is a heterogenous set of disorders characterized by joint laxity, hyperelasticity of the skin, and other defects in collagen synthesis. A variety of defects have been identified in different types of collagen as well as enzymes that facilitate collagen cross-linking. Marfan syndrome is characterized by a triad of features: long, thin extremities (with arachnodactyly and loose joints), reduced vision as a result of ectopia lentis, and aortic aneurysms. Defects in the fibrillin gene are responsible for this syndrome. Alport syndrome is caused by mutations in type IV collagen, resulting in the most common phenotype of X-linked inheritance, hematuria, sensorineural deafness, and lenticonus. McArdle's disease is a defect in glycogenolysis that results from myophosphorylase deficiency.

I-103. **The answer is D.** *(Chap. 355)* Lysosomes are subcellular organelles that contain specific hydrolyases that allow the processing and degradation of proteins, nucleic acids, carbohydrates, and lipids. Lysosomal storage diseases result from mutations in various genes for these hydrolyases. Clinical symptoms result from the accumulation of the undegraded macromolecule. Tay-Sachs disease is caused by a deficiency of hexosaminidase A. Buildup of G_{M2} gangliosides results in a phenotype that is characterized by a fatal progressive neurodegenerative disease. In the infantile form, these patients have macrocephaly, loss of motor skills, an increased startle reaction, and a macular cherry red spot. The juvenile-onset form presents with ataxia and progressive dementia that result in death by age 15. The adult-onset form is characterized by clumsiness in childhood, progressive motor weakness in adolescence, and neurocognitive decline. Death occurs in early adulthood. Survival to the third or fourth decade is rare. Splenomegaly is uncommon. The disease is seen most commonly in Ashkenazi Jews, with a carrier frequency of about 1 in 30. Inheritance is autosomal recessive.

I-104. **The answer is D.** *(Chap. 355)* Gaucher disease is an autosomal recessive lysosomal storage disorder caused by decreased activity of acid β-glucosidase. Nearly 200 mutations have been described. Type 1 Gaucher disease can present from childhood to young adulthood. The average age at diagnosis is 20 years in white people. Clinical features result from an accumulation of lipid-laden macrophages, termed Gaucher cells, throughout the body. Hepatosplenomegaly is present in virtually all symptomatic patients. Bone marrow involvement is common, with subsequent infarction, ischemia, and necrosis. Anemia and thrombocytopenias may occur. Bone pain is common. Although the liver and spleen may become massive, severe liver dysfunction is very rare. The disease is most common in Ashkenazi Jewish populations. The diagnosis is made by measuring enzyme activity. Enzyme therapy is currently the treatment of choice in significantly affected patients. Other therapies include symptomatic management of the blood cytopenias and joint replacement surgery for bone injury. Type 2 Gaucher disease is a rare, severe central nervous system (CNS) disease that leads to death in infancy. Type 3 disease is nearly identical to type 1 disease except that the course is more rapidly progressive.

I-105. **The answer is A.** *(Chap. 62)* The information provided in the pedigree is adequate to determine the mode of a single-gene inheritance pattern. The example provided is typical of patients with hemophilia A or Duchenne's muscular dystrophy. Other examples exist. X-linked recessive inheritance is marked by the fact that the incidence of the trait is much higher in males than in females. The genetic trait is passed from an affected male through all his daughters to, on average, half their sons. The trait is never transmitted directly from father to son. The trait may be transmitted through a series of carrier females; if that occurs, the affected males are related to each other through the female, as in this case.

I-106. **The answer is A.** *(Chap. 62)* Many common diseases are known to "run in families" yet are not inherited in a simple Mendelian fashion. It is likely that the expression of these disorders depends on a family of genes that can impart a certain degree of risk and then be modified by subsequent environmental factors. The risk of the development of disease in a relative of an affected person varies with the degree of relationship; first-degree relatives (parents, siblings, and offspring) have the highest risk, which in itself varies with the specific disease. Many of these multifactorial genetic diseases are inherited in a greater frequency in persons with certain HLA (major histocompatibility system) types. For example, there is a tenfold increased risk of celiac sprue (gluten-sensitive enteropathy) in persons who have HLA-B8. This genotype also imparts an increased risk for chronic active hepatitis, myasthenia gravis, and Addison's disease. The incidence of diabetes mellitus is much higher in those expressing HLA-D3 and HLA-D4. Spondyloarthropathies, psoriatic arthritis (HLA-B27), hyperthyroidism (HLA-DR3), and multiple sclerosis (HLA-DR2) are other examples of diseases with histocompatibility predispositions. By contrast, Wilson's disease and cystic fibrosis are inherited in an autosomal recessive fashion, and adult polycystic kidney disease and neurofibromatosis are among the disorders inherited in an autosomal dominant manner.

I-107. **The answer is C.** *(Chap. 19)* Fever of unknown origin (FUO) is defined as the presence of fevers to >38.3°C (101.0°F) on several occasions occurring for >3 weeks without a defined cause after appropriate investigation into potential causes have failed to yield a diagnosis. Initial laboratory investigation into an FUO should include a complete blood count with differential, peripheral blood smear, ESR, C-reactive protein, electrolytes, creatinine, calcium, liver function tests, urinalysis, and muscle enzymes. In addition, specific testing for a variety of infections should be performed, including VDRL for syphilis, HIV, CMV, EBV, PPD testing, and blood, sputum, and urine cultures if appropriate. Finally, the workup should include evaluation for inflammatory disorders. These tests include antinuclear antibodies, rheumatoid factor, ferritin, iron, and transferrin. In several large studies, infectious etiologies are the most commonly identified source of FUO. In the earlier studies, infectious etiologies accounted for 32–36% of all FUO. In more recent studies, up to 30% of individuals will not have an identified cause of FUO, and infectious etiologies continue to comprise 25% of all FUO. The most common infection causing FUO is extrapulmonary tuberculosis. Viral and fungal etiologies are also common. In addition, intraabdominal, retroperitoneal, renal, and paraspinal abscesses should be considered. In earlier studies, neoplasm was the second most common cause of FUO. However, given the improvements in imaging and diagnostic techniques, neoplasm accounts for fewer cases of FUO than previously described. Presently the second most common cause of FUO is noninfectious inflammatory disorders. In the elderly, giant cell arteritis can present as an FUO, as can many other inflammatory disease such as polymyositis, Behçet's disease, and adult Still's disease. Drug fever and hereditary periodic fever syndromes are grouped in the "miscellaneous" category and are among the least common causes of prolonged fever of uncertain origin.

I-108. **The answer is C.** *(Chap. 58; R Crapo et al.)* Chronic hypoxia, seen in people acclimated to high altitudes, causes a shift in the oxygen dissociation curve to the right (decreased affinity) causing more oxygen to be released in tissues deprived of oxygen. This is achieved by increased red blood cell production of 2,3-diphosphoglycerate (2,3-DPG). Four factors decrease the affinity of hemoglobin for oxygen: high temperature, increased partial pressure of carbon dioxide (the Bohr effect), increased levels of 2,3-DPG, increase in acidity. The opposite changes in these four factors increase hemoglobin affinity for oxygen and impair delivery of oxygen to peripheral tissues. Healthy men acclimated to altitude (1400 m) have an average pH/Pa_{CO_2} of 7.43/34 mmHg and healthy women 7.44/33 mmHg. Hemoglobin concentration will increase due to the stimulatory effect of hypoxia on erythropoietin production.

I-109. **The answer is E.** *(Chap. e3)* Minority patients have poorer health outcomes from many preventable and treatable conditions such as cardiovascular disease, asthma, diabetes, cancer, and others. The causes of these differences are multifactorial and include social determinants (education, socioeconomic status, environment) and access to care (which often leads to more serious illness before seeking care). However, there are also clearly described racial differences in quality of care once patients enter the health care system. These differences have been found in cardiovascular, oncologic, renal, diabetic, and palliative care. Eliminating these differences will require systematic changes in health system factors, provider level factors, and patient level factors.

I-110. **The answer is B.** *(Chap. e6)* To be able to differentiate among the disorders that cause memory loss, it should be determined whether the patient has nondeclarative or declarative memory loss. A simple way to think of the differences between nondeclarative and declarative memory is to consider the difference between "knowing how" (nondeclarative) and "knowing who or what" (declarative). Nondeclarative memory loss refers to loss of skills, habits, or learned behaviors that can be expressed without an awareness of what was learned. Procedural memory is a type of nondeclarative memory and may involve motor, perceptual, or cognitive processes. Examples of nondeclarative procedural memory include remembering how to tie one's shoes (motor), responding to the tea kettle whistling on the stove (perceptual), or increasing ability to complete a puzzle (cognitive). Nondeclarative memory involves several brain areas, including the amygdala, basal ganglia, cerebellum, and sensory cortex. Declarative memory refers to the conscious memory for facts and events and is divided into two categories: semantic memory and episodic memory. Semantic memory refers to general knowledge about the world without specifically recalling how or when the information was learned. An example of semantic memory is the recollection that a wristwatch is an instrument for keeping time. Vocabulary and the knowledge of associations between verbal concepts comprise a large portion of semantic memory. Episodic memory allows one to recall specific personal experiences. Examples of episodic memory include ability to recall the birthday of a spouse, to recognize a photo from one's wedding, or recall the events at one's high school graduation. The areas of the brain involved in declarative memory include the hippocampus, entorhinal cortex, mamillary bodies, and thalamus.

I-111.   **The answer is F.** *(Chap. 60)* This patient's lymphadenopathy is benign. Inguinal nodes <2 cm are common in the population at large and need no further work up provided that there is no other evidence of disseminated infection or tumor, and that the nodes have qualities that do not suggest tumor (not hard or matted). A practical approach would be to measure the nodes or even photograph them if visible, and follow them serially over time. Occasionally, inguinal lymph nodes can be associated with sexually transmitted diseases. However, these are usually ipsilateral and tender, and evaluation for this would include bimanual examination and appropriate cultures, not necessarily pelvic ultrasound. Total-body CT scan would be indicated if other pathologic nodes suggestive of lymphoma or granulomatous disease are present in other anatomic locations. Bone marrow biopsy would be indicated only if a diagnosis of lymphoma is made first.

I-112.   **The answer is E.** *(Chap. 60)* Hard, matted, nontender lymph nodes are worrisome for tumor and should always prompt a workup, including excisional biopsy, if possible, and examination for a primary source depending on the location of the nodes. Supraclavicular lymphadenopathy should always be considered abnormal, particularly when documented on the left side. A thorough investigation for cancer, particularly with a primary gastrointestinal source, is necessary. Splenomegaly associated with diffuse adenopathy can be associated with tumor, particularly lymphoma, but is most often associated with systemic infections, such as mononucleosis, cytomegalovirus, or HIV, that often cause diffuse lymphadenopathy. Generalized lymphadenopathy and splenomegaly may be found in autoimmune diseases such as systemic lupus erythematosus or mixed connective tissue disease. Tender adenopathy of the cervical anterior chain is nearly always associated with infection of the head and neck, most commonly a viral upper respiratory infection.

I-113.   **The answer is C.** *(Chap. 60)* Portal hypertension causes splenomegaly via passive congestion of the spleen. It generally causes only mild enlargement of the spleen as expanded varices provide some decompression for elevated portal pressures. Myelofibrosis necessitates extramedullary hematopoiesis in the spleen, liver, and even other sites such as the peritoneum, leading to massive splenomegaly due to myeloid hyperproduction. Autoimmune hemolytic anemia requires the spleen to dispose of massive amounts of damaged red blood cells, leading to reticuloendothelial hyperplasia and frequently an extremely large spleen. Chronic myelogenous leukemia and other leukemias/lymphomas can lead to massive splenomegaly due to infiltration with an abnormal clone of cells. If a patient with cirrhosis or right-heart failure has massive splenomegaly, a cause other than passive congestion should be considered.

I-114.   **The answer is A.** *(Chap. 60)* The presence of Howell-Jolly bodies (nuclear remnants), Heinz bodies (denatured hemoglobin), basophilic stippling, and nucleated red blood cells in the peripheral blood implies that the spleen is not properly clearing senescent or damaged red blood cells from the circulation. This usually occurs because of surgical splenectomy but is also possible when there is diffuse infiltration of the spleen with malignant cells. Hemolytic anemia can have various peripheral smear findings depending on the etiology of the hemolysis. Spherocytes and bite cells are an example of damaged red cells that might appear due to autoimmune hemolytic anemia and oxidative damage, respectively. DIC is characterized by schistocytes and thrombocytopenia on smear, with elevated INR and activated partial thromboplastin time as well. However, in these conditions, damaged red cells are still cleared effectively by the spleen. Transformation to acute leukemia does not lead to splenic damage.

I-115. **The answer is A.** *(Chap. 60)* Splenectomy leads to an increased risk of overwhelming postsplenectomy sepsis, an infection that carries an extremely high mortality rate. The most commonly implicated organisms are encapsulated. *Streptococcus pneumoniae, Haemophilus influenzae* and sometime gram-negative enteric organisms are most frequently isolated. There is no known increased risk for any viral infections. Vaccination for *S. pneumoniae, H. influenzae,* and *Neisseria meningitidis* is indicated for any patient who may undergo splenectomy. The vaccines should be given at least 2 weeks before surgery. The highest risk of sepsis occurs in patients under 20 because the spleen is responsible for first-pass immunity and younger patients are more likely to have primary exposure to implicated organisms. The risk is highest during the first 3 years after splenectomy and persists at a lower rate until death.

I-116. **The answer is A.** *(Chap. 49)* Erectile dysfunction increases with age but is not considered a normal part of the aging process. This patient has evidence of atherosclerosis, which is the most common organic cause of erectile dysfunction in males. Medications account for 25% of cases of erectile dysfunction: diuretics, beta blockers and other antihypertensives being common culprits. Psychogenic erectile dysfunction can cause or be caused by organic erectile dysfunction. We are given no indication that this patient is experiencing a relationship conflict or that he has developed performance anxiety. This patient is not clinically hypogonadal.

I-117. **The answer is D.** *(Chap. 49)* This patient has vasculogenic erectile dysfunction. Sildenafil, tadalafil, and vardenafil are the only approved and effective agents for erectile dysfunction due to psychogenic, diabetic, or vasculogenic causes or resulting from postradical prostatectomy and spinal cord injury. As such, they should be considered as first-line therapy. If the patient were to fail to respond to oral agents, intraurethral vasoactive substances are a reasonable next choice. Implantation of a penile prosthesis would be of consideration if intraurethral or intracavernosal injections failed. Sex therapy will not address the organic dysfunction that this patient has, as evidenced by the lack of nocturnal erections.

I-118. **The answer is C.** *(Chap. 49)* Female sexual dysfunction (FSD) includes disorders of desire, arousal, pain, and muted orgasm. The risk factors for FSD are similar to those in men including cardiovascular disease, endocrine diseases, neurologic disorders, and smoking. The female sexual response requires the presence of estrogens and possibly androgens. While the neurotransmission for clitoral corporal engorgement are the same as for men and include nitric oxide, the use of PDE-5 inhibitors for FSD has not been proven efficacious and should be discouraged until proof is available that they are effective. PDE-5 inhibitors have not been shown to be of more or less benefit in pre- or postmenopausal women. For FSD, behavioral and nonpharmacologic therapies including lifestyle modification, medication adjustment, and use of lubricants should be a first step.

I-119. **The answer is B.** *(Chap. 41)* Patients with unintentional weight loss of >5% of the total body weight over a 6- to 12-month period should prompt an evaluation. In the elderly, weight loss is an independent predictor of morbidity and mortality. Studies in the elderly have found mortality rates of 10–15%/year in patients with significant unintentional weight loss. It is important to confirm the weight loss and the duration of time over which it occurred. The causes of weight loss are protean and usually become apparent after a careful evaluation and directed testing. A thorough review of systems should be performed including constitutional, respiratory, gastrointestinal, and psychiatric. Travel history and risk factors for HIV are also important. Medications and supplements should be reviewed. The physical examination must include an examination of the skin, oropharynx, thyroid gland, lymphatic system, abdomen, rectum, prostate, neurologic system, and pelvis. A reasonable laboratory approach would include an initial phase of testing including the tests outlined in this scenario. In the absence of signs or symptoms, close follow-up rather than undirected testing is appropriate. Total-body scanning with PET or CT has not been shown to be effective as screening tests without a clinical indication.

I-120. **The answer is A.** *(Chaps. 56 and 311)* Drugs can trigger inflammatory mediators (histamine, leukotrienes, etc.) directly; i.e., the *pharmacoimmune concept*. These "anaphylactoid" responses are not IgE-mediated. NSAIDS, aspirin, and radiocontrast media are frequent causes of pharmacologically mediated anaphylactoid reactions. Given that this is an investigational drug, it is improbable that patients in this study have taken this drug before. T cell clones have been obtained after pharmacologically mediated anaphylactoid reactions, with a majority being CD4+. A constitutively IgE receptor would not manifest solely after drug exposure.

I-121. **The answer is D.** *(Chap. 214)* Anthrax is caused by the gram-positive spore-forming rod *Bacillus anthrax*. Anthrax spores may be the prototypical disease of bioterrorism. Although not spread person to person, inhalational anthrax has a high mortality, a low infective dose (five spores), and may be spread widely with aerosols after bioengineering. It is well-documented that anthrax spores were produced and stored as potential bioweapons. In 2001, the United States was exposed to anthrax spores delivered as a powder in letters. Of 11 patients with inhalation anthrax, 5 died. All 11 patients with cutaneous anthrax survived. Because anthrax spores can remain dormant in the respiratory tract for 6 weeks, the incubation period can be quite long and post-exposure antibiotics are recommended for 60 days. Trials of a recombinant vaccine are underway.

I-122. **The answer is D.** *(Chap. 214)* The three major clinical forms of anthrax are gastrointestinal (GI), cutaneous, and inhalational. GI anthrax results from eating contaminated meat and is an unlikely bioweapon. Cutaneous anthrax results from contact with the spores and results in a black eschar lesion. Cutaneous anthrax had a 20% mortality before antibiotics became available. Inhalational anthrax typically presents with the most deadly form and is the most likely bioweapon. The spores are phagocytosed by alveolar macrophages and transported to the mediastinum. Subsequent germination, toxin elaboration, and hematogenous spread cause septic shock. A characteristic radiographic finding is mediastinal widening and pleural effusion. Prompt initiation of antibiotics is essential as mortality is likely 100% without specific treatment. Inhalational anthrax is not known to be contagious. Provided that there is no concern for release of another highly infectious agent such as smallpox, only routine precautions are warranted.

I-123. **The answer is F.** *(Chap. 214)* Smallpox has been proposed as a potential bioweapon. It is essential that clinicians be able to recognize this infection clinically and distinguish it from the common infection with varicella. Infection with smallpox occurs principally with close contact, although saliva droplets or aerosols may also spread disease. Approximately 12–14 days after exposure, the patient develops high fever, malaise, nausea, vomiting, headache, and a maculopapular rash that begins on the face and extremities and spreads (centripetally) to the trunk with lesions at the same stage of development at any given location. This is in contrast to the rash of varicella (chickenpox), which begins on the face and trunk and spreads (centrifugally) to the extremities with lesions at all stages of development at any given location. Smallpox is associated with a 10–30% mortality. Vaccination with vaccinia (cowpox) is effective, even if given during the incubation period.

I-124. **The answer is C.** *(Chap. 214)* Tularemia, caused by the small nonmotile gram-negative coccobacillus *Francisella tularensis*, has been proposed as a potential bioweapon (CDC category A) because of its high degree of environmental infectiousness, potential for aerolization, and ability to cause severe pneumonia. It is not as lethal as anthrax or plague (*Yersinia pestis*). Infection with *F. tularensis* is most common in rural areas where small mammals serve as a reservoir. Human infections may occur from tick or mosquito bites or from contact with infected animals while hunting. The isolation of this pathogen in two patients without obvious exposure risk factors should prompt concern that a terrorist has intentionally aerosolized *F. tularensis* as an agent of bioterror. It is highly infectious, with as few as 10 organisms causing infection, and outbreaks have been reported in microbiology laboratory workers streaking Petri dishes. However, it is not infectious person-to-person. Streptomycin, doxycycline, gentamicin, chloramphenicol, and ciprofloxacin are likely effective agents; however, given the possibility of genetically altered organisms, broad-spectrum antibiotics are indicated pending sensitivity testing. In outbreaks, tularemia pneumonia has a mortality of 30–60% in untreated patients and <2% with appropriate therapy.

I-125.   **The answer is C.** *(Chap. 389)* The most common physical effects of smoking marijuana are conjunctival infection and tachycardia; however, tolerance for the tachycardia develops quickly among habitual users. Smoking marijuana can precipitate angina in those with a history of coronary artery disease, and such patients should be advised to abstain from smoking marijuana or using cannabis compounds. This effect may be more pronounced with smoking marijuana than cigarettes. Because chronic use of marijuana typically involves deep inhalation and prolonged retention of marijuana smoke, chronic smokers may develop chronic bronchial irritation and impaired single-breath carbon monoxide diffusion capacity (DL_{CO}). Decreased sperm count, impaired sperm motility, and morphologic abnormalities of spermatozoa have been reported. Prospective studies demonstrated a correlation between impaired fetal growth and development with heavy marijuana use during pregnancy.

I-126.   **The answer is B.** *(Chap. 389)* Although LSD abuse has been a well-known public health hazard, the use of LSD may be increasing in some communities in the Unites States among adolescents and young adults. LSD causes a variety of bizarre perceptual changes that can last for up to 18 h. Panic episodes due to LSD use ("bad trip") are the most frequent medical emergency associated with LSD. These episodes may last up to 24 h and are best treated in a specialized psychiatric setting. Marijuana intoxication causes a feeling of euphoria and is associated with some impairment in cognition similar to alcohol intoxication. Heroin intoxication usually produces a feeling of euphoria and intoxication; panic attacks during usage are uncommon. Methamphetamine intoxication produces feelings of euphoria and decreases the fatigue associated with difficult life situations. Psychosis is possible with the ingestion of most illicit substances, depending on the user and the environmental setting; however, the classic panic attack associated with the "bad trip" of LSD is distinct in the predominance of paranoia and fear of imminent doom.

I-127.   **The answer is E.** *(Chap. e35)* "Body packing" is a common practice among members of the illicit drug trade for transport of illicit drugs across international borders. Human "mules" swallow sealed packages of illicit drugs in special bags to conceal the drug from drug enforcement officials. Because these bags may rupture while in the gastrointestinal tract, all persons who are unconscious at airports, or who develop symptoms after returning from a country where drug trafficking is common, should be evaluated for this particular contingency. Initial examination is a cursory orifice examination, but abdominal imaging and bowel lavage are necessary in many cases. Confirmed cases need to be followed closely as further absorption of the drug is possible. Blood cultures and echocardiogram are only necessary if infective endocarditis is suspected. However, this patient has no fevers or indication of active drug abuse. CSF analysis would be necessary only if no obvious cause of the patient's mental status change were available. As her respiratory rate is now elevated rather than low, her mental status is normal, and her oxygen saturations are high, there is little reason to expect CO_2 retention or hypoxemia. A blood gas can likely be avoided unless her clinical status changes.

I-128.   **The answer is D.** *(Chap. e35)* Sympathetic toxidromes share many features including increased pulse, blood pressure, neuromuscular activity, tremulousness, delirium, and agitation. In many cases, these syndromes can be subclassified according to other features or relative strengths of the above symptoms. Sympathomimetics like cocaine and amphetamines cause extreme elevations in vital signs and organ damage due to peripheral vasoconstriction, usually in the absence of hallucinations. Benzodiazepine and alcohol withdrawal syndromes present similarly but hallucinations, and often seizures, are common in these conditions. Hot, dry, flushed skin, urinary retention, and absent bowel sounds characterize anticholinergic syndromes associated with antihistamines, antipsychotics, antiparkinsonian agents, muscle relaxants, and cyclic antidepressants. Nystagmus is a unique feature of ketamine and phencyclidine overdose.

I-129.   **The answer is E.** *(Chap. e35)* Opiate overdose falls broadly into a toxidrome character-ized by physiologic depression and sedation. If a history is obtained suggesting a toxic in-gestion or injection, then the diagnosis is straightforward. However, this history is often absent and it can be a challenge initially to differentiate opiate toxicity from other central nervous system (CNS) and physiologic depressants. Therefore, naloxone should always be given as a diagnostic and therapeutic trial under circumstances of unexplained altered mental status, especially in the presence of coma or seizures. An immediate clinical im-provement characterizes opiate overdose. In opiate overdose, abnormal vital signs occur exclusively as a result of central respiratory depression and the accompanying hypoxemia. Low blood pressure in an alert patient should prompt a search for an alternative explana-tion for the hypotension. An anion gap metabolic acidosis with normal lactate is seen in syndromes such as methanol or ethylene glycol ingestion: mental status change usually precedes vital sign changes, and vital signs are often discordant as a result of physiologic adjustments to the severity of the acidosis. Mydriasis is a result of stimulant use. Miosis is associated with CNS depression. Sweating and drooling are manifestations of cholinergic agents such as muscarinic and micotinic agonists.

I-130.   **The answer is A.** *(Chap. e35)* Lithium interferes with cell membrane ion transport, leading to nephrogenic diabetes insipidus and falsely elevated chloride. This can cause the appearance of low anion gap metabolic acidosis. Sequelae include nausea, vomiting, ataxia, encephalopathy, coma, seizures, arrhythmia, hyperthermia, permanent move-ment disorder, and/or encephalopathy. Severe cases are treated with bowel irrigation, en-doscopic removal of long-acting formulations, hydration, and sometimes hemodialysis. Care should be taken because toxicity occurs at lower levels in chronic toxicity compared to acute toxicity. Salicylate toxicity leads to a normal osmolal gap as well as an elevated anion gap metabolic acidosis, respiratory alkalosis, and sometimes normal anion gap metabolic acidosis. Methanol toxicity is associated with blindness and is characterized by an increased anion gap metabolic acidosis, with normal lactate and ketones, and a high osmolal gap. Propylene glycol toxicity causes an increased anion gap metabolic acidosis with elevated lactate and a high osmolal gap. The only electrolyte abnormalities associ-ated with opiate overdose are compensatory to a primary respiratory acidosis.

I-131.   **The answer is B.** *(Chap. e35)* The clinical ramifications of this question are critical. Drug effects begin earlier, peak later, and last longer in the context of overdose, compared to commonly referenced values. Therefore, if a patient has a known ingestion of a toxic dose of a dangerous substance and symptoms have not yet begun, then aggressive gut de-contamination should ensue, because symptoms are apt to ensue rapidly. The late peak and longer duration of action are important as well. A common error in practice is for patients to be released or watched less carefully after reversal of toxicity associated with an opiate agonist or benzodiazepine. However, the duration of activity of the offending toxic agent often exceeds the half-life of the antagonists, naloxone or flumazenil, requir-ing the administration of subsequent doses several hours later to prevent further central nervous system or physiologic depression.

I-132.   **The answer is E** *(Chap. e35)* Management of the toxin-induced seizure includes ad-dressing the underlying cause of the seizure, antiepileptic therapy, reversal of the toxin ef-fect, and supportive management. In this patient, lithium toxicity has led to diabetes insipidus and encephalopathy. The patient was unlikely to take in free water due to his in-capacitated state, and as a result developed hypernatremia. The hypernatremia and lith-ium toxicity are contributing to his seizure and should be addressed with careful free water replacement and bowel irrigation, plus hemodialysis. As he is not protecting his airway, supportive management will need to include endotracheal intubation. Antisei-zure prophylaxis with first-line agent, a benzodiazepine, has failed, and therefore he should be treated with a barbiturate as well as a benzodiazepine. Benzodiazepines should be continued as they work by a different mechanism than barbiturates in preventing sei-zures. Phenytoin is contraindicated for the use of toxic seizures due to worse outcomes documented in clinical trials for this indication.

I-133. **The answer is E.** *(Chap. e35)* Gastric decontamination is controversial because there are few data to support or refute its use more than an hour after ingestion. It remains a very common practice in most hospitals. Syrup of ipecac is no longer endorsed for in-hospital use and is controversial even for home use, though its safety profile is well documented, and therefore it likely poses little harm for ingestions when the history is clear and the indication strong. Activated charcoal is generally the decontamination method of choice as it is the least aversive and least invasive option available. It is effective in decreasing systemic absorption if given within an hour of poison ingestion. It may be effective even later after ingestion for drugs with significant anticholinergic effect (e.g., tricyclic antidepressants). Considerations are poor visibility of the gastrointestinal tract on endoscopy following charcoal ingestion, and perhaps decreased absorption of oral drugs. Gastric lavage is the most invasive option and is effective, but it is occasionally associated with tracheal intubation and bowel-wall perforation. It is also the least comfortable option for the patient. Moreover, aspiration risk is highest in those undergoing gastric lavage. All three of the most common options for decontamination carry at least a 1% risk of an aspiration event, which warrants special consideration in the patient with mental status change.

I-134. **The answer is C.** *(Chap. 60)* To keep body weight stable, energy intake must match energy output. Energy output has two main determinants: resting energy expenditure and physical activity. Other, less clinically important determinants include energy expenditure to digest food and thermogenesis from shivering. Resting energy expenditure can be calculated and is $900 + 10w$ (where w = weight) in males and $700 + 7w$ in females. This calculation is then modified for physical activity level. The main determinant of resting energy expenditure is lean body mass.

II. NUTRITION

QUESTIONS

DIRECTIONS: Choose the **one best** response to each question.

II-1. A 19-year-old woman with anorexia nervosa undergoes surgery for acute appendicitis. The postoperative course is complicated by acute respiratory distress syndrome, and she remains intubated for 10 days. She develops wound dehiscence on postoperative day 10. Laboratory data show a white blood cell count of 4000/μL, hematocrit 35%, albumin 2.1 g/dL, total protein 5.8 g/dL, transferrin 54 mg/dL, and iron-binding capacity 88 mg/dL. You are considering initiating nutritional therapy on hospital day 11. Which of the following is true regarding the etiology and treatment of malnutrition in this patient?

A. She has marasmus, and nutritional support should be started slowly.
B. She has kwashiorkor, and nutritional support should be aggressive.
C. She has marasmic kwashiorkor, kwashiorkor predominant, and nutritional support should be aggressive.
D. She has marasmic kwashiorkor, marasmus predominant, and nutritional support should be slow.

II-2. You are seeing a patient in follow-up 2 weeks after hospitalization. The patient is recovering from nosocomial pneumonia due to a resistant *Pseudomonas* spp. His hospital course was complicated by a deep venous thrombosis. The patient is currently on IV piperacillin/tazobactam and tobramycin via a tunneled catheter, warfarin, lisinopril, hydrochlorothiazide, and metoprolol. Laboratory data this morning show an INR of 8.2. At hospital discharge his INR was stable at 2.5. He has no history of liver disease. What is the most likely cause of the elevated INR?

A. The patient has inadvertently overdosed.
B. The patient has developed a recurrent deep venous thrombosis, which has affected the laboratory data.
C. The patient is deficient in vitamin K and needs supplementation.
D. The warfarin prescription was written incorrectly at the time of discharge.

II-3. A 51-year-old alcoholic man is admitted to the hospital for upper gastrointestinal bleeding. From further history and physical examination, it becomes apparent that his bleeding is from gingival membranes. He is intoxicated and complains of fatigue. Reviewing his chart you find that he had a hemarthrosis evacuated 6 months ago and has been lost to follow-up since then. He takes no medications. Laboratory data show platelets of 250,000, INR of 0.9. He has a diffuse hemorrhagic eruption on his legs (Figure II-3, Color Atlas).

What is the recommended treatment for this patient's underlying disorder?

A. Folate
B. Niacin
C. Thiamine
D. Vitamin C
E. Vitamin K

II-4. While working in the intensive care unit, you admit a 57-year-old woman with acute pancreatitis and oliguric renal failure. Respiratory rate is 26 breaths/min, heart rate is 125 beats/min, and temperature is 37.2°C. Physical examination shows marked abdominal tenderness with normoactive bowel sounds. A CT scan shows an inflamed pancreas without hemorrhage. You calculate her APACHE-I score to be 28. When deciding on when to initiate nutritional replacement in this patient, which of the following statements is true?

A. Bowel rest is the cornerstone of treatment for acute pancreatitis.
B. Administering parenteral nutrition within 24 h will decrease the risk of infection and mortality.
C. Enteral feeding supports gut function by secretion of gastrointestinal hormones that stimulate gut trophic activity.
D. In severe systemic response to inflammation, feeding can be withheld initially because the patient is likely to have adequate, spontaneous oral intake in the first 7 days.

II-5. The resting energy expenditure is a rough estimate of total caloric needs in a state of energy balance. Of these two patients with stable weights, which person has the highest resting energy expenditure (REE): Patient A, a 40-year-old man who weighs 90 kg and is sedentary, or Patient B, a 40-year-old man who weighs 70 kg and is very active?

     A.   40-year-old man who weighs 90 kg and is sedentary
     B.   40-year-old man who weighs 70 kg and is very active
     C.   REE is the same
     D.   Not enough information given to calculate the REE

II-6. All of the following clinical features are common in patients with anorexia nervosa *except*

     A.   Avoid food-related occupations
     B.   Distorted body image
     C.   Engage in binge eating
     D.   Exercise extensively
     E.   Rarely complain of hunger
     F.   Socially withdrawn

II-7. You diagnose anorexia nervosa in one of your new clinic patients. When coordinating a treatment program with the psychiatrist, what characteristics should prompt consideration for inpatient treatment instead of scheduling an outpatient assessment?

     A.   Amenorrhea
     B.   Exaggeration of food intake
     C.   Irrational fear of gaining weight
     D.   Purging behavior
     E.   Weight <75% of expected body weight

II-8. It is hospital day 16 for a 49-year-old homeless patient who is recovering from alcohol withdrawal and delirium tremens. She spent the first 9 days of this hospitalization in the intensive care unit but is now awake, alert, and conversant. She has a healing decubitus ulcer, and her body mass index is 19 kg/m². Laboratory data show an albumin of 2.9 g/dL and a prothrombin time of 18 s (normal range). Is this patient malnourished?

     A.   Cannot be determined, need more information.
     B.   No. Given her heavy alcohol intake, her prothrombin time is expected to be delayed.
     C.   No. She has a low resting energy expenditure and her intact mental state argues against malnutrition.
     D.   Yes, this degree of hypoalbuminemia is uncommon in cirrhosis and is likely due to malnutrition.

II-9. A 42-year-old male patient wants your opinion about vitamin E supplements. He has read that taking high doses of vitamin E can improve his sexual performance and slow the aging process. He is not vitamin E deficient. You explain to him that these claims are not based on good evidence. What other potential side effect should he be concerned about?

     A.   Deep venous thrombosis
     B.   Hemorrhage

II-9. *(Continued)*
     C.   Night blindness
     D.   Peripheral neuropathy
     E.   Retinopathy

II-10. Doing rounds in the oncology center, you are see a patient with carcinoid syndrome. Due to the increased conversion of tryptophan to serotonin, this patient has developed niacin deficiency. All of the following are components of the pellagra syndrome *except*

     A.   dermatitis
     B.   dementia
     C.   diarrhea
     D.   dyslipidemia
     E.   glossitis

II-11. An 86-year-old woman with chronic obstructive pulmonary disease (COPD), congestive heart failure, and insulin-requiring type 2 diabetes mellitus is admitted to the intensive care unit with an exacerbation of her COPD. She is intubated and treated with glucocorticoids and nebulized albuterol. She is also continued on her glargine insulin, aspirin, pravastatin, furosemide, enalapril, and metoprolol. On hospital day 8, parenteral nutrition is begun via catheter in the subclavian vein. Her insulin requirements increase on hospital day 9 due to episodes of hyperglycemia. On hospital day 10, she develops rales and an increasing oxygen requirement. A chest radiograph shows bilateral pulmonary edema. Laboratory data show hypokalemia, hypomagnesemia, and hypophosphatemia and a normal creatinine. Her weight has increased by 3 kg since admission. Urine sodium is <10 meq/dL. All of the following changes in her nutritional regimen will improve her volume status *except*

     A.   combination of glucose and fat in the parenteral nutrition mixture
     B.   decreasing the sodium content of the mixture to <40 meq per day
     C.   increasing the protein content of the parenteral nutrition mixture
     D.   reducing the overall glucose content

II-12. A new study has been published showing a benefit of 25 mg/day of vitamin X. The recommended estimated average requirement of vitamin X is 10 mg/day, 2 standard deviations below the amount published in the study. The tolerable upper limit of vitamin X is unknown. Your patient wants to know if it is safe to consume 25 mg/day of vitamin X. Which is the most appropriate answer?

     A.   Two standard deviations above the estimated average requirement defines the tolerable upper limit.
     B.   25 mg/day is probably too much vitamin X in 1 day.
     C.   25 mg/day is statistically in a safe range of the estimated average requirement.
     D.   The study was not designed to assess safety and therefore should not influence practice.

II-13. An elevation in which of the following hormones is consistent with the effects of anorexia nervosa?

A. Cortisol
B. Gonadotropin-releasing hormone (GnRH)
C. Leptin
D. Thyroxine (T_4)
E. Thyroid-stimulating hormone (TSH)

II-14. Which of the following statements regarding anorexia nervosa (AN) and bulimia nervosa (BN) is true?

A. Patients with the purging subtype of BN tend to be heavier than those with the nonpurging subtype.
B. Patients with the restricting subtype of AN are more emotionally labile than those with the purging subtype.
C. Patients with the restricting subtype of AN are more likely to abuse illicit drugs than those with the purging subtype.
D. The mortality of BN is lower than that of AN.

II-15. You are seeing a pediatric patient from Djibouti in consultation who was admitted with a constellation of symptoms including diarrhea, alopecia, muscle wasting, depression, and a rash involving the face, extremities, and perineum. The child has hypogonadism and dwarfism. You astutely make the diagnosis of zinc deficiency, and laboratory test confirm this (zinc level <70 µL/dL). What other clinical findings is this patient likely to manifest?

A. Dissecting aortic aneurysm
B. Hypochromic anemia
C. Hypoglycemia
D. Hypopigmented hair
E. Macrocytosis

II-16. You are rotating on a medical trip to impoverished areas of China. You are examining an 8-year-old child whose mother complains of him being clumsy and sickly. He has had many episodes of diarrheal illnesses and pneumonia. His "clumsiness" is most pronounced in the evening when he has to go outside and do his chores. On examination, you notice conjunctival dryness with white patches of keratinized epithelium on the sclera. What is the cause of this child's symptoms?

A. Autoimmune neutropenia
B. Congenital rubella
C. Spinocerebellar ataxia (SCA) type 1
D. Vitamin A deficiency
E. Vitamin B_1 deficiency

II-17. After being stranded alone in the mountains for 8 days, a 26-year-old hiker is brought to the hospital for evaluation of a right femoral neck fracture. He has not

II-17. *(Continued)*
had anything to eat or drink for the past 6 days. Vital signs are within normal limits. Weight is 79.5 kg, which is 1.8 kg less than he weighed 6 months ago. Laboratory data show a creatinine of 2.5 mg/dL, blood urea nitrogen of 52 mg/dL, glucose 96 mg/dL, albumin 4.1 mg/dL, chloride 105 meq/L, and ferritin on 173 ng/mL. Which of the following statements is true regarding his risk of malnourishment?

A. He has protein-calorie malnutrition due to the rate of weight loss.
B. He has protein-calorie malnutrition due to his elevated ferritin.
C. He is at risk, but a normal individual can tolerate 7 days of starvation.
D. He is not malnourished because he is not hypoglycemic after 6 days of no food or water.

II-18. You are doing rounds in the intensive care unit on an intubated patient who is recovering from a stroke and has diabetic gastroparesis. When suctioning the patient in the morning, she coughs profusely, with thick green secretions. You are concerned about the possibility of aspiration pneumonia. All of the following measures are useful in preventing aspiration pneumonia in an intubated patient *except*

A. combined enteral and parenteral nutrition
B. elevating the head of the bed to 30°
C. physician-directed methods for formula advancement
D. post-ligament of Treitz feeding

II-19. Which of these features represents a critical distinction between anorexia nervosa and bulimia nervosa?

A. Binge eating
B. Electrolyte abnormalities
C. Self-induced vomiting
D. Underweight

II-20. You are counseling a patient who is recovering from long-standing anorexia nervosa (AN). She is a 22-year-old woman who suffered the effects of AN for 8 years with a nadir body mass index of 17 kg/m^2 and many laboratory abnormalities during that time. Which of the following characteristics of AN is least likely to improve despite successful lasting treatment of the disorder?

A. Amenorrhea
B. Delayed gastric emptying
C. Lanugo
D. Low bone mass
E. Salivary gland enlargement

II. NUTRITION

ANSWERS

II-1. **The answer is C.** *(Chap. 72)* The two major types of protein energy malnutrition are marasmus and kwashiorkor; differentiating the two is extremely important in the malnourished patient since this directly effects your therapy. This patient has marasmic kwashiorkor due to the impact of her anorexia nervosa, the acute stressor of the surgery, and the 10 days of starvation. This patient has chronic starvation (marasmus) as well as the major sine qua non of kwashiorkor; i.e., reduction of levels of serum proteins. She is kwashiorkor predominant because of the acute starvation and the severely low levels of serum proteins. Vigorous nutritional therapy is indicated for kwashiorkor.

TABLE II-1   Comparison of Marasmus and Kwashiorkor

	Marasmus	Kwashiorkor[a]
Clinical setting	↓ Energy intake	↓ Protein intake during stress state
Time course to develop	Months or years	Weeks
Clinical features	Starved appearance	Well-nourished appearance
	Weight <80% standard for height	Easy hair pluckability[b]
	Triceps skinfold <3 mm	Edema
	Mid-arm muscle circumference <15 cm	
Laboratory findings	Creatinine-height index <60% standard	Serum albumin <2.8 g/dL
		Total iron-binding capacity <200 μg/dL
		Lymphocytes <1500/μL
		Anergy
Clinical course	Reasonably preserved responsiveness to short-term stress	Infections
		Poor wound healing, decubitus ulcers, skin breakdown
Mortality	Low unless related to underlying disease	High
Diagnostic criteria	Triceps skinfold <3 mm	Serum albumin <2.8 g/dL
	Mid-arm muscle circumference <15 cm	At least one of the following:
		Poor wound healing, decubitus ulcers, or skin breakdown
		Easy hair pluckability[b]
		Edema

[a]The findings used to diagnose kwashiorkor must be unexplained by other causes.
[b]Tested by *firmly* pulling a lock of hair from the top (not the sides or back), grasping with the thumb and forefinger. An average of three or more hairs removed easily and painlessly is considered abnormal hair pluckability.

II-2. **The answer is C.** *(Chap. 71)* There are two natural sources of vitamin K. Vitamin K_1 comes from vegetable and animal sources. Vitamin K_2 is synthesized by enteric bacterial flora and is found in hepatic tissue. Vitamin K deficiency in adults can be seen with chronic small-intestinal disease, in those with obstructed biliary tracts, after small-bowel resection, or in those on broad-spectrum antibiotics. As a result of reducing gut bacteria, antibiotics can precipitate vitamin K deficiency. Overdose and medication error are plausible explanations but are less likely to be the root cause given the antibiotic exposure. Acute venous thromboses can deplete levels of coagulant proteins (especially protein C and protein S), but the INR should not be affected.

II-3. The answer is D. *(Chap. 71)* This patient has the classic perifollicular hemorrhagic rash of scurvy (vitamin C deficiency). In the United States, scurvy is primarily a disease of alcoholics and the elderly who consume <10 mg/d of vitamin C. In addition to nonspecific symptoms of fatigue, these patients also have impaired ability to form mature connective tissue and can bleed into various sites, including the skin and gingiva. A normal INR excludes symptomatic vitamin K deficiency. Thiamine, niacin, and folate deficiencies are also seen in patients with alcoholism. Thiamine deficiency may cause a peripheral neuropathy (beri-beri). Folate deficiency causes macrocytic anemia and thrombocytopenia. Niacin deficiency causes pellagra, which is characterized by glossitis and a pigmented, scaling rash that may be particularly noticeable in sun exposed areas.

II-4. The answer is C. *(Chap. 73)* In the past, bowel rest was the cornerstone of treatment; however, the value of adding minimal amounts of enteral nutrition (EN) is widely accepted. Timing of enteral therapy is important. Although administering EN can improve mortality, there is an increased risk of infection. Patients with severe SRI are unlikely to be able to take adequate, spontaneous oral intake within the first week of their hospitalization. Therefore, enteral nutrition should be considered early for severely sick patients.

II-5. The answer is B. *(Chap. 70)* For patients with stable weights, REE can be calculated if the gender, weight, and activity level are provided. For males, REE = 900 + 10w, and for females, REE = 700 + 7w, where w is weight in kilograms. The REE is then adjusted for activity level by multiplying 1.2 for sedentary, 1.4 for moderately active, and 1.8 for very active individuals. Patient A has an REE of 2160 kcal/day. Patient B has an REE of 2880 kcal/day. For a given weight, a higher level of activity increases the REE more than a 20-kg change in weight at a given level of activity.

II-6. The answer is A. *(Chap. 76)* Anorexia nervosa (AN) is much less common in men than women and is more prevalent in cultures where food is plentiful and where thinness is associated with attractiveness. Individuals who pursue occupations that place a premium on thinness, such as ballet or modeling, are at greater risk of developing anorexia nervosa. In patients with AN, as weight loss increases thoughts of food dominate mental life. AN patients may obsessively collect cookbooks and recipes and tend to be drawn to food-related occupations. These patients become socially withdrawn and may also engage in binge eating, similar to bulimia nervosa patients. AN patients rarely complain of hunger or fatigue and will exercise extensively as a means to achieve weight loss.

II-7. The answer is E. *(Chap. 76)* Based on the American Psychiatric Association's practice guidelines, inpatient treatment or partial hospitalization is indicated for patients whose weight <75% of expected for age and height, have severe metabolic disturbances (e.g., electrolyte disturbances, bradycardia, hypotension), or who have serious concomitant psychiatric problems (e.g., suicidal ideation, substance abuse). There should be a low threshold for inpatient treatment if there has been rapid weight loss or if weight <80% of expected. Amenorrhea, exaggeration of food intake, and fear of gaining weight are part of the diagnostic criteria for AN, and purging is not uncommon in this population. Weight restoration to 90% of predicted weight is the goal of nutritional therapy.

II-8. The answer is A. *(Chap. 72)* Interactions between illness and nutrition are complex, therefore many physical and laboratory findings reflect both underlying disease and nutritional status. The nutritional evaluation of a patient requires an integration of history, physical examination, anthropometrics, and laboratory studies. The finding of isolated hypoalbuminemia may be due to her underlying liver disease and does not necessarily indicate malnutrition. This patient is at high risk for malnutrition, but her current status may reflect malnutrition or sequelae of chronic alcoholism.

II-9.   The answer is B.   *(Chap. 71)*   High doses of vitamin E (>800 mg/d) may reduce platelet aggregation and interfere with vitamin K metabolism. Doses >400 mg/d may increase mortality from any cause. Vitamin E excess is not related to increased risk of venous thrombosis. Peripheral neuropathy and a pigmented retinopathy may be seen in vitamin E deficiency. Vitamin A deficiency is a cause of night blindness.

II-10.   The answer is D.   *(Chap. 71)*   Pellagra (niacin deficiency) is most commonly a disorder among people eating corn-based diets but can also be seen in alcoholics. Tryptophan is converted to niacin with an efficiency of 60:1 by weight. Therefore, in a patient with congenital defects in tryptophan absorption or with increased conversion of tryptophan to serotonin, niacin deficiency can develop. The early symptoms of pellagra include anorexia, irritability, abdominal pain and vomiting, and glossitis. Vaginitis and esophagitis may also occur. The four Ds of pellagra are *d*ermatitis, *d*iarrhea, and *d*ementia leading to *d*eath. Dyslipidemia is not a part of the pellagra syndrome.

II-11.   The answer is C.   *(Chap. 73)*   The most common metabolic problems related to parenteral nutrition (PN) are fluid overload and hyperglycemia. Hypertonic dextrose stimulates a much higher insulin level than normal feeding, which is evident on hospital day 9 in this scenario. Hyperinsulinemia stimulates antinatriuretic and antidiuretic hormone, which leads to sodium and fluid retention as well as increased intracellular transport of potassium, magnesium, and phosphorus. It is not uncommon to see an increase in weight and a low urine sodium in patients with normal renal function. Providing sodium in limited amounts of 40 meq/day and the use of both glucose and fat in the PN mixture will help reduce fluid retention. Reducing the overall glucose content will also abate the need for higher insulin level. The fluid retention in this scenario is not mediated by low protein levels.

II-12.   The answer is C.   *(Chap. 70)*   The estimated average requirement (EAR) is the amount of a nutrient estimated to be adequate for half of the individuals of a specific age and sex. It is not useful clinically for estimating nutritional adequacy because it is a median requirement for a group; 50% of the individuals in a group fall below the requirement and 50% fall above it. A person taking the EAR of a vitamin has a 50% risk of inadequate intake. The recommended dietary allowances (RDA) is defined statistically as 2 standard deviations above the EAR to ensure that the needs of most individuals are met. In this case the study used a dosage of 2 standard deviations above the EAR, which would be the RDA. Data on the tolerable upper limit of a vitamin are usually inadequate to establish a value for upper limit of tolerability. The absence of a published tolerable upper limit does not imply that the risks are nonexistent.

II-13.   The answer is A.   *(Chap. 76)*   Regulation of virtually every endocrine system is disturbed in patients with anorexia nervosa (AN). Hypothalamic amenorrhea reflects diminished production of GnRH. Serum leptin levels are reduced due to decreased mass of adipose tissue, and this is thought to be the mediator of the other neuroendocrine abnormalities associated with AN. Thyroid function tests resemble the pattern seen in euthyroid sick syndrome (low-normal or depressed TSH and T_4, depressed T_3, increased reverse T_3). Serum cortisol and 24-h urine free cortisol are generally elevated without the expected clinical consequences of hypercortisolism.

II-14.   The answer is D.   *(Chap. 76)*   The mortality of AN is ~5% per decade and is much lower in patients with BN. This is probably mediated by the weight loss and malnutrition associated with AN. There are two subtypes of BN: purging and nonpurging. Patients with the nonpurging subtype tend to be heavier and are less prone to electrolyte disturbances. There are also two mutually exclusive subtypes of AN: restricting and purging. Patients with the purging subtype are more emotionally labile and tend to have other problems with impulse control such as illicit drug abuse.

II-15.   The answer is D.   *(Chap. 71)*   Hypozincemia is most commonly due to poor oral intake of zinc, although some medications can also inhibit zinc absorption (e.g., sodium valproate, penicillamine, ethambutol). Severe chronic zinc deficiency has been described among children from Middle Eastern countries as a cause of hypogonadism and dwarfism. Hypopigmented hair is also a part of this syndrome. Hypochromic anemia can be seen in a number of vitamin deficiency/excess disorders, including zinc toxicity and copper deficiency. Copper deficiency is also associated with dissecting aortic aneurysm. Hypoglycemia does not correlate with hypozincemia. Macrocytosis is associated with folate and vitamin B_{12} deficiency.

II-16. **The answer is D.** *(Chap. 71)* Vitamin A deficiency remains a problem of children with chronically poor diets in parts of Asia, Africa, and China. This child has xerophthalmia with evidence of mild night blindness. He also has Bitot's spots (white patches on the sclera). Vitamin A deficiency also impairs the host's ability to fight infection. Mortality amongst vitamin A–deficient children is substantially higher when infected with diarrhea, dysentery, measles, malaria, or respiratory disease. Supplementation improves the mortality. SCA type 1 does not have any associated ophthalmologic findings. Autoimmune neutropenia may account for the repeated bouts of infection, but the constellation of Bitot's spots and recurrent infection argues against this as the cause. Congenital rubella causes congenital cataracts, not Bitot's spots. Vitamin B_1 (thiamine) deficiency causes beri-beri, which is associated with high output cardiac failure or peripheral neuropathy.

II-17. **The answer is C.** *(Chap. 72)* The energy stores in a healthy 70-kg man include ~15 kg as fat, 6 kg as protein, and 500 mg as glycogen. During the first day of a fast, most energy needs are met by consumption of liver glycogen. During longer fasting, resting energy expenditure will decrease by up to 25% (provided there is no ongoing inflammation). In the presence of water intake and no inflammation, a normal individual may fast for months. A well-nourished individual can tolerate ~7 days of starvation while experiencing a systemic response to inflammation. The hiker in this scenario has starved for 6 days and, except for mild acute renal failure, he has compensated well for his starvation. Greater than 10% weight loss in 6 months represents significant protein-calorie malnutrition. This person's ferritin is only mildly elevated, although a true systemic response to inflammation (SRI) does increase the rate of lean tissue loss. Moreover, he has no other indicators that he is experiencing the systemic inflammatory response syndrome (SIRS). SRI often causes hyperglycemia, not hypoglycemia.

II-18. **The answer is C.** *(Chap. 73)* Tracheal suctioning induces coughing and gastric regurgitation and cuffs on endotracheal tubes seldom protect against aspiration. Effective preventive measures include elevating the head of the bed to 30°, nurse-directed algorithms for formula advancement, combining enteral and parenteral feeding, and using postligament of Treitz feeding. Recent studies have suggested that constant suction above the endotracheal cuff may reduce ventilator-associated pneumonia.

II-19. **The answer is D.** *(Chap. 76)* Anorexia nervosa (AN) and bulimia nervosa (BN) are distinct clinical entities but share certain features. Many patients with BN have a history of anorexia, and patients with AN engage in binge eating and abnormal compensatory behaviors such as purging. The critical distinction between AN and BN depends on body weight: patients with AN are significantly underweight, whereas patients with BN have normal weight or are overweight. The presence of electrolyte disturbances confers an increased morbidity for both disorders.

II-20. **The answer is D.** *(Chap. 76)* Approximately 25–50% of patients with anorexia nervosa (AN) recover fully with few physiologic or psychological sequelae. However, many patients have persistent difficulties with weight maintenance, depression, and eating disturbances. Approximately 5% of patients die per decade, usually due to the physical effects of chronic starvation or from suicide. Virtually all of the physiologic derangements associated with anorexia nervosa will improve with weight gain. One exception is the loss of bone mass, which may not recover fully when AN occurs during adolescence (i.e., during peak bone mass formation). Psychological health also improves with successful treatment, although these patients remain at risk for depression, recurrence, and development of bulimia nervosa.

III. ONCOLOGY AND HEMATOLOGY

QUESTIONS

DIRECTIONS: Choose the **one best** response to each question.

III-1. A 73-year-old male presents to the clinic with 3 months of increasing back pain. He localizes the pain to the lumbar spine and states that the pain is worst at night while he is lying in bed. It is improved during the day with mobilization. Past history is notable only for hypertension and remote cigarette smoking. Physical examination is normal. Laboratory studies are notable for an elevated alkaline phosphatase. A lumbar radiogram shows a lytic lesion in the L3 vertebra. Which of the following malignancies is most likely?

A. Gastric carcinoma
B. Non-small cell lung cancer
C. Osteosarcoma
D. Pancreatic carcinoma
E. Thyroid carcinoma

III-2. Patients from which of the following regions need not be screened for glucose-6-phosphate dehydrogenase (G6PD) deficiency when starting a drug that carries a risk for G6PD mediated hemolysis?

A. Brazil
B. Russia
C. Southeast Asia
D. Southern Europe
E. Sub-Saharan Africa
F. None of the above

III-3. All the following are vitamin K–dependent coagulation factors *except*

A. factor X
B. factor VII
C. protein C
D. protein S
E. factor VIII

III-4. A 31-year-old male with hemophilia A is admitted with persistent gross hematuria. He denies recent trauma or any history of genitourinary pathology. The examination is unremarkable. Hematocrit is 28%. All the following are treatments for hemophilia A *except*

A. desmopressin (DDAVP)
B. fresh-frozen plasma (FFP)

III-4. *(Continued)*
C. cryoprecipitate
D. recombinant factor VIII
E. plasmapheresis

III-5. Which of the following statements regarding incidence of and risk factors for hepatocellular carcinoma is true?

A. A chemical toxin produced by *Aspergillus* species, aflatoxin B has a strong association with development of hepatocellular carcinoma and can be found in stored grains in hot, humid places.
B. In the United States, the incidence of hepatocellular carcinoma is decreasing.
C. Nonalcoholic steatohepatitis is not associated with an increased risk for hepatocellular carcinogen.
D. Fewer than 5% of individuals diagnosed with hepatocellular carcinoma in the United States do not have underlying cirrhosis.
E. The risk of developing hepatocellular carcinoma in individuals with hepatitis C infection is 50%.

III-6. You are asked to review the peripheral blood smear from a patient with anemia. Serum lactate dehydrogenase is elevated and there is hemoglobinuria. This patient is likely to have which physical examination finding? (See Figure III-6, Color Atlas.)

A. Goiter
B. Heme-positive stools
C. Mechanical second heart sound
D. Splenomegaly
E. Thickened calvarium

III-7. All of the enzyme deficiencies that lead to porphyrias are inherited either as autosomal dominant (AD) or autosomal recessive (AR) traits with one exception. Which of the following most commonly occurs sporadically?

A. 5-ALA dehydratase-deficient porphyria
B. Acute intermittent porphyria
C. Erythropoietic porphyria
D. Porphyria cutanea tarda
E. Variegate porphyria

III-8. A 55-year-old female presents with progressive incoordination. Physical examination is remarkable for nystagmus, mild dysarthria, and past-pointing on finger-to-nose testing. She also has an unsteady gait. MRI reveals atrophy of both lobes of the cerebellum. Serologic evaluation reveals the presence of anti-Yo antibody. Which of the following is the most likely cause of this clinical syndrome?

A.   Non-small cell cancer of the lung
B.   Small-cell cancer of the lung
C.   Breast cancer
D.   Non-Hodgkin's lymphoma
E.   Colon cancer

III-9. A 36-year-old African-American woman with systemic lupus erythematosus presents with the acute onset of lethargy and jaundice. On initial evaluation, she is tachycardic, hypotensive, appears pale, is dyspneic, and is somewhat difficult to arouse. Physical examination reveals splenomegaly. Her initial hemoglobin is 6 g/dL, white blood cell count is 6300/μL, and platelets are 294,000/μL. Her total bilirubin is 4 g/dL, reticulocyte count is 18%, and haptoglobin is not detectable. Renal function is normal, as is urinalysis. What would you expect on her peripheral blood smear?

A.   Macrocytosis and PMN's with hypersegmented nuclei
B.   Microspherocytes
C.   Schistocytes
D.   Sickle cells
E.   Target cells

III-10. You are investigating the cause for a patient's anemia. He is a 50-year-old man who was found to have a hematocrit of 25% on routine evaluation. His hematocrit was 47% 1 year ago. Mean corpuscular volume is 80, mean corpuscular hemoglobin concentration is 25, mean corpuscular hemoglobin is 25. Reticulocyte count is 5%. Review of the peripheral blood smear shows marked numbers of polychromatophilic macrocytes. Ferritin is 340 μg/L. What is the cause of this patient's anemia?

A.   Defective erythroid marrow proliferation
B.   Extravascular hemolysis
C.   Intravascular hemolysis
D.   Iron-deficiency anemia
E.   Occult gastrointestinal bleeding

III-11. All the following are associated with pure red cell aplasia *except*

A.   anterior mediastinal masses
B.   connective tissue disorders
C.   giant pronormoblasts
D.   low erythropoietin levels
E.   parvovirus B19 infection

III-12. A 73-year-old man is admitted to the hospital with 3 weeks of malaise and fevers. His past medical history is notable only for hypertension controlled with a thiazide diuretic. He smokes one pack of cigarettes per day and

III-12. *(Continued)*
works as an attorney. His physical examination is notable only for a new systolic heart murmur heard best in the mitral region. His laboratory examination is notable for mild anemia, an elevated white blood cell count, and occasional red blood cells on clean catch urine. Blood cultures grow *Streptococcus bovis* and echocardiogram shows a <1-cm vegetation on the mitral valve. What additional evaluation is indicated for this patient?

A.   Colonoscopy
B.   Head CT scan
C.   Pulmonary embolism protocol CT scan
D.   Renal biopsy
E.   Toxicology screen

III-13. A 58-year-old woman presents to the emergency room complaining of jaundice. She first noticed a yellowish discoloration of her skin about 3 days ago. It has become progressively worse since that time. In association with the development of jaundice, she also has noticed clay-colored stools and pruritus. There has been no associated abdominal pain, fever, chills, or night sweats. She has a past medical history of alcohol abuse, but has been abstinent for the past 10 years. She has no known history of cirrhosis. On physical examination, she is afebrile with normal vital signs. She is jaundiced. The bowel sounds are normal. The abdomen is soft and nontender. There is no distention. The liver span is 12 cm to percussion and is palpable at the right costal margin. The spleen tip is not palpable. Liver function testing reveals an AST of 122 IU/L, ALT of 168 IU/L, alkaline phosphatase of 483 U/L, total bilirubin of 22.1 mg/dL, and direct bilirubin of 19.2 mg/dL. On right upper quadrant ultrasound, the gallbladder cannot be visualized, and there is dilatation of the intrahepatic bile ducts but not the common bile duct. What is the most likely diagnosis?

A.   Cholangiocarcinoma
B.   Cholecystitis
C.   Gallbladder cancer
D.   Hepatocellular carcinoma
E.   Pancreatic cancer

III-14. An 81-year-old male is admitted to the hospital for altered mental status. He was found at home, confused and lethargic, by his son. His past medical history is significant for metastatic prostate cancer. The patient's medications include periodic intramuscular goserelin injections. On examination he is afebrile. Blood pressure is 110/50 mmHg, and the pulse rate is 110 beats/min. He is lethargic and minimally responsive to sternal rub. He has bitemporal wasting, and his mucous membranes are dry. On neurologic examination he is obtunded. The patient has an intact gag reflex and withdraws to pain in all four extremities. Rectal tone is normal. Laboratory values are significant for a creatinine of 4.2 mg/dL, a calcium level of 12.4 meq/L, and an albumin of 2.6 g/dL. All the following are appropriate initial management steps *except*

III-14. *(Continued)*

A. normal saline
B. pamidronate
C. furosemide when the patient is euvolemic
D. calcitonin
E. dexamethasone

III-15. Which of the following statements describes the relationship between testicular tumors and serum markers?

A. Pure seminomas produce α fetoprotein (AFP) or beta human chorionic gonadotropin (β-hCG) in more than 90% of cases.
B. More than 40% of nonseminomatous germ cell tumors produce no cell markers.
C. Both β-hCG and AFP should be measured in following the progress of a tumor.
D. Measurement of tumor markers the day after surgery for localized disease is useful in determining completeness of the resection.
E. β-hCG is limited in its usefulness as a marker because it is identical to human luteinizing hormone.

III-16. A woman with advanced breast cancer being treated with tamoxifen presents to the emergency department with nausea and vomiting. She has been tolerating her treatment well but in the last 3 days noticed nausea, vomiting, and abdominal pain. Her symptoms are not related to food intake, and she is having normal bowel movements. She has no fevers or rashes. Her medications include tamoxifen, alendronate, megestrol acetate, and a multivitamin. Abdominal examination reveals very mild tenderness diffusely, and there is no rebound tenderness. Bowel sounds are normal. Plain radiographs and a CT scan of the abdomen are unremarkable. Laboratory analysis reveals a normal white blood cell count. Sodium is 130 meq/L, potassium 4.9 meq/L, chloride 99 meq/L, bicarbonate 29 meq/L, BUN 15 mg/dL, creatinine 0.7 mg/dL. What is the next most appropriate step in this patient's management?

A. Antiemetics prn
B. Laparoscopy
C. Serum cortisol
D. Small-bowel follow through
E. Upper endoscopy

III-17. A healthy 62-year-old woman returns to your clinic after undergoing routine colonoscopy. Findings included two 1.3-cm sessile (flat-based), villous adenomas in her ascending colon that were removed during the procedure. What is the next step in management?

A. Colonoscopy in 3 months
B. Colonoscopy in 3 years
C. Colonoscopy in 10 years
D. CT scan of the abdomen
E. Partial colectomy
F. Reassurance

III-18. Which of the following statements regarding polycythemia vera is correct?

A. An elevated plasma erythropoietin level excludes the diagnosis.
B. Transformation to acute leukemia is common.
C. Thrombocytosis correlates strongly with thrombotic risk.
D. Aspirin should be prescribed to all these patients to reduce thrombotic risk.
E. Phlebotomy is used only after hydroxyurea and interferon have been tried.

III-19. A 52-year-old female is evaluated for abdominal swelling with a computed tomogram that shows ascites and likely peritoneal studding of tumor but no other abnormality. Paracentesis shows adenocarcinoma but cannot be further differentiated by the pathologist. A thorough physical examination, including breast and pelvic examination, shows no abnormality. CA-125 levels are elevated. Pelvic ultrasound and mammography are normal. Which of the following statements is true?

A. Compared with other women with known ovarian cancer at a similar stage, this patient can be expected to have a less than average survival.
B. Debulking surgery is indicated.
C. Surgical debulking plus cisplatin and paclitaxel is indicated.
D. Bilateral mastectomy and bilateral oophorectomy will improve survival.
E. Fewer than 1% of patients with this disorder will remain disease-free 2 years after treatment.

III-20. A 34-year-old female with a past medical history of sickle cell anemia presents with a 5-day history of fatigue, lethargy, and shortness of breath. She denies chest pain or bone pain. She has had no recent travel. Of note, the patient's 4-year-old daughter had a "cold" 2 weeks before the presentation. On examination she has pale conjunctiva, is anicteric, and is mildly tachycardic. Abdominal examination is unremarkable. Laboratories show a hemoglobin of 3 g/dL; her baseline is 8 g/dL. The white blood cell count and platelets are normal. Reticulocyte count is undetectable. Total bilirubin is 1.4 mg/dL. Lactic dehydrogenase is at the upper limits of the normal range. Peripheral blood smear shows a few sickled cells but a total absence of reticulocytes. The patient is given a transfusion of 2 units of packed red blood cells and admitted to the hospital. A bone marrow biopsy shows a normal myeloid series but an absence of erythroid precursors. Cytogenetics are normal. What is the most appropriate next management step?

A. Make arrangements for exchange transfusion.
B. Tissue type her siblings for a possible bone marrow transplant.
C. Check parvovirus titers.

III-20. *(Continued)*
   D.   Start prednisone and cyclosporine.
   E.   Start broad-spectrum antibiotics.

III-21. A 22-year-old pregnant woman of northern European descent presents 3 months into her first pregnancy with extreme fatigue, pallor, and icterus. She reports being previously healthy. On evaluation her hemoglobin is 8 g/dL, reticulocyte count is 9%, indirect bilirubin is 4.9 mg/dL, and serum haptoglobin is not detectable. Her physical examination is notable for splenomegaly and a normal 3-month uterus. Peripheral smear is shown below. What is the most likely diagnosis? (See Figure III-21, Color Atlas.)

   A.   Colonic polyp
   B.   G6PD deficiency
   C.   Hereditary spherocytosis
   D.   Parvovirus B19 infection
   E.   Thrombotic thrombocytopenic purpura

III-22. A patient with acute lymphoid leukemia (ALL) is admitted with respiratory distress and chest pain. The patient reports 1 day of shortness of breath not associated with cough. There have been no sick contacts, and before the onset of the respiratory symptoms, the patient only recalls fatigue. A chest radiograph shows faint diffuse interstitial infiltrates without pulmonary edema. The cardiac silhouette is normal. An arterial blood gas shows a $Pa_{O_2} = 54$ mmHg, while the pulse oximetry is 97% on room air. A carbon monoxide level is normal. All of the following laboratory abnormalities are expected in this patient *except*

   A.   bcr-abl mutation
   B.   blast count >100,000/μL
   C.   elevated lactate dehydrogenase levels
   D.   increased blood viscosity
   E.   methemoglobinemia

III-23. A 48-year-old male is referred for evaluation by an acute care center because of a nodule on chest radiography. Three weeks ago he was diagnosed with pneumonia after reporting 3 days of fever, cough, and sputum production. The chest radiogram showed a small right lower lobe alveolar infiltrate and a left upper lobe 1.5-cm round nodule. He was treated with antibiotics and is now asymptomatic. A repeat chest radiogram shows that the right lower lobe pneumonia is resolved, but the nodule is still present. He is asymptomatic. He smoked one pack of cigarettes per day for 25 years and quit 3 years ago. He never had a prior chest radiogram. CT scan shows that the nodule is 1.5 by 1.7 cm and is located centrally in the left upper lobe, has no calcification, and has slightly scalloped edges. There is no mediastinal adenopathy or pleural effusion. Which of the following is the appropriate next step in his management?

   A.   Bronchoscopy
   B.   Mediastinoscopy

III-23. *(Continued)*
   C.   MRI scan
   D. ^{18}FDG PET scan
   E.   Repeat chest CT in 6 months

III-24. All the following types of cancer commonly metastasize to the central nervous system (CNS) *except*

   A.   ovarian
   B.   breast
   C.   hypernephroma
   D.   melanoma
   E.   acute lymphoblastic leukemia (ALL)

III-25. A 54-year-old woman with atrial fibrillation is anticoagulated with warfarin, 5 mg daily. She developed a urinary tract infection that her primary care physician has treated with ciprofloxacin, 250 mg orally twice daily for 7 days. She presents to the emergency room today complaining of blood in her urine and easy bruising. Her physical examination shows ecchymoses on her arms. Her urine is bloody in appearance, but no clots are present. After flushing the bladder with 100 mL of sterile saline, the urine returns with a slight pink hue only. A urinalysis shows 3–5 white blood cells per high power field and many red blood cells per high power field. There are no bacteria present. The international normalized ratio (INR) is 7.0. What is the best approach to treatment of this patient's coagulopathy?

   A.   Administer vitamin K 10 mg IV.
   B.   Administer vitamin K 2 mg SC.
   C.   Administer vitamin K 1 mg sublingually.
   D.   Hold further warfarin doses until the INR falls to 2.0.
   E.   Transfuse four units of fresh-frozen plasma.

III-26. Which of the following statements about cardiac toxicity from cancer treatment is true?

   A.   Doxorubicin-based cardiac toxicity is idiosyncratic and dose-independent.
   B.   Anthracycline-induced congestive heart failure is reversible with time and control of risk factors.
   C.   Mediastinal irradiation often results in acute pericarditis during the first few weeks of treatment.
   D.   Chronic constrictive pericarditis often manifests symptomatically up to 10 years after treatment.
   E.   The incidence of coronary atherosclerosis in patients who have a history of mediastinal irradiation is the same as that in age-matched controls.

III-27. A 23-year-old woman is diagnosed with a lower extremity deep venous thrombosis. Which of the following medical conditions represents a contraindication to therapy with low-molecular-weight heparin (LMWH)?

   A.   Pregnancy
   B.   Obesity
   C.   Dialysis-dependent renal failure
   D.   Uncontrolled diabetes mellitus
   E.   Jaundice

III-28. Which of the following pairs of chemotherapy and complication is incorrect?

   A. Daunorubicin—CHF

   B. Bleomycin—interstitial fibrosis

   C. Cyclophosphamide—hematuria

   D. Cisplatin—liver failure

   E. Ifosfamide—Fanconi syndrome

III-29. A 70-year-old man is admitted to the cardiac care unit for complaints of chest pressure occurring at rest radiating to his left arm with associated diaphoresis and presyncope. His admission electrocardiogram (ECG) showed ST depressions in V4–V6. The chest pain and ECG changes resolve with sublingual nitroglycerin. He is treated with IV heparin, aspirin, metoprolol, and lisinopril. His cardiac catheterization shows 90% occlusion of the left anterior descending artery, 80% occlusion of the distal circumflex artery, and 99% occlusion of the right coronary artery. He remains in the cardiac care unit awaiting coronary artery bypass. He has a history of rheumatic heart disease and underwent mechanical mitral valve replacement at age 58. On admission, his hemoglobin is 12.2 g/dL, hematocrit 37.1%, white blood cell (WBC) count 9800/μL, and platelet count 240,000/μL. His creatinine is 1.7 mg/dL. On the fourth hospital day, his hemoglobin is 10.0, hematocrit 31%, WBC count 7600/μL, and platelet count 112,000/μL. His creatinine has risen to 2.9 mg/dL after the cardiac catheterization. What is the most appropriate treatment of the patient at this time?

   A. Continue heparin and give a platelet transfusion.

   B. Discontinue heparin infusion and start argatroban.

   C. Discontinue heparin and start lepirudin.

   D. Discontinue heparin and start warfarin.

   E. Send serum to assess for the presence of heparin–platelet factor 4 (PF4) IgG antibody and continue heparin.

III-30. A 24-year-old woman presents to the emergency room complaining of a red, tender rash that has been spreading across her arms and legs over the past 2 days. She also describes severe diffuse muscle pain that has worsened over a week's time. She woke up feeling as though she could not catch her breath and has developed a dry cough over the past several days. She is without any significant medical history but recalls that she had similar symptoms several years ago, and was told she was having an allergic reaction. Her symptoms abated with an oral glucocorticoid taper. She takes no prescription medications but takes a number of over-the-counter nutritional supplements daily. She cannot describe any allergic trigger to her previous episode or her current one. Her family history is unremarkable, and her close contacts are not ill. She works in an office, has no pets, and has not travelled internationally. Her laboratory results are remarkable for a leukocyte count of 12,100 cells/μL and a total eosinophil count of 1100/μL. Which of the following is the most likely cause of her symptoms?

III-30. *(Continued)*

   A. Early stage of systemic lupus erythematosus

   B. Gluten allergy

   C. Ingestion of L-tryptophan

   D. Lactose intolerance

   E. Recent viral upper respiratory tract infection

III-31. A woman wants your advice regarding Papanicolaou smears. She is 36 years old and is monogamous with her husband since they were married 3 years ago. She has had normal Pap smears every year for the past 6 years. She would like to avoid the yearly test. What is your advice to this patient, based on the current screening guidelines?

   A. She may discontinue screening at age 50 if she has had normal yearly Pap smears for the previous 10 years.

   B. She may extend the screening interval to once every 2–3 years.

   C. She may extend the screening interval to once every 5 years if she agrees to use barrier protection.

   D. She may discontinue Pap screening if she receives the human papilloma virus (HPV) vaccine.

   E. The only indication to cease Pap testing is if she were to have a total hysterectomy.

III-32. The evaluation in a newly diagnosed case of acute lymphoid leukemia (ALL) should routinely include all of the following *except*

   A. bone marrow biopsy

   B. cell-surface phenotyping

   C. complete metabolic panel

   D. cytogenetic testing

   E. lumbar puncture

   F. plasma viscosity

III-33. Which of the following statements about lead-time bias occurrence is true?

   A. A test does not influence the natural history of the disease; patients are merely diagnosed at an earlier date.

   B. Slow-growing, less aggressive cancers are detected during screening; aggressive cancers are not detected by screening, due to death.

   C. Screening identifies abnormalities that would never have caused a problem during a person's lifetime.

   D. The screened population differs significantly from the general population in that they are healthier.

   E. A test detects disease at an earlier and more curable stage of disease.

III-34. Which of the following is sufficient to make a definitive diagnosis of porphyria?

   A. Appropriate clinical scenario including positive family history

   B. Evidence of an enzyme deficiency or gene defect

   C. Laboratory measurements in blood indicating accumulation of porphyrin precursors

III-34. *(Continued)*

D. Laboratory measurements in urine indicating accumulation of porphyrin precursors at the time of symptoms

E. Laboratory measurements in stool indicating accumulation of porphyrin precursors at the time of symptoms

III-35. All but which of the following statements about the lupus anticoagulant (LA) are true?

A. Lupus anticoagulants typically prolong the aPTT.

B. A 1:1 mixing study will not correct in the presence of lupus anticoagulants.

C. Bleeding episodes in patients with lupus anticoagulants may be severe and life-threatening.

D. Female patients may experience recurrent midtrimester abortions.

E. Lupus anticoagulants may occur in the absence of other signs of systemic lupus erythematosus (SLE).

III-36. The most common inherited prothrombotic disorder is

A. activated protein C resistance

B. prothrombin gene mutation

C. protein C deficiency

D. protein S deficiency

E. antithrombin deficiency

III-37. A 34-year-old woman presents for evaluation of left lower extremity swelling and pain. She is obese and 8 weeks postpartum. She recently traveled 6 h by airplane to visit her parents with her infant. She has had no dyspnea, palpitations, or syncope. She is currently on no medications except iron tablets. She is otherwise healthy. Her vitals signs are: heart rate 86 beats/min, blood pressure 110/80 mm/Hg, temperature 37.0°C, and respiratory rate 12 breaths/min. Her weight is 98 kg, and height is 170 cm. The left lower extremity is swollen, tender, and warm to touch. A Homan's sign is present, but there are no palpable cords. A lower extremity Doppler shows a thrombosis in the common and superficial femoral veins of the left leg. You are considering outpatient treatment with enoxaparin. All of the following statements regarding low-molecular-weight heparins (LMWH) are true *except*

A. In patients with uncomplicated deep venous thrombosis (DVT), LMWH is a safe and effective alternative to IV heparin and is associated with reduced health care costs compared to IV heparin.

B. LMWH can be safely used in pregnancy, but factor Xa levels should be monitored to ensure adequate anticoagulation.

C. Monitoring of factor Xa levels is unnecessary in most patients as there is a predictable dose-dependent anticoagulation effect.

D. There is a decrease in the risk of development of heparin-induced thrombocytopenia with use of LMWH.

E. This patient's recent pregnancy is a contraindication to use of LMWH because there is a greater risk of bleeding with LWMH compared to IV heparin.

III-38. A 65-year-old man is brought to the emergency room by ambulance after his daughter found him to be incoherent earlier today. She last spoke with him yesterday, and at that time, he was complaining of 2 days of myalgias, headache, and fever. He had attributed it to an upper respiratory tract infection and did not seek evaluation from his primary care physician. Today, he did not answer when she called his home, and she found him lying in his bed smelling of urine. He was minimally arousable but appeared to be moving all of his extremities. His past medical history is significant for hypertension, hypercholesterolemia, and chronic obstructive pulmonary disease. He was evaluated 2 weeks previously for a transient ischemic attack after an episode where he had numbness and weakness of his left arm and leg that resolved over 6 h without intervention. His current medications include aspirin, 81 mg daily, clopidogrel, 75 mg daily, atenolol, 100 mg daily, atorvastatin, 20 mg daily, and tiotropium, once daily. He is allergic to lisinopril, which caused angioedema. He is a former smoker and drinks alcohol rarely.

On physical examination, he is obtunded and minimally arousable. He is febrile with a temperature of 38.9°C. His blood pressure is 159/96 mmHg, and heart rate is 98 beats/min. He is breathing at a rate of 24 breaths/min with a room air oxygen saturation of 95%. He has minimal scleral icterus. The oropharynx reveals dry mucous membranes. His cardiovascular, pulmonary, and abdominal examinations are normal. There are no rashes. His neurologic examination is difficult to obtain. There are no cranial nerve findings. He resists movement of his extremities but has normal strength. Deep tendon reflexes are brisk, 3+ and equal.

The laboratory values are as follows: hemoglobin 9.3 g/dL, hematocrit 29.1%, white blood cell count 14,000/μL, and platelets 42,000/μL. The differential demonstrates 83% neutrophils, 2% band forms, 6% lymphocytes, and 9% monocytes. The sodium is 145 meq/L, potassium 3.8 meq/L, chloride 113 meq/L, bicarbonate 19 meq/L, blood urea nitrogen 68 mg/dL, and creatinine 3.4 mg/dL. The bilirubin is 2.4 mg/dL, and lactate dehydrogenase is 450 U/L. A peripheral blood smear shows diminished platelets and many schistocytes. What is the next most appropriate step in this patient's care?

A. Discontinue clopidogrel.

B. Discontinue clopidogrel and initiate plasmapheresis.

C. Initiate therapy with intravenous immunoglobulin.

D. Obtain a head CT scan and initiate treatment with factor VIIa, if subarachnoid hemorrhage is seen.

E. Perform a lumbar puncture and start broad-spectrum antibiotic coverage with ceftazidime and vancomycin.

III-39. A primary tumor of which of these organs is the *least likely* to metastasize to bone?

A. Breast

B. Colon

III-39. *(Continued)*

   C. Kidney

   D. Lung

   E. Prostate

III-40. The triad of portal vein thrombosis, hemolysis, and pancytopenia suggests which of the following diagnoses?

   A. Acute promyelocytic leukemia

   B. Hemolytic-uremic syndrome (HUS)

   C. Leptospirosis

   D. Paroxysmal nocturnal hemoglobinuria (PNH)

   E. Thrombotic thrombocytopenia purpura (TTP)

III-41. A 68-year-old man seeks evaluation for fatigue, weight loss, and early satiety that have been present for about 4 months. On physical examination, his spleen is noted to be markedly enlarged. It is firm to touch and crosses the midline. The lower edge of the spleen reaches to the pelvis. His hemoglobin is 11.1 g/dL, and hematocrit is 33.7%. The leukocyte count is 6200/μL, and platelet count is 220,000/μL. The white cell count differential is 75% PMNs, 8% myelocytes, 4% metamyelocytes, 8% lymphocytes, 3% monocytes, and 2% eosinophils. The peripheral blood smear shows teardrop cells, nucleated red blood cells, and immature granulocytes. Rheumatoid factor is positive. A bone marrow biopsy is attempted, but no cells are able to be aspirated. No evidence of leukemia or lymphoma is found. What is the most likely cause of the splenomegaly?

   A. Chronic idiopathic myelofibrosis

   B. Chronic myelogenous leukemia

   C. Rheumatoid arthritis

   D. Systemic lupus erythematosus

   E. Tuberculosis

III-42. The most common cause of high serum calcium in a patient with a known cancer is

   A. ectopic production of parathyroid hormone

   B. direct destruction of bone by tumor cells

   C. local production of tumor necrosis factor and IL-6 by bony metastasis

   D. high levels of 1,25-hydroxyvitamin D

   E. production of parathyroid hormone–like substance

III-43. A 72-year-old man with chronic obstructive pulmonary disease and stable coronary disease presents to the emergency room with several days of worsening productive cough, fevers, malaise, and diffuse muscle aches. A chest x-ray demonstrates a new lobar infiltrate. Laboratory measurements reveal a total white blood cell count of 12,100 cells/μL, with a neutrophilic predominance of 86% and 8% band forms. He is diagnosed with community-acquired pneumonia, and antibiotic treatment is initiated. Under normal, or "nonstress," conditions, what percentage of the total body neutrophils are present in the circulation?

III-43. *(Continued)*

   A. 2%

   B. 10%

   C. 25%

   D. 40%

   E. 90%

III-44. All of the following laboratory values are consistent with an intravascular hemolytic anemia *except*

   A. increased haptoglobin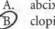

   B. increased lactate dehydrogenase (LDH)

   C. increased reticulocyte count

   D. increased unconjugated bilirubin

   E. increased urine hemosiderin

III-45. All the following match the anticoagulant with its correct mechanism of action *except*

   A. abciximab—GpIIb/IIIa receptor inhibition

   B. clopidogrel—inhibition of thromboxane A_2 release

   C. fondaparinux—inhibition of factor Xa

   D. argatroban—thrombin inhibition

   E. warfarin—vitamin K—dependent carboxylation of coagulation factors

III-46. All the following are late complications of bone marrow transplant preparative regimens *except*

   A. growth retardation

   B. azoospermia

   C. hypothyroidism

   D. cataracts

   E. dementia

III-47. Which of the following best describes the mechanism of action of clopidogrel?

   A. Activates antithrombin and inhibits clotting enzymes

   B. Binds to the activated GPIIb/IIIa receptor on the platelet surface to block binding of adhesive molecules

   C. Inhibits cyclooxygenase 1 (COX-1) on platelets to decrease production of thromboxane A_2

   D. Inhibits phosphodiesterase to block the breakdown of cyclic adenosine monophosphate (cAMP) to inhibit platelet activation

   E. Irreversibly blocks $P2Y_{12}$ to prevent adenosine diphosphate (ADP)–induced platelet aggregation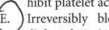

III-48. A 45-year-old man is evaluated by his primary care physician for complaints of early satiety and weight loss. On physical examination, his spleen is palpable 10 cm below the left costal margin and is mildly tender to palpation. His laboratory studies show a leukocyte count of 125,000/μL with a differential of 80% neutrophils, 9% bands, 3% myelocytes, 3% metamyelocytes, 1% blasts, 1% lymphocytes, 1% eosinophils, and 1% basophils. Hemoglobin is 8.4 g/dL, hematocrit 26.8%, and platelet count 668,000/μL. A bone marrow biopsy demonstrates increased cellularity with an increased myeloid to eryth-

III-48. *(Continued)*

roid ratio. Which of the following cytogenetic abnormalities is most likely to be found in this patient?

A. Deletion of a portion of the long arm of chromosome 5, del(5q)
B. Inversion of chromosome 16, inv(16)
C. Reciprocal translocation between chromosomes 9 and 22 (Philadelphia chromosome)
D. Translocations of the long arms of chromosomes 15 and 17
E. Trisomy 12

III-49. A 35-year-old patient comes into your office with persistent iron deficiency anemia. His past medical history is significant for end-stage renal disease on hemodialysis, hypertension, and rheumatoid arthritis. His medications include calcium acetate, a multivitamin, nifedipine, aspirin, iron sulfate, and omeprazole. His hemoglobin 6 months ago was 8 mg/dL. One week ago, it was 7.9 mg/dL. His ferritin is 8 mg/dL. He reports no bright red blood per rectum, and his stool guaiac examinations have been repeatedly negative over the past 6 months. What is the most likely cause of this patient's iron deficiency anemia?

A. Celiac sprue
B. Colon cancer
C. Hemorrhoids
D. Medication effect
E. Peptic ulcer disease

III-50. A 32-year-old male presents complaining of a testicular mass. On examination you palpate a 1-by 2-cm painless mass on the surface of the left testicle. A chest x-ray shows no lesions, and a CT scan of the abdomen and pelvis shows no evidence of retroperitoneal adenopathy. The α fetoprotein (AFP) level is elevated at 400 ng/mL. Beta human chorionic gonadotropin (β-hCG) is normal, as is LDH. You send the patient for an orchiectomy. The pathology comes back as seminoma limited to the testis alone. The AFP level declines to normal at an appropriate interval. What is the appropriate management at this point?

A. Radiation to the retroperitoneal lymph nodes
B. Adjuvant chemotherapy
C. Hormonal therapy
D. Retroperitoneal lymph node dissection (RPLND)
E. Positron emission tomography (PET) scan

III-51. All of the following statements regarding tobacco usage and cessation are correct *except*

A. Most Americans who quit do so on their own without involvement in an organized cessation program.
B. Over 80% of adult Americans who smoke began before the age of 18.
C. Smokeless tobacco is associated with gum and dental disease, not cancer.

III-51. *(Continued)*

D. Tobacco cessation messages and programs are more effective for light smokers than for heavy smokers.
E. Tobacco use is the most modifiable cancer risk factor.

III-52. A 29-year-old male is found on routine chest radiography for life insurance to have right hilar adenopathy. He is otherwise healthy. Besides biopsy of the lymph nodes, which of the following is indicated?

A. Angiotensin-converting enzyme (ACE) level
B. β-hCG
C. Thyroid stimulating hormone (TSH)
D. PSA
E. C-reactive protein

III-53. Which of the following is correct regarding small-cell lung cancer compared with non-small cell lung cancer?

A. Small-cell lung cancer is more radiosensitive.
B. Small-cell lung cancer is less chemosensitive.
C. Small-cell lung cancer is more likely to present peripherally in the lung.
D. Small-cell lung cancer is derived from an alveolar cell.
E. Bone marrow involvement is more common in non-small cell lung cancer.

III-54. Which of the following statements regarding esophageal cancer is true?

A. Cigarette smoking and heavy alcohol intake are synergistic risk factors for adenocarcinoma.
B. Chronic gastric reflux is a risk factor for development of esophageal squamous cell carcinoma.
C. Esophageal cancer is most common in the middle third of the esophagus.
D. Incidence of squamous cell carcinoma has decreased over the past 30 years while adenocarcinoma continues to increase.
E. The prognosis for patients with adenocarcinoma is consistently better than for those with squamous cell carcinoma.
F. All of the above are true.

III-55. All the following conditions are associated with an increased incidence of cancer *except*

A. Down's syndrome
B. Fanconi's anemia
C. Von Hippel–Lindau syndrome
D. neurofibromatosis
E. fragile X syndrome

III-56. A 50-year-old female presents to your clinic for evaluation of an elevated platelet count. The latest complete blood count is white blood cells (WBC) 7,000/mm³, hematocrit 34%, and platelets 600,000/mm³. All the following are common causes of thrombocytosis *except*

A. iron-deficiency anemia

III-56. *(Continued)*

- B. essential thrombocytosis
- C. chronic myeloid leukemia
- D. myelodysplasia
- E. pernicious anemia

III-57. A 76-year-old man presents to an urgent care clinic with pain in his left leg for 4 days. He also describes swelling in his left ankle, which has made it difficult for him to ambulate. He is an active smoker and has a medical history remarkable for gastroesophageal reflux disease, prior deep venous thrombosis (DVT) 9 months ago that resolved, and well-controlled hypertension. Physical examination is revealing for 2+ edema in his left ankle. A D-dimer is ordered and is elevated. Which of the following makes D-dimer less predictive of DVT in this patient?

- A. Age >70
- B. History of active tobacco use
- C. Lack of suggestive clinical symptoms
- D. Negative Homan's sign on examination
- E. Previous DVT in the past year

III-58. A patient with longstanding HIV infection, alcoholism, and asthma is seen in the emergency room for 1–2 days of severe wheezing. He has not been taking any medicines for months. He is admitted to the hospital and treated with nebulized therapy and systemic glucocorticoids. His CD4 count is 8 and viral load is >750,000. His total white blood cell (WBC) count is 3200 cells /μL with 90% neutrophils. He is accepted into an inpatient substance abuse rehabilitation program and before discharge is started on opportunistic infection prophylaxis, bronchodilators, a prednisone taper over 2 weeks, ranitidine, and highly-active antiretroviral therapy. The rehabilitation center pages you 2 weeks later; a routine laboratory check reveals a total WBC count of 900 cells/μL with 5% neutrophils. Which of the following new drugs would most likely explain this patient's neutropenia?

- A. Darunavir
- B. Efavirenz
- C. Ranitidine
- D. Prednisone
- E. Trimethoprim-sulfamethoxazole

III-59. Which of the following symptoms is most suggestive of an esophageal mass?

- A. Early satiety
- B. Liquid phase dysphagia only
- C. Odynophagia with chest pain
- D. Oropharyngeal dysphagia
- E. Solid phase dysphagia progressing to liquid phase dysphagia

III-60. All of the following have been associated with development of a lymphoid malignancy *except*

III-60. *(Continued)*

- A. celiac sprue
- B. *Helicobacter pylori* infection
- C. hepatitis B infection
- D. HIV infection
- E. human herpes virus 8 (HHV8) infection
- F. inherited immunodeficiency syndromes

III-61. A 31-year-old female is referred to your clinic for an evaluation of anemia. She describes a 2-month history of fatigue. She denies abdominal pain but notes that her abdomen has become slightly more distended in recent weeks. Past medical history is otherwise unremarkable. The patient's parents are alive, and she has three healthy siblings. Physical examination is significant for pale conjunctiva and a palpable spleen 4 cm below the left costal margin. Hematocrit is 31% and bilirubin is normal. The reticulocyte percentage is low. Haptoglobin and lactic dehydrogenase (LDH) are normal. A peripheral blood smear shows numerous teardrop-shaped red cells, nucleated red cells, and occasional myelocytes. A bone marrow aspirate is unsuccessful, but a biopsy shows a hypercellular marrow with trilineage hyperplasia and findings consistent with the presumed diagnosis of chronic idiopathic myelofibrosis. You transfuse her to a hematocrit of 40%. What is the most appropriate next management step?

- A. Administer erythropoietin.
- B. Follow up in 6 months.
- C. Institute combined-modality chemotherapy.
- D. Perform HLA matching of her siblings.
- E. Perform a splenectomy.

III-62. All the following are suggestive of iron deficiency anemia *except*

- A. koilonychia
- B. pica
- C. decreased serum ferritin
- D. decreased total iron-binding capacity (TIBC)
- E. low reticulocyte response

III-63. Which source of stem cell is *incorrectly* paired with the challenge associated with their clinical application?

- A. Bone marrow mesenchymal stem cells: Transplanted cells may not differentiate into the desired cell type
- B. Embryonic stem cells: High potential to form teratomas
- C. Organ-specific multipotent stem cells: Difficult to isolate from tissues other than bone marrow
- D. Umbilical cord blood stem cells: Graft-versus-host disease

III-64. You are seeing a patient in follow-up in whom you have begun an evaluation for an elevated hematocrit. You suspect polycythemia vera based on a history of aquagenic pruritus and splenomegaly. Which set of laboratory tests are consistent with the diagnosis of polycythemia vera?

III-64. *(Continued)*

  A. Elevated red blood cell mass, high serum erythropoietin levels, normal oxygen saturation
  B. Elevated red blood cell mass, low serum erythropoietin levels, normal oxygen saturation
  C. Normal red blood cell mass, high serum erythropoietin levels, low arterial oxygen saturation
  D. Normal red blood cell mass, low serum erythropoietin levels, low arterial oxygen saturation

III-65. A 59-year-old man is admitted with a painful, blistering rash on the dorsal aspects of both hands. He has a medical history of alcoholism and admits to a recent relapse and has been drinking heavily over the past week. He is admitted and stabilized. A diagnosis of porphyria cutanea tarda (PCT) is made based on increased circulating porphyrins in the blood and decreased URO-decarboxylase activity. He is discharged to a rehabilitation facility and follows up in your clinic 2 weeks later. He has been abstinent from alcohol but his rash has persisted, and now he also has some blistering on the legs and feet. Which of the following treatment modalities is most appropriate?

  A. Hydroxyurea
  B. IV iron infusion weekly while following serum iron levels
  C. Oral iron plus vitamin C
  D. The rash of PCT can take months to resolve; the patient should continue to abstain from alcohol and be followed closely
  E. Weekly phlebotomy until ferritin normalizes

III-66. Which of the following hemolytic anemias can be classified as extracorpuscular?

  A. Elliptocytosis
  B. Paroxysmal nocturnal hemoglobinuria
  C. Pyruvate kinase deficiency
  D. Sickle cell anemia
  E. Thrombotic thrombocytopenic purpura

III-67. All of the following are obstacles to the more widespread application of stem cells for regenerative medicine *except*

  A. controlling the migration of transplanted stem cells
  B. identifying diseases suitable for stem cell based therapies
  C. identifying the pathways for differentiating stem cells into specific cell types
  D. overcoming ethical concerns over their harvest and use
  E. predicting the response of cells to the environment of the diseased organ

III-68. You are asked to consult on a 34-year-old male with thrombocytopenia. He sustained a motor vehicle collision 10 days ago, resulting in shock, internal bleeding, and acute renal failure. An exploratory laparotomy was performed that showed a ruptured spleen requiring a

III-68. *(Continued)*

splenectomy. He also underwent an open reduction and internal fixation of the left femur. The platelet count was 260,000 cells/μL on admission. Today it is 68,000 cells/μL. His medications are oxacillin, morphine, and subcutaneous heparin. On examination the vital signs are stable. The examination is significant for an abdominal scar that is clean and healing. The patient's left leg is in a large cast and is elevated. The right leg is swollen from the calf downward. Ultrasound of the right leg shows a deep venous thrombosis. Antiheparin antibodies are positive. Creatinine is 3.2 mg/dL. What is the most appropriate next management step?

  A. Discontinue heparin.
  B. Stop heparin and start enoxaparin.
  C. Stop heparin and start argatroban.
  D. Stop heparin and start lepirudin.
  E. Observe the patient.

III-69. A 64-year-old man with chronic lymphoid leukemia (CLL) and chronic hepatitis C presents for his yearly follow-up. His white blood cell count is stable at 83000/μL, but his hematocrit has dropped from 35% to 26% and his platelet count also dropped from 178,000/μL to 69,000/μL. His initial evaluation should include all of the following *except*

  A. AST, ALT, and prothrombin time
  B. bone marrow biopsy
  C. Coomb's test
  D. peripheral blood smear
  E. physical examination

III-70. A 64-year-old man with Child-Pugh class B cirrhosis presents to his gastroenterologist complaining of weight loss and a feeling of abdominal fullness. He was diagnosed with hepatitis C cirrhosis 5 years previously. It is thought that the patient developed with hepatitis C following a blood transfusion 20 years ago after a car accident. His initial presentation with cirrhosis was volume overload and ascites. He has been successfully managed with sodium restriction, spironolactone, and furosemide. He has no other significant medical history. On examination today, his liver is enlarged and firm. No ascites is present. A helical CT of the abdomen shows a single tumor in the right lobe of the liver measuring 4 cm in diameter. The location of the mass is near the main portal pedicles. There is no evidence of vascular invasion or metastatic lesions. The α fetoprotein level is 384 ng/mL. Biopsy of the mass is diagnostic for hepatocellular carcinoma. What is the best approach for treatment?

  A. Liver transplantation
  B. Radiofrequency ablation
  C. Resection of the right hepatic lobe
  D. Systemic chemotherapy
  E. Transarterial chemoembolization

III-71. Which of the following should prompt investigation for hereditary nonpolyposis colon cancer screening in a 32-year-old man?

    A. Father, paternal aunt, and paternal cousin with colon cancer with ages of diagnosis of 54, 68, and 37 years, respectively

    B. Innumerable polyps visualized on routine colonoscopy

    C. Mucocutaneous pigmentation

    D. New diagnosis of ulcerative colitis

    E. None of the above

III-72. Which of the following carries the best disease prognosis with appropriate treatment?

    A. Burkitt's lymphoma

    B. Diffuse large B cell lymphoma

    C. Follicular lymphoma

    D. Mantle cell lymphoma

    E. Nodular sclerosing Hodgkin's disease

III-73. You are asked to consult on a 31-year-old male with prolonged bleeding after an oral surgery procedure. He has no prior history of bleeding diathesis or family history of bleeding disorders. The patient's past medical history is remarkable for infection with the human immunodeficiency virus, with a CD4 count of 51/mL^3. The examination is remarkable only for spotty lymphadenopathy. The platelet count is 230,000 cells/mL. His international normalized ratio (INR) is 1.5. Activated partial thromboplastin time is 40 s. Peripheral blood smear shows no schistocytes and is otherwise unremarkable. A 1:1 mixing study corrects both conditions immediately and after a 2-h incubation. Fibrinogen level is normal. Thrombin time is prolonged. What is the diagnosis?

    A. Disseminated intravascular coagulation (DIC)

    B. Dysfibrinogenemia

    C. Factor V deficiency

    D. Liver disease

    E. Factor XIII deficiency

III-74. Chemoprevention strategies for cancer have met with varying levels of success. Which of the following pairings correctly identifies an effective chemoprevention strategy with its target effect?

    A. Aspirin: colon cancer

    B. β-Carotene: lung cancer

    C. Calcium: adenomatous gastrointestinal polyps

    D. Isotretinoin: oral leukoplakia

    E. Tamoxifen: endometrial cancer

III-75. A 48-year-old woman is admitted to the hospital with anemia and thrombocytopenia after complaining of profound fatigue. Her initial hemoglobin is 8.5 g/dL, hematocrit 25.7%, and platelet count 42,000/μL. Her leukocyte count is 9540/μL, but 8% blast forms are noted on peripheral smear. A chromosomal analysis shows a recip-

III-75. *(Continued)*
rocal translocation of the long arms of chromosomes 15 and 17, t(15;17), and a diagnosis of acute promyelocytic leukemia is made. The induction regimen of this patient should include which of the following drugs:

    A. All-*trans*-retinoic acid (ATRA, or triretinoin)

    B. Arsenic

    C. Cyclophosphamide, daunorubicin, vinblastine, and prednisone

    D. Rituximab

    E. Whole-body irradiation

III-76. The patient above is started on the appropriate induction regimen. Two weeks following initiation of treatment, the patient develops acute onset of shortness of breath, fever, and chest pain. Her chest radiograph shows bilateral alveolar infiltrates and moderate bilateral pleural effusions. Her leukocyte count is now 22,300/μL, and she has a neutrophil count of 78%, bands of 15%, and lymphocytes 7%. She undergoes bronchoscopy with lavage that shows no bacterial, fungal, or viral organisms. What is the most likely diagnosis in this patient?

    A. Arsenic poisoning

    B. Bacterial pneumonia

    C. Cytomegalovirus pneumonia

    D. Radiation pneumonitis

    E. Retinoic acid syndrome

III-77. A 76-year-old man is admitted to the hospital with complaints of fatigue for 4 months and fever for the past 1 week. His temperature has been as high as 38.3°C at home. During this time, he intermittently has had a 5.5-kg weight loss, severe bruising with minimal trauma, and an aching sensation in his bones. He last saw his primary care physician 2 months ago and was diagnosed with anemia of unclear etiology at that time. He has a history of a previous left middle cerebral artery cerebrovascular accident which has left him with decreased functional status. At baseline, he is able to ambulate in his home with the use of a walker and is dependent upon a caregiver for assistance with his activities of daily living. His vital signs are: blood pressure 158/86 mmHg, heart rate 98 beats/min, respiratory rate 18 breaths/min, Sa$_{O_2}$ 95%, and temperature 38°C. He appears cachectic with temporal muscle wasting. He has petechiae on his hard palate. He has no lymph node enlargement. On cardiovascular examination, there is a II/VI systolic ejection murmur present. His lungs are clear. The liver is enlarged and palpable 6 cm below the right costal margin. In addition, the spleen is also enlarged, with a palpable spleen tip felt about 4 cm below the left costal margin. There are multiple hematomas and petechiae present in the extremities. Laboratory examination reveals the following: hemoglobin 5.1 g/dL, hematocrit 15%, platelets 12,000/μL, and white blood cell (WBC) count 168,000/μL with 45% blast forms, 30% neutrophils, 20% lymphocytes, and 5% monocytes. Re-

III-77. *(Continued)*

view of the peripheral blood smear confirms acute myeloid leukemia (M1 subtype, myeloblastic leukemia without maturation) with complex chromosomal abnormalities on cytogenetics. All of the following confer a poor prognosis for this patient *except*

A.   advanced age
B.   complex chromosomal abnormalities on cytogenetics
C.   hemoglobin <7 g/dL
D.   prolonged interval between symptom onset and diagnosis
E.   WBC count >100,000/μL

III-78. A new screening test for thyroid cancer has been introduced into the population. In the first year, 1000 positive tests lead to correct identification of thyroid cancer in the screened population. Over the next year, 250 cases of thyroid cancer are detected among those who initially had a negative test. What is the sensitivity of this new screening test?

A.   25%
B.   67%
C.   80%
D.   Not enough information to calculate

III-79. A 56-year-old patient inquires about screening for colon cancer. He has no risk factors for colon cancer, other than age. Which of the following statements is true regarding which screening test you recommend for this patient?

A.   50% of patients with a positive fecal occult blood testing have colon cancer.
B.   One-time colonoscopy detects more advanced lesions than one-time fecal occult blood testing with sigmoidoscopy.
C.   Perforation rates for sigmoidoscopy and colonoscopy are equivalent.
D.   Sigmoidoscopy has not been shown to reduce mortality.
E.   Virtual colonoscopy is as effective as endoscopic colonoscopy for detecting polyps <5 mm in size.

III-80. A 65-year-old man seeks evaluation for nasal congestion, headaches, and dysphagia, most notably when he lies supine for sleeping. These symptoms have been slowly worsening for the past month. He has no nasal discharge or fevers. On review of systems, he reports recent hoarseness and dizziness. His past medical history is significant only for mild hypertension. He worked as a roofing contractor and smoked one pack/day of cigarettes since age 16. On physical examination, you note facial edema. His oropharynx is also mildly edematous, and the tonsils are unremarkable. His external and internal jugular veins are engorged bilaterally, and there are prominent veins on the anterior chest. Chest percussion reveals dullness in the right base with decreased tactile fremitus. A chest radiograph shows a right upper lung mass that on

III-80. *(Continued)*

biopsy is consistent with non-small cell lung cancer. All of the following treatments may help this patient's symptoms *except*

A.   chemotherapy
B.   diuretics
C.   glucocorticoids
D.   radiation therapy
E.   venous stenting

III-81. All of the following statements regarding the epidemiology of and risk factors for acute myeloid leukemias are true *except*

A.   Anticancer drugs such as alkylating agents and topoisomerase II inhibitors are the leading cause of drug-associated myeloid leukemias.
B.   Individuals exposed to high-dose radiation are at risk for acute myeloid leukemia whereas individuals treated with therapeutic radiation are not unless they are also treated with alkylating agents.
C.   Men have a higher incidence of acute myeloid leukemia than women.
D.   The incidence of acute myeloid leukemia is greatest in individuals <20 years.
E.   Trisomy 21 (Down syndrome) is associated with an increased risk of acute myeloid leukemia.

III-82. A 42-year-old man presented to the hospital with right upper quadrant pain. He was found to have multiple masses in the liver that were found to be malignant on H&E staining of a biopsy sample. Your initial history, physical examination and laboratory tests, including prostate-specific antigen, are unrevealing. Lung, abdominal, and pelvic CT scans are unremarkable. He is an otherwise healthy individual with no chronic medical problems. Which immunohistochemical markers should be obtained from the biopsy tissue?

A.   α Fetoprotein
B.   Cytokeratin
C.   Leukocyte common antigen
D.   Thyroglobulin
E.   Thyroid transcription factor 1

III-83. A 56-year-old woman is diagnosed with chronic myelogenous leukemia, Philadelphia chromosome–positive. Her presenting leukocyte count was 127,000/μL, and her differential shows <2% circulating blasts. Her hematocrit is 21.1% at diagnosis. She is asymptomatic except for fatigue. She has no siblings. What is the best initial therapy for this patient?

A.   Allogeneic bone marrow transplant
B.   Autologous stem cell transplant
C.   Imatinib mesylate
D.   Interferon-α
E.   Leukapheresis.

III-84. All the following are associated with a reduced lifetime risk of developing breast cancer *except*

A. absence of a history of maternal nursing
B. first full-term pregnancy before age 18 years
C. menarche after age 15 years
D. natural menopause before age 42 years
E. surgical menopause before age 42 years

III-85. All the following cause prolongation of the activated partial thromboplastin time (aPTT) that does not correct with a 1:1 mixture with pooled plasma *except*

A. lupus anticoagulant
B. factor VIII inhibitor
C. heparin
D. factor VII inhibitor
E. factor IX inhibitor

III-86. A 53-year-old woman seeks evaluation from her primary care physician regarding primary prevention of cardiovascular disease and stroke. She has a past medical history of type 2 diabetes mellitus for the past 5 years with a known hemoglobin A1C of 7.2%. She does not have hypertension or known coronary artery disease. She has been obese throughout adulthood, and her BMI is 33.6 kg/m^2. She is currently perimenopausal with irregular bleeding that last occurred 3 months ago. She is taking metformin, 1000 mg twice daily. She has been intolerant of ibuprofen in the past due to gastrointestinal upset. She previously smoked one pack of cigarettes daily from the ages of 18 to 38. She drinks a glass of wine with dinner. Her family history is significant for myocardial infarction in her father at age 58, paternal uncle at age 67, and paternal grandmother at age 62. On the maternal side, her mother died of a stroke at age 62. She is concerned that she should be taking a daily aspirin as primary prevention of cardiovascular disease and stroke but is also concerned about potential side effects. Which of the following statements regarding aspirin therapy is true?

A. Aspirin is indicated for primary prevention of cardiovascular disease because she has a strong family history and has a history of diabetes mellitus.
B. Aspirin is only indicated for secondary prevention of cardiovascular and cerebrovascular disease in women.
C. Because she is not postmenopausal, aspirin therapy is not recommended as it will increase menstrual bleeding without significantly decreasing the risk of cardiovascular disease.
D. Her adverse reaction to ibuprofen prevents use of aspirin because there is a high degree of cross-reactivity, and she is at risk for development of bronchospasm with aspirin use.
E. The risk of major bleeding related to use of aspirin is 1–3% per year, but use of an enteric-coated or buffered aspirin will eliminate this risk.

III-87. A 22-year-old man comes into clinic because of a swollen leg. He does not remember any trauma to the leg, but the pain and swelling began 3 weeks ago in the anterior shin area of his left foot. He is a college student and is active in sports daily. A radiograph of the right leg shows a destructive lesion with a "moth-eaten" appearance extending into the soft tissue and a spiculated periosteal reaction. Codman's triangle (a cuff of periosteal bone formation at the margin of the bone and soft tissue mass) is present. What is the most likely diagnosis and optimal therapy for this lesion?

A. Chondrosarcoma; chemotherapy alone is curative
B. Chondrosarcoma; radiation with limited surgical resection
C. Osteosarcoma; preoperative chemotherapy followed by limb-sparing surgery
D. Osteosarcoma; radiation therapy
E. Plasma cell tumor; chemotherapy

III-88. Which of the following statements is true?

A. Factor VIII deficiency is characterized clinically by bleeding into soft tissues, muscles, and weightbearing joints.
B. Congenital factor VIII deficiency is inherited in an autosomal recessive fashion.
C. Factor VIII deficiency results in prolongation of the prothrombin time.
D. Factor VIII complexes with Hageman factor, allowing for a longer half-life.
E. Factor VIII has a half-life of nearly 24 h.

III-89. All of the following statements regarding gastric carcinoma are true *except*

A. Linitis plastica is an infiltrative form of gastric lymphoma with no defined margins that carries a poorer prognosis than intestinal-type lesions.
B. Reduction of tumor bulk with surgery is the best therapeutic option for gastric adenocarcinoma, if surgically feasible.
C. The long-term ingestion of high concentrations of nitrates in dried, smoked, or salted foods is associated with higher rates of gastric cancer.
D. The presence of palpable, firm peri-umbilical nodules is a poor prognostic sign.
E. Ulcerative lesions in the distal stomach should always undergo brush sampling and biopsy to rule out adenocarcinoma.

III-90. Which of the following statements correctly describes characteristics of stem cells?

A. Ability to differentiate into a variety of mature cells types
B. Capacity for self-renewal
C. Generate, maintain, and repair tissue
D. A and C
E. A and B
F. All of the above

III-91. Which of the following statements regarding malignant spinal cord compression (MSCC) is true?

A. Less than 50% of patients who are treated while ambulatory will remain ambulatory.
B. Neurologic abnormalities on physical examination are sufficient to initiate high-dose glucocorticoids.
C. Neurologic findings often appear before pain.
D. Renal cell carcinoma is the most common cause of MSCC.
E. The lumbosacral spine is the most commonly affected site.

III-92. All the following are characteristic of tumor lysis syndrome *except*

A. hyperkalemia
B. hypercalcemia
C. lactic acidosis
D. hyperphosphatemia
E. hyperuricemia

III-93. A 22-year-old woman comes to the emergency department complaining of 12 h of shortness of breath. The symptoms began towards the end of a long car ride home from college. She has no past medical history and her only medication is an oral contraceptive. She smokes occasionally but the frequency has increased recently because of examinations. On physical examination, she is afebrile with respiratory rate of 22 breaths/min, blood pressure 120/80 mmHg, heart rate 110 beats/min, Sa_{O_2} (room air) 92%. The rest of her physical examination is normal. A chest radiograph and complete blood count are normal. Her serum pregnancy test is negative. Which of the following is the indicated management strategy?

A. Check D-dimer and, if normal, discharge with nonsteroidal anti-inflammatory therapy.
B. Check D-dimer and, if normal, obtain lower extremity ultrasound.
C. Check D-dimer and, if abnormal, treat for deep venous thrombosis/pulmonary embolism (DVT/PE).
D. Check D-dimer and, if abnormal, obtain contrast multislice CT of chest.
E. Obtain contrast multislice CT of chest.

III-94. The patient described above is found to have a right pulmonary embolus. She is started on low-molecular-weight heparin and warfarin. What is the goal international normalized ratio (INR) and the duration of therapy?

A. INR 3.5; 1 month
B. INR 2.5; 3 months
C. INR 3.5; 3 months
D. INR 2.5; 6 months
E. INR 3.5; 6 months
F. INR 2.5; lifetime

III-95. A patient asks you about the utility of performing monthly breast self-examination (BSE). Which of the following statements is correct regarding the utility of and recommendations regarding breast self-examination?

A. Breast self-examination reduces mortality only in women who undergo breast biopsy.
B. Most screening societies recommend performing BSE monthly for women >20 years.
C. Self-examination leads to increased biopsy rate.
D. Very few breast cancers are first detected by patients.
E. Breast self-examination leads to improved survival from breast cancer.

III-96. Which of the following tumor characteristics confers a poor prognosis in patients with breast cancer?

A. Estrogen receptor-positive
B. Good nuclear grade
C. Low proportion of cells in S-phase
D. Overexpression of *erbB2* (*HER-2/neu*)
E. Progesterone receptor-positive

III-97. Which of the following serum laboratory tests is most useful for predicting return of renal function in a patient with tumor lysis syndrome and acute renal failure?

A. Creatinine
B. Phosphate
C. Potassium
D. Serum pH
E. Uric acid

III-98. Fondaparinux may be used to treat all of the following patients *except*

A. A 33-year-old woman weighing 48 kg presents with a pulmonary embolus 2 months after a motor vehicle accident that resulted in a fractured femur.
B. A 46-year-old man with hypertension and focal segmental glomerulosclerosis with a baseline creatinine of 3.3 mg/dL presents with a left lower extremity deep venous thrombosis. He weighs 82 kg.
C. A 57-year-old woman had an aortic valve replacement 7 days ago. The platelet count preoperatively was 320,000/μL. On day 7, the platelet count is 122,000/μL.
D. A 60-year-old man presents to the hospital with chest pain and ST-segment depression in leads II, III, and aV_F on electrocardiogram. Troponin I level is 2.32 ng/mL.
E. A 68-year-old man has undergone an uncomplicated right total hip replacement.

III-99. A 26-year-old female who is 4 months pregnant is seen for a standard evaluation. She reports feeling well with decreasing nausea over the last 1 month. The physical examination is normal except for the presence of a 1.5-cm hard nodule in the upper outer quadrant of the right breast. She does not recall the nodule being present

III-99. *(Continued)*

previously and has not performed self-examination since be coming pregnant. Which of the following is the next most appropriate action?

A. Aspiration of the nodule
B. Mammogram after delivery
C. Prescription of oral progesterone therapy
D. Recommendation of genetic testing for *BRCA-1*
E. Repeat physical examination after delivery

III-100. Aplastic anemia has been associated with all of the following *except*

A. carbamazepine therapy
B. methimazole therapy
C. non-steroidal inflammatory drugs
D. parvovirus B19 infection
E. seronegative hepatitis

III-101. A 23-year-old man presents with diffuse bruising. He otherwise feels well. He takes no medications, does not use dietary supplements, and does not use illicit drugs. His past medical history is negative for any prior illnesses. He is a college student and works as a barista in a coffee shop. A blood count reveals an absolute neutrophil count of 780/µL, hematocrit of 18% and platelet count of 21,000/µL. Bone marrow biopsy reveals hypocellularity with a fatty marrow. Chromosome studies of peripheral blood and bone marrow cells are performed which exclude Fanconi's anemia and myelodysplastic syndrome. The patient has a fully histocompatible brother. Which of the following is the best therapy?

A. Anti-thymocyte globulin plus cyclosporine
B. Glucocorticoids
C. Growth factors
D. Hematopoietic stem cell transplant
E. Red blood cell and platelet transfusion

III-102. A 46-year-old woman presents with new onset ascites and severe abdominal pain: a hepatic Doppler examination reveals hepatic vein thrombosis. She also reports tea colored urine on occasion, particularly in the morning, as well as recurrent worsening abdominal pain. On further evaluation, she is found to have an undetectable serum haptoglobin, elevated serum lactase dehydrogenase, hemoglobinuria and an elevated reticulocyte count. A peripheral smear shows no schistocytes. What is the most likely diagnosis?

A. Adenocarcinoma of the ovary
B. Antiphospholipid syndrome
C. Aplastic anemia
D. Factor V Leiden deficiency
E. Paroxysmal nocturnal hemoglobinuria

III-103. A Sudanese refugee is brought to see you in clinic for abdominal pain. He has had intermittent fevers for months and has lost considerable weight. He was previously a guard for a refugee camp in the Sudan and worked the night shift

III-103. *(Continued)*

exclusively. On examination, he is severely malnourished with temporal wasting. He has massive splenomegaly but no palpable lymphadenopathy. Oropharynx shows no thrush. Laboratory data reveal an anemia, neutropenia, and thrombocytopenia. Skin examination shows no discrete lesions but you and the patient notice that the skin appears gray throughout. Malaria smears are negative and HIV testing is negative. Chest X-ray is normal. What is the most likely diagnosis?

A. Cirrhosis
B. Kala-azar (visceral leishmaniasis)
C. Kaposi's sarcoma
D. Miliary tuberculosis
E. Sickle cell anemia

III-104. A 16-year-old male has recurrent thigh hematomas. He has been active in sports all of his life and has had 3 episodes of limb-threatening bleeding with compartment syndrome. A family history is notable for a maternal grandfather with a similar bleeding history. Paternal family history is not available. Laboratory analysis in clinic reveals a normal platelet count, a normal activated partial thromboplastin time (22 s) and a prolonged prothrombin time (25 s). He takes no medications. What is the most likely reason for his coagulation disorder?

A. Factor VIII deficiency
B. Factor VII deficiency
C. Factor IX deficiency
D. Prothrombin deficiency
E. Surreptitious warfarin ingestion

III-105. A 52-year-old man is admitted with recurrent hemarthroses of his knees. He is an electrician who is still working but over the last year has had recurrent hemarthroses requiring surgical evacuation. Before one year ago, he had no medical problems. He has no other past medical history and seldom sees a physician. He smokes tobacco regularly. His platelet count is normal, erythrocyte sedimentation rate is 55 mm/hr, hemoglobin is 9 mg/dL and albumin is 3.1 mg/dL. Coagulation studies show a prolonged activated partial thromboplastin time (aPTT) and a normal prothrombin time (PT). Adding plasma from a normal subject does not correct the aPTT. What is the cause of his recurrent hemarthroses?

A. Acquired inhibitor
B. Factor VIII deficiency
C. Factor IX deficiency
D. Secondary syphilis
E. Vitamin C deficiency

III-106. During a pre-employment physical and laboratory evaluation, a 20-year-old male is noted to have a prolonged activated prothromblastin time (aPTT). On review of systems, he denies a history of recurrent mucosal bleeding and has never had an issue with other major

III-106. *(Continued)*

bleeding. He has never had any major physical trauma. A family history is limited because he does not know his biologic family history. Mixing studies correct the aPTT when normal serum is used. You suspect an inherited hemorrhagic disease such as hemophilia. Which other laboratory abnormality would you most likely expect to find if this patient has hemophilia?

A. Low Factor VIII activity
B. Low factor IX activity
C. Prolonged bleeding time
D. Prolonged prothrombin time
E. Prolonged thrombin time

III-107. You are evaluating a 45-year-old man with an acute upper GI bleed in the emergency department. He reports increasing abdominal girth over the past 3 months associated with fatigue and anorexia. He has not noticed any lower extremity edema. His past medical history is significant for hemophilia A diagnosed as a child with recurrent elbow hemarthroses in the past. He has been receiving infusions of factor VIII for most of his life, and received his last injection earlier that day. His blood pressure is 85/45 mmHg with a heart rate of 115/min. His abdominal examination is tense with a positive fluid wave. Hematocrit is 21%. Renal function and urinalysis is normal. His aPTT is minimally prolonged, his INR is 2.7, platelets are normal. Which of the following is most likely to yield a diagnosis for the cause of his GI bleeding?

A. Factor VIII activity level
B. *H. pylori* antibody test
C. Hepatitis B surface antigen
D. Hepatitis C RNA
E. Mesenteric angiogram

III-108. You are managing a patient with suspected disseminated intravascular coagulopathy (DIC). The patient has end-stage liver disease awaiting liver transplantation and was recently in the intensive care unit with *E. coli* bacterial peritonitis. You suspect DIC based on a new upper gastroin-

III-108. *(Continued)*

testinal bleed in the setting of oozing from venipuncture sites. Platelet count is 43000/μL, INR is 2.5, hemoglobin is 6 mg/dL and D-dimer is elevated to 4.5. What is the best way to distinguish between new-onset DIC and chronic liver disease?

A. Blood culture
B. Elevated fibrinogen degradation products
C. Prolonged aPTT
D. Reduced platelet count
E. Serial laboratory analysis

III-109. A 38-year-old woman is referred for evaluation of an elevated hemoglobin and hematocrit that was discovered during an evaluation of recurrent headaches. Until about 8 months previously, she was in good health, but developed increasingly persistent headaches with intermittent vertigo and tinnitus. She was originally prescribed sumatriptan for presumed migraine headaches, but did not experience relief of her symptoms. A CT scan of the brain showed no evidence of mass lesion. During evaluation of her headaches, she was found to have a hemoglobin of 17.3 g/dL, and a hematocrit of 52%. Her only other symptom is diffuse itching after hot showers. She is a non-smoker. She has no history pulmonary or cardiac disease. On physical examination, she appears well. Her BMI is 22.3 kg/m². Vitals signs are BP 148/84 mmHg, HR 86/min, RR 12/min, Sa$_{O_2}$ 99% on room air. She is afebrile. The physical examination including full neurologic examination is normal. There are no heart murmurs. There is no splenomegaly. Peripheral pulses are normal. Laboratory studies confirm elevated hemoglobin and hematocrit. She also has a platelet count of 650,000/μL. Leukocyte count is 12,600/μL with a normal differential. Which of the following tests should be performed next in the evaluation of this patient?

A. Bone marrow biopsy
B. Erythropoietin level
C. Genetic testing for JAK2 V617F mutation
D. Leukocyte alkaline phosphatase
E. Red cell mass and plasma volume determination

III. ONCOLOGY AND HEMATOLOGY

ANSWERS

III-1. The answer is B. *(Chap. 94)* Bone pain resulting from metastatic lesions may be difficult to distinguish from degenerative disease, osteoporosis, or disk disease in the elderly. Generally, these patients present with insidious worsening localized pain without fevers or signs of infection. In contrast to pain related to disk disease, the pain of metastatic disease is worse when the patient is lying down or at night. Neurologic symptoms related to metastatic disease constitute an emergency. Lung, breast, and prostate cancers account for approximately 80% of bone metastases. Thyroid carcinoma, renal cell carcinoma, lymphoma, and bladder carcinoma may also metastasize to bone. Metastatic lesions may be lytic or blastic. Most cancers cause a combination of both, although prostate cancer is predominantly blastic. Either lesion may cause hypercalcemia, although lytic lesions more commonly do this. Lytic lesions are best detected with plain radiography. Blastic lesions are prominent on radionuclide bone scans. Treatment and prognosis depend on the underlying malignancy. Bisphosphonates may reduce hypercalcemia, relieve pain, and limit bone resorption.

III-2. The answer is B. *(Chap. 101)* Red blood cells utilize glutathione produced by the hexose monophosphate shunt to compensate for increased production of reactive oxygen species (oxidant stress), usually induced by drugs or toxins. Defects in G6PD are the most common congenital hexose monophosphate shunt defect. If the red blood cell (RBC) is unable to maintain an adequate level of glutathione during oxidant stress, hemoglobin precipitates in the RBC, producing Heinz bodies. Because the G6PD gene is on the X chromosome, almost all afflicted patients are males. G6PD deficiency is widely distributed throughout regions that are currently or were once highly malarial endemic. It is common in males of African, African-American, Sardinian, and Sephardic descent. In most persons with G6PD deficiency, there is no evidence of symptomatic disease. However, infection, ingestion of fava beans, or exposure to an oxidative agent (drug or toxin) can trigger an acute hemolytic event. Bite cells, Heinz bodies, and bizarre poikilocytes may be evident on smear. The drugs that most commonly precipitate a G6PD crisis include dapsone, sulfamethoxazole, primaquine, and nitrofurantoin. The anemia is often severe with rapid onset after drug ingestion, and renal failure can occur.

III-3. The answer is E. *(Chaps. 110 and 111)* Vitamin K is a fat-soluble vitamin that plays an essential role in hemostasis. It is absorbed in the small intestine and stored in the liver. It serves as a cofactor in the enzymatic carboxylation of glutamic acid residues on prothrombin-complex proteins. The three major causes of vitamin K deficiency are poor dietary intake, intestinal malabsorption, and liver disease. The prothrombin complex proteins (factors II, VII, IX, and X and protein C and protein S) all decrease with vitamin K deficiency. Factor VII and protein C have the shortest half-lives of these factors and therefore decrease first. Therefore, vitamin K deficiency manifests with prolongation of the prothrombin time first. With severe deficiency, the aPTT will be prolonged as well. Factor VIII is not influenced by vitamin K.

III-4. The answer is E. *(Chaps. 110 and 111)* Hemophilia A results from a deficiency of factor VIII. Replacement of factor VIII is the centerpiece of treatment. Cessation of aspirin or nonsteroidal anti-inflammatory drugs (NSAIDs) is highly recommended. FFP contains pooled plasma from human sources. Cryoprecipitate refers to FFP that is cooled, resulting in the precipitation of material at the bottom of the plasma. This product contains about half the factor VIII activity of FFP in a tenth of the volume. Both agents are therefore reasonable treatment options. DDAVP causes the release of a number of factors and von Willebrand factor from the liver and endothelial cells. This may be useful for patients with mild hemophilia. Recombinant or purified factor VIII (i.e., Humate P) is indicated in patients with more severe bleeding. Therapy may be required for weeks, with levels of factor VIII kept at 50%, for postsurgical or severe bleeding. Plasmapheresis has no role in the treatment of hemophilia A.

III-5.   The answer is A.   *(Chap. 88)*   Hepatocellular carcinoma (HCC) is one of the commonest cancers worldwide with the highest incidence in Southeast Asia and sub-Saharan Africa. However, the incidence of HCC in the United States is rapidly increasing and is thought to be related to an increase in the number of individuals infected with hepatitis C. At present, an estimated 4 million individuals are infected with hepatitis C, of whom 10% have cirrhosis. Of those who develop cirrhosis due to hepatitis C, ~5% will develop HCC. Other common risk factors for development of HCC include cirrhosis from any cause, chronic hepatitis B or C infection, alcoholism, nonalcoholic steatohepatitis, aflatoxin B exposure, and primary biliary cirrhosis. Aflatoxin B is a mycotoxin produced by *Aspergillus* species that is found in stored grains in hot and humid places. It is the best studied and most potent naturally occurring carcinogen associated with HCC. In the United States, ~20% of individuals diagnosed with HCC do not have cirrhosis. In these individuals, the etiology of HCC is unknown, and the natural history is not well defined.

III-6.   The answer is C.   *(Chap. 58)*   This blood smear shows fragmented red blood cells of varying size and shape. In the presence of a foreign body within the circulation (prosthetic heart valve, vascular graft), red blood cells can become destroyed. Such intravascular hemolysis will also cause serum lactate dehydrogenase to be elevated and hemoglobinuria. In isolated extravascular hemolysis, there is no hemoglobin or hemosiderin released into the urine. The characteristic peripheral blood smear in splenomegaly is the presence of Howell-Jolly bodies (nuclear remnants within red blood cells). Certain diseases are associated with extramedullary hematopoiesis (e.g., chronic hemolytic anemias), which can be detected by an enlarged spleen, thickened calvarium, myelofibrosis, or hepatomegaly. The peripheral blood smear may show tear-drop cells or nucleated red blood cells. Hypothyroidism is associated with macrocytosis, which is not demonstrated here. Chronic gastrointestinal blood loss will cause microcytosis, not schistocytes.

III-7.   The answer is D.   *(Chap. 352)*   Porphyria cutanea tarda (PCT) is the most common porphyria and usually arises from a sporadic gene mutation leading to a deficiency of the enzyme uroporphyrinogen decarboxylase. Despite being a hepatic porphyria, it usually presents with blistering skin lesions on the back of the hands. These lesions lead to areas of atrophy and scarring after resolution. Neurologic symptoms are absent. Any condition that increases hepatic iron will exacerbate PCT. PCT is associated with alcoholism, hepatitis C, estrogens, elevated serum iron, and HIV infection. Rare forms of PCT are familial. 5-ALA dehydratase-deficient porphyria is inherited in autosomal recessive fashion. Acute intermittent porphyria, erythropoietic porphyria, and variegate porphyria are autosomal dominant.

III-8.   The answer is C.   *(Chap. 97; Sillevis Smith et al.)*   One of the better characterized paraneoplastic neurologic syndromes is cerebellar ataxia caused by Purkinje cell drop-out in the cerebellum; it is manifested by dysarthria, limb and gait ataxia, and nystagmus. Radiologic imaging reveals cerebellar atrophy. Many antibodies have been associated with this syndrome, including anti-Yo, anti-Tr, and antibodies to the glutamate receptor. Although lung cancer, particularly small-cell cancer, accounts for a large number of patients with neoplasm-associated cerebellar ataxia, those with the syndrome who display anti-Yo antibodies in the serum typically have breast or ovarian cancer.

III-9.   The answer is B.   *(Chaps. 101 and 313)*   This patient's lupus and her rapid development of truly life-threatening hemolytic anemia are both very suggestive of autoimmune hemolytic anemia. Diagnosis is made by a positive Coomb's test documenting antibodies to the red cell membrane, but smear will often show microspherocytes, indicative of the damage incurred to the red cells in the spleen. Schistocytes are typical for microangiopathic hemolytic anemias such as hemolytic-uremic syndrome (HUS) or thrombocytopenic thrombotic purpura (TTP). The lack of thrombocytopenia makes these diagnoses considerably less plausible. Macrocytosis and PMN's with hypersegmented nuclei are very suggestive of vitamin B_{12} deficiency, which causes a more chronic, non-life-threatening anemia. Target cells are seen in liver disease and thalassemias. Sickle cell anemia is associated with aplastic crises, but she has no known diagnosis of sickle cell disease and is showing evidence of erythropoietin response based on the presence of elevated reticulocyte count.

III-10. **The answer is A.** *(Chap. 58)* An accurate reticulocyte count is a critical component of the laboratory workup of anemia. There are two corrections that need to be made to the reticulocyte count when it is being used to estimate the marrow's response to anemia. The first correction adjusts the reticulocyte count for the number of circulating red cells (i.e., the percentage of reticulocytes may be increased although the absolute number is unchanged). The absolute reticulocyte count = reticulocyte count * (hematocrit/expected hematocrit). Second, when there is evidence of prematurely released reticulocytes on the blood smear (polychromatophilia), prolonged maturation in the serum may cause a falsely high estimate of daily red blood cell production. Correction is achieved by dividing by a "maturation time correction," usually 2 if the hematocrit is between 25% and 35%. In this example, the reticulocyte production index is: 5 * (25/45)/2, or 1.4. If a reticulocyte production index is <2 in the face of anemia, a defect in erythroid marrow proliferation must be present. Gastrointestinal bleeding should be considered in this demographic; however, a low reticulocyte count with normal iron stores argues strongly for a defect in erythroid proliferation. A ferritin >200 µg/L indicates that there are some iron stores present. Clues for extravascular hemolysis include an elevated lactate dehydrogenase, spherocytes on the peripheral blood smear, and hepatosplenomegaly. Intravascular hemolysis (disseminated intravascular coagulation, mechanical heart valve, thrombotic thrombocytopenic purpura) will show schistocytes on peripheral smear.

III-11. **The answer is D.** *(Chap. 102)* Pure red cell aplasia is a normochromic, normocytic anemia with absent erythroblasts on the bone marrow, hence the diminished number or lack of reticulocytes. The bone marrow shows red cell aplasia and the presence of giant pronormoblasts. Several conditions have been associated with pure red cell aplasia, including viral infections such as B19 parvovirus (which can have cytopathic bone marrow changes), HIV, EBV, HTLV, and hepatitis B virus; malignancies such as thymomas and lymphoma (which often present with an anterior mediastinal mass); connective tissue disorders such as SLE and rheumatoid arthritis (RA); pregnancy; drugs; and hereditary disorders. Erythropoietin levels are elevated because of the anemia.

III-12. **The answer is A.** *(Chap. 87)* This patient has *Streptococcus bovis* endocarditis. For unknown reasons, individuals who develop endocarditis or septicemia from this fecal organism have a high frequency of having occult colorectal carcinomas. Upper gastrointestinal tumors have been described as well. All patients with *S. bovis* endocarditis should receive colonoscopy after stabilization. Tobacco use has been linked to the development of colorectal adenomas, particularly after >35 years of tobacco use, again for unknown reasons. Patients with illicit drug use (diagnosed by toxicology screen) are at risk of endocarditis due to *Staphylococcus aureus*. A head CT scan looking for embolic lesions is not necessary in the absence of physical findings or large vegetations that are prone to embolize. Patients with endocarditis often have renal abnormalities, including microscopic hematuria from immune complex deposition, but a renal biopsy to evaluate for glomerulonephritis is not indicated in the presence of documented endocarditis. A pulmonary embolus, while certainly a possible event during hospitalization, would not be associated with the acute presentation of *S. bovis* endocarditis.

III-13. **The answer is A.** *(Chap. 88)* This patient is presenting with painless jaundice and acholic stools. On right upper quadrant ultrasound, the gallbladder cannot be visualized, suggesting collapse of the gallbladder. In addition, there is dilatation of the intrahepatic bile ducts, but not the common bile duct, suggesting a tumor at the bifurcation of the common bile duct.

This tumor is a type of cholangiocarcinoma called a *Klatskin tumor*. The incidence of cholangiocarcinoma appears to be increasing. In general, the cause of most cholangiocarcinoma is unknown, but there is an increased risk in primary sclerosing cholangitis, liver flukes, alcoholic liver disease, and any cause of chronic biliary injury. Cholangiocarcinoma typically presents as painless jaundice. Imaging usually shows dilatation of the bile ducts, and the extent of dilatation depends upon the site of obstruction. Diagnosis is usually made during endoscopic retrograde cholangiopancreatography (ERCP), which defines the biliary tree and allows a biopsy to be taken. Hilar cholangiocarcinoma is resectable in about 30% of patients, and the mean survival is ~24 months. Cholecystitis is typically associated with fever, chills, and abdominal pain. The degree of jaundice would not be expected to be as high as is seen in this patient. Gallbladder cancer should present with a gallbladder mass rather than a collapsed gallbladder, and chronic right upper quadrant pain is usually present. Hepatocellular carcinoma may be associated with painless jaundice but is not associated with dilatation of intrahepatic bile ducts and the marked elevation in alkaline phosphatase. Malignancy at the head of the pancreas may present in a similar fashion but should not result in gallbladder collapse. In addition, the common bile duct should be markedly dilated.

III-14. The answer is E. *(Chaps. 96 and 347)* Hypercalcemia is a common oncologic complication of metastatic cancer. Symptoms include confusion, lethargy, change in mental status, fatigue, polyuria, and constipation. Regardless of the underlying disease, the treatment is similar. These patients are often dehydrated, as hypercalcemia may cause a nephrogenic diabetes insipidus, and are often unable to take fluids orally. Therefore, the primary management entails reestablishment of euvolemia. Often hypercalcemia will resolve with hydration alone. Bisphosphonates are another mainstay of therapy as they stabilize osteoclast resorption of calcium from the bone. However, their effects may take 1 to 2 days to manifest. Care must be taken in cases of renal insufficiency as rapid administration of pamidronate may exacerbate renal failure. Once euvolemia is achieved, furosemide may be given to increase calciuresis. Nasal or subcutaneous calcitonin further aids the shift of calcium out of the intravascular space. Glucocorticoids may be useful in patients with lymphoid malignancies as the mechanism of hypercalcemia in those conditions is often related to excess hydroxylation of vitamin D. However, in this patient with prostate cancer, dexamethasone will have little effect on the calcium level and may exacerbate the altered mental status.

III-15. The answer is C. *(Chap. 92)* Ninety percent of persons with nonseminomatous germ cell tumors produce either AFP or β-hCG; in contrast, persons with pure seminomas usually produce neither. These tumor markers are present for some time after surgery; if the presurgical levels are high, 30 days or more may be required before meaningful postsurgical levels can be obtained. The half-lives of AFP and β-hCG are 6 days and 1 day, respectively. After treatment, unequal reduction of β-hCG and AFP may occur, suggesting that the two markers are synthesized by heterogeneous clones of cells within the tumor; thus, both markers should be followed. β-hCG is similar to luteinizing hormone except for its distinctive beta subunit.

III-16. The answer is C. *(Chap. 270)* Abdominal pain can be a sign of an oncologic emergency, both obstructive or metabolic. The differential diagnosis is broad; however, when there is obstruction, constipation and colicky abdominal pain are prominent. The pain may also be exacerbated postprandially. Normal imaging, moreover, suggests the abnormality is metabolic or may be due to peritoneal metastases too small to be seen on standard imaging. Adrenal insufficiency is suggested by mild hyponatremia and hyperkalemia, the history of breast cancer and use of megestrol acetate. Adrenal insufficiency may go unrecognized because the symptoms such as nausea, vomiting, orthostasis, or hypotension may be mistakenly attributed to progressive cancer or to therapy.

III-17. The answer is B. *(Chap. 87)* Most colorectal cancers arise from adenomatous polyps. Only adenomas are premalignant, and only a minority of these lesions becomes malignant. Most polyps are asymptomatic, causing occult bleeding in <5% of patients. Sessile (flat-based) polyps are more likely to become malignant than pedunculated (stalked) polyps. Histologically, villous adenomas are more likely to become malignant than tubular adenomas. The risk of containing invasive carcinoma in the polyp increases with size with

<2% in polyps <1.5 cm, 2–10% in polyps 1.5–2.5 cm, and 10% in polyps >2. 5 cm. This patient had two polyps that were high-risk based on histology (villous) and appearance (sessile) but only moderate risk by size (<1.5 cm). Polyps, particularly those >2.5 cm in size, sometimes contain cancer cells but usually progress to cancer quite slowly over a ~5-year period. Patients with adenomatous polyps should have a follow-up colonoscopy or radiographic study in 3 years. If no polyps are found on initial study, the test (endoscopic or radiographic) should be repeated in 10 years. CT scan is only warranted for staging if there is a diagnosis of colon cancer, not for the presence of polyps alone.

III-18. **The answer is A.** *(Chap. 103)* Polycythemia vera (PV) is a clonal disorder that involves a multipotent hematopoietic progenitor cell. Clinically, it is characterized by a proliferation of red blood cells, granulocytes, and platelets. The precise etiology is unknown. Erythropoiesis is regulated by the hormone erythropoietin. Hypoxia is the physiologic stimulus that increases the number of cells that produce erythropoietin. Erythropoietin may be elevated in patients with hormone-secreting tumors. Levels are usually "normal" in patients with hypoxic erythrocytosis. In polycythemia vera, however, because erythrocytosis occurs independently of erythropoietin, levels of the hormone are usually low. Therefore, an elevated level is *not* consistent with the diagnosis. Polycythemia is a chronic, indolent disease with a low rate of transformation to acute leukemia, especially in the absence of treatment with radiation or hydroxyurea. Thrombotic complications are the main risk for PV and correlate with the erythrocytosis. Thrombocytosis, although sometimes prominent, does not correlate with the risk of thrombotic complications. Salicylates are useful in treating erythromelalgia but are not indicated in asymptomatic patients. There is no evidence that thrombotic risk is significantly lowered with their use in patients whose hematocrits are appropriately controlled with phlebotomy. Phlebotomy is the mainstay of treatment. Induction of a state of iron deficiency is critical to prevent a reexpansion of the red blood cell mass. Chemotherapeutics and other agents are useful in cases of symptomatic splenomegaly. Their use is limited by side effects, and there is a risk of leukemogenesis with hydroxyurea.

III-19. **The answer is C.** *(Chap. 95)* The patient presents with symptoms suggestive of ovarian cancer. Although her peritoneal fluid is positive for adenocarcinoma, further speciation cannot be done. Surprisingly, the physical examination and imaging do not show a primary source. Although the differential diagnosis of this patient's disorder includes gastric cancer or another gastrointestinal malignancy and breast cancer, peritoneal carcinomatosis most commonly is due to ovarian cancer in women, even when the ovaries are normal at surgery. Elevated CA-125 levels or the presence of psammoma bodies is further suggestive of an ovarian origin, and such patients should receive surgical debulking and carboplatin or cisplatin plus paclitaxel. Patients with this presentation have a similar stage-specific survival compared with other patients with known ovarian cancer. Ten percent of patients with this disorder, also known as primary peritoneal papillary serous carcinoma, will remain disease-free 2 years after treatment.

III-20. **The answer is C.** *(Chap. 102)* Pure red cell aplasia (PRCA) is a condition characterized by the absence of reticulocytes and erythroid precursors. A variety of conditions may cause PRCA. It may be idiopathic. It may be associated with certain medications, such as trimethoprim-sulfamethoxazole (TMP-SMX) and phenytoin. It can be associated with a variety of neoplasms, either as a precursor to a hematologic malignancy such as leukemia or myelodysplasia or as part of an autoimmune phenomenon, as in the case of thymoma. Infections also may cause a pure red cell aplasia. Parvovirus B19 is a single-strand DNA virus that is associated with erythema infectiosum, or fifth disease in children. It is also associated with arthropathy and a flulike illness in adults. It is thought to attack the P antigen on proerythroblasts directly. Patients with a chronic hemolytic anemia, such as sickle cell disease, or with an immunodeficiency are less able to tolerate a transient drop in reticulocytes as their red blood cells do not survive in the peripheral blood for an adequate period. In this patient, her daughter had an illness before the appearance of her symptoms. It is reasonable to check her parvovirus IgM titers. If they are positive, a dose of intravenous immunoglobulin is indicated. Because her laboratories and smear are not suggestive of dramatic sickling, an exchange transfusion is not indicated. Immunosuppression with prednisone and/or cyclosporine may be indicated if another etiology of the PRCA is identified. However, that would not be the next step. Similarly, a bone marrow transplant might be a consideration in a young patient with myelodysplasia or leukemia, but there is no evidence of that at this time. Antibiotics have no role in light of her normal white blood cell count and the lack of evidence for a bacterial infection.

III-21.   The answer C.   *(Chap. 101)*   Hereditary spherocytosis is a heterogeneous red cell membranopathy that can be either congenital (usually autosomal dominant) or acquired; it is characterized by predominantly extravascular hemolysis in the spleen due to defects in membrane structural proteins. This spleen-mediated hemolysis leads to the conversion of classic biconcave red blood cells on smear to spherocytes. Splenomegaly is common. This disorder can be severe, depending on the site of mutation, but is often overlooked until some stressor such as pregnancy leads to a multifactorial anemia, or an infection such as parvovirus B19 transiently eliminates red cell production altogether. The peripheral blood smear shows microspherocytes, small densely staining red blood cells that have lost their central pallor. Acute treatment is with transfusion. G6PD deficiency is a cause of hemolysis that is usually triggered by the presence of an offending oxidative agent. The peripheral blood smear may show Heinz bodies. Parvovirus infection may cause a pure red cell aplasia. The presence of active reticulocytosis and laboratory findings consistent with hemolysis are not compatible with that diagnosis. Chronic gastrointestinal blood loss, such as due to a colonic polyp, would cause a microcytic, hypochromic anemia without evidence of hemolysis (indirect bilirubin, haptoglobin abnormalities).

III-22.   The answer is E.   *(Chap. 270)*   Hyperleukocytosis is a potentially fatal complication of acute leukemia when the blast count is >100,000/μL. Complications of the syndrome are mediated by hyperviscosity, tumor aggregates causing slow blood flow, and invasion of the primitive leukemic cells, which cause hemorrhage. The brain and lungs are most commonly involved. The pulmonary syndrome may lead to respiratory distress and progressive respiratory failure. Chest radiographs may show either alveolar or interstitial infiltrates. A common finding in patients with markedly elevated immature white blood cell counts is low arterial oxygen tension on arterial blood gas with a normal pulse oximetry. This may actually be due to pseudohypoxemia, because white blood cells rapidly consume plasma oxygen during the delay between collecting arterial blood and measuring oxygen tension, causing a spuriously low measured oxygen tension. Placing the arterial blood gas immediately in ice will prevent the pseudohypoxemia. The bcr-abl mutation is found in up to 25% of patients with ALL. In addition, as tumor cells lyse, lactate dehydrogenase levels can rise rapidly. Methemoglobinemia is usually due to exposure to oxidizing agents such as antibiotics or local anesthetics. Respiratory symptoms may develop when methemoglobin levels are >10–15% (depending on hemoglobin concentration). Typically arterial Pa_{O_2} is normal and measured Sa_{O_2} is inappropriately reduced because pulse oximetry is inaccurate with high levels of methemoglobin.

III-23.   The answer is D.   *(Chap. 85; Ost et al.)*   The evaluation of a solitary pulmonary nodule (SPN) remains a combination of art and science. Approximately 50% of SPNs (less than 3.0 cm) turn out to be malignant, but studies have found a range between 10 and 70%, depending on patient selection. If the SPN is malignant, surgical therapy can result in 80% 5-year survival. Most benign lesions are infectious granulomas. Spiculated or scalloped lesions are more likely to be malignant, whereas lesions with central or popcorn calcification are more likely to be benign. Masses (larger than 3.0 cm) are usually malignant. ^{18}FDG PET scanning has added a new test to the options for evaluating a SPN. PET has over 95% sensitivity and 75% specificity for identifying a malignant SPN. False negatives occur with small (less than 1 cm) tumors, bronchoalveolar carcinomas, and carcinoid tumors. False positives are usually due to inflammation. In this patient with a moderate risk of malignancy (age over 45, lesion larger than 1 cm, positive smoking history, suspicious lesion, no prior radiogram demonstrating the lesion) a PET scan would be the most reasonable choice. PET is also useful for staging disease. The diagnostic accuracy of PET for malignant mediastinal lymph nodes approaches 90%. Another option would be a transthoracic needle biopsy, with a sensitivity of 80 to 95% and a specificity of 50 to 85%. Transthoracic needle aspiration has the best results and the fewest complications (pneumothorax) with peripheral lesions versus central lesions. Bronchoscopy has a very poor yield for lesions smaller than 2 cm. Mediastinoscopy would be of little value unless PET or CT raised a suspicion of nodal disease. MRI scan will not add any information and is less able than CT to visualize lesions in the lung parenchyma. A repeat chest CT is a reasonable option for a patient with a low clinical suspicion.

III-24. The answer is A. *(Chap. 374)* About 25% of patients with cancer die with intracranial metastases. Symptoms may relate to parenchymal or leptomeningeal involvement. The signs and symptoms of metastatic brain tumor are similar to those of other intracranial expanding lesions: headache, nausea, vomiting, behavioral changes, seizures, and focal neurologic deficits. Three percent to 8% of patients with cancer develop a tumor involving the leptomeninges. These patients typically present with multifocal neurologic signs and symptoms. Signs include cranial nerve palsies, extremity weakness, paresthesias, and loss of deep tendon reflexes. CT and MRI are useful in establishing the diagnosis of intraparenchymal lesions. The treatment of choice is radiotherapy. Solitary lesions in selected patients may be resected to achieve improved disease-free survival. The diagnosis of leptomeningeal disease is made by demonstrating tumor cells in the cerebrospinal fluid (CSF). Each attempt has limited sensitivity, and so patients with clinical features suggestive of leptomeningeal disease should undergo three serial CSF samplings. Neoplastic meningitis usually occurs in the setting of uncontrolled cancer outside the CNS. Therefore, the prognosis is typically dismal, with a median survival between 10 and 12 weeks.

III-25. The answer is C. *(Chap. 112)* Warfarin is the most widely used oral anticoagulant. Its mechanism of action is to interfere with production of the vitamin K–dependent procoagulant factors (prothrombin and factors VII, IX, and X) and anticoagulant factors (proteins C and S). Warfarin accumulates in the liver when it undergoes oxidative metabolism by the CYP2C9 system. Multiple medications can interfere with the metabolism of warfarin by this system causing both over- and underdosing of warfarin. This patient has recently been treated with a fluoroquinolone antibiotic that is known to increase the prothrombin time and INR if the warfarin dose is not adjusted during treatment. When the INR is >6, there is a greater risk of development of bleeding complications. However, if no evidence of bleeding is present at presentation, it is safe to hold warfarin and allow the INR to fall gradually into the therapeutic range before reinstituting therapy (*DA Garcia: J Am Coll Cardiol 47:804, 2006; J Ansell et al: Chest 126:204S, 2004*). In this patient, however, there is evidence of minor bleeding complications warranting treatment. She likely has developed a degree of hemorrhagic cystitis due to over-anticoagulation in the setting of a urinary tract infection, which had already inflamed the bladder lining. In addition, she had developed multiple ecchymoses. Thus, treatment of the elevated INR is indicated. In the absence of life-threatening bleeding, treatment with vitamin K is indicated. When the INR falls between 4.9 and 9, an oral dose of vitamin K, 1 mg, is usually adequate to correct the INR without conferring vitamin K resistance, evidenced by decreased sensitivity to oral warfarin for an extended period. When a more rapid correction of anticoagulation is needed, vitamin K can be given by the IV or IM route. However, there is a risk of anaphylaxis, shock, and death. This can be minimized by delivering the drug slowly at a rate of ≤1 mg/min. Additionally, fresh-frozen plasma is indicated to replete coagulation factors when there is significant bleeding in the setting of an elevated INR. While the SC route for delivery of vitamin K has long been a primary route of correction, a meta-analysis has shown the SC route to be no better than placebo and inferior to the oral and IV routes, which have similar efficacy (*KJ Dezee et al.*).

III-26. The answer is D. *(Chap. e13)* Cancer is the second leading cause of mortality in the United States. Millions of Americans who are alive today have cancer in their past history. Cardiac toxicity is typically related to prior treatment with anthracycline-based chemotherapy or mediastinal irradiation. This is seen most commonly in patients who have survived Hodgkin's or non-Hodgkin's lymphoma. Anthracycline-related cardiotoxicity is dose-dependent. About 5% of patients who receive more than 550 mg/m^2 of doxorubicin will develop congestive heart failure (CHF). Rates are higher in those with other cardiac risk factors and those who have received mediastinal irradiation. Unfortunately, anthracycline-related CHF is typically not reversible. Intracellular chelators or liposomal formulations of the chemotherapy may prevent cardiotoxicity, but their impact on cure rates is unclear. Radiation has both acute and chronic effects on the heart. It may result in acute and chronic pericarditis, myocardial fibrosis, and accelerated atherosclerosis. The mean time to onset of "acute" pericarditis is 9 months after treatment, and so caretakers must be vigilant. Similarly, chronic pericarditis may manifest years later.

III-27.   **The answer is C.** *(Chap. 111)* Low-molecular-weight heparins are cleared renally, and these drugs have been described as causing significant bleeding in patients on hemodialysis. They should not be used in patients with dialysis-dependent renal failure. They are class B drugs for pregnancy and dosage is weight-based. Their utility is not affected by diabetes mellitus or hepatic dysfunction. Thrombocytopenia is a rare side effect of both unfractionated heparin and LMWH, but LMWH should not be used in someone with a documented history of heparin-induced thrombocytopenia.

III-28.   **The answer is D.** *(Chap. e13)* The focus of cancer care is cure. Many individuals who are fortunate enough to survive the malignancy will nevertheless bear chronic stigmata, both psychological and medical, of the treatment. Anthracyclines, which are used frequently in the treatment of breast cancer, Hodgkin's disease, lymphoma, and leukemia, are toxic to the myocardium and, at high doses, can lead to heart failure. Bleomycin results in pulmonary toxicity. Pulmonary fibrosis and pulmonary venoocclusive disease may result. Liver dysfunction is common with a number of chemotherapy agents. However, cisplatin primarily causes renal toxicity and acute renal failure. It may also cause neuropathy and hearing loss, but liver dysfunction is not a common complication. Ifosfamide may cause significant neurologic toxicity and renal failure. Also, it may cause a proximal tubular defect resembling Fanconi syndrome. Cyclophosphamide may result in cystitis and increases the long-term risk of bladder cancer. Administration of mesna ameliorates but does not completely eliminate this risk.

III-29.   **The answer is B.** *(Chap. 112)* The most likely diagnosis in this patient is heparin-induced thrombocytopenia (HIT), and heparin should be stopped immediately while continuing anticoagulation with the direct thrombin inhibitor, argatroban. HIT should be suspected in individuals with a fall in platelet count by >50% of pretreatment levels. Usually the fall in platelet counts occurs 5–13 days after starting heparin, but it can occur earlier if there is a prior exposure to heparin, which this patient undoubtedly has because of his mechanical mitral valve replacement. While a platelet count of <100,000/μL is highly suggestive of HIT, in most individuals, the platelet count rarely falls this low. HIT is caused by IgG antibodies directed against antigens on PF4 that are exposed when heparin binds to this protein. The IgG antibody binds simultaneously to the heparin-PF4 complex and the Fc receptor on platelet surface and causes platelet activation, resulting in a hypercoagulable state. Individuals with HIT are at increased risk of both arterial and venous thromboses, although venous thromboses are much more common. Demonstration of antibodies directed against the heparin–platelet factor complex is suggestive of, but not sufficient for, diagnosis because these antibodies may be present in the absence of clinical HIT. The serotonin release assay is the most specific test for determining if HIT is present. This assay determines the amount of serotonin released when washed platelets are exposed to patient serum and varying concentrations of heparin. In the cases of HIT, addition of patient serum to the test causes platelet activation and serotonin release due to the presence of heparin-PF4 antibodies. However, treatment of HIT should not be delayed until definitive diagnosis as there is a high risk of thrombotic events if heparin is continued. The risk of thrombotic events due to HIT is increased for about 1 month after heparin is discontinued. Thus, all patients with HIT should be continued on anticoagulation until the risk of thrombosis is decreased, regardless of whether there is additional need of ongoing anticoagulation. Patients should not be switched to low-molecular-weight heparin (LMWH). While the incidence of HIT is lower with LMWH, there is cross-reactivity with heparin-PF4 antibodies, and thrombosis can occur. Choice of anti-coagulation should be with either a direct thrombin inhibitor or a factor Xa inhibitor. The direct thrombin inhibitors include lepirudin, argatroban, and bivalirudin. In this patient, argatroban is the appropriate choice because the patient has developed acute renal failure in association with contrast dye administration for the cardiac catheterization. Argatroban is hepatically metabolized and is safe to give in renal failure, whereas lepirudin is renally metabolized. Dosage of lepirudin in renal failure is unpredictable, and lepirudin should not be used in this setting. The factor Xa inhibitors, fondaparinux or danaparoid, are also possible treatments for HIT, but due to renal metabolism, are also contraindicated in this patient. Finally, warfarin is contraindicated as sole treatment for HIT as the fall in vitamin K–dependent anticoagulant factors, especially factor C, can further increase risk of thrombosis and trigger skin necrosis.

III-30.   The answer is C. *(Chap. 61)*   This patient presents with signs and symptoms of eosino-philia-myalgia syndrome, which is triggered by ingestion of contaminants in L-tryptophan-containing products. This is a multisystem disease that can present acutely and can be fa-tal. The two clinical hallmarks are marked eosinophilia and myalgias without any obvi-ous etiology. Eosinophilic fasciitis, pneumonitis, and myocarditis may be present. Typical eosinophil counts are >1000/μL. Treatment includes withdrawal of all L-tryptophan-containing products and administration of glucocorticoids. Lactose intolerance is very common and typically presents with diarrhea and gas pains temporally related to inges-tion of lactose-containing foods. While systemic lupus erythematosus can present in myriad ways, eosinophilia and myalgias are atypical of this illness. Celiac disease, also known as gluten-sensitive enteropathy, is characterized by malabsorption and weight loss and can present with non-gastrointestinal symptoms; these classically include arthritis and central nervous system disturbance. The case above would not be compatible with celiac disease.

III-31.   The answer is B. *(Chap. 78)*   The American Cancer Society recommends yearly Pap testing beginning at age 21 or 3 years after first intercourse. The United States Preven-tive Services Task Force (USPSTF) recommends Pap testing every 1–3 years for women ages 18–65. At age 30, women who have had 3 successive years of normal test results may extend the screening interval to 2–3 years. An upper age limit at which screening ceases to be effective is unknown, however, women >70 years may choose to stop testing if they have had normal Pap smears for the previous 10 years. Women who have no cervical remnant (i.e., with total hysterectomy) do not require Pap smear testing. Current recommendations advise continued Pap screening even after receiv-ing HPV vaccination given that the vaccine does not protect against all forms of hu-man papilloma virus that cause cervical cancer. The vaccine protects against the strains that cause about 70% of the cervical cancers.

III-32.   The answer is F. *(Chap. 105)*   Viscosity testing is typically reserved for cases of multiple myeloma where paraproteins (particularly IgM) can lead to vascular sludging and subse-quent tissue ischemia. ALL can lead to end-organ abnormalities in kidney and liver there-fore routine chemistry tests are indicated. A lumbar puncture must be performed in cases of newly diagnosed ALL to rule out spread of disease to the central nervous system. Bone marrow biopsy reveals the degree of marrow infiltration and is often necessary for classi-fication of the tumor. Immunologic cell-surface marker testing often identifies the cell lineage involved and the type of tumor, information that is often impossible to discern from morphologic interpretation alone. Cytogenetic testing provides key prognostic in-formation on the disease natural history.

III-33.   The answer is A. *(Chap. 78)*   Lead-time bias, length-time bias, selection bias, overdiag-nosis bias, and avoidance bias can make a screening test appear to improve outcomes when it does not. When lead-time bias occurs, survival appears increased, but life is not truly prolonged. The test only lengthens the time that the patient, the physician, or the investigator is aware of the disease. When length-time bias occurs, aggressive cancers are not detected during screening, presumably due to the higher mortality from these cancers and the length of the screening interval. Selection bias can occur when the test population is either healthier or at higher risk for developing the condition than the general public. Overdiagnosis bias, such as with some indolent forms of prostate cancer, detects conditions that will never cause significant mortality or morbidity during a person's lifetime. The goal of screening is to detect disease at an earlier and more curable stage.

III-34. The answer is B. *(Chap. 352)* The porphyrias are a group of metabolic disorders resulting from a specific enzyme deficiency in the heme synthesis pathway. All are inherited except porphyria cutanea tarda (PCT), which is usually sporadic. The porphyrias are classified as erythropoietic or hepatic, depending on the primary site of overproduction or accumulation of porphyrins or precursors. The predominant symptoms of the hepatic porphyrias (e.g., acute intermittent porphyria, PCT) are neurologic including pain, neuropathy, and mental disturbances. The erythropoietic porphyrias usually present with cutaneous photosensitivity at birth. However, PCT, which is a hepatic porphyria, usually presents with skin lesions. The genetic mutations that cause each type of porphyria have been elucidated, and demonstration of a specific gene defect or resulting enzyme deficiency is required for definitive diagnosis. Clinical symptoms of porphyria are notoriously nonspecific with great overlap. Laboratory measurements of fecal, urinary, or plasma protoporphyrins, porphobilinogens, or porphyrins during a crisis will help guide diagnosis but require further testing for confirmation. The symptoms of many of the porphyrias are exacerbated by a large number and wide variety of drugs.

III-35. The answer is C. *(Chaps. 110 and 111)* Lupus anticoagulants cause prolongation of coagulation tests by binding to phospholipids. Although most often encountered in patients with SLE, they may develop in normal individuals. The diagnosis is first suggested by prolongation of coagulation tests. Failure to correct with incubation with normal plasma confirms the presence of a circulating inhibitor. Contrary to the name, patients with LA activity have normal hemostasis and are not predisposed to bleeding. Instead, they are at risk for venous and arterial thromboembolisms. Patients with a history of recurrent unplanned abortions or thrombosis should undergo lifelong anticoagulation. The presence of lupus anticoagulants or anticardiolipin antibodies without a history of thrombosis may be observed as many of these patients will not go on to develop a thrombotic event.

III-36. The answer is A. *(Chaps. 110 and 111)* Factor V Leiden refers to a point mutation in the factor V gene (arginine to glutamine at position 506). This makes the molecule resistant to degradation by activated protein C. This disorder alone may account for up to 25% of inherited prothrombotic states, making it the most common of these disorders. Heterozygosity for this mutation increases an individual's lifetime risk of venous thromboembolism sevenfold. A homozygote has a 20-fold increased risk of thrombosis. Prothrombin gene mutation is probably the second most common condition that causes "hypercoagulability." Antithrombin, protein C, and protein S deficiencies are more rare. Antithrombin complexes with activated coagulation proteins and blocks their biologic activity. Deficiency in antithrombin therefore promotes prolonged activity of coagulation proteins, resulting in thrombosis. Similarly, protein C and protein S are involved in the proteolysis of factors Va and VIIIa, which shuts off fibrin formation. Because proteins C and S are dependent on vitamin K for carboxylation, administration of warfarin anticoagulants may lower the level of proteins C and S more quickly relative to factors II, VII, IX, and X, thereby promoting coagulation. Patients with protein C deficiency may develop warfarin-related skin necrosis.

III-37. The answer is E. *(Chap. 112)* Low-molecular-weight heparins have become widely used in the management of uncomplicated DVT and pulmonary embolus due to their ease of administration and predictable anticoagulant effects. LMWH is derived from unfractionated heparin by chemical or enzymatic depolymerization that results in smaller fragments of heparin, weighing approximately one-third the mean molecular mass of un-fractionated heparin. The mechanism of action of the LMWH is different from that of heparin in that the anticoagulant effect of LMWH is related to its ability to potentiate factor Xa inhibition via activating antithrombin. While heparin does have the ability to potentiate factor Xa, heparin primarily acts as a cofactor to activate antithrombin and binding antithrombin to thrombin. In order to activate antithrombin, an 18-unit poly-saccharide chain is required. With a mean molecular mass of 5000 kD, the average pentasaccharide chain of LMWH is only 17 units, and thus over half the LMWH molecules lack the ability to bridge antithrombin to thrombin. A further difference between LMWH and unfractionated heparin is that LMWH is less bound to proteins in plasma, resulting in >90% bioavailability after SC injection. Thus, LMWHs have a more predictable anti-coagulant response and a longer half-life. Because of the pharmacokinetics of LMWH, most individuals do not require monitoring of factor Xa levels to ensure adequate antico-agulation, allowing for outpatient treatment of uncomplicated DVT and pulmonary em-bolus. When outcomes are compared with heparin, LMWHs are equally effective for treatment, but there is substantial health care savings when outpatient treatment is used. Furthermore, studies have demonstrated that serious bleeding events are less likely to oc-cur with LMWH than with unfractionated heparin. Thrombocytopenia is also less likely to occur with LMWH compared to unfractionated heparin. A meta-analysis of 5275 pa-tients on 13 studies suggested that the rates of thrombocytopenia in patients on unfrac-tionated heparin and LMWH may actually be similar (*Morris et al., 2007*). Caution should be taken, however, when using LMWH in individuals who are obese, pregnant, or have renal insufficiency. In these instances, monitoring of factor Xa levels is required to ensure adequacy of dosing without evidence of drug accumulation.

III-38. **The answer is B.** *(Chap. 112; CL Bennett.)* The patient has evidence of thrombotic thrombocytopenic purpura (TTP) from clopidogrel manifested as altered mental status, fever, acute renal failure, thrombocytopenia, and microangiopathic hemolytic anemia. The peripheral blood smear show anisocytosis with schistocytes and platelet clumping consistent with this disease. Clopidogrel is a thienopyridine antiplatelet agent that is known to be associated with life-threatening hematologic effects, including neutropenia, TTP, and aplastic anemia. The true incidence of TTP associated with thienopyridine use is unknown, but it occurs with both clopidogrel and ticlopidine use. When compared to ticlopidine, TTP associated with clopidogrel use occurs earlier (often within 2 weeks) and tends to be less responsive to therapy with plasmapheresis. In addition, individuals with TTP associated with clopidogrel generally have a higher platelet count and creatinine and their TTP is less likely to be associated with ADAMTS13 deficiency, a von Willebrand fac-tor–cleaving protease implicated in the pathogenesis of idiopathic TTP. The mortality of TTP associated with thienopyridines is approximately 25–30%.

III-39. **The answer is B.** *(Chap. 94)* Metastatic tumors of bone are more common than pri-mary bone tumors. Prostate, breast, and lung primaries account for 80% of all bone me-tastases. Tumors from the kidney, bladder, and thyroid and lymphomas and sarcomas also commonly metastasize to bone. Metastases usually spread hematogenously. In de-creasing order, the most common sites of bone metastases include vertebrae, proximal fe-mur, pelvis, ribs, sternum, proximal humerus, and skull. Pain is the most common symptom. Hypercalcemia may occur with bone destruction. Lesions may be osteolytic, osteoblastic, or both. Osteoblastic lesions are associated with a higher level of alkaline phosphatase.

III-40. **The answer is D.** *(Chap. 101)* Each of the listed diagnoses has a rather characteristic set of laboratory findings that are virtually diagnostic for the disease once the disease has progressed to a severe stage. Both HUS and TTP cause hemolysis and thrombocytopenia, as well as fevers. Cerebrovascular events and mental status change occur more commonly in TTP, and renal failure is more common in HUS. Severe leptospirosis, or Weil's disease, is notable for fevers, hyperbilirubinemia, and renal failure. Conjunctival suffusion is an-other helpful clue. Acute promyelocytic leukemia is notable for anemia, thrombocytopenia, and either elevated or decreased white blood cell count, all in the presence of disseminated intravascular coagulation. PNH is a rare disorder characterized by hemolytic anemia (particularly at night), venous thrombosis, and deficient hematopoiesis. It is a stem cell–derived intracorpuscular defect. Anemia is usually moderate in severity, and there is often concomitant granulocytopenia and thrombocytopenia. Venous thrombosis occurs much more commonly than in the population at large. The intraabdominal veins are often involved, and patients may present with Budd-Chiari syndrome. Cerebral sinus thrombosis is a common cause of death in patients with PNH. The presence of pancytopenia and hemolysis should raise suspicion for this diagnosis, even before the development of a venous thrombosis. In the past PNH was diagnosed by abnormalities on the Ham or sucrose lysis test; however, currently flow cytometry analysis of glycosylphosphatidylinositol (GPI) linked proteins (such as CD55 and CD59) on red blood cells and granulocytes is recommended.

III-41. **The answer is A.** *(Chap. 103)* Chronic idiopathic myelofibrosis (IMF) is the least common myeloproliferative disorder and is considered a diagnosis of exclusion after other causes of myelofibrosis have been ruled out. The typical patient with IMF presents in the sixth decade, and the disorder is asymptomatic in many patients. Fevers, fatigue, night sweats, and weight loss may occur in IMF whereas these symptoms are rare in other myeloproliferative disorders. However, no signs or symptoms are specific for the diagnosis of IMF. Often marked splenomegaly is present and may extend across the midline and to the pelvic brim. A peripheral blood smear demonstrates the typical findings of myelofibrosis including teardrop-shaped red blood cells, nucleated red blood cells, myelocytes, and metamyelocytes that are indicative of extramedullary hematopoiesis. Anemia is usually mild, and platelet and leukocyte counts are often normal. Bone marrow aspirate is frequently unsuccessful because the extent of marrow fibrosis makes aspiration impossible. When a bone marrow biopsy is performed, it demonstrates hypercellular marrow with trilineage hyperplasia and increased number of megakaryocytes with large dysplastic nuclei. Interestingly, individuals with IMF often have associated autoantibodies, including rheumatoid factor, antinuclear antibodies, or a positive Coomb's tests. To diagnose someone as having IMF, it must be shown that they do not have another myeloproliferative disorder or hematologic malignancy that is the cause of myelofibrosis. The most common disorders that present in a similar fashion to IMF are polycythemia vera and chronic myelogenous leukemia. Other nonmalignant disorders that can cause myelofibrosis include HIV infection, hyperparathyroidism, renal osteodystrophy, systemic lupus erythematosus, tuberculosis, and marrow replacement in other cancers such as prostate or breast cancer. In the patient described here, there is no other identifiable cause of myelofibrosis; thus chronic idiopathic myelofibrosis can be diagnosed.

III-42. **The answer is E.** *(Chaps. 96 and 270)* Although it once was thought that most cases of hypercalcemia of malignancy are due to a direct resorption of bone by the tumor, it is now recognized that 80% of such instances occur because of the production of a protein called parathyroid hormone reactive protein (PTHrP) by the tumor. PTHrP shares 80% homology in the first 13 terminal amino acids with native parathyroid hormone. The aberrantly produced molecule is essentially functionally identical to native parathyroid hormone in that it causes renal calcium conservation, osteoclast activation and bone resorption, renal phosphate wasting, and increased levels of urinary cyclic adenine monophosphate (cAMP). Only about 20% of cases of the hypercalcemia malignancy are due to local production of substances, such as transforming growth factor and IL-1 or IL-6, which cause bone resorption at the local level and release of calcium from bony stores. Although aggressive hydration with saline and administration of a loop diuretic are helpful in the short-term management of patients with the hypercalcemia of malignancy, the most important therapy is the administration of a bisphosphonate, such as pamidronate, that will control the laboratory abnormalities and the associated symptoms in the vast majority of these patients. Symptoms of hypercalcemia are nonspecific and include fatigue, lethargy, polyuria, nausea, vomiting, and decreased mental acuity.

III-43. **The answer is A.** *(Chap. 61)* Under normal or nonstress conditions, roughly 90% of the neutrophil pool is in the bone marrow, 2–3% in the circulation, and the remainder in the tissues. The circulating pool includes the freely flowing cells in the bloodstream and the others are marginated in close proximity to the endothelium. Most of the marginated pool is in the lung, which has a vascular endothelium surface area. Margination in the postcapillary venules is mediated by selectins that cause a low-affinity neutrophil–endothelial cell interaction that mediates "rolling" of the neutrophils along the endothelium. A variety of signals including interleukin 1, tumor necrosis factor α, and other chemokines can cause leukocytes to proliferate and leave the marrow and enter the circulation. Neutrophil integrins mediate the stickiness of neutrophils to endothelium and are important for chemokine-induced cell activation. Infection causes a marked increase in bone marrow production of neutrophils that marginate and enter tissue. Acute glucocorticoids increase neutrophil count by mobilizing cells from the bone marrow and marginated pool.

III-44. **The answer is A.** *(Chap. 101)* Haptoglobin is an α globulin normally present in serum. It binds specifically to the globin portion of hemoglobin, and the complex is cleared by the mononuclear cell phagocytosis. Haptoglobin is reduced in all hemolytic anemias as it binds free hemoglobin. It can also be reduced in cirrhosis and so is not diagnostic of hemolysis outside of the correct clinical context. Assuming a normal marrow and iron stores, the reticulocyte count will be elevated as well to try to compensate for the increased red cell destruction of hemolysis. Release of intracellular contents from the red cell (including hemoglobin and LDH) induces heme metabolism, producing unconjugated bilirubinemia. If the haptoglobin system is overwhelmed, the kidney will filter free hemoglobin and reabsorb it in the proximal tubule for storage of iron by ferritin and hemosiderin. Hemosiderin in the urine is a marker of filtered hemoglobin by the kidneys. In massive hemolysis, free hemoglobin may be excreted in urine.

III-45. **The answer is B.** *(Chap. 112)* Antiplatelet and anticoagulant agents act by a variety of mechanisms. Platelet aggregation is dependent initially on the binding of von Willebrand factor and platelet glycoprotein IB. This initiates the release of a variety of molecules, including thromboxane A_2 and adenosine diphosphate (ADP), resulting in platelet aggregation. Glycoprotein IIB/IIIa receptors recognize the amino acid sequence that is present in adhesive proteins such as fibrinogen. Coagulation occurs by a convergence of different pathways on the prothrombinase complex, which mediates the conversion of fibrinogen to fibrin, thus forming the clot. Factor Xa and factor Va are two of the essential components of the prothrombinase complex. Abciximab is a monoclonal antibody of human and murine protein that binds to GpIIb/IIIa. It and other inhibitors have been studied extensively in patients with unstable angina, patients with MI, and those undergoing percutaneous coronary intervention. Clopidogrel acts by inhibiting ADP-induced platelet aggregation. It has been evaluated in many of the same settings either in place of or in conjunction with aspirin. Heparin acts to bind factor Xa and activate antithrombin. Low-molecular-weight heparins primarily act through anti–factor Xa activity. Fondaparinux is a synthetic pentasaccharide that causes selective indirect inhibition of factor Xa. Lepirudin and argatroban are direct thrombin inhibitors. They are indicated in patients with heparin-induced thrombocytopenia. Warfarin acts by inhibiting vitamin K–dependent carboxylation of factors II, VII, IX, and X.

III-46. **The answer is E.** *(Chap. 108)* In addition to chronic GHVD, there are late complications of bone marrow transplantation that result from the chemotherapy and radiotherapy preparative regimen. Children may experience decreased growth velocity and delay in the development of secondary sex characteristics. Hormone replacement may be necessary. Gonadal dysfunction is common. Men frequently become azoospermic, and women develop ovarian failure. Patients who receive total body irradiation are at risk for cataract formation and thyroid dysfunction. Although cognitive dysfunction may occur in the peritransplant period for many reasons, there is no definitive evidence that dementia occurs at an increased frequency.

III-47. **The answer is E.** *(Chap. 112)* Clopidogrel and ticlopidine are the two currently available members of the thienopyridine class of antiplatelet agents. As demonstrated in the figure below, the mechanism of action of these agents is to prevent ADP-induced platelet aggregation by irreversibly inhibiting the $P2Y_{12}$ receptor. Both agents are prodrugs that require hepatic activation by the cytochrome P450 system; in the usual dose they require several days to reach maximal effectiveness. Clopidogrel is a more potent agent than ticlopidine with fewer associated side effects, and thus it has replaced ticlopidine in clinical practice.

Other antiplatelet drugs act at other sites in the cascade that leads to platelet aggregation. Aspirin is the most commonly used antiplatelet agent. At the usual doses, aspirin inhibits COX-1 to prevent the production of thromboxane A_2, a potent platelet agonist. Dipyridamole is a weak platelet inhibitor alone and acts as a phosphodiesterase inhibitor. In addition, dipyridamole blocks the uptake of adenosine by platelets. When combined with aspirin, dipyridamole has been shown to decrease the risk of stroke, but because it acts as a vasodilator, there is concern that it might increase the risk of cardiac events in severe coronary artery disease. A final class of antiplatelet agents is the glycoprotein IIb/IIIa inhibitors, which include abciximab, eptifibatide, and tirofiban. Each of these agents has a slightly different site of action, but all decrease the ability of platelets to bind adhesive molecules such as fibrinogen and von Willebrand factor. Thus, these agents decrease platelet aggregation. Abciximab is a monoclonal antibody directed against the activated form of GPIIb/IIIa. Tirofiban and eptifibatide are small synthetic molecules that bind to various sites of the GPIIb/IIIa receptor to decrease platelet aggregation.

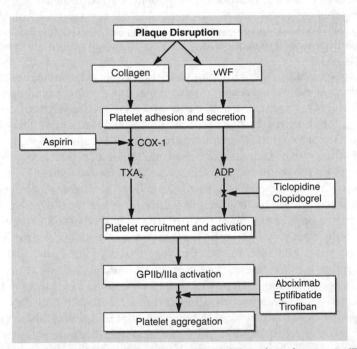

FIGURE III-47   Site of action of antiplatelet drugs. Aspirin inhibits thromboxane A_2 (TXA_2) synthesis by irreversibly acetylating cyclooxygenase-1 (COX-1). Reduced TXA_2 release attenuates platelet activation and recruitment to the site of vascular injury. Ticlopidine and clopidogrel irreversibly block $P2Y_{12}$, a key ADP receptor on the platelet surface. Therefore, these agents also attenuate platelet recruitment. Abciximab, eptifibatide, and tirofiban inhibit the final common pathway of platelet aggregation by blocking fibrinogen binding to activated glycoprotein (GP) IIb/IIIa.

III-48. **The answer is C.** *(Chap. 104)* This patient presents with typical findings of chronic myelogenous leukemia (CML) which has an incidence of 1.5 per 100,000 people yearly. The typical age of onset is in the mid-forties and there is a slight male predominance. Half of individuals are asymptomatic at the time of diagnosis. If symptoms are present, they are typically nonspecific and include fatigue and weight loss. Occasionally patients will have symptoms related to splenic enlargement such as early satiety and left upper quadrant pain. Laboratory findings are suggestive of CML. A high leukocyte count of 100,000/µL is typical, with a predominant granulocytic differential, including neutrophils, myelocytes, metamyelocytes, and band forms. The circulating blast count should be <5%. Anemia and thrombocytosis are also common. The bone marrow demonstrates nonspecific increase in cellularity with an increase in the myeloid to erythroid ratio. The definitive diagnosis of CML is usually made by demonstrating the presence of the Philadelphia chromosome, a reciprocal translocation between chromosomes 9 and 22. This cytogenetic abnormality is present in 90–95% of individuals with CML and can be found by fluorescent in situ hybridization (FISH) or by cytogenetics. This translocation results in the fusion of the *bcr* gene with the *abl* gene. The bcr-abl fusion protein results in constitutive activation of abl tyrosine kinase enzyme that prevents apoptosis and leads to increased survival of the cells containing the mutation. Ultimately, untreated CML develops into an accelerated phase with increasing numbers of mutations and leads to acute blast crisis. The deletion of the long arm of chromosome 5 is present in some acute myeloid leukemias and is associated with older age at diagnosis. The inversion of chromosome 16 is typically present in acute myelomonocytic leukemia (M4 subtype). The translocation of the long arms of chromosomes 15 and 17 is the mutation associated with acute promyelocytic anemia that results in arrest of cellular differentiation that can be treated with pharmacologic doses of ATRA. Finally, trisomy 12 is one of several mutations that may result in the development of chronic lymphocytic leukemia.

III-49. **The answer is D.** *(Chap. 70)* In a young person with no family history and without signs or symptoms suggesting a bleeding colonic lesion, colon cancer would be very unlikely. Similarly, although peptic ulcer disease and celiac sprue can cause iron deficiency by hemorrhage and malabsorption, respectively, he has neither symptoms nor stool findings consistent with gastrointestinal blood loss. Impaired iron absorption is commonly caused by dietary composition. High amounts of calcium or lead or the lack of ascorbic acid or amino acids in the meal can impair iron absorption. Calcium can cause a substantial decrease in iron absorption. This patient should be advised to make sure he does not take his iron tablet at the same time as his calcium tablet.

III-50. **The answer is D.** *(Chap. 92)* Testicular cancer occurs most commonly in the second and third decades of life. The treatment depends on the underlying pathology and the stage of the disease. Germ cell tumors are divided into seminomatous and nonseminomatous subtypes. Although the pathology of this patient's tumor was seminoma, the presence of AFP is suggestive of occult nonseminomatous components. If there are any nonseminomatous components, the treatment follows that of a nonseminomatous germ cell tumor. This patient therefore has a clinical stage I nonseminomatous germ cell tumor. As his AFP returned to normal after orchiectomy, there is no obvious occult disease. However, between 20 and 50% of these patients will have disease in the retroperitoneal lymph nodes. Because numerous trials have indicated no survival difference in this cohort between observation and RPLND and because of the potential side effects of RPLND, either approach is reasonable. Radiation therapy is the appropriate choice for stage I and stage II seminoma. It has no role in nonseminomatous lesions. Adjuvant chemotherapy is not indicated in early-stage testicular cancer. Hormonal therapy is effective for prostate cancer and receptor positive breast cancer but has no role in testicular cancer. PET scan has no currently defined clinical role.

III-51. **The answer is C.** *(Chap. 78)* Tobacco use is the most modifiable risk factor for cardiovascular disease, respiratory disease, and cancer. Smokers have a 33% lifetime chance of dying from a smoking-related cause. While tobacco is associated with more cardiovascular deaths than cancer deaths, it is associated with malignancies in the mouth, lung, esophagus, kidney, bladder, pancreas, and stomach. The degree of smoke exposure as well as the degree of inhalation is correlated with risk of lung cancer mortality. Smokeless tobacco is the fastest growing part of the tobacco industry and carries with it a substantial risk for dental and gingival disease as well as oral and esophageal cancers. Most American smokers begin before 18 years of age. The COMMIT trial showed that a cessation message and cessation programs were effective for light tobacco smokers, whereas heavy smokers were more likely to need counseling, behavioral strategies, or pharmacologic adjuncts. Most Americans who quit smoking cigarettes, however, do so without involvement in a cessation program.

III-52. **The answer is B.** *(Chap. 95)* The patient is a young man with asymmetric hilar adenopathy. The differential diagnosis would include lymphoma, testicular cancer, and, less likely, tuberculosis or histoplasmosis. Because of his young age, testicular examination and ultrasonography would be indicated, as would measurement of β-hCG and AFP, which are generally markedly elevated. In men with carcinoma of unknown primary source, AFP and β-hCG should be checked as the presence of testicular cancer portends an improved prognosis compared with possible primary sources. Biopsy would show lymphoma. The ACE level may be elevated but is not diagnostic of sarcoidosis. Thyroid disorders are not likely to present with unilateral hilar adenopathy. Finally, PSA is not indicated in this age category, and C-reactive protein would not differentiate any of the disorders mentioned above. Biopsy is the most important diagnostic procedure.

III-53. **The answer is A.** *(Chap. 85)* Approximately 20% of all lung cancers are small-cell cancers. These tumors tend to present centrally, be derived from neuroendocrine tissues, and be much more chemo-and radiosensitive than non-small cell cancer. Histologic subtypes of non-small cell cancer include adenocarcinoma (which has a more often peripheral presentation), large cell cancer, bronchoalveolar cell cancer, and squamous cell (or bronchogenic) lung cancer. All histologic types of lung cancer are associated with smoking. In the relatively uncommon patient who presents with a small non-small cell primary lesion and no lymph node involvement, surgery alone may be curative. Patients with small-cell lung cancer are divided into two staging groups: those with limited disease who have tumors generally confined to one hemithorax encompassable by a single radiation port and all others who are said to have extensive disease. About 20 percent of patients who present with limited-stage small-cell lung cancer are curable with a combination of radiation therapy and chemotherapy, with cisplatin and etoposide being the two most active agents.

III-54. **The answer is D.** *(Chap. 87)* In the United States, esophageal cancers are either squamous cell carcinomas or adenocarcinomas. Esophageal cancer is a deadly cancer with a very high mortality rate, regardless of cell type. This is because diagnosis is usually made well after patients develop symptoms, meaning that the mass is often large with frequent spread to the mediastinum and paraaortic lymph nodes, by the time that endoscopy is considered for diagnosis. Smoking and alcohol consumption are synergistic risks for squamous cell carcinoma, not adenocarcinoma. Other risks for squamous cell carcinoma include nitrites, smoked opiates, mucosal injury (including ingestion of hot tea), and achalasia. The major risk for adenocarcinoma is chronic gastric reflux, gastric metaplasia of the esophagus (Barrett's esophagus). These adenocarcinomas account for 60% of esophageal carcinomas and behave like gastric carcinomas. In recent years, the incidence of squamous carcinoma of the esophagus has declined while the incidence of adenocarcinoma has increased, particularly in white men. Approximately 10% of esophageal carcinomas arise in the upper third, 35% in the middle third, and 55% in the lower third. Fewer than 5% of patients with esophageal carcinoma survive 5 years. There is no consistent advantage of one cell type over another. Surgery, radiation therapy, and chemotherapy are all options, but usually these interventions are palliative.

III-55. **The answer is E.** *(Chap. 79)* A small proportion of cancers occur in patients with a genetic predisposition. Roughly 100 syndromes of familial cancer have been reported. Recognition allows for genetic counseling and increased cancer surveillance. Down's syndrome, or trisomy 21, is characterized clinically by a variety of features, including moderate to severe learning disability, facial and musculoskeletal deformities, duodenal atresia, congenital heart defects, and an increased risk of acute leukemia. Fanconi's anemia is a condition that is associated with defects in DNA repair. There is a higher incidence of cancer, with leukemia and myelodysplasia being the most common cancers. Von Hippel–Lindau syndrome is associated with hemangioblastomas, renal cysts, pancreatic cysts and carcinomas, and renal cell cancer. Neurofibromatosis (NF) type I and type II are both associated with increased tumor formation. NF II is more associated with a schwannoma. Both carry a risk of malignant peripheral nerve sheath tumors. Fragile X is a condition associated with chromosomal instability of the X chromosome. These patients have mental retardation, typical morphologic features including macroorchidism and prognathia, behavioral problems, and occasionally seizures. Increased cancer incidence has not been described.

III-56. **The answer is E.** *(Chap. 103)* Thrombocytosis may be "primary" or "secondary." Essential thrombocytosis is a myeloproliferative disorder that involves a multipotent hematopoietic progenitor cell. Unfortunately, there is no clonal marker that can reliably distinguish it from more common nonclonal, reactive forms of thrombocytosis. Therefore, the diagnosis is one of exclusion. Common causes of secondary thrombocytosis include infection, inflammatory conditions, malignancy, iron deficiency, hemorrhage, and postsurgical states. Other myeloproliferative disorders, such as CML and myelofibrosis, may result in thrombocytosis. Similarly, myelodysplastic syndromes, particularly the 5q-syndrome, may cause thrombocytosis. Pernicious anemia caused by vitamin B_{12} deficiency does not typically cause thrombocytosis. However, correction of B_{12} deficiency or folate deficiency may cause a "rebound" thrombocytosis. Similarly, cessation of chronic ethanol use may also cause a rebound thrombocytosis.

III-57. **The answer is A.** *(Chap. 111)* D-Dimer is a degradation product of cross-linked fibrin and is elevated in conditions of ongoing thrombosis. Low concentrations of D-dimer are considered to indicate the absence of thrombosis. Patients over the age of 70 will frequently have elevated D-dimers in the absence of thrombosis, making this test less predictive of acute disease. Clinical symptoms are often not present in patients with DVT and do not affect interpretation of a D-dimer. Tobacco use, while frequently considered a risk factor for DVT, and previous DVT should not affect the predictive value of D-dimer. Homan's sign, calf pain elicited by dorsiflexion of the foot, is not predictive of DVT and is unrelated to D-dimer.

III-58. **The answer is E.** *(Chap. 61)* Many drugs can lead to neutropenia, most commonly via retarding neutrophil production in the bone marrow. Of the list above, trimethoprim-sulfamethoxazole is the most likely culprit. Other common causes of drug-induced neutropenia include alkylating agents such as cyclophosphamide or busulfan, antimetabolites including methotrexate and 5-flucytosine, penicillin and sulfonamide antibiotics, antithyroid drugs, antipsychotics, and anti-inflammatory agents. Prednisone, when used systemically, often causes an increase in the circulating neutrophil count as it leads to demargination of neutrophils and bone marrow stimulation. Ranitidine, an H_2 blocker, is a well-described cause of thrombocytopenia but has not been implicated in neutropenia. Efavirenz is a non-nucleoside reverse transcriptase inhibitor whose main side effects include a morbilliform rash and central nervous system effects including strange dreams and confusion. The presence of these symptoms does not require drug cessation. Darunavir is a new protease inhibitor that is well tolerated. Common side effects include a maculopapular rash and lipodystrophy, a class effect for all protease inhibitors.

III-59. **The answer is E.** *(Chap. 87)* Although esophageal masses and cancer can lead to several types of dysphagia, the most common complaint is solid food dysphagia that worsens to the point that liquids are also hard to swallow. Such a complaint warrants upper endoscopy, particularly if the patient falls in a high-risk group for esophageal cancer, with careful examination of the stomach, trachea, and larynx. Odynophagia with chest pain is more reminiscent of ulcerative disease of the esophagus due to either infection, such as cytomegalovirus or *Candida*, or pill esophagitis. Spasm causes severe pain as well, but this may occur independent of swallowing. Liquid phase dysphagia often implies a functional disorder of the esophagus rather than a mass-like obstruction. A barium swallowing study or cine-esophagram in conjunction with a thorough history and physical examination may prove diagnostic. Oropharyngeal dysphagia usually localizes disease quite specifically to the oropharynx. Early satiety is often due to gastric obstruction or extrinsic compression of the stomach (splenomegaly is a common reason for this), or to a functional gastric disorder such as gastroparesis.

III-60. **The answer is C.** *(Chap. 105)* Hepatitis B and C are both common causes of cirrhosis and are strongly associated with the development of hepatocellular carcinoma. Hepatitis C, but not hepatitis B, can also lead to a lymphoplasmacytic lymphoma, often in the spleen, that resolves with cure of hepatitis C. Other infections are commonly implicated as causes of lymphoma. Epstein-Barr virus has been associated with a large number of lymphoid malignancies including posttransplant lymphoproliferative disease (PTLD), Hodgkin's disease, central nervous system lymphoma, and Burkitt's lymphoma. *H. pylori* is necessary and sufficient for gastric mucosa-associated lymphoid tissue lymphoma development, and cure can be achieved with eradication of the organism in some cases. HHV8 is a known cause of body cavity lymphoma, including primary pleural lymphoma. Celiac sprue has been associated with gastrointestinal tract lymphoma. Many collagen vascular diseases and their treatments (tumor necrosis factor α inhibitors) have also been associated with lymphomas, as have acquired and inherited immunodeficiencies.

III-61. **The answer is D.** *(Chaps. 102 and 103)* Chronic idiopathic myelofibrosis is a clonal disorder of a multipotent hematopoietic progenitor cell of unknown etiology that is characterized by marrow fibrosis, myeloid metaplasia, extramedullary hematopoiesis, and splenomegaly. The peripheral blood smear reflects the features of extramedullary hematopoiesis, with teardrop-shaped red cells, immature myeloid cells, and abnormal platelets. Leukocytes and platelets may both be elevated. The median survival is poor at only 5 years. These patients eventually succumb to increasing organomegaly, infection, and possible transformation to acute leukemia. There is no specific therapy for chronic idiopathic myelofibrosis. Erythropoietin has not been shown to be consistently effective and may exacerbate splenomegaly. Supportive care with red blood cell transfusions is necessary as anemia worsens. Chemotherapy has no role in changing the natural history of the disease. Some newer agents, such as interferon and thalidomide, may play a role, but their place is not clear. Splenectomy may be necessary in symptomatic patients with massive splenomegaly. However, extramedullary hematopoiesis may worsen with rebound thrombocytosis and compensatory hepatomegaly. The only potential curative modality is allogeneic bone marrow transplantation. Morbidity and mortality are high, particularly in older patients. In light of this patient's young age and the presence of three healthy siblings, HLA matching of her siblings is the most reasonable step.

III-62. **The answer is D.** *(Chap. 98)* Iron deficiency anemia is a condition in which there is anemia and clear evidence of iron deficiency. Initially, a state of negative iron balance occurs during which iron stores become slowly depleted. Serum ferritin may decrease, and the presence of stainable iron on bone marrow preparation decreases. When iron stores are depleted, serum iron begins to fall. TIBC starts to increase, reflecting the presence of circulating unbound transferrin. Once the transferrin saturation falls to 15 to 20%, hemoglobin synthesis is impaired. The peripheral blood smear reveals the presence of microcytic and hypochromic red cells. Reticulocytes may also become hypochromic. Reticulocyte numbers are reduced relative to the level of anemia, reflecting a hypoproduction anemia secondary to iron deficiency. Clinically, these patients exhibit the usual signs of anemia: fatigue, pallor, and reduced exercise capacity. Cheilosis and koilonychia are signs of advanced tissue iron deficiency. Some patients may experience pica, a desire to ingest certain materials, such as ice (pagophagia) and clay (geophagia).

III-63. **The answer is D.** *(Chap. 67)* Regardless of the source of stem cells used in regenerative strategies, a number of generic and specific problems must be overcome before successful clinical applications are available. Embryonic stem cells tend to develop abnormal karyotypes and have the potential to form teratomas. Umbilical cord blood stem cells have less graft-versus-host disease than marrow-derived stem cells and are less likely to be contaminated by the herpes virus. Organ-specific multipotent stem cells are easy to isolate from the marrow but are difficult to isolate from tissues such as the heart and brain. Early studies of bone marrow mesenchymal stem cells have shown that the transplanted cells fuse with cells resident in the organ.

III-64. The answer is B. *(Chap. 58)* The first step in diagnosing polycythemia vera is to document an elevated red blood cell (RBC) mass. A normal RBC mass suggests spurious polycythemia. Next, serum erythropoietin (EPO) levels should be measured. If EPO levels are low, the diagnosis is polycythemia vera. Confirmatory tests include JAK-2 mutation analysis, leukocytosis, and thrombocytosis. Elevated EPO levels are seen in the normal physiologic response to hypoxia as well as in autonomous production of EPO. Further steps in the workup include evaluation for hypoxia with an arterial blood gas, consideration of smoker's polycythemia (elevated carboxyhemoglobin levels) and disorders of increased hemoglobin affinity for oxygen. Low serum EPO levels with low oxygen saturation suggest inadequate renal production (renal failure). High RBC mass and high EPO levels with normal oxygen saturation may be seen with autonomous EPO production, such as in renal cell carcinoma.

III-65. The answer is E. *(Chap. 352)* Any increase in hepatic iron will exacerbate PCT, and efforts should be made to minimize iron overload. The first step in management of PCT is to identify and discontinue any potential trigger (alcohol, estrogens, iron supplements). PCT that does not respond to these conservative measures requires weekly phlebotomy with the goal of reducing hepatic iron. In the above case, conservative measures have not led to remission and phlebotomy is necessary. Serum ferritin can be used as a gauge of hepatic iron overload and should guide the course of phlebotomy. Iron infusion or oral iron supplementation would result in an exacerbation of PCT by increasing iron stores. Hydroxyurea is used to treat sickle cell disease and some forms of essential thrombocytosis; it has no role in the primary management of PCT.

III-66. The answer is E. *(Chap. 101)* Hemolytic anemias may be classified as intracorpuscular or extracorpuscular. In intracorpuscular disorders, the patient's red blood cells (RBCs) have an abnormally short life span due to an intrinsic RBC factor. In extracorpuscular disorders, the RBC has a short life span due to a nonintrinsic RBC factor. Thrombotic thrombocytopenic purpura (TTP) is an acquired disorder where red cell and platelet destruction occur not because of defects of these cell lines, but rather as a result of microangiopathy leading to destructive shear forces on the cells. Other clinical sign and symptoms include fever, mental status change, and, less commonly, renal impairment. All cases of hemolysis in conjunction with thrombocytopenia should be rapidly ruled out for TTP by evaluation of a peripheral smear for schistocytes as plasmapheresis is life-saving. Other causes of extravascular hemolytic anemia include hypersplenism, autoimmune hemolytic anemia, disseminated intravascular coagulation, and other microangiopathic hemolytic anemias. The other four disorders listed in the question all refer to some defect of the red blood cell itself that leads to hemolysis. Elliptocytosis is a membranopathy that leads to varying degrees of destruction of the red cell in the reticuloendothelial system. Sickle cell anemia is a congenital hemoglobinopathy classified by recurrent pain crises and numerous long-term sequelae that is due to a well-defined β globin mutation. Pyruvate kinase deficiency is a rare disorder of the glycolytic pathway that causes hemolytic anemia. Paroxysmal nocturnal hemoglobinuria (PNH) is a form of acquired hemolysis due to an intrinsic abnormality of the red cell. It also often causes thrombosis and cytopenias. Bone marrow failure is a feared association with PNH.

III-67. The answer is B. *(Chap. 67)* There are many attractive targets for which to use stem cells as regenerative therapies (e.g., myocardial infarction, type I diabetes, Parkinson's disease). All of the other options represent a few of the obstacles that are yet to be overcome. Stem cell therapies raise important questions about the definition of human life and have raised issues of justice and safety regarding the care of patients. It is clear that the resolution of these ethical issues will require multidisciplinary discussion between scientists, physicians, patients, lawmakers, and the general public.

III-68. The answer is C. *(Chap. 112)* Heparin-induced thrombocytopenia (HIT) is common in patients who receive heparin products. Because the risk of death is significantly increased in patients with HIT type II and thrombosis if no anticoagulation is given, observation or simply discontinuation of heparin is not an option. Although enoxaparin and other low-molecular-weight heparins have less of a propensity to cause HIT, they are cross-reactive in patients who already have HIT and thus are contraindicated. Direct thrombin inhibitors are the treatment of choice. Lepirudin is a recombinant direct thrombin inhibitor. It may be given intravenously or subcutaneously. It is excreted through the kidney and lacks an antidote. Therefore, it is relatively contraindicated in patients with renal insufficiency. Argatroban is another direct thrombin inhibitor. Because it is hepatically metabolized, it is a reasonable option in patients with HIT and renal insufficiency.

III-69.   The answer is B.   *(Chap. 105)*   Autoimmune hemolytic anemia and thrombocytopenia are common, and a peripheral blood smear and a Coomb's test help evaluate their presence. Hypersplenism is also seen in CLL as the spleen sequesters large numbers of circulating blood cells and enlarges. Hence, a careful left upper quadrant examination looking for a palpable splenic tip is the standard of care in this situation. This patient is at risk of hepatic decompensation as well, given his hepatitis C that can also cause anemia and thrombocytopenia. Bone marrow infiltration of tumor cells can lead to cytopenias in CLL. However, this is in effect a diagnosis of exclusion. Once these three possibilities are ruled out, a bone marrow biopsy is a reasonable next step. This initial evaluation before presuming spread of CLL is critical for therapy because each possibility will require different therapy (glucocorticoids or retuximab for hemolysis, hepatology referral for liver failure, and splenectomy for symptomatic hypersplenism).

III-70.   The answer is A.   *(Chap. 88)*   Currently hepatocellular carcinoma can be staged using a variety of staging systems. The TNM system set up by the American Joint Commission for Cancer has been largely replaced by either the Okuda system or the Cancer of the Liver Italian Program (CLIP) system because these systems include the presence of cirrhosis as a part of staging. This patient would have stage II disease by the TNM system because he has a single tumor >2 cm but without evidence of vascular invasion. By the CLIP system, the patient would be classified as CLIP stage I because of the presence of Child-Pugh class B cirrhosis. Primary surgical resection of a solitary mass is reserved for those individuals with stage I or II HCC or CLIP stage 0. However, because of the high rate of liver failure and mortality following surgical resection in individuals with Child-Pugh class B or C cirrhosis, these individuals are not candidates for surgical resection. Orthotopic liver transplantation (OLTX) is the treatment of choice in individuals with stage I or II disease and cirrhosis. Individuals can be referred for OLTX if there is a single mass <5 cm or three masses <3 cm and no vascular invasion is present. Radiofrequency ablation uses heat to cause necrosis of an ~7 cm zone in a non-specific manner. This technique can be used effectively in single lesions that are 3–4 cm in size. However, tumors located near the main portal pedicles can lead to bile duct injury and obstruction. Percutaneous ethanol injection (not listed) results in necrosis of the injected area and requires multiple injections. The maximum size of tumor that can be treated with percutaneous ethanol injection is 3 cm. Transarterial chemoembolization is a form of regional chemotherapy in which a variety of chemotherapeutic agents are directly injected into the hepatic artery. Two randomized trials have shown a survival advantage for transarterial chemoembolization in a highly selected subset of patients. The technique is recommended for individuals who are not candidates for orthotopic liver transplantation, including individuals with multiple medical comorbidities, more than four lesions, lymph node metastases, tumors >5 cm, and gross vascular invasion. Systemic chemotherapy has no effect on survival and has a <25% response rate. It is not recommended for most individuals with HCC. Sorafenib is a novel agent that increases median survival from 6 months to 9 months in patients with advanced disease.

III-71.   The answer is A.   *(Chap. 87)*   A strong family history of colon cancer should prompt consideration for hereditary nonpolyposis colon cancer (HNPCC), or Lynch syndrome particularly if diffuse polyposis is <u>not</u> noted on colonoscopy. HNPCC is characterized by (1) three or more relatives with histologically proven colorectal cancer, one of whom is a first-degree relative and of the other two, at least one with the diagnosis before age 50; and (2) colorectal cancer in at least two generations. The disease is an autosomal dominant trait and is associated with other tumors, including in the endometrium and ovary. The proximal colon is most frequently involved, and cancer occurs with a median age of 50 years, 15 years earlier than in sporadic colon cancer. Patients with HNPCC are recommended to receive biennial colonoscopy and pelvic ultrasound beginning at age 25. Innumerable polyps suggest the presence of one of the autosomal dominant polyposis syndromes, many of which carry a high malignant potential. These include familial adenomatous polyposis, Gardner's syndrome (associated with osteomas, fibromas, epidermoid cysts), or Turcot's syndrome (associated with brain cancer). Peutz-Jeghers syndrome is associated with mucocutaneous pigmentation and hamartomas. Tumors may develop in the ovary, breast, pancreas, and endometrium; however, malignant colon cancers are not common. Ulcerative colitis is strongly associated with development of colon cancer, but it is unusual for colon cancer to be the presenting finding in ulcerative colitis. Patients are generally symptomatic from their inflammatory bowel disease long before cancer risk develops.

III-72. **The answer is E.** *(Chap. 105)* Classical Hodgkin's disease carries a better prognosis than all types of non-Hodgkin's lymphoma. Patients with good prognostic factors can achieve cure with extended field radiation alone, while those with higher risk disease often achieve cure with high-dose chemotherapy and sometimes radiation. The chance of cure is so high (>90%) that many protocols are now considering long-term sequelae of current therapy such as carcinomas, hypothyroidism, premature coronary disease, and constrictive pericarditis in those receiving radiation therapy. Combination chemotherapy with ABVD appears to be the form of treatment with the lowest risk of late fatal complications.

III-73. **The answer is B.** *(Chap. 111)* Fibrinogen is a 340-kDa dimeric molecule made up of two sets of three covalently linked polypeptide chains. Thrombin cleaves multiple peptides to produce fibrin monomer that factor XIII stabilizes by cross-linking. Although fibrinogen is needed for platelet aggregation and fibrin formation, even severe fibrinogen deficiency such as afibrinogenemia produces mild, rare bleeding episodes, most often after surgery. Dysfibrinogenemia refers to a constellation of disorders that involve mutations that alter the release of fibrinopeptides, affect the rate of polymerization of fibrin monomers, or alter the sites of fibrin cross-linking. Dysfibrinogenemia is either inherited in an autosomal dominant fashion or acquired. Patients with liver disease, hepatomas, AIDS, and lymphoproliferative disorders may develop an acquired form of dysfibrinogenemia. The presence of altered partial thromboplastin time (PTT) and prothrombin time (PT)/INR reflects an abnormality in coagulation from the prothrombinase complex downstream to fibrin. Correction with a mixing study eliminates factor inhibition as a cause of the coagulation disorder. Other causes of prolongation of the PT and PTT include factor deficiencies in factor V or X, afibrinogenemia or dysfibrinogenemia, and consumption of coagulation factors from DIC. The absence of schistocytes from the blood smear makes DIC unlikely. The thrombin time tests the interaction with thrombin directly on fibrinogen. Its prolongation indicates an abnormality with that interaction and suggests a diagnosis of dysfibrinogenemia. Factor XIII deficiency is a bleeding disorder that manifests in childhood and is not consistent with this presentation.

III-74. **The answer is C.** *(Chap. 78)* Chemoprevention involves the use of specific natural or synthetic chemical agents to reverse, suppress, or prevent carcinogenesis before the development of invasive malignancy. Calcium, by binding to luminal free fatty acids and bile, may reduce gastrointestinal endothelium proliferation. Calcium supplementation decreases the risk of adenomatous polyps by up to 20%. Trials with cancer-incidence endpoints are currently underway. High doses of relatively toxic isotretinoin caused regression of the premalignant oral leukoplakia lesions; however, lower doses were not effective in preventing head and neck cancers. It also did not prevent second malignancies in patients cured of early stage non-small cell lung cancer. β-Carotene has been investigated for the chemoprevention of lung cancer in two trials. Both trials actually showed harm from β-carotene. Aspirin had no effect on colon cancer incidence in a 6-year trial. Cyclooxygenase-2 inhibitors have been shown to reduce recurrence rates for polyps in familial adenomatous polyposis. The effects on colon cancer in sporadic cases were initiated, but were complicated by the association of these drugs with increased cardiovascular death. Tamoxifen is used for primary prevention of breast cancer among those at very high risk. It is associated with a small increase in the risk of endometrial cancer.

III-75 and III-76. The answers are A and E. *(Chap. 104)* Treatment of acute promyelocytic leukemia (PML) is an interesting example of how understanding the function of the protein produced by the genetic abnormality can be utilized to develop a treatment for the disease. The translocation of the long arms of chromosomes 15 and 17, t(15;17), results in the production of a chimeric protein called promyelocytic leukemia (Pml)/retinoic acid receptor α (Rarα). The Pml-Rarα fusion protein suppresses gene transcription and arrests differentiation of the cells in an immature state leading to promyelocytic leukemia. Pharmacologic doses of the ligand of the Rar-α receptor, all-*trans*-retinoic acid (ATRA), stimulate the cells to resume differentiation. With use of ATRA, the leukemic cells differentiate to mature neutrophils and undergo subsequent apoptosis. This leads to treatment and remission of PML without causing the myelosuppression that is common to other chemotherapy used for treatment of leukemia. While ATRA alone can yield hematologic remission of PML, it is most often combined with traditional chemotherapeutic agents in order to generate a cytogenetic remission as well. Since introduction of ATRA into therapy of PML, complete remission and survival rates have further improved to about 75–80% at 5 years. The primary side effect of ATRA is the development of retinoic acid syndrome. The onset of retinoic acid syndrome from ATRA is usually within the first 3 weeks of treatment. Typical symptoms are chest pain, fever, and dyspnea. Hypoxia is common, and chest radiography usually shows diffuse alveolar infiltrates with pleural effusions. Pericardial effusions may also occur. The cause of retinoic acid syndrome is possibly related to the adhesion of the differentiated leukemia cells to the pulmonary endothelium or the release of cytokines by these cells to cause vascular leak. Mortality of retinoic acid syndrome is 10%. High-dose glucocorticoid therapy is usually effective in treatment of retinoic acid syndrome. Arsenic trioxide is currently indicated for the treatment of relapsed PML and is effective in up to 85% of individuals who are refractory to ATRA. Ongoing clinical trials are attempting to determine if combination therapy with ATRA and arsenic may further improve outcomes in PML. Cyclophosphamide, daunorubicin, vinblastine, and prednisone are the constituents of the combination chemotherapy commonly known as CHOP, and it is indicated for the treatment of B cell lymphomas. Rituximab is most commonly used as a treatment of B cell non-Hodgkin's lymphoma and is currently under investigation for the treatment of chronic lymphocytic leukemia and a variety of refractory autoimmune disorders, including systemic lupus erythematosus and rheumatoid arthritis. Rituximab is a monoclonal antibody directed against the CD20 cell surface molecule of B lymphocytes. Neither of these drug regimens has a role in the treatment of myeloid leukemias. Whole-body irradiation is used primarily before bone marrow transplant to ensure complete eradication of cancerous leukemic cells in the bone marrow.

III-77.   The answer is C. *(Chap. 104)* Patients with acute leukemia frequently present with nonspecific symptoms of fatigue and weight loss. In addition, weight loss and anorexia are also common. About half have had symptoms for >3 months at the time of presentation. Fever is present in only about 10% of patients at presentation, and 5% have evidence of abnormal hemostasis. On physical examination, hepatomegaly, splenomegaly, sternal tenderness, and evidence of infection or hemorrhage are common presenting signs. Laboratory studies are confirmatory with evidence of anemia, thrombocytopenia, and leukocytosis often present. The median presenting leukocyte count at presentation is 15,000/μL. About 20–40% will have presenting leukocyte counts of <5000/μL, and another 20% will have counts >100,000/μL. Review of the peripheral smear confirms leukemia in most cases. If Auer rods are seen, the diagnosis of AML is virtually certain. Thrombocytopenia (platelet count <100,000/μL) is seen in >75% of individuals with AML. Once the diagnosis of AML has been confirmed, rapid evaluation and treatment should be undertaken. The overall health of the cardiovascular, pulmonary, hepatic, and renal systems should be evaluated as chemotherapy has adverse effects that may cause organ dysfunction in any of these systems. Among the prognostic factors that predict poor outcomes in AML, age at diagnosis is one of the most important because individuals of advanced age tolerate induction chemotherapy poorly. In addition, advanced age is more likely to be associated with multiple chromosomal abnormalities that predict poorer response to chemotherapy, although some chromosomal markers predict a better response to chemotherapy. Poor performance status independent of age also decreases survival in AML. Chromosome findings at diagnosis are also very important in predicting outcomes in AML. Responsiveness to chemotherapy and survival are also worse if the leukocyte count >100,000/μL or the antecedent course of symptoms is prolonged. Anemia, leukopenia, or thrombocytopenia present for >3 months is a poor prognostic indicator. However, there is no absolute degree of anemia or thrombocytopenia that predicts worse outcomes.

III-78. **The answer is C.** *(Chap. 78)* The sensitivity of a test is a numerical description of the test's ability to detect the disease when it is present. It is the proportion of persons with the condition who also test positive. In this example, 1000 people test positive using the screening test. The number of persons who actually have the condition is 1250, yielding an 80% sensitivity.

III-79. **The answer is B.** *(Chap. 78; NEJM 349:2191, 2003)* For colon cancer screening, the three major preventive societies (i.e., American Cancer Society, The United States Preventive Services Task Force, and the Canadian Task Force on Preventive Health Care) recommend sigmoidoscopy, colonoscopy, or fecal occult blood testing (FOBT) starting at 50 years of age. Digital rectal examination is not recommended. FOBT has a high false-positive rate; 2–10% of those with a positive result have colon cancer, and ~25% have adenomas. Sigmoidoscopy has been shown to reduce mortality, and the recommended screening interval is 5 years. Sigmoidoscopy carries a perforation risk of 1/1000, while the risk with colonoscopy is three times greater. Colonoscopy detects more advanced lesions and is the screening test of choice in subjects who are at high-risk. Virtual colonoscopy using CT imaging can detect adenomatous polyps, compares favorably with endoscopic colonoscopy for polyps >8 mm in size, and may be an effective screening method in average-risk adults. It is not as sensitive as endoscopic colonoscopy for small (<5 mm) polyps.

III-80. **The answer is C.** *(Chap. 270)* Superior vena cava (SVC) syndrome is the clinical manifestation of superior vena cava obstruction with severe reduction in venous return from the head, neck, and upper extremities. Small cell and squamous cell lung cancer account for 85% of all cases of malignant superior vena cava obstruction. Common complaints include neck and facial swelling with dyspnea. Other symptoms include hoarseness, tongue swelling, headaches, nasal congestion, epistaxis, hemoptysis, dysphagia, pain, dizziness, syncope, and lethargy. Temporizing measures include diuretics, low-salt diet, oxygen, and head elevation. Glucocorticoids may be effective for shrinking the size of lymphomatous masses, but they are of no benefit in patients with primary lung cancer. Radiation therapy is the primary treatment for SVC syndrome due to non-small cell lung cancer. Chemotherapy is most effective for small cell lung cancer, lymphoma, or germ cell tumors. Some non-small cell lung tumors are responsive to novel chemotherapy agents. Intravascular stenting is effective for palliation and may be considered to prevent recurrence.

III-81. **The answer is D.** *(Chap. 104)* Acute myeloid leukemias (AML) are a group of hematologic malignancies derived from hematologic stem cells that have acquired chromosomal mutations that prevent differentiation into mature myeloid cells. The specific chromosomal abnormalities predict in which stage of differentiation the cell is arrested and are associated with the several subtypes of AML that have been identified. In the United States, >16,000 new cases of AML are diagnosed yearly, and the numbers of new cases of AML has increased in the past 10 years. Men are diagnosed with AML more frequently than women (4.6 cases per 100,000 population vs. 3.0 cases per 100,000). In addition, older age is associated with increased incidence of AML, with an incidence of 18.6 cases per 100,000 population in those >65 years. AML is uncommon in adolescents. Other known risk factors for development of AML include hereditary genetic abnormalities, radiation and chemical exposures, and drugs. The most common hereditary abnormality linked to AML is trisomy 21 (Down syndrome). Other hereditary syndromes associated with an increase of AML include diseases associated with defective DNA repair such as Fanconi anemia and ataxia telangiectasia. Survivors of the atomic bomb explosions in Japan were found to have a high incidence of AML as have survivors of other high-dose radiation exposures. However, therapeutic radiation is not associated with an increased risk of AML unless the patient was also treated concomitantly with alkylating agents. Anticancer drugs are the most common causes of drug-associated AML. Of the chemotherapeutic agents, alkylating agents and topoisomerase II inhibitors are the drugs most likely to be associated with AML.

III-82. **The answer is B.** *(Chap. 95)* Patients with cancer from an unknown primary site present a common diagnostic dilemma. Initial evaluation should include history, physical examination, appropriate imaging, and blood studies based on gender (e.g., prostate-specific antigen in men, mammography in women). Immunohistochemical staining of biopsy samples using antibodies to specific cell components may help elucidate the site of the primary tumor. Although many immunohistochemical stains are available, a logical approach is represented in the figure below. Additional tests may be helpful based on the appearance under light microscopy and/or the results of the cytokeratin stains. In cases of cancer of unknown primary, cytokeratin staining is usually the first branch point from which the tumor lineage is determined. Cytokeratin is positive in carcinoma, since all epithelial tumors contain this protein. Subsets of cytokeratin, such as CK7 and CK20, may be useful to determine the likely etiology of the primary tumor. Leukocyte common antigen, thyroglobulin, and thyroid transcription factor 1 are characteristic of lymphoma, thyroid cancer, and lung or thyroid cancer, respectively. α Fetoprotein staining is typically positive in germ cell, stomach, and liver carcinoma.

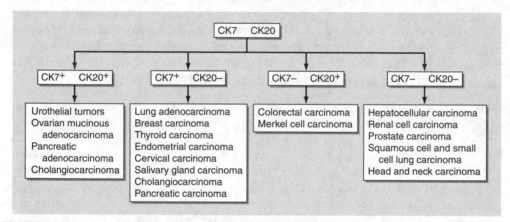

FIGURE III-82   Approach to cytokeratin (CK7 and CK20) markers used in CUP.

III-83. **The answer is C.** *(Chap. 104)* Imatinib mesylate is a tyrosine kinase inhibitor that acts to decrease the activity of the bcr-abl fusion protein that results from the reciprocal translocation of chromosomes 9 and 22 (Philadelphia chromosome). It acts as a competitive inhibitor of the abl kinase at its ATP binding site and thus leads to inhibition of tyrosine phosphorylation of proteins in *bcr-abl* signal transduction. Imatinib mesylate results in hematologic remission in 97% of treated individuals at 18 months and cytogenetic remission of 76%. This is compared to traditional chemotherapy of interferon-α and cytarabine, which resulted in hematologic remission in 69% and cytogenetic remission in only 14% of individuals. More than 87% of individuals who achieved cytogenetic remission had not developed progressive disease at 5 years. This drug taken orally has limited side effects that include nausea, fluid retention, diarrhea, and skin rash and is usually well tolerated. If individuals do not achieve hematologic remission by 3 months or complete cytogenetic remission by 12 months, it is recommended that they proceed to allogeneic bone marrow transplant. While imatinib is the best initial therapy to achieve hematologic and cytogenetic remission, individuals who have a well-matched related bone marrow donor may proceed to early allogeneic transplant, particularly if the individual is <18 years of age. This is done because younger individuals generally have better outcomes following bone marrow transplant than older individuals, and the durability of responses to imatinib mesylate is not known at this time. Interferon-α was previously the first-line chemotherapy if bone marrow transplant was not an option, but it has been replaced by imatinib mesylate. Autologous stem cell transplant is not currently used for treatment of CML as there is no reliable way to select residual normal hematopoietic progenitor cells. Clinical trials utilizing autologous stem cell transplantation are currently underway to determine if this treatment may be possible following control of disease with imatinib therapy. Leukopheresis is used for control of leukocyte counts when the patient is experiencing complications such as respiratory failure or cerebral ischemia related to the high white blood cell count.

III-84. **The answer is A.** *(Chap. 86; Collaborative Group in Hormonal Factors in Breast Cancer, 2002.)* Approximately 80 to 90% of the variation in breast cancer frequency in different countries can be attributed to differences in menarche, first pregnancy, and menopause. Women who experience menarche at age 16 have 40 to 50% the risk of breast cancer of women who experience menarche at age 12 years. Menopause, surgical or natural, occurring 10 years before the median age of 52 years reduces the risk of breast cancer by 35%. Women who have the first full-term pregnancy by age 18 have a 30 to 40% reduced risk of breast cancer compared with nulliparous women. These data taken together suggest that a substantial portion of the risk of developing breast cancer is related directly to the length of menstrual life, particularly the fraction occurring before the first full-term pregnancy. Independently of these factors, the duration of maternal nursing is associated with a reduction in breast cancer risk.

III-85. **The answer is D.** *(Chap. 110)* The aPTT involves the factors of the intrinsic pathway of coagulation. Prolongation of the aPTT reflects either a deficiency of one of these factors (factor VIII, IX, XI, XII, etc.) or inhibition of the activity of one of the factors or components of the aPTT assay (i.e., phospholipids). This may be further characterized by the "mixing study," in which the patient's plasma is mixed with pooled plasma. Correction of the aPTT reflects a deficiency of factors that are replaced by the pooled sample. Failure to correct the aPTT reflects the presence of a factor inhibitor or phospholipid inhibitor. Common causes of a failure to correct include the presence of heparin in the sample, factor inhibitors (factor VIII inhibitor being the most common), and the presence of antiphospholipid antibodies. Factor VII is involved in the extrinsic pathway of coagulation. Inhibitors to factor VII would result in prolongation of the prothrombin time.

III-86. **The answer is A.** *(Chap. 112)* Aspirin is the most widely used antiplatelet agent worldwide and is cheap and effective for both primary and secondary prevention of cardiovascular disease. Aspirin can be recommended for primary cardiovascular prevention in patients whose annual estimated risk of a cardiovascular event is >1%. This includes patients over the age of 40 who have two or more major cardiovascular risk factors and patients over age 50 with one major cardiovascular risk factor. The major risk factors in this patient who is >50 are diabetes mellitus and family history. Other contributing risk factors include obesity and a history of tobacco use, although this is not ongoing. Aspirin is equally effective in men and women, and menopausal status does not impact its efficacy. However, there is a differential effect of aspirin in men and women. In men, aspirin has a greater risk reduction on the incidence of myocardial infarction, whereas in women, there is a greater risk reduction in the occurrence of stroke. The most common side effect of aspirin is major bleeding at a rate of 1–3% yearly. Enteric-coated and buffered preparations decrease, but do not eliminate, this risk. The risk of bleeding is higher if administered concurrently with other anticoagulant or antiplatelet medications. Aspirin does not cause an increased risk of menorrhagia. Finally, aspirin should be used with caution in individuals with a history of bronchospasm in association with nonsteroidal anti-inflammatory drugs (NSAIDs) or aspirin. Usually, these patients have a history of asthma and nasal polyposis (Samter's triad). However, this patient reports only gastrointestinal upset with ibuprofen. While GI upset is a common adverse reaction with NSAIDs, it does not denote a true allergy.

III-87. **The answer is C.** *(Chap. 94)* The most common malignant tumors of bone are plasma cell tumors related to multiple myeloma. The bone lesions are lytic lesions due to increased osteoclast activity, without osteoblastic new bone formation. Of the nonhematopoietic tumors, the most common are osteosarcoma, chondrosarcoma, Ewing's sarcoma, and malignant fibrous histiocytoma. Osteosarcomas account for 45% of bone sarcomas and produce osteoid (unmineralized bone) or bone. They typically occur in children, adolescents, and adults to the third decade. The "sunburst" appearance of the lesion and Codman's triangle in this young man are indicative of an osteosarcoma. Osteosarcomas have a predilection for long bones, whereas chondrosarcomas are more often found in flat bones, especially the shoulder and pelvic girdles. Osteosarcomas are radioresistant. Long-term survival with combined chemotherapy and surgery is 60–80%. Chondrosarcomas account for 20–25% of bone sarcomas and are most common in adults in the fourth to sixth decades. They typically present indolently with pain and swelling. They are often difficult to distinguish from benign bone lesions. Most chondrosarcomas are chemoresistant, and the mainstay of therapy is resection of the primary as well as metastatic sites.

III-88.   The answer is A.   *(Chap. 110)*   Hemophilia A results from an inherited deficiency of factor VIII. The gene for factor VIII is on the X chromosome. Therefore, its X-linked inheritance pattern results in approximately 1 in 10,000 male patients being born with some level of dysfunction. Clinically, it is characterized by bleeding into soft tissues, muscles, and weight-bearing joints. Symptomatic patients usually have levels below 5%. Bleeding occurs hours or days after an injury and can involve any organ. Factor VIII is involved in the intrinsic pathway of coagulation. Therefore, deficiency usually results in abnormalities of the activated partial thromboplastin time. Factor VIII has a very short half-life of 8 to 12 h. Therefore, repeated transfusions of plasma, cryoprecipitate, or purified factor VIII must be given at least twice daily. Factor VIII complexes to von Willebrand factor, not Hageman factor.

III-89.   The answer is A.   *(Chap. 87)*   The rates of gastric cancer have declined significantly over the past 75 years. Nevertheless, there were >20,000 new cases in the United States with >10,000 deaths in 2007. Gastric cancer still has a high incidence in Japan, China, Chile, and Ireland. Epidemiologic evidence, such as the higher prevalence in lower socioeconomic groups and the maintenance of risk for individuals but not offspring migrating from a high-risk to low-risk environment, suggests an environmental exposure early in life is a risk. Risk is associated with ingestion of high nitrite foods. The nitrites may be converted to carcinogens by bacteria in partially decayed food. Chronic gastritis and achlorhydria due to *Helicobacter pylori* gastric infection may contribute to this risk. The effect of *H. pylori* eradication on risk of gastric cancer is under investigation. The combination of recognition of *H. pylori* infection, improved food preservation, and widespread availability of refrigeration may all be contributing to the declining incidence. The most common histologic type of stomach cancer is adenocarcinoma. The majority of adenocarcinomas occur in the distal stomach and appear ulcerative on contrast radiography and endoscopy. Therefore, all gastric ulcers warrant a biopsy and brushings for early detection of adenocarcinoma of the stomach. Such early lesions have the highest likelihood for surgical cure. Some 13% of gastric adenocarcinomas are diffuse-type, involve most of the stomach, and are referred to as *linitis plastica* based on poor distensibility of the stomach. Prognosis for diffuse carcinomas is worse than for intestinal type, and this disease is seen more commonly in the young. There is not a good association between this type of gastric cancer and *H. pylori* infection. For all adenocarcinomas, the presence of palpable periumbilical nodes, or Sister Mary Joseph's nodes, implies metastatic spread and confers a poor prognosis. Surgery should be considered first-line therapy for cure, or palliation/debulking if the patient is a surgical candidate. It is critical to differentiate adenocarcinoma from gastric lymphoma as lymphoma carries a much better prognosis, with *H. pylori* eradication causing regression in 75% of cases. Antimicrobial therapy should be considered before surgery, radiation, or chemotherapy in gastric lymphoma. Surgery, usually with chemotherapy, may be curative in 40–60% of patients with resistant or high-grade lymphoma.

III-90.   The answer is F.   *(Chap. 68)*   All peripheral blood cells and some cells in peripheral tissue are derived from hematopoietic stem cells. When hematopoietic stem cells are irreversibly damaged, as in severe radiation exposure, an individual cannot survive longer than a few weeks. The two cardinal features of stem cells are the ability to differentiate into a variety of mature cell types and the capacity for self-renewal. The ability to differentiate into a variety of cell types allows stem cells to participate in the maintenance and repair of tissues. In addition, the capacity for self-renewal assures an ongoing supply of stem cells to continually maintain adequate tissue function. These characteristics are the basis for the growing excitement regarding the use of stem cells for a wide array of medical conditions including (but limited to) diabetes, spinal cord injury, cardiomyopathy, hematologic disorders, and enzyme deficiencies.

III-91. **The answer is B.** *(Chap. 270)* The malignant spinal cord compression (MSCC) syndrome is defined as compression of the spinal cord and/or cauda equina by an extradural tumor mass. The minimum radiologic evidence for cord compression is compression of the theca at the level of clinical features. However, radiologic confirmation is not necessary in a patient whose physical examination suggests cord compression. These patients should receive immediate high-dose dexamethasone (24 mg IV every 6 h). Cancers that most commonly cause the MSCC syndrome include prostate, lung, and breast. Renal cell carcinoma, lymphomas and melanomas may also cause cord compression. The most commonly affected site is the thoracic spine (70% of cases), followed by the sacral spine (20%). Pain is usually present for days or months before the neurologic defects manifest. Some 75% percent of patients who are ambulatory at the time of diagnosis will remain ambulatory, whereas <10% of patients who present paraplegic will regain the ability to walk despite treatment.

III-92. **The answer is B.** *(Chap. 81)* Tumor lysis syndrome is a well recognized clinical entity that is characterized by metabolic derangements secondary to the destruction of tumor cells. Lysis of cells causes the release of intracellular pools of phosphate, potassium, and nucleic acids, leading to hyperphosphatemia and hyperuricemia. Lactic acidosis frequently develops for similar reasons. The increased urine acidity may promote the formation of uric acid nephropathy and subsequent renal failure. Hyperphosphatemia promotes a reciprocal depression in serum calcium. This hypocalcemia may result in severe neuromuscular irritability and tetany.

III-93. **The answer is E.** *(Chap. 111)* The clinical probability of PE can be delineated into likely vs. unlikely using the clinical decision rule shown in the table below. In those with a score ≤4, PE is unlikely and a D-dimer test should be performed. A normal D-dimer combined with an unlikely clinical probability of PE identifies patients who do not need further testing or anticoagulation therapy. Those with either a likely clinical probability (score >4) or an abnormal D-dimer (with unlikely clinical probability) require an imaging test to rule out PE. Currently the most attractive imaging method to detect PE is the multislice CT scan. It is accurate and, if normal, safely rules out PE. This patient has a clinical probability score of 4.5 because of her resting tachycardia and the lack of an alternative diagnosis at least as likely as PE. Therefore, there is no indication for measuring D-dimer, and she should proceed directly to multislice CT of the chest. If this cannot be performed expeditiously, she should receive one dose of low-molecular-weight heparin while awaiting the test.

TABLE III-93, 94 Long-Term Treatment with Vitamin K Antagonists for Deep Vein Thrombosis (DVT) and Pulmonary Embolism (PE)

Patient Categories	Duration, months	Comments
First episode of DVT or PE secondary to a transient (reversible) risk factor	3	Recommendation applies to both proximal and calf vein thrombosis
First episode of idiopathic DVT or PE	6–12	Continuation of anticoagulant therapy after 6–12 months may be considered
First episode of DVT or PE with a documented thrombophilic abnormality	6–12	Continuation of anticoagulant therapy after 6–12 months may be considered
First episode of DVT or PE with documented antiphospholipid or two or more thrombophilic abnormalities	12	Continuation of anticoagulant therapy after 12 months may be considered

III-94. **The answer is D.** *(Chap. 111)* The goal of treatment with vitamin K antagonists, including warfarin, is maintenance of an INR of 2–3, with a goal of 2.5. Higher intensity treatment is not more effective and has a higher bleeding risk. Lower intensity treatment is less effective, with a similar bleeding risk. The recommendations for duration of therapy for the first episode of deep venous thrombosis (DVT) or pulmonary embolism (PE) are shown in the table in the previous question. Generally, recurrent PE/DVT is treated for at least 12 months. All treatment decisions require balancing risk of recurrence or long-term sequelae with bleeding risk as well as patient preference.

III-95. **The answer is C.** *(Chap. 78)* No study of breast self-examination has shown a reduced mortality due to breast cancer, despite being associated with higher rates of biopsy. The procedure is still recommended as prudent by many organizations; however, only the American Cancer Society recommends monthly BSE in women >19 years. The United States Preventive Services Task Force (USPSTF) provides no recommendation for BSE, and the Canadian Task Force on Preventive Health Care (CTFPHC) excludes its use as a useful screening technique. A substantial fraction of breast cancers are first detected by patients. Though mortality rates have not declined as a result of BSE, the size of lumps being detected by patients have steadily gotten smaller since the 1990s.

III-96. **The answer is D.** *(Chap. 86)* Pathologic staging remains the most important determinant of overall prognosis. Other prognostic factors have an impact on survival and the choice of therapy. Tumors that lack estrogen and/or progesterone receptors are more likely to recur. The presence of estrogen receptors, particularly in postmenopausal women, is also an important factor in determining adjuvant chemotherapy. Tumors with a high growth rate are associated with early relapse. Measurement of the proportion of cells in S-phase is a measure of the growth rate. Tumors with more than the median number of cells in S-phase have a higher risk of relapse and an improved response rate to chemotherapy. Histologically, tumors with a poor nuclear grade have a higher risk of recurrence than do tumors with a good nuclear grade. At the molecular level, tumors that overexpress *erbB2* (*HER-2/neu*) or that have a mutated p53 gene portend a poorer prognosis for patients. The overexpression of *erbB2* is also useful in designing optimal treatment regimens, and a human monoclonal antibody to *erbB2* (Herceptin) has been developed.

III-97. **The answer is E.** *(Chap. 270)* Tumor lysis syndrome is characterized by hyperuricemia, hyperkalemia, hyperphosphatemia, and hypocalcemia. Metabolic acidosis occurs frequently. Acute renal failure is common, and hemodialysis should be considered early in the treatment of this problem. Effective cancer therapy kills cells, which release uric acid from the turnover of nucleic acids. In an acidic environment, uric acid can precipitate in the renal tubules, medulla, and collecting ducts leading to renal failure. Hyperphosphatemia and hyperkalemia also occur as a result of cell death. Hyperphosphatemia produces a reciprocal depression in serum calcium. Indications for hemodialysis include extreme hyperkalemia (>6.0 meq/L), hyperuricemia (>10 mg/dL), hyperphosphatemia (>10 mg/dL or rapidly increasing), or symptomatic hypocalcemia. Daily uric acid levels should be monitored; excellent renal recovery can be expected once the uric acid level is <10 mg/dL.

III-98. **The answer is B.** *(Chap. 112)* Fondaparinux is a direct factor Xa inhibitor that is a synthetic analogue of the pentasaccharide sequence found in heparin. A smaller compound than either unfractionated heparin or low-molecular-weight heparin (LMWH), fondaparinux acts by binding antithrombin and catalyzing factor Xa inhibition. At only 5 polysaccharide units, fondaparinux is too small to bridge antithrombin to thrombin and does not potentiate thrombin inhibition. Fondaparinux is given by the subcutaneous route and has 100% bioavailability without plasma protein binding. Like LMWH, it has a predictable anticoagulant effect and monitoring of factor Xa levels is not required. It is excreted unchanged in the urine. Fondaparinux is absolutely contraindicated in those with a creatinine clearance of <30 mL/min and should be used with caution in individuals with a creatinine clearance of <50 mL/min. The individual presented in scenario B has a creatinine clearance of 32 mL/min and should not receive fondaparinux.

Currently, fondaparinux is approved for prophylaxis against venous thromboembolic disease (VTE) following general surgery and orthopedic procedures. In addition, fondaparinux has been shown to be equivalent to heparin and LMWH in initial treatment of both deep venous thrombosis and pulmonary embolus. Recent studies have demonstrated equivalency with enoxaparin in the treatment of non-ST elevation acute coronary syndromes. Finally, there have been several case reports of successful use of fondaparinux in the treatment of heparin-induced thrombocytopenia as there is no cross-reactivity between it and heparin-induced thrombocytopenia antibodies.

The usual dosage of fondaparinux is 7.5 mg once daily. In individuals weighing <50 kg, the dose should be reduced to 5 mg. Likewise, in those weighing >100 kg, the dose is increased to 10 mg.

III-99.   The answer is A.   *(Chap. 86)*   During pregnancy the breast grows under the influence of estrogen, progesterone, prolactin, and human placental lactogen. However, the presence of a dominant breast nodule/mass during pregnancy should never be attributed to hormonal changes. Breast cancer develops in 1:3000 to 4000 pregnancies. The prognosis for breast cancer by stage is no different in pregnant compared with pregnant women. Nevertheless, pregnant women are often diagnosed with more advanced disease because of delay in the diagnosis. Pregnant patients with persistent lumps in the breast should be receive prompt diagnostic evaluation.

III-100.   The answer is D.   *(Chap. 102)*   Aplastic anemia is defined as pancytopenia with bone marrow hypocellularity. Aplastic anemia may be acquired, iatrogenic (chemotherapy), or genetic (e.g., Fanconi's anemia). Acquired aplastic anemia may be due to drugs or chemicals (expected toxicity or idiosyncratic effects), viral infections, immune diseases, paroxysmal nocturnal hemoglobinuria, pregnancy, or idiopathic causes. Aplastic anemia from idiosyncratic drug reactions (including those listed as well others including as quinacrine, phenytoin, sulfonamides, cimetidine) are uncommon but may be encountered given the wide usage of some of these agents. In these cases there is usually not a dose-dependent response; the reaction is idiosyncratic. Seronegative hepatitis is a cause of aplastic anemia, particularly in young men who recovered from an episode of liver inflammation 1–2 months prior. Parvovirus B19 infection most commonly causes pure red cell aplasia, particularly in patients with chronic hemolytic states and high RBC turnover (e.g., sickle cell anemia).

III-101.   The answer D.   *(Chap. 102)*   This patient has aplastic anemia. In the absence of drugs or toxins that cause bone marrow suppression, it is most likely that he has immune-mediated injury. Growth factors are not effective in the setting of a hypoplastic marrow. Transfusion should be avoided unless emergently needed to prevent the development of alloantibodies. Glucocorticoids have no efficacy in aplastic anemia. Immunosuppression with antithymocyte globulin and cyclosporine is a therapy with proven efficacy for this autoimmune disease with a response rate of up to 70%. Relapses are common and myelodysplastic syndrome or leukemia may occur in approximately 15% of treated patients. Immunosuppression is the treatment of choice for patients without suitable bone marrow transplant donors. Bone marrow transplantation is the best current therapy for young patients with matched sibling donors. Allogeneic bone marrow transplants from matched siblings result in long term survival in >80% of patients, with better results in children than adults.

III-102.   The answer is E.   *(Chap. 102)*   The combination of intravascular hemolysis (hemoglobinuria) and thrombosis in an unusual location (particularly in proximity to the abdominal viscera) should prompt a search for paroxysmal nocturnal hemoglobinuria (PNH). PNH results from an acquired mutation in stem cells resulting in the loss of a glycosylphosphatidylinositol-linked cell surface membrane proteins in a clone of granulocytes. Diagnosis is made by flow cytometry of CD55 or CD59 expression on these granulocytes. The Ham or sucrose lysis tests are no longer routinely performed. Clones of deficient cells are often detected in patients with aplastic anemia. Adenocarcinomas are strongly associated with thrombosis (Trousseau's syndrome) and may cause ascites, but hemolysis without microangiopathic hemolytic anemia makes this less likely. Other causes of a hypercoagulable state such as those listed should be examined if an evaluation for PNH is negative.

III-103. **The answer is B.** *(Chap. 205)* The differential diagnosis for a patient presenting with visceral leishmaniasis is broad and includes diseases that cause fever or organomegaly. Characteristic findings include a history of exposure to sandflies at night or darkening of the skin on physical examination. The skin discoloration is usually only seen in end-stage cachectic patients. Miliary tuberculosis is on the differential but would be unlikely with a normal chest radiograph. Cirrhosis of the liver may present this way although the persistent fevers would be uncharacteristic. The visceral form of Kaposi's sarcoma (KS) may present with a similar physical examination and can be seen in the HIV-negative patient who is otherwise malnourished or immunosuppressed. KS would be less likely than visceral leishmaniasis given the exposure history and the characteristic end-stage finding of skin discoloration. Sickle cell anemia causes autosplenectomy, not splenomegaly.

III-104. **The answer is B.** *(Chap. 110)* This patient has a coagulation disorder characterized by recurrent bleeding episodes into closed spaces with an inheritance pattern suggestive of a recessive or X-linked pattern. An isolated prolonged prothrombin time suggests Factor VII deficiency, which is inherited in an autosomal recessive pattern. The thrombin time will also be normal in these cases. While hemophilia A (factor VIII deficiency) and hemophilia B (factor IX deficiency) are the most common inherited factor deficiencies, these disorders do not cause an isolated prolonged prothrombin time. They will cause a prolongation of the aPTT with a normal PT. Both hemophilias are inherited in an X-linked pattern. Prothrombin deficiency is a rare autosomal recessive disorder that will cause prolongation of the aPTT, PT, and thrombin time. Ingestion of warfarin may also cause this clinical scenario but is less likely given the inheritance pattern.

III-105. **The answer is C.** *(Chap. 110)* An elevated aPTT with a normal PT is consistent with a functional deficiency of Factor VIII, IX, XI, XII, high molecular weight kininogen, or prekallikrein. Congenital or nutritional deficiencies of these factors will be corrected in the laboratory by the addition of serum from a normal subject. The presence of a specific antibody to a coagulation factor is termed an acquired inhibitor. Usually these are directed against Factor VIII, although acquired inhibitors to prothrombin, Factor V, Factor IX, Factor X, and Factor XI are described. Patients with acquired inhibitors are typically older adults (median age 60) with pregnancy or post-partum states being less common. No underlying disease is found in 50%. The most common underlying diseases are autoimmune diseases, malignancies (lymphoma, prostate cancer), and dermatologic diseases. Acquired factor VIII or IX inhibitors present clinically in the same fashion as congenital hemophilias. Developing the coagulation disorder later in life is more suggestive of an acquired inhibitor if there is no antecedent history of coagulopathy. Syphilis infection is a cause of a falsely abnormal aPTT but since this is a laboratory phenomenon, there is no associated clinical coagulopathy. Vitamin C deficiency may cause gingival bleeding and a perifollicular petechial rash but does not cause significant hemarthroses or a prolonged aPTT. A tobacco history and laboratory evidence of chronic illness (anemia, hypoalbuminemia) in this scenario raise the suspicion of an underlying malignancy.

III-106. **The answer is A, although B possible.** *(Chap. 110)* Hemophilia A (absent Factor VIII) and hemophilia B (absent Factor IX) are indistinguishable clinically. Hemophilia A accounts for 80% of the cases of hemophilia. It has a prevalence in the general population of 1:5000 in contrast to Hemophilia B that has a prevalence of 1:30,000. The disease phenotype correlates with the amount of residual Factor activity and can be classified as severe (<1% activity), moderate (1–5% activity) or mild (6–30% activity). The patient in this scenario is likely to have a mild form of the disease. Hemophiliacs have a normal bleeding time, platelet count, thrombin time and prothrombin time. The diagnosis is made by measuring residual factor activity. The prolonged aPTT in hemophilia will be corrected by mixing with normal plasma (that will contain the deficient Factors VIII and IX). Patients with acquired inhibitors will not correct the prolonged aPTT with normal plasma because the defect is antibody mediated.

III-107. **The answer is D.** *(Chap. 110)* This patient presents with a significant upper GI bleed with a prolonged prothrombin time. Hemophilia should not cause a prolonged prothrombin time. This and the presence of ascites raise the possibility of liver disease and cirrhosis. The contamination of blood products in the 1970s and 1980s resulted in widespread transmission of HIV and Hepatitis C within the hemophilia population receiving factor infusions. It is estimated in 2006 that >80% of hemophilia patients >20 years old are infected with hepatitis C virus. Viral inactivation steps were introduced in the 1980s and recombinant Factor VIII and IX were first produced in the 1990s. Hepatitis C is the major cause of morbidity and the second leading cause of death in patients exposed to older factor concentrates. Patients develop cirrhosis and the complications including ascites and variceal bleeding. End-stage liver disease requiring a liver transplant will be curative for the cirrhosis and the hemophilia (the liver produces Factor VIII). Hepatitis B was not transmitted in significant numbers to patients with hemophilia. Diverticular disease or peptic ulcer disease would not explain the prolonged prothrombin time. Patients with inadequately repleted Factor VIII levels are more likely to develop hemarthroses than GI bleeds and the slightly prolonged aPTT makes this unlikely.

III-108. **The answer is E.** *(Chap. 110)* The differentiation between DIC and severe liver disease is challenging. Both entities may manifest with similar laboratory findings: elevated fibrinogen degradation products, prolonged aPTT and PT, anemia, and thrombocytopenia. When suspecting DIC, these tests should be repeated over a period of 6–8 hours because abnormalities may change dramatically in patients with severe DIC. In contrast, these tests should not fluctuate as much in patients with severe liver disease. Bacterial sepsis with positive blood cultures is a common cause of DIC but is not diagnostic.

III-109. **The answer is E.** *(Chap. 103)* In a patient presenting with an elevated hemoglobin and hematocrit, the initial step in the evaluation is to determine whether erythrocytosis represents a true elevation in red cell mass or whether spurious erythrocytosis is present due to plasma volume contraction. This step may be not necessary however in those individuals with hemoglobin greater than 20 g/dL. Once absolute erythrocytosis has been determined by measurement of red cell mass and plasma volume, the cause of erythrocytosis must be determined. If there is not an obvious cause of the erythrocytosis, an erythropoietin level should be checked. An elevated erythropoietin level suggests hypoxia or autonomous production of erythropoietin as the cause of erythrocytosis. However, a normal erythropoietin level does not exclude hypoxia as a cause. A low erythropoietin level should be seen in the myeloproliferative disorder polycythemia vera (PV), the most likely cause of erythrocytosis in this patient. PV is often discovered incidentally when elevated hemoglobin is found during testing for other reasons. When symptoms are present, the most common complaints are related to hyperviscosity of the blood and include vertigo, headache, tinnitus, and transient ischemic attacks. Patients may also complain of pruritus after showering. Erythromelalgia is the term give to the symptoms complex of burning, pain and erythema in the extremities and is associated with thrombocytosis in PV. Isolated systolic hypertension and splenomegaly may be found. In addition to elevated red blood cell mass and low erythropoietin levels, other laboratory findings in PV include thrombocytosis and leukocytosis with abnormal leukocytes present. Uric acid levels and leukocyte alkaline phosphatase may be elevated, but are not diagnostic for PV. Approximately 30% of individuals with PV are homozygous for the JAK2 V617F mutation, and over 90% are heterozygous for this mutation. This mutation located on the short arm of chromosome 9 causes constitutive activation of the JAK protein, a tyrosine kinase that renders erythrocytes resistant to apoptosis and allows them to continue production independently from erythropoietin. However, not every patient with PV expresses this mutation. Thus, it is not recommended as a diagnostic test for PV at this time. Bone marrow biopsy provides no specific information in PV and is not recommended.

IV. INFECTIOUS DISEASES

QUESTIONS

DIRECTIONS: Choose the **one best** response to each question

IV-1. Which type of bite represents a potential medical emergency in an asplenic patient?

    A. Cat bite
    B. Dog bite
    C. Fish bite
    D. Human bite

IV-2. A 24-year-old man with advanced HIV infection presents to the emergency department with a tan painless nodule on the lower extremity (Figure IV-2, Color Atlas). He is afebrile and has no other lesions. He does not take antiretroviral therapy, and his last CD4+ T cell count was 20/μL. He lives with a friend who has cats and kittens. A biopsy shows lobular proliferation of blood vessels lined by enlarged endothelial cells and a mixed acute and chronic inflammatory infiltrate. Tissue stains show gramnegative bacilli. Which of the following is most likely to be effective therapy for the lesion?

    A. Azithromycin
    B. Cephazolin
    C. Interferon α
    D. Penicillin
    E. Vancomycin

IV-3. A 38-year-old homeless man presents to the emergency room with a transient ischemic attack characterized by a facial droop and left arm weakness lasting 20 min, and left upper quadrant pain. He reports intermittent subjective fevers, diaphoresis, and chills for the past 2 weeks. He has had no recent travel or contact with animals. He has taken no recent antibiotics. Physical examination reveals a slightly distressed man with disheveled appearance. His temperature is 38.2°C; heart rate is 90 beats per minute; blood pressure is 127/74 mmHg. He has poor dentition. Cardiac examination reveals an early diastolic murmur over the left 3d intercostal space. His spleen is tender and 2 cm descended below the costal margin. He has tender painful red nodules on the tips of the third finger of his right hand and on the fourth finger of his left hand that are new. He has nits evident on his clothes, consistent with body louse infection. White blood cell count is 14,500,

IV-3. (*Continued*)
with 5% band forms and 93% polymorphonuclear cells. Blood cultures are drawn followed by empirical vancomycin therapy. These cultures remain negative for growth 5 days later. He remains febrile but hemodynamically stable but does develop a new lesion on his toe similar to those on his fingers on hospital day 3. A transthoracic echocardiogram reveals a 1-cm mobile vegetation on the cusp of his aortic valve and moderate aortic regurgitation. A CT scan of the abdomen shows an enlarged spleen with wedge-shaped splenic and renal infarctions. What test should be sent to confirm the most likely diagnosis?

    A. *Bartonella* serology
    B. Epstein-Barr virus (EBV) heterophile antibody
    C. HIV polymerase chain reaction (PCR)
    D. Peripheral blood smear
    E. Q fever serology

IV-4. A 36-year-old man with HIV/AIDS (CD4+ lymphocyte count = 112/μL) develops a scaly, waxy, yellowish, patchy, crusty, pruritic rash on and around his nose. The rest of his skin examination is normal. Which of the following is the most likely diagnosis?

    A. Molluscum contagiosum
    B. Psoriasis
    C. Reactivation herpes zoster
    D. Seborrheic dermatitis

IV-5. A 28-year-old woman returns from a 6-week trip to Tanzania in March. She calls your office 2 weeks later complaining of new symptoms of fever, mild abdominal pain, and headache. She feels like she has the flu. What should you do next?

    A. Ask her to come to the clinic in the next 24 h.
    B. Emergently refer her to the emergency department.
    C. Write her a prescription for oseltamivir and call her in 24 h to ensure improvement.
    D. Write her a prescription for a respiratory fluoroquinolone.

IV-6. A 26-year-old woman comes to your clinic complaining of 3–4 weeks of a malodorous white vaginal discharge. She recently began having unprotected sexual intercourse with a new male partner. He is asymptomatic. Her only medication is oral contraceptives. Examination reveals a thin white discharge that evenly coats the vagina. Further examination of the discharge reveals that it has a pH of 5.0 and has a "fishy" odor when 10% KOH is added to the discharge. Microscopic examination reveals vaginal cells coated with coccobacillary organisms. Which of the following therapies is indicated?

A. Acyclovir, 400 mg PO tid × 7 days
B. Metronidazole, 2 g PO × 1
C. Metronidazole, 500 mg PO bid × 7 days
D. Fluconazole, 100 mg PO × 1
E. Vaginal douching

IV-7. A 51-year-old woman is diagnosed with *Plasmodium falciparum* malaria after returning from a safari in Tanzania. Her parasitemia is 6%, hematocrit is 21%, bilirubin is 7.8 mg/dL, and creatinine is 2.7 mg/dL. She is still making 60 mL of urine per hour. She rapidly becomes obtunded. Intensive care is initiated, with frequent creatinine checks, close monitoring for hypoglycemia, infusion of phenobarbital for seizure prevention, mechanical ventilation for airway protection, and exchange transfusion to address her high parasitemia. Which of the following regimens is recommended as first-line treatment for her malarial infection?

A. Chloroquine
B. Intravenous artesunate
C. Intravenous quinine
D. Intravenous quinidine
E. Mefloquine

IV-8. All of the following infections associated with sexual activity correlate with increased acquisition of HIV infection in women *except*

A. bacterial vaginosis
B. *Chlamydia*
C. gonorrhea
D. herpes simplex virus-2
E. *Trichomonas vaginalis*
F. all of the above are associated with increased acquisition

IV-9. A 9-year-old boy is brought to a pediatric emergency room by his father. He has had 2 days of headache, neck stiffness, and photophobia and this morning had a temperature of 38.9°C (102°F). He has also had several episodes of vomiting and diarrhea overnight. A lumbar puncture is performed, which reveals pleocytosis in the cerebrospinal fluid (CSF). Which of the following is true regarding enteroviruses as a cause of aseptic meningitis?

A. An elevated CSF protein rules out enteroviruses as a cause of meningitis.

IV-9. *(Continued)*
B. Enteroviruses are responsible for up to 90% of aseptic meningitis in children.
C. Lymphocytes will predominate in the CSF early on, with a shift to neutrophils at 24 h.
D. Symptoms are more severe in children than in adults.
E. They occur more commonly in the winter and spring.

IV-10. A 56-year-old man with a history of hypertension and cigarette smoking is admitted to the intensive care unit after 1 week of fever and nonproductive cough. Imaging shows a new pulmonary infiltrate, and urine antigen test for *Legionella* is positive. Each of the following is likely to be an effective antibiotic *except*

A. azithromycin
B. aztreonam
C. levofloxacin
D. tigecycline
E. trimethoprim/sulfamethoxazole

IV-11. Which of the following statements regarding HIV epidemiology in the United States is true as of 2005?

A. HIV incidence is currently decreasing among men who sleep with men.
B. Heterosexual contact accounts for the majority of current HIV cases.
C. Minority women aged 13–19 from the southeastern United States account for a growing proportion of prevalent HIV cases.
D. The proportion of cases due to high-risk heterosexual contact has decreased dramatically over the past 20 years.
E. The proportion of prevalent HIV cases due to injection drug use is currently increasing.

IV-12. A 48-year-old female presents to her physician with a 2-day history of fever, arthralgias, diarrhea, and headache. She recently returned from an ecotour in tropical sub-Saharan Africa, where she went swimming in inland rivers. Notable findings on physical examination include a temperature of 38.7°C (101.7°F); 2-cm tender mobile lymph nodes in the axilla, cervical, and femoral regions; and a palpable spleen. Her white blood cell count is 15,000/μL with 50% eosinophils. She should receive treatments with which of the following medications?

A. Chloroquine
B. Mebendazole
C. Metronidazole
D. Praziquantel
E. Thiabendazole

IV-13. A 39-year-old woman received a liver transplant 2 years ago and is maintained on prednisone, 5 mg, and cyclosporine A, 8 mg/kg per day. She has had two episodes of rejection since transplant, as well an episode of cytomegalovirus syndrome and *Nocardia* pneumonia. She in-

IV-13. (*Continued*)

tends on taking a 2-week gorilla-watching trip to Rwanda and seeks your advice regarding her health while abroad. Which of the following potential interventions is strictly contraindicated?

A. Malaria prophylaxis
B. Meningococcal vaccine
C. Rabies vaccine
D. Typhoid purified polysaccharid vaccine
E. Yellow fever vaccine

IV-14. A 17-year-old woman presents to the clinic complaining of vaginal itchiness and malodorous discharge. She is sexually active with multiple partners, and she is interested in getting tested for sexually transmitted diseases. A wet-mount microscopic examination is performed, and trichomonal parasites are identified. Which of the following statements regarding trichomoniasis is true?

A. A majority of women are asymptomatic.
B. No treatment is necessary as disease is self-limited.
C. The patient's sexual partner need not be treated.
D. Trichomoniasis can only be spread sexually.
E. Trichomoniasis is 100% sensitive to metronidazole.

IV-15. The most common clinical presentation of infection with *Babesia microti* is

A. acute hepatitis
B. chronic meningitis
C. generalized lymphadenopathy
D. overwhelming hemolysis, high-output congestive heart failure, respiratory failure, and disseminated intravascular coagulation
E. self-limited flulike illness

IV-16. When given as a first-line agent for invasive *Aspergillus* infection, voriconazole commonly causes all of the following side effects *except*

A. drug-drug interactions
B. hepatotoxicity
C. photosensitivity skin rashes
D. renal toxicity
E. visual disturbances

IV-17. A 42-year-old man with AIDS and a CD4+ lymphocyte count of 23 presents with shortness of breath and fatigue in the absence of fevers. On examination, he appears chronically ill with pale conjunctiva. Hematocrit is 16%. Mean corpuscular volume is 84. Red cell distribution width is normal. Bilirubin, lactose dehydrogenase, and haptoglobin are all within normal limits. Reticulocyte count is zero. White blood cell count is 4300, with an absolute neutrophil count of 2500. Platelet count is 105,000. Which of the following tests is most likely to produce a diagnosis?

A. Bone marrow aspirate and biopsy

IV-16. (*Continued*)

B. Iron studies
C. Parvovirus B19 IgG
D. Parvovirus B19 polymerase chain reaction (PCR)
E. Parvovirus B19 IgM
F. Peripheral blood smear

IV-18. All of the following are risk factors for the development of *Legionella* pneumonia *except*

A. glucocorticoid use
B. HIV infection
C. neutropenia
D. recent surgery
E. tobacco use

IV-19. A 38-year-old female pigeon keeper who has no significant past medical history, is taking no medications, has no allergies, and is HIV-negative presents to the emergency room with a fever, headache, and mild nuchal rigidity. Neurologic examination is normal. Head CT examination is normal. Lumbar puncture is significant for an opening pressure of 20 cmH$_2$O, white blood cell count of 15 cells/μL (90% monocytes), protein of 0.5 g/L (50 mg/mL), glucose of 2.8 mmol/L (50 mg/dL), and positive India ink stain. What is the appropriate therapy for this patient?

A. Amphotericin B for 2 weeks
B. Amphotericin B with flucytosine for 2 weeks
C. Amphotericin B for 2 weeks followed by oral fluconazole, 400 mg daily
D. Amphotericin B for 10 weeks followed by oral fluconazole, 400 mg daily for 6–12 months
E. Ceftriaxone and vancomycin for 2 weeks

IV-20. A 30-year-old female with end-stage renal disease who receives her dialysis through a tunneled catheter in her shoulder presents with fever and severe low back pain. On examination, she is uncomfortable and diaphoretic but hemodynamically stable. She has a soft 2/6 early systolic flow murmur. Her line site is red and warm with no pustular exudates. She is very tender over her lower back. Neurologically, she is completely intact. There is no evidence of Janeway lesions, Osler nodes, or Roth spots. Her white count is 16,700 with 12% bands. Immediate evaluation should include all of the following *except*

A. MRI of the lumbar spine
B. removal of her dialysis catheter
C. transthoracic echocardiogram
D. two sets of blood cultures followed by vancomycin as well as gram-negative coverage

IV-21. While attending the University of Georgia, a group of friends go on a 5-day canoeing and camping trip in rural southern Georgia. A few weeks later, one of the campers develops a serpiginous, raised, pruritic, erythematous eruption on the buttocks. Strongyloides larvae are found in his stool. Three of his companions, who are asympto-

IV-21. *(Continued)*
matic, are also found to have strongyloides larvae in their stool. Which of the following is indicated in the asymptomatic carriers?

A. Fluconazole
B. Ivermectin
C. Mebendazole
D. Mefloquine
E. Treatment only for symptomatic illness

IV-22. A 79-year-old man has had a diabetic foot ulcer overlying his third metatarsal head for 3 months but has not been compliant with his physician's request to off-load the affected foot. He presents with dull, throbbing foot pain and subjective fevers. Examination reveals a putrid-smelling wound notable also for a pus-filled 2.5 cm wide ulcer. A metal probe is used to probe the wound and it detects bone as well as a 3-cm deep cavity. Gram stain of the pus shows gram-positive cocci in chains, gram-positive rods, gram-negative diplococci, enteric-appearing gram-negative rods, tiny pleomorphic gram-negative rods, and a predominance of neutrophils. Which of the following empirical antibiotic regimens is recommended while blood and drainage cultures are processed?

A. Ampicillin/sulbactam, 1.5 g IV q4h
B. Clindamycin, 600 mg PO tid
C. Linezolid, 600 mg IV bid
D. Metronidazole, 500 mg PO qid
E. Vancomycin, 1g IV bid

IV-23. Which of the following scenarios is most likely associated with the lowest risk of HIV transmission to a health care provider after an accidental needle stick from a patient with HIV?

A. The needle is visibly contaminated with the patient's blood.
B. The needle stick injury is a deep tissue injury to the health care provider.
C. The patient whose blood is on the contaminated needle has been on antiretroviral therapy for many years with a history of resistance to many available agents but most recently has had successful viral suppression on current therapy.
D. The patient whose blood is on the contaminated needle was diagnosed with acute HIV infection 2 weeks ago.

IV-24. All of the following regarding herpes simplex virus (HSV)-2 infection are true *except*

A. Approximately one in five Americans harbors HSV-2 antibodies.
B. Asymptomatic shedding of HSV-2 in the genital tract occurs nearly as frequently in those with no symptoms as in those with ulcerative disease.

IV-24. *(Continued)*
C. Asymptomatic shedding of HSV-2 is associated with transmission of virus.
D. HSV-2 seropositivity is an independent risk factor for HIV transmission.
E. Seroprevalence rates of HSV-2 are lower in Africa than in the United States.

IV-25. What is the most common manifestation of *Coccidioides* infection in an immunocompetent host?

A. Acute pneumonia
B. Asymptomatic seroconversion
C. Hypersensitivity phenomena such as erythema nodosum
D. Meningitis
E. Self limited flulike illness

IV-26. You are a physician working on a cruise ship traveling from Miami to the Yucatán Peninsula. In the course of 24 h, 32 people are seen with acute gastrointestinal illness that is marked by vomiting and watery diarrhea. The most likely causative agent of the illness is

A. enterohemorrhagic *Escherichia coli*
B. norovirus
C. rotavirus
D. *Shigella*
E. *Salmonella*

IV-27. What is the best method for diagnosis?

A. Acute and convalescent antibody titers
B. Demonstration of Norwalk toxin in the stool
C. Electron microscopy
D. Isolation in cell culture
E. Polymerase chain reaction (PCR) to identify the Norwalk-associated calcivirus

IV-28. A 32-year-old man presents with jaundice and malaise. He is found to have acute hepatitis B with positive hepatitis B virus (HBV) DNA and E antigen. Which of the following antiviral agents are approved as part of a therapeutic regimen for mono-infection with hepatitis B?

A. Efavirenz
B. Ganciclovir
C. Lamivudine
D. Rimantadine
E. Tenofovir

IV-29. Which of the following factors is the most important determinant of the rate of disease progression from initial HIV infection to clinical diagnosis of AIDS?

A. Age
B. CD4+ lymphocyte count 6 months after infection
C. Cytomegalovirus (CMV) IgG status
D. HIV resistance panel at infection
E. HIV viral load set point 6 months after initial infection

IV-30. The standard starting regimen for acid-fast bacilli smear–positive active pulmonary tuberculosis is

A. isoniazid
B. isoniazid, rifampin
C. isoniazid, moxifloxacin, pyrazinamide, ethambutol
D. isoniazid, rifampin, pyrazinamide, ethambutol
E. rifampin, moxifloxacin, pyrazinamide, ethambutol

IV-31. All of the following are common manifestations of cytomegalovirus (CMV) infection following lung transplantation *except*

A. bronchiolitis obliterans
B. CMV esophagitis
C. CMV pneumonia
D. CMV retinitis
E. CMV syndrome (fever, malaise, cytopenias, transaminitis, and CMV viremia)

IV-32. Which of the following statements regarding severe acute respiratory syndrome (SARS) is true?

A. SARS displays poor human-to-human transmission.
B. SARS is more severe among children than adults.
C. The etiologic agent of SARS is in the Adenovirus family.
D. There have been no reported cases of SARS since 2004.
E. There is no known environmental reservoir for the virus causing SARS.

IV-33. A 72-year-old woman is admitted to the intensive care unit with respiratory failure. She has fever, obtundation, and bilateral parenchymal consolidation on chest imaging. Which of the following is true regarding the diagnosis of *Legionella* pneumonia?

A. Acute and convalescent antibodies are not helpful due to the presence of multiple serotypes.
B. *Legionella* can never be seen on a Gram stain.
C. *Legionella* cultures grow rapidly on the proper media.
D. *Legionella* urinary antigen maintains utility after antibiotic use.
E. Polymerase chain reaction (PCR) for *Legionella* DNA is the "gold standard" diagnostic test.

IV-34. Which of the following has resulted in a significant decrease in the incidence of trichinellosis in the United States?

A. Adequate therapy that allows for eradication of infection in index cases before person-to-person spread can occur
B. Earlier diagnosis due to a new culture assay
C. Federal laws limiting the import of foreign cattle
D. Laws prohibiting the feeding of uncooked garbage to pigs
E. Requirements for hand-washing by commercial kitchen staff who handle raw meat

IV-35. A 23-year-old woman is newly diagnosed with genital herpes simplex virus (HSV)-2 infection. What can you tell her that the chance of reactivation disease will be during the first year after infection?

A. 5%
B. 25%
C. 50%
D. 75%
E. 90%

IV-36. The most common cause of traveler's diarrhea in Mexico is

A. *Campylobacter jejuni*
B. *Entamoeba histolytica*
C. enterotoxigenic *Escherichia coli*
D. *Giardia lamblia*
E. *Vibrio cholerae*

IV-37. A patient comes to clinic and describes progressive muscle weakness over several weeks. He has also experienced nausea, vomiting, and diarrhea. One month ago he had been completely healthy and describes a bear hunting trip in Alaska, where they ate some of the game they killed. Soon after he returned, his gastrointestinal (GI) symptoms began, followed by muscle weakness in his jaw and neck that has now spread to his arms and lower back. Examination confirms decreased muscle strength in the upper extremities and neck. He also has slowed extraocular movements. Laboratory examination shows panic values for elevated eosinophils and serum creatine phosphokinase. Which of the following organisms is most likely the cause of his symptoms?

A. *Campylobacter*
B. Cytomegalovirus
C. *Giardia*
D. *Taenia solium*
E. *Trichinella*

IV-38. Abacavir is a nucleoside transcription inhibitor that carries which side effect unique for HIV antiretroviral agents?

A. Fanconi's anemia
B. Granulocytopenia
C. Lactic acidosis
D. Lipoatrophy
E. Severe hypersensitivity reaction

IV-39. A 30-year-old healthy woman presents to the hospital with severe dyspnea, confusion, productive cough, and fevers. She had been ill 1 week prior with a flulike illness characterized by fever, myalgias, headache, and malaise. Her illness almost entirely improved without medical intervention until 36 h ago, when she developed new rigors followed by progression of the respiratory symptoms. On initial examination, her temperature is 39.6°C, pulse is 130 beats per minute, blood pressure is 95/60 mmHg, respiratory rate is 40, and oxygen saturation is 88% on 100% face

IV-39. *(Continued)*

mask. On examination she is clammy, confused, and very dyspneic. Lung examination reveals amphoric breath sounds over her left lower lung fields. She is intubated and resuscitated with fluid and antibiotics. Chest CT scan reveals necrosis of her left lower lobe. Blood and sputum cultures grow *Staphylococcus aureus*. This isolate is likely to be resistant to which of the following antibiotics?

A. Doxycycline
B. Linezolid
C. Methicillin
D. Trimethoprim/sulfamethoxazole (TMP/SMX)
E. Vancomycin

IV-40. *Helicobacter pylori* colonization is implicated in all of the following conditions *except*

A. duodenal ulcer disease
B. gastric adenocarcinoma
C. gastric mucosa-associated lymphoid tissue (MALT) lymphoma
D. gastroesophageal reflux disease
E. peptic ulcer disease

IV-41. A 24-year-old woman presents with diffuse arthralgias and morning stiffness in her hands, knees, and wrists. Two weeks earlier she had a self-limited febrile illness notable for a red facial rash and lacy reticular rash on her extremities. On examination, her bilateral wrists, metacarpophalangeal joints, and proximal interphalangeal joints are warm and slightly boggy. What test is most likely to reveal her diagnosis?

A. Antinuclear antibody
B. *Chlamydia trachomatis* ligase chain reaction of the urine
C. Joint aspiration for crystals and culture
D. Parvovirus B19 IgM
E. Rheumatoid factor

IV-42. *Candida albicans* is isolated from the following patients. Rate the likelihood in order from *greatest to least* that the positive culture represents true infection rather than contaminant or noninfectious colonization?

Patient X: A 63-year-old man admitted to the intensive care unit (ICU) with pneumonia who has recurrent fevers after receiving 5 days of levofloxacin for pneumonia. A urinalysis drawn from a Foley catheter shows positive leukocyte esterase, negative nitrite, 15 white blood cells/hpf, 10 red blood cells/hpf, and 10 epithelial cells/hpf. Urine culture grows *Candida albicans*.
Patient Y: A 38-year-old female on hemodialysis presents with low-grade fevers and malaise. Peripheral blood cultures grow *Candida albicans* in one out of a total of three sets of blood cultures in the aerobic bottle only.
Patient Z: A 68-year-old man presents with a 2-day history of fever, productive cough, and malaise. Chest roentgenogram reveals a left lower lobe infiltrate. A sputum Gram stain shows many PMNs, few epithelial

IV-42. *(Continued)*

cells, moderate gram-positive cocci in chains, and yeast consistent with *Candida*.

A. Patient X > patient Z > patient Y
B. Patient Y > patient Z > patient X
C. Patient Y > patient X > patient Z
D. Patient X > patient Y > patient Z
E. Patient Z > patient X > patient Y

IV-43. Which of the following statements regarding *Clostridium difficile*–associated disease relapses is true?

A. A first recurrence does not imply greater risk of further recurrences.
B. Most recurrences are due to antibiotic resistance.
C. Recurrent *C. difficile*–associated disease has been associated with a higher risk of colon cancer.
D. Recurrent disease is associated with serious complications.
E. Testing for clearance of *C. difficile* is warranted after treating recurrences.

IV-44. A 38-year-old man with HIV/AIDS presents with 4 weeks of diarrhea, fever, and weight loss. Which of the following tests makes the diagnosis of cytomegalovirus (CMV) colitis?

A. CMV IgG
B. Colonoscopy with biopsy
C. Serum CMV polymerase chain reaction (PCR)
D. Stool CMV antigen
E. Stool CMV culture

IV-45. In the inpatient setting, extended-spectrum β-lactamase (ESBL)-producing gram-negative infections are most likely to occur after frequent use of which of the following classes of antibiotics?

A. Carbapenems
B. Macrolides
C. Quinolones
D. Third-generation cephalosporins

IV-46. A 46-year-old veterinary researcher who frequently operates on rats presents to the emergency room with jaundice and scant hemoptysis. She recalls having a fairly deep cut on her hand during an operation about 14 days prior. She has had no recent travel or other animal exposures. Her illness started ~9 days prior with fever, chills, severe headache, intense myalgias, and nausea. She also noted bilateral conjunctival injection. Thinking that she had influenza infection, she stayed home from work and started to feel better 5 days into the illness. However, within a day her symptoms had returned with worsening headache, and soon thereafter she developed jaundice. On initial evaluation, her temperature is 38.6°C, pulse is 105 beats per minute, and blood pressure is 156/89 mmHg with O$_2$ saturations of 92% on room air. She appears acutely ill and is both icteric and profoundly jaundiced. Her liver is enlarged and tender, but there are no pal-

IV-46. *(Continued)*

pable masses and she has no splenomegaly. Laboratory results are notable for a BUN of 64, creatinine of 3.6, total bilirubin of 64.8 (direct 59.2), AST = 84, ALT = 103, alkaline phosphatase = 384, white blood cell (WBC) count is 11,000 with 13% bands and 80% polymorphonuclear forms, hematocrit of 33%, and platelets = 142. Urinalysis reveals 20 WBCs/hpf, 3+ protein, and granular casts. Coagulation studies are within normal limits. Lumbar puncture reveals a sterile pleocytosis. CT scan of the chest shows diffuse flame-like infiltrates consistent with pulmonary hemorrhage. What is the likely diagnosis?

A. Acute interstitial pneumonitis
B. Acute myeloid leukemia
C. Polyarteritis nodosum
D. Rat bite fever (*Streptobacillus moniliformis* infection)
E. Weil's syndrome (*Leptospira interrogans* infection)

IV-47. A 17-year-old boy in Arkansas presents to a clinic in August with fever, headache, myalgias, nausea, and anorexia 8 days after returning from a 1-week camping trip. Physical examination is remarkable for a temperature of 38.6°C and a generally fatigued but nontoxic appearing, well-developed young man. He does not have a rash, and orthostatic vital sign measurements are negative. What would be a reasonable course of action?

A. Initiate ceftriaxone, 1g IM × 1
B. Initiate doxycycline, 100 mg PO bid
C. Initiate oseltamivir, 75 mg PO qd
D. Reassure the patient and order a heterophile antibody titer (Monospot)
E. Reassure the patient and order rickettsial serologies

IV-48. A 26-year-old woman presents to the emergency department with fever, chills, backache, and malaise. She reports a habit of active IV drug use; last use was 2 days ago. Her vital signs show a temperature of 38.4°C, heart rate of 106/minute, respiratory rate of 22/minute, blood pressure of 114/61 mmHg, and oxygen saturation of 98% on 2 L per nasal cannula. A chest x-ray and subsequent chest CT scan demonstrate multiple peripheral nodular infiltrates with cavitation. Blood cultures are sent to the laboratory and are pending. At this point in the workup, how many minor criteria are met from the Duke criteria for the clinical diagnosis of infective endocarditis?

A. 0
B. 1
C. 2
D. 3
E. 5

IV-49. Which of the following is true regarding influenza prophylaxis?

A. Patients receiving an intramuscular influenza vaccine should be warned of the increased risk of Guillain-Barré syndrome.

IV-49. *(Continued)*

B. Patients with hypersensitivity to eggs should not receive the intramuscular vaccine.
C. The intramuscular influenza vaccine is a live, attenuated strain of influenza that is based on isolates from the previous year's strains of influenza A and B.
D. The intramuscular influenza vaccine should not be given to immunocompromised hosts.
E. The intranasal spray, "Flu-mist," is an inactivated virus preparation based on the previous year's strains of influenza A and B.

IV-50. Which of the following is the most common manifestation of initial (primary) herpes simplex virus (HSV)-1 infection?

A. Asymptomatic infection
B. Genital ulcers
C. Gingivostomatitis and pharyngitis
D. Orolabial ulcers
E. Trigeminal neuralgia

IV-51. A patient presents to the clinic complaining of nausea, vomiting, crampy abdominal pain, and markedly increased flatus. The patient has not experienced any diarrhea or vomiting but notes that he has been belching more than usual and he describes a "sulfur-like" odor when he does so. He returned from a 3-week trip to Peru and Ecuador several days ago and notes that his symptoms began about a week ago. Giardiasis is considered in the differential. Which of the following is true regarding *Giardia*?

A. Boiling water prior to ingestion will not kill *Giardia* cysts.
B. *Giardia* is a disease of developing nations; if this patient had not travelled, there would be no likelihood of giardiasis.
C. Hematogenous dissemination and eosinophilia are common.

D. Ingestion of as few as 10 cysts can cause human disease.
E. Lack of diarrhea makes the diagnosis of *Giardia* very unlikely.

IV-52. An 18-year-old man presents with a firm, nontender lesion around his anal orifice. The lesion is about 1.5 cm in diameter and has a cartilaginous feel on clinical examination. The patient reports that it has progressed to this stage from a small papule. It is not tender. He reports recent unprotected anal intercourse. Bacterial culture of the lesion is negative. A rapid plasmin reagin (RPR) test is also negative. Therapeutic interventions should include

A. IM ceftriaxone, 1g
B. IM penicillin G benzathine, 2.4 million U
C. oral acyclovir, 200 mg 5 times per day
D. observation
E. surgical resection with biopsy

IV-53. A 17-year-old woman with a medical history of mild intermittent asthma presents to your clinic in February with several days of cough, fever, malaise, and myalgias. She notes that her symptoms started 3 days earlier with a headache and fatigue, and that several students and teachers at her high school have been diagnosed recently with "the flu." She did not receive a flu shot this year. Which of the following medication treatment plans is the best option for this patient?

A. Aspirin and a cough suppressant with codeine
B. Oseltamivir, 75 mg PO bid for 5 days
C. Rimantadine, 100 mg PO bid for 1 week
D. Symptom-based therapy with over-the-counter agents
E. Zanamivir, 10 mg inhaled bid for 5 days

IV-54. One month after receiving a 14-day course of omeprazole, clarithromycin, and amoxicillin for *Helicobacter pylori*–associated gastric ulcer disease, a 44-year-old woman still has mild dyspepsia and pain after meals. What is the appropriate next step in management?

A. Empirical long-term proton pump inhibitor therapy
B. Endoscopy with biopsy to rule out gastric adenocarcinoma
C. *H. pylori* serology testing
D. Reassurance
E. Second-line therapy for *H. pylori* with omeprazole, bismuth subsalicylate, tetracycline, and metronidazole
F. Urea breath test

IV-55. Which of the following medications used as antimycobacterial drugs require dose reduction for patients with an estimated glomerular filtration rate <30 mL/min?

A. Isoniazid
B. Pyrazinamide
C. Rifabutin
D. Rifampin
E. Streptomycin

IV-56. Which of the following statements regarding the currently licensed human papillomavirus (HPV) vaccine (Gardasil) is true?

A. It does not protect against genital warts.
B. It is an inactivated live virus vaccine.
C. It is targeted towards all oncogenic strains of HPV but is only 70% effective at decreasing infection in an individual.
D. Once sexually active, women will derive little protective benefit from the vaccine.
E. Vaccinees should continue to receive standard Pap smear testing.

IV-57. A 25-year-old woman presents with 1 day of fever to 38.3°C (101°F), sore throat, dysphagia, and a number of grayish-white papulovesicular lesions on the soft palate, uvula, and anterior pillars of the tonsils (Figure IV-57, Color Atlas). The patient is most likely infected with which of the following?

IV-57. (Continued)
A. *Candida albicans*
B. Coxsackievirus
C. Herpesvirus
D. HIV
E. *Staphylococcus lugdunensis*

IV-58. There is wide concern among many members of the general public regarding which of the following vaccines as a potential cause of autism?

A. DTap (diphtheria and tetanus toxoid and acellular pertussis) vaccine
B. Hepatitis B vaccine
C. Hib (*Haemophilus influenza* type b) vaccine
D. Human papilloma virus (HPV) vaccine
E. Measles-mumps-rubella (MMR) vaccine

IV-59. A 19-year-old female from Guatemala presents to your office for a routine screening physical examination. At age 4 years she was diagnosed with acute rheumatic fever. She does not recall the specifics of her illness and remembers only that she was required to be on bed rest for 6 months. She has remained on penicillin V orally at a dose of 250 mg bid since that time. She asks if she can safely discontinue this medication. She has had only one other flare of her disease, at age 8, when she stopped taking penicillin at the time of her emigration to the United States. She is currently working as a day care provider. Her physical examination is notable for normal point of maximal impulse (PMI) with a grade III/VI holosystolic murmur that is heard best at the apex of the heart and radiates to the axilla. What do you advise the patient to do?

A. An echocardiogram should be performed to determine the extent of valvular damage before deciding if penicillin can be discontinued.
B. Penicillin prophylaxis can be discontinued because she has had no flares in 5 years.
C. She should change her dosing regimen to IM benzathine penicillin every 8 weeks.
D. She should continue on penicillin indefinitely as she had a previous recurrence, has presumed rheumatic heart disease, and is working in a field with high occupational exposure to group A streptococcus.
E. She should replace penicillin prophylaxis with polyvalent pneumococcal vaccine every 5 years.

IV-60. In a patient with bacterial endocarditis, which of the following echocardiographic lesions is most likely to lead to embolization?

A. 5-mm mitral valve vegetation
B. 5-mm tricuspid valve vegetation
C. 11-mm aortic valve vegetation
D. 11-mm mitral valve vegetation
E. 11-mm tricuspid valve vegetation

IV-61. Testing for latent *Mycobacterium tuberculosis* infection is indicated in HIV patients at the time of initial diagnosis for all of the following reasons *except*

A. Active tuberculosis treatment success rates are lower in HIV-infected patients compared to HIV-uninfected patients.
B. Drug interactions between drug regimens for active tuberculosis therapy and highly active antiretroviral therapy are challenging to manage.
C. HIV-associated active tuberculosis is more likely to be extrapulmonary and can be diagnostically challenging.
D. HIV-infected patients with active tuberculosis have high 6-month HIV-related mortality rates.
E. The rate of progression from latent tuberculosis to active tuberculosis is higher in HIV-infected persons compared to HIV-uninfected persons.

IV-62. A 19-year-old man presents to the emergency department with 4 days of watery diarrhea, nausea, vomiting, and low-grade fever. He recalls no unusual meals, sick contacts, or travel. He is hydrated with IV fluid, given antiemetics and discharged home after feeling much better. Three days later two out of three blood cultures are positive for *Clostridium perfringens*. He is called at home and says that he feels fine and is back to work. What should your next instruction to the patient be?

A. Return for IV penicillin therapy
B. Return for IV penicillin therapy plus echocardiogram
C. Return for IV penicillin therapy plus colonoscopy
D. Return for surveillance blood culture
E. Reassurance

IV-63. All of the following are clinical manifestations of *Ascaris lumbricoides* infection *except*

A. asymptomatic carriage
B. fever, headache, photophobia, nuchal rigidity, and eosinophilia
C. nonproductive cough and pleurisy with eosinophilia
D. right upper quadrant pain and fever
E. small-bowel obstruction

IV-64. In the developed world, seroprevalence of *Helicobacter pylori* infection is currently

A. decreasing
B. increasing
C. staying the same
D. unknown

IV-65. An 87-year-old nursing home resident is brought by ambulance to a local emergency room. He is obtunded and ill-appearing. Per nursing home staff, the patient has experienced low-grade temperatures, poor appetite, and lethargy over several days. A lumbar puncture is performed, and the Gram stain returns gram-positive rods

IV-65. *(Continued)*
and many white blood cells. *Listeria* meningitis is diagnosed and appropriate antibiotics are begun. Which of the following best describes a clinical difference between *Listeria* and other causes of bacterial meningitis?

A. More frequent nuchal rigidity.
B. More neutrophils are present on the cerebrospinal fluid (CSF) differential.
C. Photophobia is more common.
D. Presentation is often more subacute.
E. White blood cell (WBC) count is often more elevated in the CSF.

IV-66. Which of the following antibiotics has the weakest association with the development of *Clostridium difficile*–associated disease?

A. Ceftriaxone
B. Ciprofloxacin
C. Clindamycin
D. Moxifloxacin
E. Piperacillin/tazobactam

IV-67. All of the following statements regarding human T cell lymphotropic virus-I (HTLV-I) infection are true *except*

A. Acute T cell leukemia is associated with HTLV-I infection.
B. HTLV-I endemic regions include southern Japan, the Caribbean, and South America.
C. HTLV-I infection is associated with a gradual decline in T cell function and immunosuppression.
D. HTLV-I is transmitted parenterally, sexually, and from mother to child.
E. Tropical spastic paraparesis is associated with HTLV-I infection.

IV-68. A 33-year-old woman is undergoing consolidation chemotherapy for acute myelocytic leukemia with cytarabine plus daunorubicin. She developed a fever 5 days prior which has persisted despite the addition of cefepime and vancomycin to her prophylactic antibiotic regimen of norfloxacin, fluconazole, and acyclovir. Other than diaphoresis and chills during her periodic fevers, she remains largely asymptomatic except for a general sense of malaise and nausea associated with her chemotherapy, as well as oral pain due to mucositis. She remains neutropenic despite administration of hematopoietic growth factors. Blood, urine, and sputum cultures all remain negative. What is the next step in her management?

A. Addition of metronidazole
B. Addition of tobramycin
C. Change fluconazole to caspofungin
D. Chest roentgenogram
E. High-resolution CT plus serum galactomannan enzyme immunoassay

IV-69. Which of the following organisms is most likely to cause infection of a shunt implanted for the treatment of hydrocephalus?

A. *Bacteroides fragilis*
B. *Corynebacterium diphtheriae*
C. *Escherichia coli*
D. *Staphylococcus aureus*
E. *Staphylococcus epidermidis*

IV-70. A 3-year-old boy is brought by his parents to clinic. They state that he has experienced fevers, anorexia, weight loss, and, most recently, has started wheezing at night. He had been completely healthy until these symptoms started 2 months ago. The family had travelled through Europe several months prior and reported no unusual exposures or exotic foods. They have a puppy at home. On examination, the child is ill-appearing and is noted to have hepatosplenomegaly. Laboratory results show a panic value of 82% eosinophils. Total white blood cells are elevated. A complete blood count is repeated to rule out a laboratory error and eosinophils are 78%. Which of the following is the most likely organism or process?

A. *Cysticercus*
B. Giardiasis
C. *Staphylococcus lugdunensis*
D. Toxocariasis
E. Trichinellosis

IV-71. An otherwise healthy 5-year-old child presents with low-grade fevers, sore throat, and red, itchy eyes. He attends summer camp, where several other campers were ill. On examination, the patient is noted to have pharyngitis and bilateral conjunctivitis. Which of the following is the most likely etiologic agent?

A. Adenovirus
B. Enterovirus
C. Influenza virus
D. Metapneumovirus
E. Rhinovirus

IV-72. A 35-year-old male is seen 6 months after a cadaveric renal allograft. The patient has been on azathioprine and prednisone since that procedure. He has felt poorly for the past week with fever to 38.6°C (101.5°F), anorexia, and a cough productive of thick sputum. Chest x-ray reveals a left lower lobe (5 cm) nodule with central cavitation. Examination of the sputum reveals long, crooked, branching, beaded gram-positive filaments. The most appropriate initial therapy would include the administration of which of the following antibiotics?

A. Ceftazidime
B. Erythromycin
C. Penicillin
D. Sulfisoxazole
E. Tobramycin

IV-73. A 53-year-old male with a history of alcoholism presents with an enlarging mass at the angle of the jaw. The patient describes the mass slowly enlarging over a period of 6 weeks with occasional associated pain. He has also noted intermittent fevers throughout this period. Recently, he has developed yellowish drainage from the inferior portion of the mass. He takes no medications and has no other past history. He drinks six beers daily. On physical examination, the patient has a temperature of 37.9°C (100.2°F). His dentition is poor. There is diffuse soft tissue swelling and induration at the angle of the mandible on the left. It is mildly tender, and no discrete mass is palpable. The area of swelling is ~8 × 8 cm. An aspirate is sent for Gram stain and culture. The culture initially grows *Eikenella corrodens*. After 7 days you receive a call reporting growth of a gram-positive bacillus branching at acute angles on anaerobic media. What organism is causing this man's clinical presentation?

A. *Actinomyces*
B. *Eikenella corrodens*
C. *Mucormycosis*
D. *Nocardia*
E. *Peptostreptococcus*

IV-74. What is the most appropriate therapy for this patient?

A. Amphotericin B
B. Itraconazole
C. Penicillin
D. Surgical debridement
E. Tobramycin

IV-75. A 40-year-old male smoker with a history of asthma is admitted to the inpatient medical service with fever, cough, brownish-green sputum, and malaise. Physical examination shows a respiratory rate of 15, no use of accessory muscles of breathing, and bilateral polyphonic wheezes throughout the lung fields. There is no clubbing or skin lesions. You consider a diagnosis of allergic bronchopulmonary aspergillosis. All the following clinical features are consistent with allergic bronchopulmonary aspergillosis *except*

A. bilateral, peripheral cavitary lung infiltrates
B. elevated serum IgE
C. peripheral eosinophilia
D. positive serum antibodies to *Aspergillus* species
E. positive skin testing for *Aspergillus* species

IV-76. All of the following factors increase the risk for *Clostridium difficile*–associated disease *except*

A. antacids
B. antecedent antibiotics
C. *C. difficile* colonization
D. enteral tube feeds
E. increasing length of hospital stay
F. older age

IV-77. A 19-year-old man presents to an urgent care clinic with urethral discharge. He reports three new female sexual partners over the past 2 months. What should his management be?

A. Nucleic acid amplification test for *Neisseria gonorrhoeae* and *Chlamydia trachomatis* and return to clinic in 2 days
B. Cefpodoxime, 400 mg PO × 1, and azithromycin, 1g PO × 1 for the patient and his partners
C. Nucleic acid amplification test for *N. gonorrhoeae* and *C. trachomatis plus* cefpodoxime, 400 mg PO × 1, and azithromycin, 1 g PO × 1, for the patient
D. Nucleic acid amplification test for *N. gonorrhoeae* and *C. trachomatis plus* cefpodoxime, 400 mg PO × 1, and azithromycin, 1g PO × 1, for the patient and his recent partners
E. Nucleic acid amplification test for *N. gonorrhoeae* and *C. trachomatis plus* cefpodoxime, 400 mg PO × 1, azithromycin, 1g PO × 1, and flagyl, 2 g PO × 1, for the patient and his partners

IV-78. During the first 2 weeks following solid organ transplantation, which family of infection is most common?

A. Cytomegalovirus (CMV) and Epstein-Barr virus (EBV) reactivation
B. Humoral immunodeficiency–associated infections (e.g., meningococcemia, invasive *Streptococcus pneumoniae* infection)
C. Neutropenia-associated infection (e.g., aspergillosis, candidemia)
D. T cell deficiency–associated infections (e.g., *Pneumocystis jiroveci*, nocardiosis, cryptococcosis)
E. Typical hospital-acquired infections (e.g., central line infection, hospital-acquired pneumonia, urinary tract infection)

IV-79. A 19-year-old college student is brought to the emergency department by friends from his dormitory for confusion and altered mental status. They state that many colleagues have upper respiratory tract infections. He does not use alcohol or illicit drugs. His physical examination is notable for confusion, fever, and a rigid neck. Cerebrospinal fluid (CSF) examination reveals a white blood cell count of 1800 cells/μL with 98% neutrophils, glucose of 1.9 mmol/L (35 mg/dL), and protein of 1.0 g/L (100 mg/dL). Which of the following antibiotic regimens is most appropriate as initial therapy?

A. Ampicillin plus vancomycin
B. Ampicillin plus gentamicin
C. Cefazolin plus doxycycline
D. Cefotaxime plus doxycycline
E. Cefotaxime plus vancomycin

IV-80. In addition to antibiotics, which of the following adjunctive therapies should be administered to improve the chance of a favorable neurologic outcome?

IV-80. *(Continued)*
A. Dexamethasone
B. Dilantin
C. Gabapentin
D. L-Dopa
E. Parenteral nutrition

IV-81. Which of the following viruses is the leading cause of respiratory disease in infants and children?

A. Adenovirus
B. Enterovirus
C. Human respiratory syncytial virus
D. Parainfluenza virus
E. Rhinovirus

IV-82. Several family members present to a local emergency room 2 days after a large family summer picnic where deli meats and salads were served. They all complain of profuse diarrhea, headaches, fevers, and myalgias. Their symptoms began ~24 h after the picnic. It appears that everyone who ate Aunt Emma's bologna surprise was afflicted. Routine cultures of blood and stool are negative to date. Which of the following is true regarding *Listeria* gastroenteritis?

A. Antibiotic treatment is not necessary for uncomplicated cases.
B. Carriers are asymptomatic but can easily spread infection via the fecal-oral route.
C. Gastrointestinal (GI) illness can result from ingestion of a single organism.
D. Illness is toxin-mediated, and organisms are not present at the time of infection.
E. Person-to-person spread is a common cause of outbreaks.

IV-83. Which clinical entity is the most difficult to distinguish from osteomyelitis in a diabetic foot on any currently available medical imaging (plain film, CT, MRI, ultrasound, and three-phase bone scan)?

A. Abscess
B. Cellulitis
C. Fracture
D. Neuropathic osteopathy
E. Tumor

IV-84. The human enterovirus family includes poliovirus, coxsackieviruses, enteroviruses, and echovirus. Which of the following statements regarding viral infection with one of the members of this group is true?

A. Among children infected with poliovirus, paralysis is common.
B. Enteroviruses cannot be transmitted via blood transfusions and insect bites.
C. In utero exposure to maternal enteroviral antibodies is not protective.

IV-84. *(Continued)*

  D. Infections are most common in adolescents and adults, though serious illness is most common in young children.

  E. Paralysis from poliovirus infection was more commonly seen in developing countries.

IV-85. Which of the following sexually transmitted infections (STIs) is the most common in the United States?

  A. Gonorrhea

  B. Herpes simplex virus (HSV) 2 infection

  C. HIV-1 infection

  D. Human papilloma virus infection

  E. Syphilis

IV-86. A 38-year-old woman presents to the emergency department with severe abdominal pain. She has no past medical or surgical history. She recalls no recent history of abdominal discomfort, diarrhea, melena, bright red blood per rectum, nausea, or vomiting prior to this acute episode. She ate ceviche (lime-marinated raw fish) at a Peruvian restaurant 3 h prior to presentation. On examination, she is in terrible distress and has dry heaves. Temperature is 37.6°C; heart rate is 128 beats per minute; blood pressure is 174/92 mmHg. Examination is notable for an extremely tender abdomen with guarding and rebound tenderness. Bowel sounds are present and hyperactive. Rectal examination is normal and guaiac test is negative. Pelvic examination is unremarkable. White blood cell count is 6738/μL; hematocrit is 42%. A complete metabolic panel and lipase and amylase levels are all within normal limits. CT of the abdomen shows no abnormality. What is the next step in her management?

  A. CT angiogram of the abdomen

  B. Pelvic ultrasonography

  C. Proton pump inhibitor therapy and observation

  D. Right upper quadrant ultrasonography

  E. Upper endoscopy

IV-87. Which of the following clinical features can be used to rule out malaria in favor of another tropical febrile illness in a returning traveler?

  A. Diarrhea

  B. Lack of paroxysmal nature of the fevers

  C. Lack of splenomegaly

  D. Severe myalgias and retroorbital headache

  E. None of the above

IV-88. Which of the following serology patterns places a transplant recipient at the lowest risk of developing cytomegalovirus (CMV) infection after renal transplantation?

  A. Donor CMV IgG negative, recipient CMV IgG negative

  B. Donor CMV IgG negative, recipient CMV IgG positive

  C. Donor CMV IgG positive, recipient CMV IgG negative

  D. Donor CMV IgG positive, recipient CMV IgG positive

  E. The risk is equal regardless of serology results

IV-89. Which of the following statements regarding liver abscesses is true?

  A. Amebic liver abscess should be ruled out only by direct sampling and culture of pus.

  B. Alkaline phosphatase is the most likely liver function test to be abnormal in the presence of a liver abscess.

  C. *Candida* species are most commonly isolated from patients with abscesses that develop as a result of peritoneal or pelvic pathology.

  D. Patients with liver abscesses nearly always have right upper quadrant pain.

  E. All of the above are true.

IV-90. All of the following antifungal medications may be used for the treatment of *Candida albicans* fungemia *except*

  A. amphotericin B

  B. caspofungin

  C. fluconazole

  D. terbinafine

  E. voriconazole

IV-91. A 40-year-old male is admitted to the hospital with 2–3 weeks of fever, tender lymph nodes, and right upper quadrant abdominal pain. He reports progressive weight loss and malaise over a year. On examination, he is found to be febrile and frail with temporal wasting and oral thrush. Matted, tender anterior cervical lymphadenopathy <1 cm and tender hepatomegaly are noted. He is diagnosed with AIDS (CD4+ lymphocyte count = 12/μL and HIV RNA 650,000 copies/mL). Blood cultures grow *Mycobacterium avium*. He is started on rifabutin and clarithromycin, as well as dapsone for *Pneumocystis* prophylaxis, and discharged home 2 weeks later after his fevers subside. He follows up with an HIV provider 4 weeks later and is started on tenofovir, emtricitabine and efavirenz. Two weeks later he returns to clinic with fevers, neck pain, and abdominal pain. His temperature is 39.2°C, heart rate is 110 beats per minute, blood pressure is 110/64 mmHg, and oxygen saturations are normal. His cervical nodes are now 2 centimeters in size and extremely tender, and one has fistulized to his skin and is draining yellow pus that is acid-fast bacillus stain–positive. His hepatomegaly is pronounced and tender. What is the *most likely* explanation for his presentation?

  A. Cryptococcal meningitis

  B. HIV treatment failure

  C. Immune reconstitution syndrome to *Mycobacterium avium*

  D. Kaposi's sarcoma

  E. *Mycobacterium avium* treatment failure due to drug resistance

IV-92. Which of the following statements regarding prevention of human respiratory syncytial virus (HRSV) infection in children is true?

IV-92. *(Continued)*

A. All children who are admitted to the hospital more than twice a year should be vaccinated against HRSV.

B. Barrier precautions remain the only effective means of prevention.

C. Children should be vaccinated at birth.

D. Inactivated, whole-virus vaccine should be considered in children <2 years old.

E. RSV immune globulin should be given monthly to children <2 years old who were born prematurely.

IV-93. A 52-year-old woman with alcoholic cirrhosis, portal hypertension, esophageal varices, and history of hepatic encephalopathy presents to the hospital with confusion over several days. Her husband remarks that the patient has been adherent to her medicines. These medicines include labetalol, furosemide, aldactone, and lactulose. Physical examination is notable for temperature of 38.3°C, heart rate of 115 bpm, blood pressure of 105/62 mmHg, respiratory rate of 12 breaths per minute, and oxygen saturation of 96% on room air. The patient is extremely drowsy, only intermittently able to answer questions, and disoriented. She has slight asterixis. Lungs are clear. Cardiac examination is unremarkable. Her abdomen is distended and tense but nontender. She has 3+ lower extremity edema extending to her thighs. She is guaiac negative. Her cranial nerves and extremity strength are symmetric and normal. Laboratory studies reveal a leukocyte count of 4830/μL, hematocrit = 33% (baseline = 30%), and platelet count of 94,000/μL. Basic metabolic panel is unremarkable. What is an essential component of the diagnostic workup?

A. CT scan of the head

B. Esophagastroduodenoscopy

C. Paracentesis

D. Therapeutic trial of lactulose

E. Serum ammonia level

IV-94. A 64-year-old female is admitted to the hospital with altered mental status. She recently returned from a summer white-water rafting trip in Colorado. Her husband reports increasing confusion, alternating lethargy and agitation, and visual hallucinations over the past 3 days. There is no history of drug abuse or psychiatric illness. She takes no medications. Her physical examination is notable for a temperature of 39°C (102.2°F), myoclonic jerks, and hyperreflexia. She is delirious and oriented to person only when aroused. There is no nuchal rigidity. Cerebrospinal fluid (CSF) examination reveals clear fluid with a white blood cell count of 15 cells/μL with 100% lymphocytes, protein of 1.0 g/L (100 mg/dL), and glucose of 4.4 mmol/L (80 mg/dL). Gram stain of the CSF shows no organisms. You suspect infection with West Nile virus. Which of the following studies will be most useful in making that diagnosis?

A. CSF culture

B. CSF IgM antibodies

IV-94. *(Continued)*

C. CNS MRI

D. CSF PCR

E. Stool culture

IV-95. Which of the following represents a rare but serious extrapulmonary complication of influenza infection?

A. Diffuse eczematous rash

B. Myositis

C. Oligoarthritis

D. Purulent conjunctivitis

E. Secondary bacterial pneumonia caused by *Staphylococcus aureus*

IV-96. You are a physician for an undergraduate university health clinic in Arizona. You have evaluated three students with similar complaints of fever, malaise, diffuse arthralgias, cough without hemoptysis, and chest discomfort, and one of the patients has a skin rash on her extremities consistent with erythema multiforme. Chest radiography is similar in all three, with hilar adenopathy and small pleural effusions. Upon further questioning you learn that all three students are in the same archaeology class and participated in an excavation 1 week ago. Your leading diagnosis is

A. mononucleosis

B. primary pulmonary aspergillosis

C. primary pulmonary coccidioidomycosis

D. primary pulmonary histoplasmosis

E. streptococcal pneumonia

IV-97. A 34-year-old recent immigrant from Burundi presents with fever, headache, severe myalgias, photophobia, conjunctival injection, and prostration. He lived in a refugee camp for the previous 10 years. In the camp, he was treated for several unknown febrile illnesses. Since arriving in the United States 7 years ago, he has worked as a computer analyst and lived only in a metropolitan Northwest city with no significant travel. Initial blood cultures are negative. Five days into the illness he develops hypotension, pneumonitis, encephalopathy, and gangrene of his distal digits as well as a petechial, hemorrhagic rash over his entire body except for his face. A biopsy of his rash reveals immunohistochemical changes consistent with a rickettsial infection. Which of the following rickettsial pathogens is most likely in this patient?

A. *Coxiella burnetii* (Q fever)

B. *Rickettsia africae* (African tick-borne fever)

C. *Rickettsia prowazekii* (Louse-borne typhus)

D. *Rickettsia rickettsii* (Rocky Mountain spotted fever)

E. *Rickettsia typhi* (Murine typhus)

IV-98. You are the on-call physician practicing in a suburban community. You receive a call from a 28-year-old female with a past medical history significant for sarcoidosis who is currently on no medications. She is complaining of the acute onset of crampy diffuse abdom-

IV-98. (Continued)

inal pain and multiple episodes of emesis that are non-bloody. She has not had any light-headedness with standing or loss of consciousness. When questioned further, the patient states that her last meal was 5 h previously, when she joined her friends for lunch at a local Chinese restaurant. She ate from the buffet, which included multiple poultry dishes and fried rice. What should you do for this patient?

A. Ask the patient to go to the nearest emergency department for resuscitation with IV fluids.
B. Initiate antibiotic therapy with azithromycin.
C. Reassure the patient that her illness is self-limited and no further treatment is necessary if she can maintain adequate hydration.
D. Refer the patient for CT to assess for appendicitis.
E. Refer the patient for admission for IV vancomycin and ceftriaxone because of her immunocompromised state resulting from sarcoidosis.

IV-99. *Borrelia burgdorferi* serology testing is indicated for which of the following patients, all of whom reside in Lyme-endemic regions?

A. A 19-year-old female camp counselor who presents with her second episode of an inflamed, red and tender left knee and right ankle
B. A 23-year-old male house painter who presents with a primary erythema migrans lesion at the site of a witnessed tick bite
C. A 36-year-old female state park ranger who presents with a malar rash, diffuse arthralgias/arthritis of her shoulders, knees, metacarpophalangeal and proximal interphalangeal joints; pericarditis; and acute glomerulonephritis
D. A 42-year-old woman with chronic fatigue, myalgias, and arthralgias
E. A 46-year-old male gardener who presents with fevers, malaise, migratory arthralgias/myalgias, and three erythema migrans lesions

IV-100. A 39-year-old injection drug user with a history of right-sided endocarditis and HIV infection notes back pain and fevers over the past week. He had an abscess recently on his right arm that he drained on his own. He is part of a needle-exchange program and always cleans his arm before shooting heroin into the vein in his antecubital fossa. On physical examination, he has a temperature of 38.1°C, heart rate of 124 beats per minute, and blood pressure of 75/30 mmHg. He is in a great deal of distress and is slightly confused. He has a 4/6 left lower sternal border murmur that varies with the respiratory cycle. His jugular venous pressure is monophasic and to the jaw when seated at 90 degrees. Lung examination is clear. Abdomen is benign. He is very tender over his lower spine. His extremities are warm. Leg strength is 5/5 on the right, with 4/5 left hip flexion and extension, 3/5 left knee

IV-100. (Continued)

flexion and extension, and 3/5 left foot extension. His Babinski reflex is upgoing on the left and downgoing on the right. What is the next step in management?

A. Avoidance of antibiotics until more definitive culture data is obtained; serial neurologic examinations
B. Urgent MRI and neurosurgical consultation; vancomycin after blood cultures are drawn
C. Urgent MRI and neurosurgical consultation; vancomycin plus cefepime after blood cultures are drawn
D. Urgent MRI and neurosurgical consultation; avoidance of antibiotics until more definitive culture data are obtained
E. Vancomycin plus cefepime after blood cultures are drawn; serial neurologic examinations

IV-101. An HIV-positive patient with a CD4 count of 110/μL who is not taking any medications presents to an urgent care center with complaints of a headache for the past week. He also notes nausea and intermittently blurred vision. Examination is notable for normal vital signs without fever but mild papilledema. Head CT does not show dilated ventricles. The definitive diagnostic test for this patient is

A. cerebrospinal fluid (CSF) culture
B. MRI with gadolinium imaging
C. ophthalmologic examination including visual field testing
D. serum cryptococcal antigen testing
E. urine culture

IV-102. Which of the following favors a diagnosis of acute bacterial epididymitis?

A. A solid nontender testicular mass
B. Absence of blood flow on Doppler examination
C. Concurrent urethral discharge
D. Elevation of the testicle within the scrotal sac
E. Lack of response to ceftriaxone plus doxycycline therapy

IV-103. A 19-year-old woman comes to your office after being bitten by a bat on the ear while camping in a primitive shelter. She is unable to produce a vaccination record. On physical examination, she is afebrile and appears well. There are two small puncture marks on the pinna of her left ear. What is an appropriate vaccination strategy in this context?

A. Intravenous ribavirin
B. No vaccination
C. Rabies immunoglobulins
D. Rabies inactivated virus vaccine
E. Rabies inactivated virus vaccine plus immunoglobulins

IV-104. A 26-year-old woman during a clinic is found to have a positive rapid plasmin reagin test (1:4) and a positive fluorescent treponemal antibody-absorption test

IV-104. *(Continued)*

(FTA-ABS). She has never been treated for syphilis. She recalls a large painless ulcer on her labia 9 months prior, followed about 2 months later by a diffuse rash and oral lesions that also resolved. She has had five sexual contacts in the past year. In addition to treating the patient, all of the following additional interventions should be considered *except*

A. echocardiogram looking at the aortic arch
B. HIV counseling and testing
C. pregnancy testing
D. screening and treatment of all recent sexual contacts
E. screening for other sexually transmitted diseases (STDs)

IV-105. Per-coital rate of HIV acquisition in a man who has unprotected sexual intercourse with an HIV-infected female partner is likely to increase under which of the following circumstances?

A. Acute HIV infection in the female partner
B. Female herpes simplex virus (HSV)-2 positive serostatus
C. Male nongonococcal urethritis at the time of intercourse
D. Uncircumcised male status
E. All of the above

IV-106. All of the following are associated with increased risk of pelvic inflammatory disease (PID) *except*

A. bacterial vaginosis
B. history of salpingitis
C. intrauterine device
D. recent sexual exposure to a man with urethritis
E. symptoms beginning on days 14–21 of the menstrual cycle

IV-107. Current Centers for Disease Control and Prevention (CDC) recommendations are that screening for HIV be performed in which of the following?

A. All high-risk groups (injection drug users, men who have sex with men, and high-risk heterosexual women)
B. All U.S. adults
C. Injection drug users
D. Men who have sex with men
E. Women who have sex with more than two men per year

IV-108. A 26-year-old woman presents late in the third trimester of her pregnancy with high fevers, myalgias, backache, and malaise. She is admitted and started on empirical broad-spectrum antibiotics. Blood cultures return positive for *Listeria monocytogenes*. She delivers a 5-lb infant 24 h after admission. Which of the following statements regarding antibiotic treatment for this infection is true?

A. Clindamycin should be used in patients with penicillin allergy.

IV-108. *(Continued)*

B. Neonates should receive weight-based ampicillin and gentamicin.
C. Penicillin plus gentamicin is first-line therapy for the mother.
D. Quinolones should be used for *Listeria* bacteremia in late-stage pregnancy.
E. Trimethoprim-sulfamethoxazole has no efficacy against *Listeria*.

IV-109. Glucocorticoids have been shown to be of benefit for treatment for all of the following infections *except*

A. *Aspergillus fumigatus* pneumonia
B. *Mycobacterium tuberculosis* pericarditis
C. *Pneumocystis carinii* pneumonia
D. severe typhoid fever
E. *Streptococcus pneumoniae* meningitis

IV-110. A 23-year-old previously healthy female letter carrier works in a suburb in which the presence of rabid foxes and skunks has been documented. She is bitten by a bat, which then flies away. Initial examination reveals a clean break in the skin in the right upper forearm. She has no history of receiving treatment for rabies and is unsure about vaccination against tetanus. The physician should

A. clean the wound with a 20% soap solution
B. clean the wound with a 20% soap solution and administer tetanus toxoid
C. clean the wound with a 20% soap solution, administer tetanus toxoid, and administer human rabies immune globulin intramuscularly
D. clean the wound with a 20% soap solution, administer tetanus toxoid, administer human rabies immune globulin IM, and administer human diploid cell vaccine
E. clean the wound with a 20% soap solution and administer human diploid cell vaccine

IV-111. In a patient who has undergone a traumatic splenectomy, what test can be ordered to establish lack of splenic function?

A. CT scan of the abdomen
B. Neutrophil migration studies
C. Peripheral blood flow cytometry
D. Peripheral blood smear

IV-112. A patient is admitted with fevers, malaise, and diffuse joint pains. His initial blood cultures reveal methicillin-resistant *Staphylococcus aureus* (MRSA) in all culture bottles. He has no arthritis on examination, and his renal function is normal. Echocardiogram shows a 5-mm vegetation on the aortic valve. He is initiated on IV vancomycin at 15 mg/kg every 12 h. Four days later the patient remains febrile and cultures remain positive for MRSA. In addition to a search for embolic foci of infection, which of the following changes would you make to his treatment regimen?

IV-112. *(Continued)*

A. No change

B. Add gentamicin

C. Add rifampin

D. Check the vancomycin serum peak and trough levels and consider tid dosing

E. Discontinue vancomycin, start daptomycin

IV-113. A 23-year-old woman develops cytomegalovirus (CMV) pneumonitis 5 months after a lung transplant. She developed severe side effects from ganciclovir while receiving prophylaxis. Foscarnet is prescribed for this episode. Which of the following side effects is most likely?

A. Bone marrow suppression

B. Electrolyte wasting

C. Embryotoxic

D. Lethargy and tremors

E. Hyperkalemia

IV-114. A 38-year-old woman is seen in clinic for a decrease in cognitive and executive function. Her husband is concerned because she is no longer able to pay bills, keep appointments, or remember important dates. She also seems to derive considerably less pleasure from caring for her children and her hobbies. She is unable to concentrate for long enough to enjoy movies. This is a clear change from her functional status 6 months prior. A workup reveals a positive HIV antibody by enzyme immunoassay and Western blot. Her CD4+ lymphocyte count is 378/μL with a viral load of 78,000/mL. She is afebrile with normal vital signs. Her affect is blunted, and she seems disinterested in the medical interview. Neurologic examination for strength, sensation, cerebellar function and cranial nerve function is nonfocal. Fundoscopic examination is normal. Mini-Mental Status Examination score is 22/30. A serum rapid plasmin reagin (RPR) test is negative. MRI of the brain shows only cerebral atrophy disproportionate to her age but no focal lesions. What is the next step in her management?

A. Antiretroviral therapy

B. Cerebrospinal fluid (CSF) JV virus polymerase chain reaction (PCR)

C. CSF mycobacterial PCR

D. CSF VDRL test

E. Serum cryptococcal antigen

F. *Toxoplasma* IgG

IV-115. A 72-year-old male is admitted to the hospital with bacteremia and pyelonephritis. He is HIV-negative and has no other significant past medical history. Two weeks into his treatment with antibiotics a fever evaluation reveals a blood culture positive for *Candida albicans*. Examination is unremarkable. White blood cell count is normal. The central venous catheter is removed, and systemic antifungal agents are initiated. What further evaluation is recommended?

IV-115. *(Continued)*

A. Abdominal CT scan to evaluate for abscess

B. Chest x-ray

C. Funduscopic examination

D. Repeat blood cultures

E. Transthoracic echocardiogram

IV-116. A 40-year-old man with HIV (CD4+ lymphocyte count = 180, viral load = 1000 copies/mL) was treated for secondary syphilis based on generalized painless lymphadenopathy, a diffuse maculopapular rash that included his palms and soles, and a preceding primary genital chancre. He reported no neurologic or ophthalmic symptoms at the time and received one dose of IM penicillin G benzathine. At the time of diagnosis, his rapid plasmin reagin (RPR) titer was 1:64 and fluorescent treponemal antibody-absorption (FTA-ABS) test was positive. He follows up a year later and is found to have an RPR titer of 1:64 and his FTA-ABS remains positive. What is the appropriate intervention at this time?

A. Aqueous penicillin G 24 mU/d IV given as 4 mU q4h × 10 days

B. Doxycycline, 100 mg PO bid

C. Lumbar puncture

D. Penicillin desensitization

E. Penicillin G benzathine 2.4 mU IM weekly × 3 doses

IV-117. A 26-year-old female college student presents with tender epitrochlear and axillary tender, firm, 3-cm lymph nodes on her left side. She has a 0.5-cm painless nodule on her left second finger. She reports low-grade fever and malaise over 2 weeks. She enjoys gardening, exotic fish collecting, and owns several pets including fish, kittens, and a puppy. She is sexually active with one partner. She traveled extensively throughout rural Southeast Asia 2 years before her current illness. The differential diagnosis includes all of the following *except*

A. *Bartonella henselae* infection

B. lymphoma

C. *Sporothrix schenkii* infection

D. *Staphylococcal* infection

IV-118. A person with liver disease caused by *Schistosoma mansoni* would be most likely to have

A. ascites

B. esophageal varices

C. gynecomastia

D. jaundice

E. spider nevi

IV-119. A previously healthy 28-year-old male describes several episodes of fever, myalgia, and headache that have been followed by abdominal pain and diarrhea. He has experienced up to 10 bowel movements per day. Physical examination is unremarkable. Laboratory findings are notable only for a slightly elevated leukocyte

IV-119. (Continued)

count and an elevated erythrocyte sedimentation rate. Wright's stain of a fecal sample reveals the presence of neutrophils. Colonoscopy reveals inflamed mucosa. Biopsy of an affected area discloses mucosal infiltration with neutrophils, monocytes, and eosinophils; epithelial damage, including loss of mucus; glandular degeneration; and crypt abscesses. The patient notes that several months ago he was at a church barbecue where several people contracted a diarrheal illness. Although this patient could have inflammatory bowel disease, which of the following pathogens is most likely to be responsible for his illness?

A. *Campylobacter*
B. *Escherichia coli*
C. Norwalk agent
D. *Staphylococcus aureus*
E. *Salmonella*

IV-120. Deficits in the complement membrane attack complex (C5-8) are associated with recurrent infections of what variety?

A. *Pseudomonas aeruginosa*
B. Catalase-positive bacteria
C. *Streptococcus pneumoniae*
D. *Salmonella* spp.
E. *Neisseria meningitis*

IV-121. A previously healthy 17-year-old woman presents in early October with profound fatigue and malaise, as well as fevers, headache, nuchal rigidity, diffuse arthralgias, and a rash. She lives in a small town in Massachusetts and spent her summer as a camp counselor at a local day camp. She participated in daily hikes in the woods but did not travel outside of the area during the course of the summer. Physical examination reveals a well-developed young woman who appears extremely fatigued but not in extremis. Her temperature is 37.4°C; pulse is 86 beats per minute; blood pressure is 96/54 mmHg; respiratory rate is 12 breaths per minute. Physical examination documents clear breath sounds, no cardiac rub or murmur, normal bowel sounds, a nontender abdomen, no organomegaly, and no evidence of synovitis. Several cutaneous lesions are noted on her lower extremities, bilateral axillae, right thigh, and left groin (Figure IV-121, Color Atlas). All of the following are possible complications of her current disease state *except*

A. Bell's palsy
B. large joint oligoarticular arthritis
C. meningitis
D. progressive dementia
E. third-degree heart block

IV-122. In the patient described above, which of the following is appropriate therapy?

IV-122. (Continued)

A. Azithromycin, 500 mg PO daily
B. Ceftriaxone, 2 g IV daily
C. Cephalexin, 500 mg PO bid
D. Doxycycline, 100 mg PO bid
E. Vancomycin, 1 g IV bid

IV-123. Which of the following represents an emergent (same day) indication for cardiac surgery in a patient with infective endocarditis?

A. Culture-proven fungal endocarditis
B. Culture-proven resistant organism with septic pulmonary emboli
C. Prosthetic valve endocarditis 4 months after surgery
D. Sinus of Valsalva abscess ruptured into right heart
E. *Staphylococcus lugdunensis* in a patient with previous history of endocarditis

IV-124. Which of the following pathogens are cardiac transplant patients at unique risk for acquiring from the donor heart early after transplant when compared to other solid organ transplant patients?

A. *Cryptococcus neoformans*
B. Cytomegalovirus
C. *Pneumocystis jiroveci*
D. *Staphylococcus aureus*
E. *Toxoplasma gondii*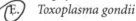

IV-125. A 68-year-old woman has been in the medical intensive care unit for 10 days with a chronic obstructive pulmonary disease flare and pneumonia, including the initial 6 days on a mechanical ventilator. She just finished a course of moxifloxacin and glucocorticoid taper when she develops abdominal discomfort over 2 days. Vital signs reveal a temperature of 38.2°C, heart rate of 94 beats per minute, blood pressure of 162/94 mmHg, respiratory rate of 18 per minute, and oxygen saturation of 90%. On examination, she is in moderate distress. She is not using accessory muscles but is tachypneic. She has a slight bilateral wheeze with good air movement. Heart sounds are distant and unchanged. Her abdomen is moderately distended and tense, with scant bowel sounds present. There is no guarding or rebound, but she is tender throughout. Review of her records reveals no bowel movement over the past 72 h and no stool is palpable in the rectal vault. White blood cell count has increased from 7100/μL to 38,000/μL over the past 2 days. Abdominal plain film shows what is read as a probable ileus in the right lower quadrant. Aside from nasogastric (NG) tube placement with suction and NPO status, which of the following should your management also include?

A. Intravenous immunoglobulin (IVIg)
B. Metronidazole, 500 mg IV tid
C. Piperacillin/tazobactam, 3.37 g IV q6h
D. Restart moxifloxacin, 400 PO qd
E. Vancomycin, 500 mg PO qid

IV-126. A 25-year-old woman presents to the clinic complaining of several days of worsening burning and pain with urination. She describes an increase in urinary frequency and suprapubic tenderness but no fever or back pain. She has no past medical history with the exception of two prior episodes similar to this in the past 2 years. Urine analysis shows moderate white blood cells. Which of the following is the most likely causative agent of her current symptoms?

A. *Candida*
B. *Escherichia coli*
C. *Enterobacter*
D. *Klebsiella*
E. *Proteus*

IV-127. A 42-year-old man with poorly controlled diabetes (HbA1C = 13.3%) presents with thigh pain and fever over several weeks. Physical examination reveals erythema and warmth over the thigh with notable woody, nonpitting edema. There are no cutaneous ulcers. CT of the thigh reveals several abscesses located between the muscle fibers of the thigh. Orthopedics is consulted to drain and culture the abscesses. Which of the following is the most likely pathogen?

A. *Clostridium perfringens*
B. Group A *Streptococcus*
C. Polymicrobial flora
D. *Staphylococcus aureus*
E. *Streptococcus milleri*

IV-128. Regarding the epidemiology of influenza viruses, which of the following is true?

A. Antigenic drift requires a change in both hemagglutinin (H) and neuraminidase (N) antigens.
B. Antigenic shift is defined by an exchange of hemagglutinin (H) and neuraminidase (N) antigens between influenza A and influenza B viruses.
C. Avian influenza outbreaks in humans occur when human influenza A viruses undergo antigenic shifts with influenza A from poultry.
D. Influenza C virus infections, while uncommon, are more virulent on a population basis due to its increased ability to undergo antigenic shift.
E. The lethality associated with avian influenza is related to its ability to spread via person-to-person contact.

IV-129. A 62-year-old man returns from a vacation to Arizona with fever, pleurisy, and a nonproductive cough. All of the following factors on history and laboratory examination favor a diagnosis of pulmonary coccidioidomycosis rather than community-acquired pneumonia *except*

A. eosinophilia
B. erythema nodosum
C. mediastinal lymphadenopathy on chest roentgenogram
D. positive *Coccidioides* complement fixation titer
E. travel limited to Northern Arizona (Grand Canyon area)

IV-130. A 36-year-old man with a history of hypertension presents complaining of a 3-year history of constant fatigue, diffuse myalgias, and memory deficits. He also notes trouble with routine tasks at work. He was diagnosed with Lyme disease 4 years ago and was briefly admitted to a cardiac care unit for transient third-degree heart block. Symptoms at that time included fever, malaise, arthralgias, diffuse erythema migrans, and facial nerve palsy. He received ceftriaxone, 2 g/d for 28 days, and had complete resolution of symptoms for several months but then developed his new constellation of problems that have gradually worsened over time. Physical examination is totally within normal limits. Which is the appropriate next step in management?

A. *Borrelia burgdorferi* enzyme-linked immunosorbent assay
B. Ceftriaxone, 2 g daily × 1 month
C. Doxycycline, 100 mg PO daily for life
D. Prednisone, 60 mg PO daily
E. Symptomatic treatment

IV-131. A sputum culture from a patient with cystic fibrosis showing which of the following organisms has been associated with a rapid decline in pulmonary function and a poor clinical prognosis?

A. *Burkholderia cepacia*
B. *Pseudomonas aeruginosa*
C. *Staphylococcus aureus*
D. *Staphylococcus epidermidis*
E. *Stenotrophomonas maltophilia*

IV-132. Empirical antibiotic therapy for continuous ambulatory peritoneal dialysis (CAPD) patients with peritonitis should be directed towards which organisms?

A. Enteric gram-negative rods
B. Enteric gram-negative rods and yeast
C. Gram-positive cocci
D. Gram-positive cocci plus enteric gram-negative rods
E. Gram-positive cocci plus enteric gram-negative rods plus yeast

IV-133. Indinavir is a protease inhibitor that carries which side effect unique for HIV antiretroviral agents?

A. Abnormal dreams
B. Benign hyperbilirubinemia
C. Hepatic necrosis in pregnant women
D. Nephrolithiasis
E. Pancreatitis

IV-134. A 28-year-old woman presents with fevers, headache, diaphoresis, and abdominal pain 2 days after returning from an aid mission to the coast of Papua New Guinea. Several of her fellow aid workers developed malaria while abroad, and she stopped her doxycycline prophylaxis due to a photosensitivity reaction 5 days prior. You send blood cultures, routine labs, and a thick and thin smear to evalu-

IV-134. *(Continued)*

ate the source of her fevers. Which of the following statements is accurate in reference to diagnosis of malaria?

A. A thick smear is performed to increase sensitivity in comparison to a thin smear but can only be performed in centers with experienced laboratory personnel and has a longer processing time.

B. Careful analysis of the thin blood film allows for prognostication based on estimation of parasitemia and morphology of the erythrocytes.

C. In the absence of rapid diagnostic information, empirical treatment for malaria should be strongly considered.

D. Morphology on blood smear is the current criterion used to differentiate the four species of *Plasmodium* that infect humans.

E. All of the above are true.

IV-135. A 34-year-old injection drug user presents with a 2-day history of slurred speech, blurry vision that is worse with bilateral gaze deviation, dry mouth, and difficulty swallowing both liquids and solids. He states that his arms feel weak as well but denies any sensory deficits. He has had no recent illness but does describe a chronic ulcer on his left lower leg that has felt slightly warm and tender of late. He frequently injects heroin into the edges of the ulcer. On review of systems, he reports mild shortness of breath but denies any gastrointestinal symptoms, urinary retention, or loss of bowel or bladder continence. Physical examination reveals a frustrated, nontoxic appearing man who is alert and oriented but noticeably dysarthric. He is afebrile with stable vital signs. Cranial nerve examination reveals bilateral cranial nerve six deficits and an inability to maintain medial gaze in both eyes. He has mild bilateral ptosis, and both pupils are reactive but sluggish. His strength is 5/5 in all extremities except for his shoulder shrug, which is 4/5. Sensory examination and deep tendon reflexes are within normal limits in all four extremities. His oropharynx is dry. Cardiopulmonary and abdominal examinations are normal. He has a 4 cm × 5 cm well-granulated lower extremity ulcer with redness, warmth, and erythema noted on the upper margin of the ulcer. What is the treatment of choice?

A. Glucocorticoids

B. Equine antitoxin to *Clostridium botulinum* neurotoxin

C. Intravenous heparin

D. Naltrexone

E. Plasmapheresis

IV-136. In an HIV-infected patient, *Isospora belli* infection is different from *Cryptosporidium* infection in which of the following ways?

A. *Isospora* causes a more fulminant diarrheal syndrome leading to rapid dehydration and even death in the absence of rapid rehydration.

IV-136. *(Continued)*

B. *Isospora* infection may cause biliary tract disease, whereas cryptosporidiosis is strictly limited to the lumen of the small and large bowel.

C. *Isospora* is more likely to infect immunocompetent hosts than *Cryptosporidium*.

D. *Isospora* is less challenging to treat and generally responds well to trimethoprim/sulfamethoxazole treatment.

E. *Isospora* occasionally causes large outbreaks among the general population.

IV-137. In a patient with known HIV infection, all of the following are an AIDS-defining criterion *except*

A. active pulmonary tuberculosis

B. CD4+ lymphocyte count < 200/μL

C. cryptococcal meningitis

D. cytomegalovirus (CMV) retinitis

E. disseminated *Mycobacterial avium* complex (MAI/MAC) infection

F. herpes zoster infection involving more than one dermatome

G. Kaposi's sarcoma

H. *Pneumocystis jiroveci* pneumonia

IV-138. A 27-year-old man presents to your clinic with 2 weeks of sore throat, malaise, myalgias, night sweats, fevers, and chills. He visited an urgent care center and was told that he likely had the flu. He was told that he had a "negative test for mono." The patient is homosexual, states that he is in a monogamous relationship and has unprotected receptive and insertive anal and oral intercourse with one partner. He had several partners prior to his current partner 4 years ago but none recently. He reports a negative HIV-1 test 2 years ago and recalls being diagnosed with *Chlamydia* infection 4 years ago. He is otherwise healthy with no medical problems. You wish to rule out the diagnosis of acute HIV. Which blood test should you order?

A. CD4+ lymphocyte count

B. HIV enzyme immunoassay (EIA)/Western blot combination testing

C. HIV resistance panel

D. HIV RNA by polymerase chain reaction (PCR)

E. HIV RNA by ultrasensitive PCR

IV-139. A 20-year-old female is 36 weeks pregnant and presents for her first evaluation. She is diagnosed with *Chlamydia trachomatis* infection of the cervix. Upon delivery, what complication is her infant most at risk for?

A. Jaundice

B. Hydrocephalus

C. Hutchinson triad

D. Conjunctivitis

E. Sensorineural deafness

IV-140. A 29-year-old man is being initiated on HIV anti-retroviral therapy (ART) because of a rising viral RNA. He has no significant past medical or psychiatric history and has never received ART. His viral resistance screening shows no likely resistance mutations. Which of the following is now considered an acceptable first-line regimen of ART for patients being newly treated for HIV infection who have no viral resistance and no other medical or psychiatric problems?

A. Stavudine (d4T), didanosine (ddI), efavirenz (EFV)
B. Tenofovir (TDF), emtricitabine (FTC), efavirenz (EFV)
C. Tenofovir (TDF), emtricitabine (FTC), indinavir
D. Tenofovir (TDF), lopinavir/ritonavir, atazanavir
E. Zidovudine (AZT), lamivudine (3TC), abacavir (ABC)

IV-141. All of the following clinical findings are consistent with the diagnosis of molluscum contagiosum *except*

A. involvement of the genitals
B. involvement of the soles of the feet
C. lack of inflammation or necrosis at the site of the rash
D. rash associated with an eczematous eruption
E. rash spontaneously resolving over 3–4 months

IV-142. A 45-year-old woman with known HIV infection and medical nonadherence to therapy is admitted to the hospital with 2–3 weeks of increasing dyspnea on exertion and malaise. Chest radiograph shows bilateral alveolar infiltrates and induced sputum is positive for *Pneumocystis jiroveci*. Which of the following clinical conditions is an indication for administration of adjunct glucocorticoids?

A. Acute respiratory distress syndrome
B. CD4+ lymphocyte count < 100/μL
C. No clinical improvement 5 days into therapy
D. Pneumothorax
E. Room air Pa$_{O_2}$ <70 mmHg

IV-143. Caspofungin is a first-line agent for which of the following conditions?

A. Candidemia
B. Histoplasmosis
C. Invasive aspergillosis
D. Mucormycosis
E. Paracoccidiomycosis

IV-144. A 19-year-old college student presents to the emergency room with crampy abdominal pain and watery diarrhea that has worsened over 3 days. He recently returned from a volunteer trip to Mexico. He has no past medical history and felt well throughout the trip. Stool examination shows small cysts containing four nuclei, and stool antigen immunoassay is positive for *Giardia*. Which of the following is an effective treatment regimen?

IV-144. *(Continued)*
A. Albendazole
B. Clindamycin
C. Giardiasis is self-limited and requires no antibiotic therapy
D. Metronidazole
E. Paromomycin
F. Tinidazole

IV-145. A 76-year-old woman is brought in to clinic by her son. She complains of a chronic nonproductive cough and fatigue. Her son adds that she has had low-grade fevers, progressive weight loss over months, and "just doesn't seem like herself." A chest CT reveals bronchiectasis and small (<5 mm) nodules scattered throughout the lung parenchyma. She had a distant history of treated tuberculosis. A sputum sample is obtained, as are blood cultures. Two weeks later, both culture sets grow acid fast bacilli consistent with *Mycobacterium avium* complex. Which of the following is the best treatment option?

A. Bronchodilators and pulmonary toilet
B. Clarithromycin and ethambutol
C. Clarithromycin and rifampin
D. Moxifloxacin and rifampin
E. Pyrazinamide, isoniazid, rifampin, and ethambutol

IV-146. Sensitive and specific serum or urine diagnostic tests exist for all of the following invasive fungal infections *except*

A. blastomycosis
B. coccidioidomycosis
C. cryptococcosis
D. histoplasmosis

IV-147. What is the most common side effect of oral ribavirin when used with pegylated interferon for the treatment of hepatitis C?

A. Drug-associated lupus
B. Hemolytic anemia
C. Hyperthyroidism
D. Leukopenia
E. Rash

IV-148. A previously unvaccinated health care worker incurs a needle stick from a patient with known active hepatitis B infection. What is the appropriate management for the health care worker?

A. Hepatitis B immunoglobulins
B. Hepatitis B vaccine
C. Hepatitis B vaccine plus hepatitis B immunoglobulins
D. Hepatitis B vaccine plus lamivudine
E. Lamivudine plus tenofovir

IV-149. Which of the following is not a common feature of severe *Plasmodium falciparum* malaria?

IV-149. *(Continued)*

   A. Acute tubular necrosis
   B. Hematocrit <15%
   C. Hepatic necrosis
   D. Hypoglycemia
   E. Obtundation

IV-150. A 55-year-old male is admitted to the hospital with aspiration pneumonia. Over the past 8 months he has had a relentless neurologic decline characterized by dementia with severe memory loss and decline in intellectual function. These symptoms were preceded by 2–3 months of labile mood, weight loss, and headache. Currently he is awake but unable to answer questions. Neurologic examination is notable for normal cranial nerves and sensation. He has marked myoclonus provoked by startle or bright lights, but it also occurs spontaneously during sleep. Prior evaluation revealed normal serum chemistries, negative serologic tests for syphilis, and normal cerebrospinal fluid (CSF) studies. Head CT scan is normal. The infectious agent that caused his neurologic syndrome is most likely a

   A. DNA virus
   B. fungus
   C. protein-lacking nucleic acid
   D. protozoan
   E. RNA virus

IV-151. A previously healthy 19-year-old man presents with several days of headache, cough with scant sputum, and fever of 38.6°C. On examination, pharyngeal erythema is noted and lung fields are clear. Chest radiograph reveals focal bronchopneumonia in the lower lobes. His hematocrit is 24.7%, down from a baseline measure of 46%. The only other laboratory abnormality is an indirect bilirubin of 3.4. A peripheral smear reveals no abnormalities. A cold agglutinin titer is measured at 1:64. What is the most likely infectious agent?

   A. *Coxiella burnetii*
   B. *Legionella pneumophila*
   C. Methicillin-resistant *Staphylococcus aureus*
   D. *Mycoplasma pneumoniae*
   E. *Streptococcus pneumoniae*

IV-152. A 79-year-old Filipino-American man with diabetes mellitus, coronary artery disease, and emphysema develops the acute onset of low back pain and night sweats. Ten days prior, he underwent a prolonged lithotripsy procedure for septic ureteral stones. He was treated for a positive PPD 23 years ago. He moved to the United States 20 years ago and was a rice farmer in the Philippines prior to moving. Examination reveals tenderness over the lumbar spine. He has 5/5 strength in his lower extremities. MRI shows findings consistent with osteomyelitis of L3 and L4, with narrowing of the disc space and a small contiguous epidural abscess that is not compressing his spinal

IV-152. *(Continued)*

cord. A needle culture of the epidural abscess drawn prior to administration of antibiotics will most likely reveal which of the following?

   A. *Brucella melitensis*
   B. *Escherichia coli*
   C. *Mycobacterium tuberculosis*
   D. *Staphylococcus aureus*
   E. Polymicrobial content with gram-positive cocci in chains, enteric gram-negative rods, and anaerobic pleomorphic forms

IV-153. A 64-year-old man in Wisconsin develops a high fever and malaise over 2 days. He has spent his weekends over the past month chopping wood in his backyard. Initial laboratory examination reveals a neutrophil count of 1000/μL, platelet count of 84,000/μL, AST of 140 U/L, and ALT of 183 U/L. A peripheral blood smear reveals prominent morulae in neutrophils. What is the most likely diagnosis?

   A. Human granulocytotropic anaplasmosis
   B. Human monocytotropic ehrlichiosis
   C. Lyme disease
   D. Rocky Mountain spotted fever
   E. Systemic lupus erythematosus

IV-154. A 26-year-old asthmatic continues to have coughing fits and dyspnea despite numerous steroid tapers and frequent use of albuterol over the past few months. Persistent infiltrates are seen on chest roentgenogram. A pulmonary consultation suggests an evaluation for allergic bronchopulmonary aspergillosis. What is the diagnostic test of choice?

   A. Bronchoalveolar lavage (BAL) with fungal culture
   B. Galactomannan enzyme immunoassay (EIA)
   C. High-resolution CT
   D. Pulmonary function tests
   E. Serum IgE level

IV-155. A patient who has undergone prosthetic valve surgery 6 weeks ago is readmitted with signs and symptoms consistent with infective endocarditis. Which of the following is the most likely etiologic organism?

   A. *Candida albicans*
   B. Coagulase-negative staphylococci
   C. *Enterococcus*
   D. *Escherichia coli*
   E. *Pseudomonas aeruginosa*

IV-156. A 28-year-old man is diagnosed with HIV infection during a clinic visit. He has no symptoms of opportunistic infection. His CD4+ lymphocyte count is 150/μL. All of the following are approved regimens for primary prophylaxis against *Pneumocystis jiroveci* infection *except*

   A. aerosolized pentamidine, 300 mg monthly

IV-156. *(Continued)*

  B.   atovaquone, 1500 mg PO daily

  C.   clindamycin, 900 mg PO q8h, plus primaquine, 30 mg PO daily

  D.   dapsone, 100 mg PO daily

  E.   trimethoprim/sulfamethoxazole, 1 single-strength tablet PO daily

IV-157. During the late 1990s, there was a resurgence of all of the following bacterial sexually transmitted infections (STIs) among homosexual men *except*

  A.   chlamydia

  B.   gonorrhea

  C.   lymphogranuloma venereum

  D.   syphilis

  E.   all of the above had a resurgence

IV-158. A 47-year-old woman with known HIV/AIDS (CD4+ lymphocyte = 106/μL and viral load = 35,000/mL) presents with painful growths on the side of her tongue (Figure IV-158, Color Atlas). What is the most likely diagnosis?

  A.   Aphthous ulcers

  B.   Hairy leukoplakia

  C.   Herpes stomatitis

  D.   Oral candidiasis

  E.   Oral Kaposi's sarcoma

IV-159. A 45-year-old patient with HIV/AIDS presents to the emergency department. He complains of a rash that has been slowly spreading up his right arm and is now evident on his chest and back. The rash consists of small nodules that have a reddish-blue appearance. Some of them are ulcerated, but there is minimal fluctuance or drainage. He is unsure when these began. He notes no foreign travel or unusual exposures. He is homeless and unemployed, but occasionally gets work as a day laborer doing landscaping and digging. A culture of a skin lesion grows a *Mycobacterium* in 5 days. Which of the following is the most likely organism?

  A.   *M. abscessus*

  B.   *M. avium*

  C.   *M. kansasii*

  D.   *M. marinum*

  E.   *M. ulcerans*

IV-160. A 25-year-old male is seen in the emergency department for symptoms of fevers and abdominal swelling, early satiety, and weight loss. His symptoms began abruptly 2 weeks ago. He was previously healthy and is taking no medications. He denies illicit drug use and recently immigrated to the United States from Bangladesh. On physical examination, temperature is 39.0°C (102.2°F) and pulse is 120, with normal blood pressure and respiratory rate. The remainder of the exam is notable for cachexia and a distended abdomen with a

IV-160. *(Continued)*

massively enlarged spleen. The spleen is tender and soft. The liver is not palpable. Mild peripheral adenopathy is present. Which of the following statements is correct regarding this patient with presumed kala azar leishmaniasis?

  A.   He probably has normal cell counts on peripheral blood smear.

  B.   *Leishmania donovani* is not endemic in Bangladesh.

  C.   Leishmania-specific cell-mediated immunity probably is present.

  D.   Splenic aspiration offers the highest diagnostic yield.

  E.   Treatment can be delayed until the diagnosis is confirmed.

IV-161. All of the following are examples of an indication for checking an HIV-resistance genotype *except*

  A.   A 23-year-old man presents to the clinic with a new diagnosis of HIV infection.

  B.   A 34-year-old man with HIV-1 infection was started on antiretroviral therapy (ART) [tenofovir (TDF), emtricitabine (FTC), efavirenz (EFV)] 1 month ago. At that time his CD4+ lymphocyte count was 213/μL and HIV-1 viral load was 65,000 (4.8 log). On recheck 1 month later, his HIV-1 viral load is 37,000 (4.6 log). He states that he is taking his medicine 100% of the time.

  C.   A 42-year-old man with HIV/AIDS who was started on ART [TDF, FTC, and ritonavir-boosted atazanavir (ATV/r)] 1 year ago was lost to follow-up. Originally his HIV-1 viral load was 197,000 (5.3 log) and CD4+ lymphocyte count was 11/μL. He was 100% compliant with his pills until he ran out of medicines 2 months ago. Viral load on recheck is 184,000 (log 5.3) with CD4+ lymphocyte count of 138/μL.

  D.   A 52-year-old woman who has had full viral suppression (HIV-1 viral load <30/mL) and 100% medical compliance on ART [zidovudine (AZT), lamivudine (3TC), EFV] for 2 years has relapsed on IV heroin over the past 3 months. She states that she continued to take her ART with "a few missed doses here and there". Repeat viral load is 3800/mL and CD4+ lymphocyte count is stable at 413/μL.

IV-162. A 41-year-old man with hepatitis C–associated ascites presents with acute abdominal pain. Physical examination is notable for temperature of 38.3°C, heart rate of 115 beats per minute, blood pressure of 88/48 mmHg, respiratory rate of 16 breaths per minute, and oxygen saturation of 99% on room air. The patient is in moderate discomfort and is lying still. He is alert and oriented. Lungs are clear. Cardiac examination is unremarkable. His abdomen is diffusely tender with distant bowel sounds, mild guarding, and no rebound tenderness. Laboratory studies reveal a leukocyte count of 11,630/μL

IV-162. (Continued)

with 94% neutrophils, hematocrit of 29%, and platelet count of 24,000/μL. Paracentesis reveals 658 PMNs/μL, total protein 1.2 g/dL, glucose 24 mg/dL, and gram stain showing gram-negative rods, gram-positive cocci in chains, gram-positive rods, and yeast forms. All of the following are indicated *except*

A. abdominal radiograph
B. broad-spectrum antibiotics
C. drotrecogin alfa
D. intravenous fluid
E. surgical consultation

IV-163. Patients with which of the following have the *lowest* risk of invasive pulmonary *Aspergillus* infection?

A. Allogeneic stem cell transplant with graft-vs-host disease
B. HIV infection
C. Long-standing high-dose glucocorticoids
D. Post-solid organ transplant with multiple episodes of rejection
E. Relapsed/uncontrolled leukemia

IV-164. All the following patient characteristics are included in the calculation of the Pneumonia Patient Outcomes Research Team (PORT) score that is used in the evaluation of patients with community-acquired pneumonia *except*

A. age
B. coexisting illness
C. laboratory findings
D. radiographic findings
E. smoking history

IV-165. Rifampin lowers serum levels of all of the following medicines *except*

A. amiodarone
B. anticonvulsants
C. oyclosporine
D. hormonal contraceptives
E. protease inhibitors
F. warfarin

IV-166. Which single clinical feature has the most specificity in differentiating *Pseudomonas aeruginosa* sepsis from other causes of severe sepsis in a hospitalized patient?

A. Ecthyma gangrenosum
B. Hospitalization for severe burn
C. Profound bandemia
D. Recent antibiotic exposure
E. Recent mechanical ventilation for >14 days

IV-167. Which of the following statements regarding varicella-zoster infection after hematopoietic stem cell transplant is true?

IV-167. (Continued)

A. Acyclovir prophylaxis is not warranted for patients with positive varicella-zoster virus serologies pretransplant as the rate of zoster reactivation is low following transplantation.
B. Herpes zoster resistance is a common problem, and a change from acyclovir to foscarnet is often required.
C. Multidermatomal and disseminated zoster can occur in transplant patients who do not receive appropriate antiviral therapy.
D. Zoster occurs more commonly following autologous transplant of stem cells than allogeneic transplant of stem cells.
E. Zoster occurs most frequently during the first month after transplant.

IV-168. All of the following factors influence the likelihood of transmitting active tuberculosis *except*

A. duration of contact with an infected person
B. environment in which contact occurs
C. presence of extrapulmonary tuberculosis
D. presence of laryngeal tuberculosis
E. probability of contact with an infectious person

IV-169. Which of the following individuals with a known history of prior latent tuberculosis infection (without therapy) has the greatest likelihood of developing reactivation tuberculosis?

A. A 28-year-old woman with anorexia nervosa, a body mass index of 16 kg/m², and a serum albumin of 2.3 g/dL
B. A 36-year-old intravenous drug user who does not have HIV but is homeless
C. A 42-year-old man who is HIV-positive with a CD4 count of 350/μL on highly active antiretroviral therapy
D. A 68-year-old man who worked as a stone mason for many years and has silicosis
E. A 73-year-old man who was infected while stationed in Korea in 1958

IV-170. A 42-year-old Nigerian man comes to the emergency room because of fevers, fatigue, weight loss, and cough for 3 weeks. He complains of fevers and a 4.5-kg weight loss. He describes his sputum as yellow in color. It has rarely been blood streaked. He emigrated to the United States 1 year ago and is an undocumented alien. He has never been treated for tuberculosis, has never had a purified protein derivative (PPD) skin test placed, and does not recall receiving BCG vaccination. He denies HIV risk factors. He is married and reports no ill contacts. He smokes a pack of cigarettes daily and drinks a pint of vodka on a daily basis. On physical examination, he appears chronically ill with temporal wasting. His body mass index is 21 kg/m². Vital signs are: blood pressure 122/68 mmHg, heart rate 89 beats/min, respiratory rate 22 breaths/min, SaO₂ 95% on room air, and temperature

IV-170. *(Continued)*

37.9°C. There are amphoric breath sounds posteriorly in the right upper lung field with a few scattered crackles in this area. No clubbing is present. The examination is otherwise unremarkable. A portion of the CT scan of his lungs is shown.

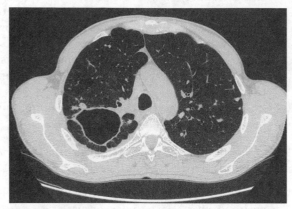

FIGURE IV-170

A stain for acid-fast bacilli is negative. What is the most appropriate approach to the ongoing care of this patient?

A.   Admit the patient on airborne isolation until three expectorated sputums show no evidence of acid-fast bacilli.

B.   Admit the patient without isolation as he is unlikely to be infectious with a negative acid-fast smear.

C.   Perform a biopsy of the lesion and consult oncology.

D.   Place a PPD test on his forearm and have him return for evaluation in 3 days.

E.   Start a 6-week course of antibiotic treatment for anaerobic bacterial abscess.

IV-171. A 50-year-old man is admitted to the hospital for active pulmonary tuberculosis with a positive sputum acid-fast bacilli smear. He is HIV positive with a CD4 count of 85/μL and is not on highly active antiretroviral therapy. In addition to pulmonary disease, he is found to have disease in the L4 vertebral body. What is the most appropriate initial therapy?

A.   Isoniazid, rifampin, ethambutol, and pyrazinamide

B.   Isoniazid, rifampin, ethambutol, and pyrazinamide; initiate antiretroviral therapy

C.   Isoniazid, rifampin, ethambutol, pyrazinamide, and streptomycin

D.   Isoniazid, rifampin, and ethambutol

E.   Withhold therapy until sensitivities are available.

IV-172. All of the following individuals receiving tuberculin skin purified protein derivative (PPD) reactions should be treated for latent tuberculosis *except*

A.   A 23-year-old injection drug user who is HIV negative has a 12-mm PPD reaction.

IV-172. *(Continued)*

B.   A 38-year-old fourth grade teacher has a 7-mm PPD reaction and no known exposures to active tuberculosis. She has never been tested with a PPD previously.

C.   A 43-year-old individual in the Peace Corps working in Sub-Saharan Africa has a 10-mm PPD reaction. 18 months ago, the PPD reaction was 3 mm.

D.   A 55-year-old man who is HIV positive has a negative PPD. His partner was recently diagnosed with cavitary tuberculosis.

E.   A 72-year-old man who is receiving chemotherapy for non-Hodgkin's lymphoma has a 16-mm PPD reaction.

IV-173. A 34-year-old man seeks the advice of his primary care physician because of an asymptomatic rash on his chest. There are coalescing light brown to salmon-colored macules present on the chest. A scraping of the lesions is viewed after a wet preparation with 10% potassium hydroxide solution. There are both hyphal and spore forms present, giving the slide an appearance of "spaghetti and meatballs." In addition, the lesions fluoresce to a yellow-green appearance under a Wood's lamp. Tinea versicolor is diagnosed. Which of the following microorganisms is responsible for this skin infection?

A.   *Fusarium solani*

B.   *Malassezia furfur*

C.   *Sporothrix schenkii*

D.   *Trichophyton rubrum*

IV-174. A 68-year-old woman seeks evaluation for an ulcerative lesion on her right hand. She reports the area on the back of her right hand was initially red and not painful. There appeared to be a puncture wound in the center of the area, and she thought she had a simple scratch acquired while gardening. Over the next several days, the lesion became verrucous and ulcerated. Now, the patient has noticed several nodular areas along the arm, one of which ulcerated and began draining a serous fluid today. She is also noted to have an enlarged and tender epitrochlear lymph node on the right arm. A biopsy of the edge of the lesion shows ovoid and cigar-shaped yeasts. Sporotrichosis is diagnosed. What is the most appropriate therapy for this patient?

A.   Amphotericin B intravenously

B.   Caspofungin intravenously

C.   Clotrimazole topically

D.   Itraconazole orally

E.   Selenium sulfide topically

IV-175. A 44-year-old man presents to the emergency room for evaluation of a severe sore throat. His symptoms began this morning with mild irritation on swallowing and have gotten progressively severe over the course of 12 h. He has been experiencing a fever to as high as 39°C at home and also reports progressive shortness of breath. He denies antecedent

IV-175. *(Continued)*

rhinorrhea or tooth or jaw pain. He has had no ill contacts. On physical examination, the patient appears flushed and in respiratory distress with use of accessory muscles of respiration. Inspiratory stridor is present. He is sitting leaning forward and is drooling with his neck extended. His vital signs are as follows: temperature 39.5°C, blood pressure 116/60 mmHg, heart rate 118 beats/min, respiratory rate 24 breaths/min, Sa$_{O_2}$ 95% on room air. Examination of his oropharynx shows erythema of the posterior oropharynx without exudates or tonsillar enlargement. The uvula is midline. There is no sinus tenderness and no cervical lymphadenopathy. His lung fields are clear to auscultation, and cardiovascular examination reveals a regular tachycardia with a II/VI systolic ejection murmur heard at the upper right sternal border. Abdominal, extremity, and neurologic examinations are normal. Laboratory studies reveal a white blood cell count of 17,000 μL with a differential of 87% neutrophil, 8% band forms, 4% lymphocytes, and 1% monocytes. Hemoglobin is 13.4 g/dL with a hematocrit of 44.2%. An arterial blood gas on room air has a pH of 7.32, a Pa$_{CO_2}$ of 48 mmHg, and Pa$_{O_2}$ of 92 mmHg. A lateral neck film shows an edematous epiglottis. What is the next most appropriate step in evaluation and treatment of this individual?

A. Ampicillin, 500 mg IV q6h
B. Ceftriaxone, 1 g IV q24h
C. Endotracheal intubation and ampicillin, 500 mg IV q6h
D. Endotracheal intubation, ceftriaxone, 1 g IV q24h, and clindamycin, 600 mg IV q6h
E. Laryngoscopy and close observation

IV-176. A 45-year-old man from western Kentucky presents to the emergency room in September complaining of fevers, headaches, and muscle pains. He recently had been on a camping trip with several friends during which they hunted for their food, including fish, squirrels, and rabbits. He did not recall any tick bites during the trip, but does recall having several mosquito bites. For the past week, he has had an ulceration on his right hand with redness and pain surrounding it. He also has noticed some pain and swelling near his right elbow. None of the friends he camped with have been similarly ill. His vital signs are: blood pressure 106/65 mmHg, heart rate 116 beats/min, respiratory rate 24 breaths/min, and temperature 38.7°C. His oxygen saturation is 93% on room air. He appears mildly tachypneic and flushed. His conjunctiva are not injected and his mucous membranes are dry. The chest examination reveals crackles in the right mid-lung field and left base. His heart rate is tachycardic but regular. There is a II/VI systolic ejection murmur heard best at the lower left sternal border. His abdominal examination is unremarkable. On the right hand, there is an erythematous ulcer with a punched-out center covered by a black eschar. He has no cervical lymphadenopathy, but there are markedly enlarged and tender lymph nodes in the right axillae and epitrochlear regions. The epitrochlear node has some fluc-

IV-176. *(Continued)*

tuance with palpation. A chest x-ray shows fluffy bilateral alveolar infiltrates. Over the first 12 h of his hospitalization, the patient becomes progressively hypotensive and hypoxic, requiring intubation and mechanical ventilation. What is the most appropriate therapy for this patient?

A. Ampicillin, 2 g IV q6h
B. Ceftriaxone, 1 g IV daily
C. Ciprofloxacin, 400 mg IV twice daily
D. Doxycycline, 100 mg IV twice daily
E. Gentamicin, 5 mg/kg twice daily

IV-177. A 24-year-old man seeks evaluation for painless penile ulcerations. He noted the first lesion about 2 weeks ago, and since that time, two adjacent areas have also developed ulceration. He states that there has been blood staining his underwear from slight oozing of the ulcers. He has no past medical history and takes no medication. He returned 5 weeks ago from a vacation in Brazil where he did have unprotected sexual intercourse with a local woman. He denies other high-risk sexual behaviors and has never had sex with prostitutes. He was last tested for HIV 2 years ago. He has never had a chlamydial or gonococcal infection. On examination, there are three well-defined red, friable lesions measuring 5 mm or less on the penile shaft. They bleed easily with any manipulation. There is no pain with palpation. There is shotty inguinal lymphadenopathy. On biopsy of one lesion, there is a prominent intracytoplasmic inclusion of bipolar organisms in an enlarged mononuclear cell. Additionally, there is epithelial cell proliferation with an increased number of plasma cells and few neutrophils. A rapid plasma reagin test is negative. Cultures grow no organisms. What is the most likely causative organism?

A. *Calymmatobacterium granulomatis* (donovanosis)
B. *Chlamydia trachomatis* (lymphogranuloma venereum)
C. *Haemophilus ducreyi* (chancroid)
D. *Leishmania amazonensis* (cutaneous leishmaniasis)
E. *Treponema pallidum* (secondary syphilis)

IV-178. A 75-year-old patient presents with fevers and wasting. He describes fatigue and malaise over the past several months and is concerned that he has been losing weight. On examination, he is noted to have a low-grade fever and a soft diastolic heart murmur is appreciated. Laboratory tests reveal a normocytic, normochromic anemia. Three separate blood cultures grow *Cardiobacterium hominis*. Which of the following statements is true about this patient's clinical condition?

A. Antibiotics are not likely to improve his condition.
B. Echocardiogram will likely be normal.
C. He has a form of endocarditis with a high risk of emboli.
D. He will likely need surgery.
E. The positive blood cultures are likely a skin contaminant.

IV-179. A 38-year-old woman with frequent hospital admissions related to alcoholism comes to the emergency room after being bitten by a dog. There are open wounds on her arms and right hand that are purulent and have necrotic borders. She is hypotensive and is admitted to the intensive care unit. She is found to have disseminated intravascular coagulation and soon develops multiorgan failure. Which of the following is the most likely organism to have caused her rapid decline?

A. *Aeromonas* spp.
B. *Capnocytophaga* spp.
C. *Eikenella* spp.
D. *Haemophilus* spp.
E. *Staphylococcus* spp.

IV-180. A 39-year-old healthy man plans to travel to Malaysia and comes to clinic for appropriate vaccinations. He cannot recall which vaccines he has had in the past, but reports having had "all the usual ones" in childhood. Which of the following represents the most common vaccine-preventable infection in travelers?

A. Influenza
B. Measles
C. Rabies
D. Tetanus
E. Yellow fever

IV-181. A 19-year-old man plans on traveling through Central America by bus. He comes to clinic interested in travel advice and any vaccinations he may need. He has no medical history and takes no medicines. In addition to DEET and mosquito netting, which of the following recommendations would be important for prophylaxis against malaria?

A. Atovaquone
B. Chloroquine
C. Doxycycline
D. Mefloquine
E. Primaquine

IV-182. Which of the following is the most common source of fever in travelers returning from Southeast Asia?

A. Dengue fever
B. Malaria
C. Mononucleosis
D. Salmonella
E. Yellow fever

IV-183. A 54-year-old woman presents to the emergency room complaining of pain and redness of her left face and cheek. The area of redness began abruptly yesterday. At that time, the area was about 5 mm² near the nasolabial fold. There was rapid progression of the redness to an area that is now about 5 cm². In addition, she is complaining of intense pain in this area. On examination, there is a

IV-183. *(Continued)*
well-demarcated 5 cm² area of erythema along her left nasolabial fold. The borders are raised and indurated. The entire area is very tender to touch. Over the next 24 h, the affected area begins to develop a flaccid bullae. What is the most appropriate treatment for this patient?

A. Acyclovir
B. Clindamycin
C. Clindamycin and penicillin
D. Penicillin
E. Trimethoprim and sulfamethoxazole

IV-184. A 68-year-old man is brought to the emergency room with altered mental status, fever, and leg pain. His wife reports that he first complained of pain in his leg yesterday, and there was some slight redness in this area. Over the night, he developed a fever to as high as 39.8°C and became obtunded this morning. At that point, his family brought him to the emergency room. Upon arrival, he is unresponsive to voice and withdraws to pain. The vital signs are: blood pressure 88/40 mmHg, heart rate 126 beats/min, respiratory rate 28 breaths/min, temperature 39.3°C, and Sa_{O_2} 95% on room air. Examination of the right leg shows diffuse swelling with brawny edema. The patient grimaces in pain when the area is touched. There are several bullae filled with dark blue to purple fluid. Laboratory studies show: pH 7.22, Pa_{CO_2} 28 mmHg, Pa_{O_2} 93 mmHg. The creatinine is 3.2 mg/dL. White blood cell count is elevated at 22,660/μL with a differential of 70% polymorphonuclear cells, 28% band forms, and 2% lymphocytes. A bulla is aspirated and the Gram stain shows gram-positive cocci in chains. What is the most appropriate therapy for this patient?

A. Ampicillin, clindamycin, and gentamicin
B. Clindamycin and penicillin
C. Clindamycin, penicillin, and surgical debridement
D. Penicillin and surgical debridement
E. Vancomycin, penicillin, and surgical debridement

IV-185. In the urgent care clinic, you are evaluating a 47-year-old woman with poorly controlled diabetes who has a chief complaint of "sinusitis." She does not have a history of atopy. She first noticed a headache 2 days ago and now feels very congested in her upper nasal passages. She has hyperesthesia over her nasal bridge as well and is inquiring about antibiotics to treat her infection. She has a bloody nasal discharge with occasional black specks. On examination, the sinuses are full and tender. She has a temperature of 38.3°C. Oral examination shows a black eschar on the roof of her mouth surrounded by discolored hyperemic areas on the palate. What is the most appropriate intervention at this time?

A. Ciprofloxacin and quarantine for possible anthrax
B. ENT consultation if no improvement with oral antibiotics
C. Immediate biopsy of the involved areas and lipid amphotericin

IV-185. *(Continued)*

   D.   Immediate biopsy of the lesion and voriconazole
   E.   Intranasal decongestants and close follow-up

IV-186. A 63-year-old man from Mississippi comes to your office for evaluation of a chronic sore on his thigh. He has an open sore on his anterior thigh that has been draining purulent material for many months. The thigh is non-tender but is warm to touch. The material is purulent and foul-smelling. He has been given multiple antibiotic courses and recently finished a course of itraconazole without relief of his symptoms. He has an intact neurovascular examination of his lower extremities. His erythrocyte sedimentation rate is 64, white blood cell

IV-186. *(Continued)*

count is 15,000/μL and hemoglobin is 8 mg/dL. A plain radiograph of the affected thigh shows a periosteal reaction of the femur with osteopenia. There is suggestion of a sinus tract between the femur and the skin. A Gram stain of the pus shows broad-based budding yeast and you make a presumptive diagnosis of blastomyces osteomyelitis. What is the treatment of choice for this patient?

   A.   Amphotericin B
   B.   Caspofungin
   C.   Itraconazole
   D.   Moxifloxacin
   E.   Voriconazole

IV. INFECTIOUS DISEASES

ANSWERS

IV-1. The answer is B. *(Chap. 115)* Cat bites are the most likely animal bites to lead to cellulitis due to deep inoculation and the frequent presence of *Pasteurella multicoda*. In the immunocompetent host, only cat bites warrant empirical antibiotics. Often the first dose is given parenterally. Ampicillin/sulbactam followed by oral amoxicillin/clavulanate is effective empirical therapy for cat bites. However, in the asplenic patient, a dog bite can lead to rapid overwhelming sepsis as a result of *Capnocytophaga canimorsus* bacteremia. These patients should be followed closely and given third-generation cephalosporins early in the course of infection. Empirical therapy should also be considered for dog bites in the elderly, for deep bites, and for bites on the hand.

IV-2. The answer is A. *(Chap. 153)* This patient has bacillary angiomatosis due to cutaneous infection with *Bartonella quintana* or *B. henselae*. Kittens are the likely source of the infection in this case. Bacillary angiomatosis occurs in HIV-infected patients with CD4+ T cell counts <100/μL. The cutaneous lesions of bacillary angiomatosis are typically painless cutaneous lesions but may appear as subcutaneous nodules, ulcerated plaques, or verrucous growths. They may be single or multiple. The differential diagnosis includes Kaposi's sarcoma, pyogenic granuloma, and tumors. Biopsy findings are as described in this case, and the diagnosis is best made with histology. Treatment is with azithromycin or doxycycline. Oxacillin or vancomycin is the treatment for staphylococcal or streptococcal skin infections.

IV-3. The answer is A. *(Chap. 153)* This patient has culture-negative endocarditis, a rare entity defined as clinical evidence of infectious endocarditis in the absence of positive blood cultures. In this case, evidence for subacute bacterial endocarditis includes valvular regurgitation, an aortic valve vegetation, and embolic phenomena on the extremities, spleen, and kidneys. A common reason for negative blood cultures is prior antibiotics. In the absence of this, the two most common pathogens (both of which are technically difficult to isolate in blood culture bottles) are Q fever, or *Coxiella burnetii* (typically associated with close contact with livestock), and *Bartonella*. In this case, the patient's homelessness and body louse infestation are clues for *Bartonella quintana* infection. Diagnosis is made by blood culture about 25% of the time. Otherwise, direct PCR of valvular tissue, if available, or acute and convalescent serologies are diagnostic options. Empirical therapy for culture-negative endocarditis usually includes ceftriaxone and gentamicin, with or without doxycycline. For confirmed *Bartonella* endocarditis, optimal therapy is gentamicin plus doxycycline. EBV and HIV do not cause endocarditis. A peripheral blood smear would not be diagnostic.

IV-4. The answer is D. *(Chap. 182)* Dermatologic problems occur in >90% of patients with HIV infection. Seborrheic dermatitis is perhaps the most common rash in HIV patients, affecting up to 50% of patients. The prevalence increases with falling CD4+ T cell count. The rash involves the scalp and the face, appearing as described in the question. Therapy is standard topical treatment, although often a topical antifungal is added because of concomitant infection with *Pityrosporum*. Herpes zoster reactivation is painful and dermatomal, with progression of papules to vesicles to small pustules and then crusting. Molluscum contagiosum typically appears as one or many small pearly umbilicated asymptomatic papules occurring anywhere on the body. They can be a significant cosmetic issue in patients with AIDS. Psoriasis is not more common in patients with HIV infection but may be more severe and generalized. It would be uncommon to involve the face only.

IV-5. **The answer is B.** *(Chaps. 115 and 203)* Any returning traveler to a region where *Plasmodium falciparum* is endemic who develops a fever warrants emergent evaluation for the most common and dangerous infection in the returning traveler: malaria. *P. falciparum* is the potentially fatal form of malaria that can lead to overwhelming sepsis, renal failure, and cerebral edema; it is also the most common form of malaria in Africa. This patient should be referred to the emergency department for a thick and thin smear. If a smear can't be performed and interpreted in an expeditious fashion, then empirical doxycycline and quinine should be started. Symptoms of malaria are nonspecific but include fever, headache, abdominal pain, jaundice, myalgias, and mental status change.

IV-6. **The answer is C.** *(Chap. 124)* This patient has a classic presentation and microscopic examination of bacterial vaginosis. Bacterial vaginosis, which is linked with HIV acquisition, herpes simplex virus (HSV) 2 shedding and acquisition, gonorrhea and *Chlamydia* acquisition, increased risk of preterm delivery, and subacute pelvic inflammatory disease, is unfortunately very difficult to treat. With the best available regimens, women recur at a rate of about 25%. Metronidazole, either as an oral formulation or vaginal gel, is recommended for at least 7 days for primary infection and 10–14 days for recurrence. Intravaginal clindamycin for this duration is also an option but has been associated with more anaerobic drug resistance. Treatment of male partners with metronidazole does not prevent recurrence of bacterial vaginosis. Metronidazole, 2g PO × 1, is standard treatment for *Trichomonas* but is too short a duration for bacterial vaginosis. Fluconazole is used for vaginal candidiasis. Douching has no proven role in bacterial vaginosis infection. Acyclovir is the recommended treatment for HSV-2 genital infection.

IV-7. **The answer is B.** *(Chap. 203)* Artemisinin-containing regimens are now recommended by the World Health Organization as first-line agents for *P. falciparum* malaria. In severe *P. falciparum* malaria, IV artesunate reduced mortality by 35% compared to IV quinine. Artemether and artemotil are given IM and are not as effective as artesunate. Although safer and more effective than quinine, artesunate is not available in the United States. In the United States, quinidine or quinine is used as a necessary second choice. Intravenous quinine is as effective as and safer than IV quinidine. Quinine causes fewer arrhythmias and hypotension with infusion than quinidine, but it is often not available in U.S. hospital pharmacies. Chloroquine is only effective for *P. vivax* and *P. ovale* infection and *P. falciparum* infection in certain pockets of the Middle East and Caribbean where resistance has not yet developed. Mefloquine comes only as an oral formulation. It is most commonly employed as a prophylactic agent but is also used for treatment of multidrug-resistant malaria.

IV-8. **The answer is F.** *(Chap. 124)* HIV is the leading cause of death in some developing countries. Efforts to decrease transmission include screening and treatment of sexually associated infections. All of the listed conditions have been linked with higher acquisition of HIV, based on epidemiologic studies and high biologic plausibility. Up to 50% of women of reproductive age in developing countries have bacterial vaginosis. All of the bacterial infections are curable, and treatment can decrease the frequency of genital herpes recurrences. This highlights an additional reason that primary care doctors should screen for each of these infections in female patients with detailed historic questions, genitourinary and rectal examinations, and evidence-based routine screening for these infections based on age and risk category.

IV-9. **The answer is B.** *(Chap. 184)* Enteroviruses are responsible for up to 90% of aseptic meningitis in which an etiologic agent can be identified. Symptoms are typically more severe in adults than children. Illness is more frequent in the summer and fall in temperate climates, whereas other causes of viral meningitis are more common in winter and spring. CSF analysis always shows an elevated (though usually <1000 cells/µL) white blood cell count. Early, there may be a neutrophil predominance; however, this typically shifts toward lymphocyte predominance by 24 h. CSF glucose and protein are usually normal, though the latter can sometimes be elevated. The illness is typically self-limiting and prognosis is excellent.

IV-10.   **The answer is B.**   *(Chap. 141)*   Despite antibiotic treatment, pneumonia from all causes remains a major source of mortality in the United States. Mortality from *Legionella* pneumonia varies from 0–11% in treated immunocompetent patients to ~30% if not treated effectively. Because *Legionella* is an intracellular pathogen, antibiotics that reach intracellular MICs are most likely to be effective. Newer macrolides and quinolones are antibiotics of choice and are effective as monotherapy. Doxycycline and tigecycline are active in vitro. Anecdotal reports have described successes and failures with trimethoprim/sulfamethoxazole and clindamycin. Aztreonam, most β-lactams, and cephalosporins cannot be considered effective therapy for *Legionella* pneumonia. For severe cases, rifampin may be added to azithromycin or a fluoroquinolone initially.

IV-11.   **The answer is C.**   *(Chap. 182)*   There is unfortunately a worsening HIV-1 epidemic in the Southeastern United States among heterosexual women, with an alarmingly increasing incidence in minority adolescent females. Despite fairly widespread knowledge among the U.S. populace about how HIV is spread, there has been a gradual increase in prevalence over the past decade in men who sleep with men as well as those who acquire HIV via high-risk heterosexual transmission. This last group is notable for major increases among long-term female partners of men who engage in, or previously engaged in, high-risk behavior. Men who sleep with men still account for the largest proportion of HIV cases in this country. The proportion of cases due to needle-sharing behaviors is still significant but is decreasing.

IV-12.   **The answer is D.**   *(Chaps. 201 and 212)*   This patient has Katayama fever caused by infection with *Schistosoma mansoni*. Approximately 4–8 weeks after exposure the parasite migrates through the portal and pulmonary circulations. This phase of the illness may be asymptomatic but in some cases evokes a hypersensitivity response and a serum sickness–type illness. Eosinophilia is usual. Since there is not a large enteric burden of parasites during this phase of the illness, stool studies may not be positive and serology may be helpful, particularly in patients from nonendemic areas. Praziquantel is the treatment of choice because Katayama fever may progress to include neurologic complications. Chloroquine is used for treatment of malaria; mebendazole for ascariasis, hookworm, trichinosis, and visceral larval migrans; metronidazole for amebiasis, giardiasis, and trichomoniasis; and thiabendazole for strongyloides.

IV-13.   **The answer is E.**   *(Chap. 116)*   Live attenuated viruses are generally contraindicated as vaccines for immunocompromised hosts for fear of vaccine-induced disease. The most cited example of this is smallpox vaccine resulting in disseminated vaccinia infection. However, yellow fever vaccine is another example of a live virus vaccine. The other examples listed in this example are inactivated organisms (rabies, IM typhoid) or polysaccharide (meningococcal) and are therefore noninfectious. Oral typhoid vaccine is a live attenuated strain, so the IM form is likely preferable in this host. Malaria prophylaxis currently involves chemoprophylaxis rather than vaccination. While safe from an infectious standpoint, potential interactions with cyclosporine should be monitored.

IV-14.   **The answer is D.**   *(Chap. 208)*   Trichomoniasis is transmitted via sexual contact with an infected partner. Many men are asymptomatic but may have symptoms of urethritis, epididymitis, or prostatitis. Most women will have symptoms of infection that include vaginal itching, dyspareunia, and malodorous discharge. These symptoms do not distinguish *Trichomonas* infection from other forms of vaginitis, such as bacterial vaginosis. Trichomoniasis is not a self-limited infection and should be treated for symptomatic and public health reasons. Wet-mount examination for motile trichomonads has a sensitivity of 50–60% in routine examination. Direct immunofluorescent antibody staining of secretions is more sensitive and can also be performed immediately. Culture is not widely available and takes 3–7 days. Treatment should consist of metronidazole either as a single 2-g dose or 500-mg doses twice daily for 7 days; all sexual partners should be treated. Trichomoniasis resistant to metronidazole has been reported and is managed with increased doses of metronidazole or with tinidazole.

IV-15. **The answer is E.** *(Chap. 204)* Babesiosis due to *B. microti* is transmitted to humans by the hard-bodied tick. The infection occurs mostly in coastal southern New England and eastern Long Island; however, cases have been reported in New York, Pennsylvania, Wisconsin, and Minnesota. Most cases of babesiosis are probably never recognized because the most common (25% of adults) presentation is either asymptomatic or indistinguishable from many other self-limited acute febrile illnesses. After an incubation of 1–6 weeks after a tick bite, patients may develop fever (intermittent or sustained as high as 40°C), malaise, shaking chills, myalgias, and arthralgias. Severe infection is most common in asplenic patients and the elderly and in immunosuppressed patients (HIV, malignancy, immunosuppressive medications). Patients co-infected with *Borrelia burgdorferi* (Lyme disease) are also at risk of severe infection. It is notable for an enormous parasitemia that can reach as high as 85% and is associated with hemolysis, high-output congestive heart failure, and renal and respiratory failure.

IV-16. **The answer is D.** *(Chap. 191)* Voriconazole is an azole antifungal with a broader spectrum of activity than fluconazole against *Candida* species (including *C. glabrata* and *C. krusei*) and has activity against *Aspergillus* species. It is available in oral and parenteral forms. Voriconazole's visual disturbances are common, transient, and harmless, but patients should be warned to expect them. Voriconazole interacts significantly with many other medications, including immunosuppressive agents, such as tacrolimus, that are often used in patients at risk for systemic fungal infections. Voriconazole may also cause liver toxicity and photosensitivity. Renal toxicity is an issue with amphotericin B products rather than the azoles.

IV-17. **The answer is D.** *(Chap. 177)* Immunocompromised patients occasionally can't clear parvovirus infection due to lack of T cell function. As parvovirus B19 selectively infects red cell precursors, persistent infection can lead to a prolonged red cell aplasia and persistent drop in hematocrit, with low or absent reticulocytes. Pure red cell aplasia has been reported in HIV infection, lymphoproliferative diseases, and after transplantation. Iron studies will show adequate iron but decreased utilization. The peripheral smear usually shows no abnormalities other than normocytic anemia and the absence of reticulocytes. Antibody tests are not useful in this setting as immunocompromised patients do not produce adequate antibodies against the virus. Therefore, a PCR is the most useful diagnostic test. Bone marrow biopsy may be suggestive as it will show no red cell precursors, but usually a less invasive PCR test is adequate. Immediate therapy is with red cell transfusion, followed by IV immunoglobulins, which contain adequate titers of antibody against parvovirus B19.

IV-18. **The answer is C.** *(Chap. 141)* *Legionella* is an intracellular pathogen that enters the body through aspiration or direct inhalation. Numerous prospective studies have found it is one of the four most common causes of community-acquired pneumonia with *Streptococcus pneumoniae*, *Haemophilus influenzae*, and *Chlamydia pneumoniae* accounting for 2–9% of cases. Postoperative patients are at risk due to an increased risk of aspiration. Cell-mediated immunity is the primary host defense against *Legionella*, and patients with HIV or those who take glucocorticoids are at risk based on their depressed cell-mediated immune function. Alveolar macrophages phagocytose *Legionella*. Smokers and those with chronic lung disease are at risk given their poor local immune responses and decreased ability for widespread phagocytosis. Neutrophils play a comparatively small role in the host defense against *Legionella*, and those with neutropenia are not predisposed to *Legionella* infection.

IV-19. **The answer is D.** *(Chap. 195)* The goal of therapy for cryptococcal meningoencephalitis in an HIV-negative patient is cure of the fungal infection, not simply control of symptoms. Thus, the course of IV amphotericin is recommended to be 10 weeks with negative cerebrospinal fluid (CSF) cultures, a decreasing CSF cryptococcal antigen titer, and a normalized CSF glucose value. Once this is completed and clinical response has been achieved, therapy is followed by fluconazole to complete a 6- to 12-month course. The 2-week amphotericin can be used in clinically responding HIV-positive patients, who then will require 8 weeks of fluconazole, 400 mg daily, followed by lifelong suppressive therapy with fluconazole, 200 mg daily. Flucytosine has been used to accelerate a negative culture response, but its use exposes the patient to potentially severe toxicities. Ceftriaxone and vancomycin are the recommended treatments for bacterial meningitis in an immunocompetent patient <50 years of age.

IV-20. The answer is C. *(Chap. 129)* The major clinical concern in this patient is epidural abscess or vertebral osteomyelitis, as well as line infection due to *Staphylococcus aureus*. Metastatic seeding during *S. aureus* bacteremia has been estimated to occur as often as 30% of the time. Bones, joints, kidneys, and lungs are the most common sites. Metastatic infection to the spine should be evaluated in an emergent fashion with an MRI. The dialysis catheter should also be removed as it is infected, based on clinical examination. Infective endocarditis is a major concern. This diagnosis is based on positive blood culture results and either a vegetation on echocardiogram, new pathologic murmur, or evidence of septic embolization on physical examination. A transthoracic echocardiogram is warranted in the evaluation for endocarditis (a disease that this patient is at risk for). However, it need not be ordered emergently as it will not impact management during the initial phase of hospitalization. Moreover, because the diagnosis can only be established in the presence of positive blood cultures (or in rare cases serology of a difficult-to-culture organism), a rational approach is to await positive blood cultures before ordering an echocardiogram.

IV-21. The answer is B. *(Chap. 210)* Strongyloides is the only helminth that can replicate in the human host, allowing autoinfection. Humans acquire strongyloides when larvae in fecally contaminated soil penetrate the skin or mucus membranes. The larvae migrate to the lungs via the bloodstream, break through the alveolar spaces, ascend the respiratory airways, and are swallowed to reach the small intestine where they mature into adult worms. Adult worms may penetrate the mucosa of the small intestine. Strongyloides is endemic in Southeast Asia, Sub-Saharan Africa, Brazil, and the Southern United States. Many patients with strongyloides are asymptomatic or have mild gastrointestinal symptoms or the characteristic cutaneous eruption, larval currens, as described in this case. Small-bowel obstruction may occur with early heavy infection. Eosinophilia is common with all clinical manifestations. In patients with impaired immunity, particularly glucocorticoid therapy, hyperinfection or dissemination may occur. This may lead to colitis, enteritis, meningitis, peritonitis, and acute renal failure. Bacteremia or gram-negative sepsis may develop due to bacterial translocation through disrupted enteric mucosa. Because of the risk of hyperinfection, all patients with strongyloides, even asymptomatic carriers, should be treated with ivermectin, which is more effective than albendazole. Fluconazole is used to treat candidal infections. Mebendazole is used to treat trichuriasis, enterobiasis (pinworm), ascariasis, and hookworm. Mefloquine is used for malaria prophylaxis.

IV-22. The answer is A. *(Chap. 120)* The Gram stain is polymicrobial and the putrid smell is very specific for anaerobic organisms. The diagnosis of acute osteomyelitis is also very likely based on the positive probe to bone test and wide ulcer. Broad-spectrum antibiotics are indicated. Vancomycin and linezolid cover methicillin-resistant *Staphylococcus aureus* (MRSA) and streptococcal isolates but would miss gram-negative rods and anaerobic bacteria. Metronidazole covers only anaerobes, missing gram-positives that are key in the initiation of diabetic foot infections. Clindamycin covers gram-positives and anaerobes but misses gram-negative rods. Ampicillin-sulbactam is broad spectrum and covers all three classes of organism. If the patient has a history of MRSA or MRSA risk factors, then the addition of vancomycin or linezolid is a strong consideration.

IV-23. **The answer is C.** *(Chap. 182)* The quoted risk for HIV transmission via a needle stick is 0.3%. However, this number is likely highly variable according to a number of factors. Large-bore needle sticks where infected patient blood is visible are higher risk, as are deep tissue puncture to the health care provider. The patient's degree of virologic control is generally inferred to be critical as well. Patients with a viral load <1500/mL are considerably less likely to transmit via a needle stick than those with high viral loads. An extension of this point is that during acute and end-stage HIV infection, viral loads are extremely high and contagion by needle stick is likely to be much higher. In addition, during end-stage disease, virulent viral forms predominate, which may increase the risk to an even greater extent. Each of these variables must be assessed rapidly after an accidental high-risk needle stick. Antiretroviral therapy (ART) is effective at preventing HIV transmission via needle stick if given before viral RNA incorporates into the host genome as proviral DNA. This is thought to occur within ~48 h, but under the best scenario, ART should be given within an hour of a needle stick. Circumstances are often murky, with key information such as viral load, viral resistance history, and even HIV serostatus of the patient variably available: therefore, urgent consultation with an HIV and/or occupational health specialist is imperative after a needle stick. (Hepatitis B and C transmission must also be considered.)

IV-24. **The answer is E.** *(Chap. 172)* Antibodies to HSV-2 are not routinely detected until puberty, consistent with the typical sexual transmission of the virus. Serosurveys suggest 15–20% of American adults have HSV-2 infection. However, only 10% report a history of genital lesions. Seroprevalence is similar or higher in Central America, South America, and Africa. Recent studies in African obstetric clinics have found seroprevalence rates as high as 70%. HSV-2 infection is felt to be so pervasive in the general population based on ease of transmission, both in symptomatic and asymptomatic states. Therefore, this sexually transmitted disease (STD) is significantly more common in individuals who less frequently engage in high-risk behavior than other STDs. HSV-2 is an independent risk factor for HIV acquisition and transmission. HIV virion is shed from herpetic lesions, thus promoting transmission.

IV-25. **The answer is B.** *(Chap. 193)* Coccidioidomycosis is amazingly diverse in terms of its scope of clinical presentation, as well as clinical severity. 60% of infections as determined by serologic conversion are asymptomatic. The most common clinical syndrome in the other 40% of infected patients is an acute respiratory illness characterized by fever, cough, and pleuritic pain. Skin manifestations, such as erythema nodosum, are also common with *Coccidioides* infection. *Coccidioides* infection can cause a severe and difficult-to-treat meningitis in AIDS patients, other immunocompromised patients, and occasionally immunocompetent hosts, and can occasionally cause acute respiratory distress syndrome and fatal multilobar pneumonia. *Coccidioides* is confined to the western hemisphere. Endemic regions include Southern Arizona, the Central Valley of California, and Northern Mexico, where it resides in soil. The risk of symptomatic infection increases with age.

IV-26 and IV-27. **The answers are B and E.** *(Chap. 122)* Norovirus, or the so-called Norwalk-like agent, was initially described as a cause of food-borne illness in Norwalk, Ohio, in 1968. Since that time the virus responsible has been identified as a small RNA virus of the Calciviridae family. The initial detection of the Norwalk agent was poor, relying on electron microscopy or immune electron microscopy. Using these techniques, the Norwalk agent was identified as the causative agent in 19–42% of nonbacterial diarrheal outbreaks. With the development of more sensitive molecular assays (reverse transcriptase PCR, enzyme-linked immunosorbent assay), Norwalk-like viruses are being found as increasingly frequent causes of diarrheal outbreaks. Treatment is supportive as symptoms improve within 10–51 h. Rotavirus is the most common cause of viral diarrhea in infants but is uncommon in adults. Salmonella, shigella, and *E. coli* present with more colonic and systemic manifestations.

IV-28.   The answer is C. *(Chap. 171)*   Lamivudine is a pyrimidine nucleoside analogue that has activity against HIV and hepatitis B. In acute hepatitis B, lamivudine results in suppression of HBV DNA and loss of hepatitis E antigen in 30% of patients. Tenofovir is a nucleotide analogue with activity against HIV and hepatitis B. It is not approved for initial treatment for HBV but may be used for HIV/HBV co-infection or for HBV resistant to lamivudine. Efavirenz has activity only against HIV and not hepatitis B. Ganciclovir has activity against herpes viruses and is mostly used for treatment of cytomegalovirus. Rimantadine has antiviral activity only against influenza A.

IV-29.   The answer is E. *(Chap. 182)*   Rate of progression from initial HIV infection to AIDS is likely determined by many factors, but viral load set point, measured ~2–6 months after acute infection, is the most predictive factor. Most persons have a median time of 10 years, but rapid progressors with high viral loads can develop AIDS over 5 years whereas some "long-term nonprogressors" with low viral load set points can be asymptomatic with HIV infection for decades. CD4+ lymphocyte count is a measure of how close one is to developing AIDS rather than a measure of rate of progression: it tends to be close to normal once viral load set point is achieved. Resistance of the virus is more of a determinant of response to specific therapies than disease progression in the absence of therapy. CMV serology is important as a predictor for CMV disease once a person reaches a CD4+ lymphocyte count < 50/μL.

IV-30.   The answer is D. *(Chap. 161)*   Drugs used to treat *Mycobacterium tuberculosis* are classified as first-line or second-line. First-line agents, which are proven most effective and are necessary for any short-course treatment regimen, include isoniazid, rifampin, ethambutol, and pyrazinamide. First-line supplemental agents, which are highly effective with acceptable toxicity, include rifabutin, rifapentine, and streptomycin. Second-line agents, which are either less clinically active or have greater toxicity, include para-aminosalicylic acid, ethionamide, cycloserine, amikacin, and capreomycin. The fluoroquinolones, levofloxacin and moxifloxacin, are active against *M. tuberculosis* but are not yet considered first-line therapy. While not approved for treatment of *M. tuberculosis* in the United States, promising trials are underway. Some experts consider moxifloxacin a supplemental first-line therapy. It is necessary to have at least three active agents during the 2-month induction phase of active tuberculosis therapy. Ethambutol is initially used as a fourth agent to account for the possibility of drug resistance to one of the other agents. Consolidation phase includes rifampin and isoniazid, and is 4–7 months in length, depending on anatomic location of infection as well as clearance of sputum cultures at 2 months.

IV-31.   The answer is D. *(Chaps. 126 and 175)*   CMV retinitis, a common CMV infection in HIV patients, occurs very rarely in solid organ transplant patients. CMV does affect the lung in a majority of transplant patients if either donor or recipient is CMV-seropositive pretransplant. CMV disease in transplant recipients typically develops 30–90 days posttransplant. It rarely occurs within 2 weeks of transplantation. CMV very commonly causes a pneumonitis that clinically is difficult to distinguish from acute rejection. Prior CMV infection has been associated with bronchiolitis obliterans syndrome (chronic rejection) in lung transplant recipients. As with HIV, the gastrointestinal tract is commonly involved with CMV infection. Endoscopy with biopsy showing characteristic giant cells, not serum polymerase chain reaction (PCR), is necessary to make this diagnosis. The CMV syndrome is also common in lung transplant patients. Serum CMV PCR should be sent as part of the workup for all nonspecific fevers, worsening lung function, liver function abnormalities, or falling leukocyte counts occurring more than a couple of weeks after transplant.

IV-32.   The answer is D. *(Chap. 179)*   In 2002, an outbreak of a severe systemic illness, named *severe acute respiratory syndrome*, or SARS, began in China. Ultimately 8000 cases were recorded in 28 countries. The etiologic agent proved to be a virus associated with the Coronavirus family, now named *SARS-CoV*. The natural reservoir appears to be the horseshoe bat, though human exposure may have come from domesticated animals such as the palm civet. While some patients acquired the virus from animals or the environment, the majority appear to have contracted the illness from other people. Human-to-human transmission, either by aerosol or fecal-oral routes, is efficient. Environmental transmission (water, sewage) may also have played a role, particularly in the outbreak centered in an apartment complex. In the outbreak, children had a much less severe clinical course compared to adults. In 2003 the outbreak ceased, and no new cases have arisen since 2004. Many unanswered questions linger in the wake of this illness.

IV-33. **The answer is D.** *(Chap. 141)* *Legionella* urine antigen is detectable within 3 days of symptoms and will remain positive for 2 months. It is not affected by antibiotic use. The urinary antigen test is formulated to detect only *L. pneumophilia* (which causes 80% of *Legionella* infections) but cross-reactivity with other *Legionella* species has been reported. The urinary test is sensitive and highly specific. Typically, Gram's staining of specimens from sterile sites such as pleural fluid show numerous white blood cells but no organisms. However, *Legionella* may appear as faint, pleomorphic gram-negative bacilli. *Legionella* may be cultured from sputum even when epithelial cells are present. Cultures, grown on selective media, take 3–5 days to show visible growth. Antibody detection using acute and convalescent serum is an accurate means of diagnosis. A fourfold rise is diagnostic, but this takes up to 12 weeks so is most useful for epidemiologic investigation. *Legionella* PCR has not been shown to be adequately sensitive and specific for clinical use. It is used for environmental sampling.

IV-34. **The answer is D.** *(Chap. 209)* There are roughly 12 cases of trichinellosis reported each year in the United States. Since most infections are asymptomatic, this may be an underestimate. Heavy infections can cause enteritis, periorbital edema, myositis, and, infrequently, death. This infection, caused by ingesting *Trichinella* cysts, occurs when infected meat from pigs or other carnivorous animals is eaten. Laws that prevent feeding pigs uncooked garbage have been an important public health measure in reducing *Trichinella* infection in this country. Person-to-person spread has not been described. The majority of infections are mild and resolve spontaneously.

IV-35. **The answer is E.** *(Chap. 172)* Primary genital herpes due to HSV-2 is characterized by fever, headache, malaise, inguinal lymphadenopathy, and diffuse genital lesions of varying stage. The cervix and urethra are usually involved in women. While both HSV-2 and HSV-1 can involve the genitals, the recurrence rate of HSV-2 is much higher (90% in the first year) than with HSV-1 (55% in the first year). The rate of reactivation for HSV-2 is very high. Acyclovir (or its cogeners valacyclovir and famciclovir) is effective in shortening the duration of symptoms and lesions in genital herpes. Chronic daily therapy can reduce the frequency of recurrences in those with frequent reactivation. Valacyclovir has been shown to reduce transmission of HSV-2 between sexual partners.

IV-36. **The answer is C.** *(Chap. 122)* Enterotoxigenic *E. coli* is responsible for 50% of traveler's diarrhea in Latin America and 15% in Asia. Enterotoxigenic and enteroaggregative *E. coli* are the most common isolates from persons with classic secretory traveler's diarrhea. Treatment of frequent watery stools due to presumed *E. coli* infection may be with ciprofloxacin, or because of concerns regarding increasing ciprofloxacin resistance, azithromycin. *E. histolytica* and *V. cholerae* account for smaller percentages of traveler's diarrhea in Mexico. *Campylobacter* is more common in Asia and during the winter in subtropical areas. *Giardia* is associated with contaminated water supplies and in campers who drink from freshwater streams.

IV-37. **The answer is E.** *(Chap. 209)* Trichinellosis occurs when infected meat products are eaten, most frequently pork. The organism can also be transmitted through the ingestion of meat from dogs, horses, and bears. Recent outbreaks in the United States and Canada have been related to consumption of wild game, particularly bear meat. During the first week of infection, diarrhea, nausea, and vomiting are prominent features. As the parasites migrate from the GI tract, fever and eosinophilia are often present. Larvae encyst after 2–3 weeks in muscle tissue, leading to myositis and weakness. Myocarditis and maculopapular rash are less common features of this illness. *Giardia* and *Campylobacter* are organisms that are frequently acquired by drinking contaminated water; neither will produce this pattern of disease. While both will cause GI symptoms (and *Campylobacter* will cause fever), neither will cause eosinophilia or myositis. *Taenia solium*, or pork tapeworm, shares a similar pathogenesis to *Trichinella* but does not cause myositis. Cytomegalovirus has varied presentations but none that lead to this presentation.

IV-38. The answer is E. *(Chap. 182)* Abacavir use is associated with a potentially severe hypersensitivity reaction in about 5% of patients. There is likely a genetic component, with HLA-B*5701 being a significant risk factor for hypersensitivity syndrome. Symptoms, which usually occur within 2 weeks of therapy but can take >6 weeks to emerge, include fever, maculopapular rash, fatigue, malaise, gastrointestinal symptoms, and/or dyspnea. Once a diagnosis is suspected, the drug should be stopped and never given again because rechallenge can be fatal. For this reason, both the diagnosis and patient education once the diagnosis is made must be performed thoroughly and carefully. It is important to note that two available combination pills contain abacavir (epzicom, trizivir), so patients must know to avoid these as well. Fanconi's anemia is a rare disorder associated with tenofovir. Zidovudine causes anemia and sometimes granulocytopenia. Stavudine and other nucleoside reverse transcriptase inhibitors are associated with lipoatrophy of the face and legs.

IV-39. The answer is C. *(Chap. 129)* In recent years, the emergence of "community acquired" methicillin-resistant *Staphylococcus aureus* (CA-MRSA) in numerous populations has been well documented. This pathogen most commonly leads to pyogenic infections of the skin but has also been associated with necrotizing fasciitis, infectious pyomyositis, endocarditis, and osteomyelitis. The most feared complication is a necrotizing pneumonia that often follows influenza upper respiratory infection and can affect previously healthy people. This pathogen produces the Panton-Valentine leukocidin protein that forms holes in the membranes of neutrophils as they arrive at the site of infection, and serves as marker for this pathogen. An easy way to identify this strain of MRSA is its sensitivity profile. Unlike MRSA isolates of the past, which were sensitive only to vancomycin, daptomycin, quinupristin/dalfopristin, and linezolid, CA-MRSA are almost uniformly susceptible to TMP/SMX and doxycycline as well. The organism is also usually sensitive to clindamycin. The term *community-acquired* has probably outlived its usefulness as this isolate has become the most common *S. aureus* isolate causing infection in many hospitals around the world.

IV-40. The answer is D. *(Chap. 144)* *Helicobacter pylori* is thought to colonize ~50% (30% in developed countries, >80% in developing countries) of the world's population. The organism induces a direct tissue response in the stomach, with evidence of mononuclear and polymorphonuclear infiltrates in all of those with colonization, regardless of whether or not symptoms are present. Gastric ulceration and adenocarcinoma of the stomach arise in association with this gastritis. MALT is specific to *H. pylori* infection and is due to prolonged B cell activation in the stomach. Though *H. pylori* does not directly infect the intestine, it does diminish somatostatin production, indirectly contributing to the development of duodenal ulcers. Gastroesophageal reflux disease is not caused by *H. pylori*, and some early, controversial research may suggest that it is in fact protective against this condition.

IV-41. The answer is D. *(Chap. 177)* The most likely diagnosis based on her antecedent illness with a facial rash is parvovirus infection. Parvovirus commonly leads to a diffuse symmetric arthritis in the immune phase of illness when IgM antibodies are developed. Occasionally the arthritis persists over months and can mimic rheumatoid arthritis. The acute nature of these complaints makes systemic lupus erythematosus and rheumatoid arthritis less likely. Reactive arthritis due to *Chlamydia* or a list of other bacterial pathogens tends to effect large joints such as the sacroiliac joints and spine. It is also sometimes accompanied by uveitis and urethritis. The large number of joints involved with a symmetric distribution argues against crystal or septic arthropathy.

IV-42. **The answer is C.** *(Chap. 196)* Isolation of yeast from the blood stream can virtually never be considered a contaminant. Presentation may be indolent with malaise only, or fulminant with overwhelming sepsis in the neutropenic host. All indwelling catheters need to be removed to ensure clearance of infection, and evaluation for endocarditis and endophthalmitis should be strongly considered, particularly in patients with persistently positive cultures or fever. Both of these complications of fungemia often entail surgical intervention for cure. A positive yeast culture in the urine is often difficult to interpret, particularly in patients on antibiotics and in the ICU. Most frequently, a positive culture for yeast represents contamination, even if the urinalysis suggests bladder inflammation. An attractive option is to remove the Foley catheter and recheck a culture. Antifungals are indicated if the patient appears ill, in the context of renal transplant where fungal balls can develop in the graft, and often in neutropenic patients. *Candida* pneumonia is uncommon, even in immunocompromised patients. A positive yeast culture of the sputum is usually representative of commensal oral flora and should not be managed as an infection, particularly as in this case where acute bacterial pneumonia is likely.

IV-43. **The answer is D.** *(Chap. 123)* *Clostridium difficile*–associated disease recurrences are most often due to reinfection (because patients carry similar risk factors as they did before first infection) or relapse (due to persistence of spores in the bowel). Approximately 15–30% of patients have at least one relapse. Recurrent disease has been associated with ~10% risk of serious complications including shock, megacolon, perforation, colectomy, or death at 30 days. Metronidazole resistance occurs but is actually a very rare event. Metronidazole and vancomycin have a similar efficacy in a first episode of recurrence. Repeated courses of metronidazole should be avoided due to neurotoxicity. Unfortunately, patients who recur are more likely to recur again, and many patients receive multiple cycles of antibiotics and are even candidates for more extreme measures such as intravenous immunoglobulin or fecal transplant via stool enema. Testing for clearance is not likely to be informative. A negative stool antigen would not change management, as symptomatic improvement is the true goal of therapy. A positive stool antigen and toxin test in a patient whose symptoms have improved after standard therapy implies colonization, not disease. It can therefore be needlessly discouraging to patients and again does not impact clinical management. There is no known association between *C. difficile*–associated disease and colon cancer.

IV-44. **The answer is B.** *(Chap. 182)* CMV colitis should be considered in AIDS patients with CD4+ lymphocyte count <50/μL, fevers, and diarrhea. Diarrhea is often bloody but can be watery. Initial evaluation often involves stool studies to rule out other parasitic or bacterial causes of diarrhea in AIDS patients. A standard panel will include some or all of the following depending on epidemiologic and historical data: *Clostridium difficile* stool antigen, stool culture, stool *Mycobacterium avium intracellulare* culture, stool ova and parasite examination and special stains for *Cryptosporidium, Isospora, Cyclospora* and *Microsporidium*. There is no stool or serum test that is useful for the evaluation of CMV colitis in an HIV-infected patient. A positive CMV IgG is merely a marker of past infection. If this test is negative, then the pretest probability of developing active CMV decreases substantially. Serum CMV PCR has gained utility in solid organ and bone marrow transplant patients for following treatment response for invasive CMV infection. However, in HIV-infected patients, CMV viremia correlates imprecisely with colitis. Further, because CMV is a latent-lytic herpesvirus, a positive serum PCR does not imply disease unless drawn in the right clinical context, for which there is none in HIV infection. Colonic histology is sensitive and specific for the diagnosis of CMV colitis, with large-cell inclusion bodies being diagnostic.

IV-45. **The answer is D.** *(Chap. 143)* β-lactamases are a major source of antibiotic resistance in gram-negative bacilli. Many gram-negative bacteria produce broad-spectrum β-lactamases that confer resistance to penicillins and first-generation cephalosporins. The addition of clavulanate, a β-lactamase inhibitor, to an antibiotic regimen is often enough to overcome this resistance. Extended-spectrum β-lactamases (ESBL), however, lead to resistance to all β-lactam drugs including third- and fourth-generation cephalosporins. ESBL-producing genes can be acquired by gram-negative bacteria via plasmids and are becoming increasingly prevalent in hospitals worldwide. *Klebsiella* and *Escherichia coli* are the most common bacteria that acquire ESBLs, though it can be seen in many other gram-negatives including *Serratia*, *Proteus*, *Enterobacter*, and *Citrobacter*. The most common scenario for the development of ESBL-gram negatives in the hospital is prevalent use of third-generation cephalosporins. Carbapenems should be considered first-line antibiotics for these bacteria. Macrolides and quinolones have different mechanisms of action than β-lactam antibiotics and do not apply selective pressure to generate ESBL-producing bacteria.

IV-46.   **The answer is E.** *(Chap. 164)* The patient has Weil's syndrome due to infection with *Leptospira interrogans* as evidenced by her flulike prodrome followed by profound hyperbilirubinemia with only minor hepatocellular dysfunction as well as renal failure. Rats are the most important reservoir. The organism is excreted in urine and can survive in water for months. Important sources of exposure include occupational, recreation in contaminated waters, and being homeless in contaminated living areas. Weil's represents the immune phase of the disease in its most severe form. A bleeding diathesis is common, as is pulmonary hemorrhage. The conjunctival suffusion during the initial spirochetemic phase of the disease is an important diagnostic clue. Penicillin G is appropriate therapy for severe leptospirosis, but its comparative efficacy is not yet proven in the literature. Acute myelogenous leukemia would likely cause more characteristic abnormalities in blood counts with this degree of illness. Acute interstitial pneumonitis (Haman-Rich syndrome) affects only the lung and would not be associated with the severe increases in bilirubin. Polyarteritis nodosa rarely involved the lung and would not be expected to cause such a high bilirubin, even in the setting of hepatic ischemia. Rat-bite fever causes intermittent fevers, polyarthritis, and a nonspecific rash.

IV-47.   **The answer is B.** *(Chap. 167)* Rocky Mountain spotted fever, caused by *Rickettsia rickettsii*, occurs throughout the United States, Canada, Mexico, Central America, and South America. It is transmitted by the dog tick in the eastern two-thirds of the United States and by the wood tick in the western United States. Humans are typically infected during tick season from May through September. In the preantibiotic era, the case fatality rate approached 25%. Currently the mortality remains ~5%, mostly due to delayed recognition and therapy. The incubation period after a tick bite is approximately 1 week. The initial signs and symptoms of Rocky Mountain spotted fever are entirely nonspecific, and the typical rash is often not seen in early disease. It may be difficult to distinguish from many self-limited viral syndromes. Only 60% of patients recall a tick bite, and only 3% of patients have the classic history of tick bite, fever, and rash. Therefore, assessment for this potentially deadly disease should be based on epidemiologic grounds. His recent high-risk travel period for tick bite in a highly endemic region makes this patient a high pretest probability. Empirical treatment is warranted and will not affect the diagnostic workup. A diagnostic indirect immunofluorescent antibody test will not be positive (≥1:64 titer) until 7–10 days after symptoms. The only diagnostic test that is useful during the acute illness is immunohistochemical staining for *R. rickettsii* of a biopsy from a skin rash. Doxycycline is effective therapy and should be continued until the patient is afebrile and improving clinically for 2–3 days.

IV-48.   **The answer is D.** *(Chap. 118)* This patient meets three of the five minor criteria: fever ≥38.0°C, predisposition of injection drug use, and evidence of vascular phenomena (septic pulmonary infarction on chest radiography). Two remaining minor criteria are not met or not described above: immunologic phenomena (glomerulonephritis, Osler's nodes, Roth's spots, rheumatoid factor) and microbiologic phenomena (positive blood cultures that do not meet major criteria or positive serology for an organism likely to cause endocarditis). Major criteria include positive blood cultures and evidence of endocardial involvement (echocardiographic or new valvular regurgitation). With three minor criteria and no major criteria described above, this patient should be considered to possibly have infective endocarditis, and the remainder of the workup should be pursued to rule in or out this diagnosis. A complete physical examination with particular attention to the joints, skin, and cardiovascular system and an echocardiogram would be crucial next steps for this patient.

IV-49.   The answer is B. *(Chap. 180)* There are inactivated and live, attenuated forms of influenza vaccine. The intranasal spray, marketed as "Flu-mist," is a live, attenuated virus and is not recommended for the elderly or immunocompromised patients. This vaccine has similar efficacy to the intramuscular vaccine, which is an inactivated, or "killed," preparation of the previous year's strains of influenza A and B. The intramuscular vaccine is manufactured using egg products; patients with true egg hypersensitivity should not receive it. It is safe for elderly and immunocompromised patients. In the past, influenza vaccines have been associated with Guillain-Barré syndrome. This association has not been demonstrated in the past decade, despite close surveillance. Patients do not need to be warned of this side effect.

IV-50.   The answer is C. *(Chap. 172)* Infection with HSV-1 is acquired more frequently and earlier than with HSV-2. More than 90% of adults have serologic evidence of HSV-1 infection by age 40. Primary HSV-1 usually causes pharyngitis and gingivostomatitis and most commonly occurs in children and young adults. Clinical manifestations of primary infection include fever, malaise, myalgias, and adenopathy. There are usually exudative or ulcerative lesions of the pharynx or tonsils. It may be difficult to distinguish from bacterial pharyngitis. Herpes labialis is the most common clinical manifestation of HSV-1 recurrence. Pharyngitis is uncommon with recurrence. HSV-1 resides in latency in the trigeminal ganglia, but trigeminal neuralgia is not a feature of primary infection. HSV-2 recurrence generally causes genital ulcers.

IV-51.   The answer is D. *(Chap. 208)* *Giardia lamblia* is one of the most common parasitic diseases, with worldwide distribution. It occurs in developed and developing countries. Infection follows ingestion of environmental cysts, which excyst in the small intestine releasing flagellated trophozoites. *Giardia* does not disseminate hematogenously; it remains in the small intestine. Cysts are excreted in stool, which accounts for person-to-person spread; however, they do not survive for prolonged periods in feces. Ingestion of contaminated water sources is another major form of infection. *Giardia* cysts can thrive in cold water for months. Filtering or boiling water will remove cysts. As few as 10 cysts can cause human disease, which has a broad spectrum of presentations. Most infected patients are asymptomatic. Symptoms in infected patients are due to small-intestinal dysfunction. Typical early symptoms include diarrhea, abdominal pain, bloating, nausea, vomiting, flatus, and belching. Diarrhea is a very common complaint, particularly early, but in some patients constipation will occur. Later, diarrhea may resolve, with malabsorption symptoms predominating. The presence of fever, eosinophilia, blood or mucus in stools, or colitis symptoms should suggest an alternative diagnosis. Diagnosis is made by demonstrating parasite antigens, cysts, or trophozoites in the stool.

IV-52.   The answer is B. *(Chap. 162)* The patient's clinical examination is consistent with primary syphilis and he should receive appropriate therapy. In primary syphilis, 25% of patients will have negative nontreponemal tests for syphilis (RPR or VDRL). A single dose of long-acting benzathine penicillin is the recommended treatment for primary, secondary, and early latent syphilis. Ceftriaxone is the treatment of choice for gonorrhea, but this lesion is not consistent with that diagnosis. Ceftriaxone given daily for 7–10 days is an alternative treatment for primary and secondary syphilis. Acyclovir is the drug of choice for genital herpes. Herpetic lesions are classically multiple and painful. Observation is not an option because the chancre will resolve spontaneously without treatment and the patient will remain infected and infectious.

IV-53.   The answer is D. *(Chap. 180)* The majority of influenza infections are clinically mild and self-limited. Treatment with over-the-counter cough suppressants and analgesics such as acetaminophen is often adequate. Patients who are under the age of 18 are at risk of developing Reye's syndrome if exposed to salicylates such as aspirin. The neuraminidase inhibitors oseltamivir and zanamivir have activity against influenza A and B. They can be used within 2 days of symptom onset and have been shown to reduce the duration of symptoms by a day or two. This patient has had symptoms for >48 h, therefore neither drug is likely to be effective. The patient's history of asthma is an additional contraindication to zanamivir, as this drug can precipitate bronchospasm. The M2 inhibitors, amantadine and rimantadine, have activity against influenza A only. However, in 2005 >90% of A/H3N2 viral isolates demonstrated resistance to amantadine, and these drugs are no longer recommended for use in influenza A.

IV-54. **The answer is F.** *(Chap. 144)* It is impossible to know whether the patient's continued dyspepsia is due to persistent *H. pylori* as a result of treatment failure or to some other cause. A quick noninvasive test to look for the presence of *H. pylori* is a urea breath test. This test can be done as an outpatient and gives a rapid, accurate response. Patients should not have received any proton pump inhibitors or antimicrobials in the meantime. Stool antigen test is another good option if urea breath testing is not available. If the urea breath test is positive >1 month after completion of first-line therapy, second-line therapy with a proton pump inhibitor, bismuth subsalicylate, tetracycline, and metronidazole may be indicated. If the urea breath test is negative, the remaining symptoms are unlikely due to persistent *H. pylori* infection. Serology is useful only for diagnosing infection initially, but it can remain positive and therefore misleading in those who have cleared *H. pylori*. Endoscopy is a consideration to rule out ulcer or upper gastrointestinal malignancy but is generally preferred after two failed attempts to eradicate *H. pylori*.

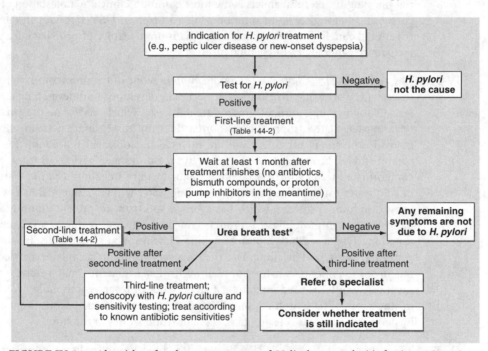

FIGURE IV-54 Algorithm for the management of *Helicobacter pylori* infection. *Occasionally, an endoscopy and a biopsy-based test are used instead of a urea breath test in follow-up after treatment. The main indication for these invasive tests is gastric ulceration; in this condition, as opposed to duodenal ulceration, it is important to check healing and to exclude underlying gastric adenocarcinoma. †Some authorities now use empirical third-line regimens, several of which have been described.

IV-55. **The answer is E.** *(Chap. 161)* Streptomycin is an aminoglycoside first-line supplemental agent for treatment of *Mycobacterium tuberculosis*, *M. marinum*, and *M. kansasii*. It is only available for IM or IV use and is not commonly utilized in the United States because of toxicity. Adverse reactions occur in 10–20% of patients. Renal toxicity and ototoxicity are most common. Ototoxicity may involve hearing and vestibular function. Like other aminoglycosides, it is eliminated almost exclusively by renal mechanisms, so drug levels must be followed along with renal function. Isoniazid and rifampin must be avoided in patients with severe hepatic toxicity. Pyrazinamide is also metabolized by liver and should be used carefully in patients with liver disease.

IV-56. **The answer is E.** *(Chap. 178)* There will soon be two available HPV vaccines. Gardasil (Merck) is currently licensed and contains HPV types 6, 11, 16, and 18; Cervarix (Glaxo-SmithKline) is pending final regulatory approval and contains HPV types 16 and 18. HPV types 6 and 11 cause 90% of anogenital warts. HPV 16 and 18 cause 70% of cervical cancers. Both vaccines consist of virus-like particles without any viral nucleic acid, therefore are not active. Both provide nearly 100% protection against two common oncogenic strains of HPV (16 and 18) but neglect to cover the other strains that cause up to 30% of cervical cancer. Because the vaccines do not protect against all oncogenic HPV serotypes, it is recommended that Pap screening of women for cervical cancer continue according to prior schedules. The vaccine should be given to girls and young women between the ages of 9 and 26 provided that they do not have evidence of infection with both HPV 16 and 18 already.

IV-57. **The answer is B.** *(Chap. 184)* These lesions are diagnostic of herpangina, which is caused by coxsackievirus A. They are typically round and discrete, which helps differentiate them from thrush caused by *Candida* species. Unlike HSV stomatitis, herpangina lesions are not associated with gingivitis. Herpangina usually presents with dysphagia, odynophagia, and fever; these lesions can persist for several weeks. The lesions do not ulcerate.

IV-58. **The answer is E.** *(Chap. 116)* Vaccines have impacted world health in an overwhelmingly positive way with the near disappearance of many infections from the developed world as a result of mass vaccination policies. Inevitably with the decline of many vaccine-preventable illnesses in modern society, fear of these diseases has been supplanted by legitimate concerns for the safety of the vaccines themselves. There has been particular attention among the public and medical field regarding the MMR vaccine due to the use of thimerosal, a mercury-containing preservative widely used in vaccines since the 1930s. Several, large-scale, carefully performed epidemiologic studies in the United States and northern Europe have shown no association between the use of these vaccines and autism or other brain development disorders. Nevertheless, autism incidence is increasing, and the proximity in age between development of autism and administration of vaccine has allowed this debate to continue in the lay press and among autism advocacy groups. World governing bodies including the Centers for Disease Control and Prevention, World Health Organization, and the Food and Drug Administration have formally rejected any causal link between vaccines and autism, but as a cautionary measure, thimerosal has been discontinued in pediatric vaccines in the United States, most notably in MMR. It is noteworthy that when vaccine coverage rates go below a certain threshold, outbreaks of vaccine-preventable illnesses invariably occur. It is important for physicians to be able to communicate this complex information accurately to patients in the current health and policy environment.

IV-59. **The answer is D.** *(Chap. 130)* Recurrent episodes of rheumatic fever are most common in the first 5 years after the initial diagnosis. Penicillin prophylaxis is recommended for at least this period. After the first 5 years secondary prophylaxis is determined on an individual basis. Ongoing prophylaxis is currently recommended for patients who have had recurrent disease, have rheumatic heart disease, or work in occupations that have a high risk for reexposure to group A streptococcal infection. Prophylactic regimens are penicillin V, PO 250 mg bid, benzathine penicillin, 1.2 million units IM every 4 weeks, and sulfadiazine, 1 g PO daily. Polyvalent pneumococcal vaccine has no cross-reactivity with group A streptococcus.

IV-60. **The answer is D.** *(Chap. 118)* While any valvular vegetation can embolize, vegetations located on the mitral valve and vegetations >10 mm are greatest risk of embolizing. Of the choices above, C, D, and E are large enough to increase the risk of embolization. However, only choice D demonstrates the risks of both size and location. Hematogenously seeded infection from an embolized vegetation may involve any organ, but particularly affects those organs with the highest blood flow. They are seen in up to 50% of patients with endocarditis. Tricuspid lesions will lead to pulmonary septic emboli, common in injection drug users. Mitral and aortic lesions can lead to embolic infections in the skin, spleen, kidneys, meninges, and skeletal system. A dreaded neurologic complication is mycotic aneurysm, focal dilations of arteries at points in the arterial wall that have been weakened by infection in the vasa vasorum or septic emboli, leading to hemorrhage.

IV-61. The answer is A. *(Chap. 182)* The purpose of testing for latent tuberculosis (with either PPD skin testing or whole-blood interferon assays) in any person is to detect latent tuberculosis infection and treat at that stage to avoid development of active tuberculosis (TB). This strategy benefits the individual patient and the greater public health. These issues are more pressing in persons with HIV infection. The progression from latent to active TB in an HIV-infected patient is estimated as high as 10% per year rather than 10% per lifetime as in the HIV-uninfected persons. In HIV-infected persons, active TB is clinically present in extrapulmonary sites (kidney, central nervous system) and can be diagnostically challenging. TB infection appears to accelerate HIV disease. The 6-month mortality rate among co-infected patients is higher than in patients with HIV-infection alone. Rifamycin derivatives, used for active TB therapy, have fairly complex drug-drug interactions with antiretroviral therapy (ART) agents often necessitating ART regimen exchange or dose adjustment. Appropriate therapy for active TB has similar efficacy rates for mycobacterial eradication in HIV-infected and HIV-uninfected persons.

IV-62. The answer is E. *(Chap. 135)* Clostridia are gram-positive spore-forming obligate anaerobes that reside normally in the gastrointestinal (GI) tract. Several clostridial species can cause severe disease. *C. perfringens*, which is the second most common clostridial species to normally colonize the GI tract, is associated with food poisoning, gas gangrene, and myonecrosis. *C. septicum* is seen often in conjunction with GI tumors. *C. sordellii* is associated with septic abortions. All can cause a fulminant overwhelming bacteremia, but this condition is rare. The fact that this patient is well several days after his acute complaints rules out this fulminant course. A more common scenario is transient, self-limited bacteremia due to transient gut translocation during an episode of gastroenteritis. There is no need to treat when this occurs, and no further workup is necessary. *Clostridium* spp. sepsis rarely causes endocarditis because overwhelming disseminated intravascular coagulation and death occur so rapidly. Screening for GI tumor is warranted when *C. septicum* is cultured from the blood or a deep wound infection.

IV-63. The answer is B. *(Chap. 210)* *Ascaris lumbricoides* is the longest nematode (15–40 cm) parasite of humans. It resides in tropical and subtropical regions. In the United States, it is found mostly in the rural Southeast. Transmission is through fecally contaminated soil. Most commonly the worm burden is low and it causes no symptoms. Clinical disease is related to larval migration to the lungs or to adult worms in the gastrointestinal tract. The most common complications occur due to a high gastrointestinal adult worm burden leading to small-bowel obstruction (most often in children with a narrow-caliber small-bowel lumen) or migration leading to obstructive complications such as cholangitis, pancreatitis, or appendicitis. Rarely, adult worms can migrate to the esophagus and be orally expelled. During the lung phase of larval migration (9–12 days after egg ingestion) patients may develop a nonproductive cough, fever, eosinophilia, and pleuritic chest pain. Eosinophilic pneumonia syndrome (Löffler's syndrome) is characterized by symptoms and lung infiltrates. Meningitis is not a known complication of ascariasis but can occur with disseminated strongyloidiasis in an immunocompromised host.

IV-64. The answer is A. *(Chap. 144)* *H. pylori* is a disease of overcrowding. Transmission has therefore decreased in the United States as the standard of living has increased. It is predicated that the percentage of duodenal ulcers due to factors other than *H. pylori* (e.g., use of nonsteroidal anti-inflammatory drugs) will increase over the upcoming decades. Controversial, but increasing, evidence suggests that *H. pylori* colonization may provide some protection from recent emerging gastrointestinal disorders, such as gastroesophageal reflux disease (and its complication, esophageal carcinoma). Therefore, the health implications of *H. pylori* eradication may not be simple.

IV-65.   The answer is D. *(Chap. 132)* *Listeria* meningitis typically affects the elderly and the chronically ill. It is frequently a more subacute (developing over days) illness than other etiologies of bacterial meningitis. It may be mistaken for aseptic meningitis. Meningeal signs, including nuchal rigidity, are less common, as is photophobia, than in other, more acute causes of bacterial meningitis. Typically WBC counts in the CSF range from 100–5000/μL with a less pronounced neutrophilia. 75% of patients will have a WBC count <1000/μL. Gram's stain is only positive in 30–40% of cases. Case fatality rates are ~20%.

IV-66.   The answer is E. *(Chap. 123)* Clindamycin, ampicillin, and cephalosporins (including ceftriaxone) were the first antibiotics associated with *C. difficile*–associated disease, and still are. More recently, broad-spectrum fluoroquinolones, including moxifloxacin and ciprofloxacin, have been associated with outbreaks of *C. difficile*, including outbreaks in some locations of a more virulent strain that has caused severe disease among elderly outpatients. For unclear reasons, β-lactams other than the later generation cephalosporins appear to carry a lesser risk of disease. Penicillin/β-lactamase combination antibiotics appear to have lower risk of *C. difficile*–associated disease than the other agents mentioned. Cases have even been reported associated with metronidazole and vancomycin administration. Nevertheless, all patients initiating antibiotics should be warned to seek care if they develop diarrhea that is severe or persists for more than a day, as all antibiotics carry some risk for *C. difficile*–associated disease.

IV-67.   The answer is C. *(Chap. 181)* HTLV-I is a retrovirus that is a chronic infection like HIV, but it does not cause similar sequelae. It was the first identified human retrovirus. Gradual decline of CD4+ lymphocyte number and function is a feature of HIV but not of HTLV-I. While many people in endemic areas have serologic evidence of infection, most do not develop disease. The two major complications of HTLV-I are tropical spastic paraparesis and acute T cell leukemia. Tropical spastic paraparesis is an upper motor neuron disease of insidious onset leading to weakness, lower extremity stiffness, urinary incontinence, and eventually a thoracic myelopathy, leading to a bedridden state in about a third of patients after 10 years. It is more common in women than men. It can easily be confused with multiple sclerosis; this is why it is important to be able to recall the geographic regions where HTLV-I is endemic when evaluating a myelopathy. Acute T cell leukemia is a difficult-to-treat leukemia that is specific to chronic HTLV-I infection. HTLV-I is thought to be transmitted in a similar fashion to HIV.

IV-68.   The answer is E. *(Chaps. 191 and 197)* The most common infection in a patient with prolonged neutropenia and fever once acute bacterial infections have been ruled out is invasive *Aspergillosis* infection. Thoracic CT and serum galactomannan testing are indicated because the initial stages of invasive disease are frequently not symptomatic. CT scan may show subtle new nodules or a halo sign (hemorrhagic infarction surrounding a nodule) that is suggestive, though not diagnostic, of this condition. *Aspergillus* antigen is detected by galactomannan release during growth of the mould. False positives are possible for both chest CT and antigen testing. However, overdiagnosis is preferable to late or missed diagnosis as this infection disseminates to the skin and brain and can be very difficult to treat at this stage. As a result, many cases are treated presumptively with serial chest CTs and galactomannan levels, rather than awaiting definitive diagnosis by culture or consistent histopathology. Galactomannan levels may be falsely elevated in the presence of β-lactam/β-lactamase combination antibiotics such as piperacillin/tazobactam. Chest roentgenogram is not sensitive for detecting early disease. Bronchoscopy with bronchoalveolar lavage is indicated for an attempt at definitive diagnosis only if abnormalities are detected on chest CT. There is no reason to suspect *Clostridium difficile* (and hence the need for metronidazole) in the absence of diarrhea. Similarly, in the absence of documented bacterial infection, there are no data to support the addition of an aminoglycoside. There is no reason to suspect fluconazole-resistant yeast infection requiring caspofungin in the absence of detectable fungemia. While caspofungin has activity against *Aspergillus*, it is approved only for salvage therapy.

IV-69.   The answer is E. *(Chaps. 129 and 131)* Probably because of its ubiquity and ability to stick to foreign surfaces, *S. epidermidis* is the most common cause of infections of central nervous system shunts as well as an important cause of infections on artificial heart valves and orthopedic prostheses. *Corynebacterium* spp. (diphtheroids), just like *S. epidermidis*, colonize the skin. When these organisms are isolated from cultures of shunts, it is often difficult to be sure if they are the cause of disease or simply contaminants. Leukocytosis in cerebrospinal fluid, consistent isolation of the same organism, and the character of a patient's symptoms are all helpful in deciding whether treatment for infection is indicated.

IV-70.   The answer is D. *(Chap. 209)* Visceral larva migrans, caused in this case by the canine roundworm *Toxocara canis*, most commonly affects young children who are exposed to canine stool. *Toxocara* eggs are ingested and begin their life cycle in the small intestine. They migrate to many tissues in the body. Particularly characteristic of this illness are hepatosplenomegaly and profound eosinophilia, at times close to 90% of the total white blood cell count. Staphylococci will not typically cause eosinophilia. Trichinellosis, caused by ingesting meat from carnivorous animals that has been infected with *Trichinella* cysts, does not cause hepatosplenomegaly and is uncommon without eating a suspicious meal. Giardiasis is characterized by profuse diarrhea and abdominal pain without systemic features or eosinophilia. Cysticercosis typically causes myalgias and can spread to the brain, where it is often asymptomatic but can lead to seizures.

IV-71.   The answer is A. *(Chap. 179)* While most of the choices listed above can cause pharyngitis in children, adenovirus classically presents with bilateral granular conjunctivitis as well as pharyngitis, and is frequently the cause of an outbreak among children who are in close contact with one another. Symptom-based and supportive therapies are indicated for all infections other than disseminated infections in immunocompromised patients. Rhinovirus infections manifest clinically as a common cold with sore throat and rhinorrhea. Human metapneumovirus (HMPV) is a recently described respiratory pathogen. Infections usually occur in winter, and antibodies are present in most children by age 5. Clinically HMPV appears similar to human respiratory syncytial virus, with upper and lower respiratory symptoms. Serious infections may occur in immunocompromised patients. Parainfluenza predominantly is a mild coldlike illness in older children and adults, presenting with hoarseness often without cough. Enteroviruses most frequently cause an acute undifferentiated febrile illness but may cause rhinitis, pharyngitis, and pneumonia.

IV-72.   The answer is D. *(Chaps. 126 and 155)* This patient is chronically immunosuppressed from his antirejection prophylactic regimen, which includes both glucocorticoids and azathioprine. However, the finding of a cavitary lesion on chest x-ray considerably narrows the possibilities and increases the likelihood of nocardial infection. The other clinical findings, including production of profuse thick sputum, fever, and constitutional symptoms, are also quite common in patients who have pulmonary nocardiosis. The Gram stain, which demonstrates filamentous branching gram-positive organisms, is characteristic. Most species of *Nocardia* are acid-fast if a weak acid is used for decolorization (e.g., modified Kinyoun method). These organisms can also be visualized by silver staining. They grow slowly in culture, and the laboratory must be alerted to the possibility of their presence on submitted specimens. Once the diagnosis, which may require an invasive approach, is made, sulfonamides are the drugs of choice. Sulfadiazine or sulfisoxazole from 6–8 g/d in four divided doses generally is administered, but doses up to 12 g/d have been given. The combination of sulfamethoxazole and trimethoprim has also been used, as have the oral alternatives minocycline and ampicillin and IV amikacin. There is little experience with the newer β-lactam antibiotics, including the third-generation cephalosporins and imipenem. Erythromycin alone is not effective, although it has been given successfully along with ampicillin. In addition to appropriate antibiotic therapy, the possibility of disseminated nocardiosis must be considered; sites include brain, skin, kidneys, bone, and muscle.

IV-73 and IV-74. The answers are A and C. *(Chap. 156)* The most common site of actinomycosis infection is the craniofacial area. Often the infection is associated with poor dentition, facial trauma, or tooth extraction. Clinically this presents as a chronic cellulitis of the face, often with drainage through sinus tracts. The infection may spread without regard for tissue planes, and adjacent bony structures may be involved. Diagnosis requires a high degree of suspicion. The drainage is frequently contaminated with other organisms, especially gram-negative rods. The characteristic sulfur granules may not be seen unless deep tissue is sampled. On Gram's stain, the characteristic appearance shows an intense gram-positive center and branching rods at the periphery. As opposed to the strictly aerobic *Nocardia* species, *Actinomyces* grows slowly in anaerobic and microaerobic conditions. Therapy requires a long course of antibiotics, even though the organism is very sensitive to penicillin therapy. This is presumed to be due to the difficulty of using antibiotics to penetrate the thick-walled masses and sulfur granules. Current recommendations are for penicillin IV for 2–6 weeks followed by oral therapy for a total of 6–12 months. Surgery should be reserved for patients who are not responsive to medical therapy.

IV-75. The answer is A. *(Chap. 197)* *Aspergillus* has many clinical manifestations. Invasive aspergillosis typically occurs in immunocompromised patients and presents as rapidly progressive pulmonary infiltrates. Infection progresses by direct extension across tissue planes. Cavitation may occur. Allergic bronchopulmonary aspergillosis (ABPA) is a different clinical entity. It often occurs in patients with preexisting asthma or cystic fibrosis. It is characterized by an allergic reaction to *Aspergillus* species. Clinically, it is characterized by intermittent wheezing, bilateral pulmonary infiltrates, brownish sputum, and peripheral eosinophilia. IgE may be elevated, suggesting an allergic process, and a specific reaction to *Aspergillus* species that is manifested by serum antibodies or skin testing is common. Although central bronchiectasis is common in ABPA, the presence of peripheral cavitary lung lesions is *not* a common feature.

IV-76. The answer is C. *(Chap. 123)* Interestingly, a number of recent studies have found that colonization is not a risk factor for disease. This may be because strains that are apt to colonize may provide some immunity to the host or are less toxigenic than disease-causing strains. In either case, this serves as a reminder that stool testing should be conducted only on symptomatic patients, as a positive test carries a totally different meaning if clinical suspicion for *C. difficile*–associated disease is low. Patients should not be considered to have *C. difficile*–associated disease based on culture results alone. Additional information to make a diagnosis in a patient with the appropriate clinical findings includes demonstrating presence of toxin A or B or demonstration of pseudomembranes at colonoscopy. Risk factors for *C. difficile*–associated disease are well defined: the most important is antecedent antibiotics, especially fluoroquinolones, cephalosporins, and clindamycin. Age, high patient acuity, enteral feedings, antacids, and length of time in a health care facility are also predictive of developing *C. difficile*–associated disease.

IV-77. The answer is D. *(Chap. 124)* Urethritis in men causes dysuria with or without discharge, usually without frequency. The most common causes of urethritis in men include *N. gonorrhoeae, C. trachomatis, Mycoplasma genitalium, Ureaplasma urealyticum, Trichomonas vaginalis,* herpes simplex virus, and possibly adenovirus. Until recently, *C. trachomatis* accounted for 30–40% of cases; however, this number may be falling. Recent studies suggest that *M. genitalium* is a common cause of non-chlamydial cases. Currently, the initial diagnosis of urethritis in men includes specific tests only for *N. gonorrhoeae* and *C. trachomatis*. Tenets of urethral discharge treatment include providing treatment for the most common causes of urethritis with the assumption that the patient may be lost to follow up. Therefore, prompt empirical treatment for gonorrhea and *Chlamydia* infections should be given on the day of presentation to the clinic. Azithromycin will also be effective for *M. genitalium*. If pus can be milked from the urethra, cultures should be sent for definitive diagnosis and to allow for contact tracing by the health department, as both of the above are reportable diseases. Urine nucleic acid amplification tests are an acceptable substitute in the absence of pus. It is also critical to provide empirical treatment for at-risk sexual contacts. If symptoms do not respond to the initial empirical therapy, patients should be reevaluated for compliance with therapy, reexposure, and *T. vaginalis* infection.

IV-78. The answer is E. *(Chap. 126)* Ultimately, solid organ transplant patients are at highest risk for infection due to T cell immunodeficiency from antirejection medicines. As a result, they are also at risk for reactivation of many of the viruses from the Herpes virus family, most notably CMV, varicella-zoster virus, and EBV. However, immediately after transplant, these deficits have not yet developed in full. Neutropenia is not common after solid organ transplantation as in bone marrow transplantation. In fact, patients are most at risk of infections typical for all hospitalized patients, including wound infections, urinary tract infection, pneumonia, *Clostridium difficile* infection, and line-associated infection. Therefore, a standard evaluation of a febrile patient in the first weeks after a solid organ transplant should include a detailed physical examination, blood and urine cultures, urinalysis, chest radiography, *C. difficile* stool antigen/toxin studies if warranted, in addition to a transplant-specific evaluation.

IV-79 and IV-80. The answers are E and A. *(Chaps. 130, 136, and 376)* In a previously healthy student, particularly one living in a dormitory, *Staphylococcus pneumoniae* and *Neisseria meningitides* are the pathogens most likely to be causing community-acquired bacterial meningitis. As a result of the increasing prevalence of penicillin- and cephalosporin-resistant streptococci, initial empirical therapy should include a third- or fourth-generation cephalosporin plus vancomycin. Dexamethasone has been shown in children and adults to decrease meningeal inflammation and unfavorable outcomes in acute bacterial meningitis. In a recent study of adults the effect on outcome was most notable in patients with *S. pneumoniae* infection. The first dose (10 mg IV) should be administered 15–20 min before or with the first dose of antibiotics and is unlikely to be of benefit unless it is begun 6 h after the initiation of antibiotics. Dexamethasone may decrease the penetration of vancomycin into the CSF.

IV-81. The answer is C. *(Chap. 179)* While rhinovirus likely represents one of the most common viral illness in humans, human respiratory syncytial virus is the most prevalent respiratory pathogen in young children and infants. Adenovirus is another common cause of the common cold and pharyngitis in children. Enteroviruses can cause an undifferentiated febrile illness and occasionally upper respiratory tract infections. Parainfluenza viruses typically cause croup or tracheobronchitis among children.

IV-82. The answer is A. *(Chap. 132)* *Listeria monocytogenes* causes GI illness via ingestion of food that has been contaminated with high concentrations of bacteria. The bacteria may survive and multiply at refrigeration temperatures, therefore deli meats, soft cheeses, hot dogs, and milk are common sources. The attack rate is very high, with close to 100% of exposed patients experiencing symptoms. Symptoms develop within 48 h of exposure, and there is no prolonged asymptomatic carrier state. Person-to-person spread (other than vertically from mother to fetus) does not appear to occur during outbreaks. While the bacteria have several virulence factors that lead to clinical symptoms, the organism, and not a specific toxin, mediates infection. A large inoculum is necessary to produce symptoms. Surveillance studies show that <5% of asymptomatic adults have positive stool cultures, and fecal-oral spread is not common. Typical symptoms, including fever, are as described in the case above. Isolated GI illness does not require antibiotics.

IV-83. The answer is D. *(Chap. 120)* Neuropathic osteopathy, or Charcot's foot, represents characteristic destruction of the joints and bones of the foot in the setting of prolonged, poorly controlled diabetes mellitus. Characteristic chronic findings on physical examination include hammer-toes and rocker bottom foot. More acutely the foot is often red and warm, with bounding pulses followed by the initial joint deformities. This condition can therefore be difficult to differentiate from cellulitis, osteomyelitis, and deep tissue infection, particularly in the presence of an ulcer. Unfortunately, all available imaging modalities can confuse osteomyelitis with the acute and chronic changes of neuropathic osteopathy as well. To add to the challenge, the presence of a Charcot's foot likely predisposes to ulceration and subsequent contiguous osteomyelitis. Generally, MRI is adequate for differentiating cellulitis and tumor; ultrasound can be useful for abscesses; MRI and plain film all helpful for fractures. Appropriate samples for microbiologic studies should be obtained to determine the presence and cause of chronic osteomyelitis.

IV-84.   The answer is B. *(Chap. 184)* Enteroviruses are single-strand RNA viruses that multiply in the gastrointestinal (GI) tract but rarely cause GI illness. Typical person-to-person spread occurs via the fecal-oral route; enteroviruses are not known to spread via blood transfusions or insect vectors. Infection is most common among infants and small children; serious illness occurs in neonates, older children, and adults. Most infections with poliovirus are symptomatic or cause a minor illness. Prior to the implementation of polio vaccines, paralysis was a rare clinical presentation of poliovirus infection and was less frequent in developing countries, likely due to earlier exposure. Paralytic disease due to polio infection is more common in older adults, pregnant women, or persons exercising strenuously or with trauma at the time of central nervous system symptoms. Exposure to maternal antibodies leads to lower risk of symptomatic neonatal infection.

IV-85.   The answer is D. *(Chap. 124)* Genital human papilloma virus is thought to be the most common sexually transmitted infection in the United States. A recent study of initially seronegative college-aged women found 60% became infected within 5 years. This underscores the importance of the recent development of effective vaccines and continued cervical cancer screening strategies. Approximately 20–25% of the U.S. population past 11–12 years old is seropositive for HSV-2. The high prevalence of this infection in the general population is due to several factors including lifelong infection, ongoing transmission during latent infection due to asymptomatic shedding of HSV-2 in the genital mucosa, and high rates of transmission within monogamous partnerships. These features are markedly different than those associated with bacterial STIs such as gonorrhea and syphilis, which require high rates of partner change to persist in subpopulations. HIV-1 infections are still concentrated within high-risk populations (men who sleep with men, injection drug users, high-risk heterosexuals, and immigrants from high prevalence regions).

IV-86.   The answer is E. *(Chap. 210)* This patient's most likely diagnosis is anisakiasis. This is a nematode infection where humans are an accidental host. It occurs hours to days after ingesting eggs that previously settled into the muscles of fish. The main risk factor for infection is eating raw fish. Presentation mimics an acute abdomen. History is critical as upper endoscopy is both diagnostic and curative. The implicated nematodes burrow into the mucosa of the stomach causing intense pain and must be manually removed by endoscope or, on rare occasion, surgery. There is no medical agent known to cure anisakiasis.

IV-87.   The answer is E. *(Chap. 203)* All febrile travelers returning from, or immigrants arriving from, *Plasmodium falciparum*–endemic regions should be assumed to have infection with this most severe form of malaria until proven otherwise. *P. falciparum* is the most common infection in returning travelers, may be fatal if not treated, and none of the listed features have sufficient predictive value to rule out malaria. Splenomegaly is a common feature of malaria but is not present in all cases. *P. vivax* and *P. ovale* infections often have paroxysmal fevers but not enough so as to carry significant predictive value; this feature is rarely present in *P. falciparum*–infected persons. Severe myalgias and retroorbital headache often appropriately prompt interest in a diagnosis of dengue fever, but these symptoms are common in malaria as well. Abdominal pain is a very common feature of malaria, and diarrhea can also occur.

IV-88.   The answer is A. *(Chaps. 126 and 175)* When the transplant donor is CMV IgG positive and recipient is negative, there is a very high risk of primary CMV infection in the recipient. However, if the recipient is IgG positive, CMV occurs as a reactivation infection. When both donor and recipient are seronegative, then the risk of any CMV infection is lowest, but not zero, as a contact with an infected host could prompt primary CMV infection. Unlike nearly all other transplant patients, many donor and recipient seronegative patients do not receive chemoprophylaxis with ganciclovir. In patients who are CMV

IgG negative and received a CMV IgG negative transplant, transfusions should be from CMV IgG negative donors or white blood cell filtered products administered to reduce the risk of primary CMV infection.

IV-89. The answer is B. *(Chap. 121)* Microbiologic data are critical in establishing the source of a liver abscess. Polymicrobial samples of pus or blood cultures with gram-negative rods, enterococcus, and anaerobes suggest an abdominal or pelvic source. Hepatosplenic candidiasis once commonly occurred in leukemia or stem cell transplant patients not receiving antifungal prophylaxis. Fungemia was thought to develop in the portal vasculature with poor clearance of yeast during neutropenia. The rejuvenation of neutrophils correlated with symptoms of hepatic abscess. Hepatosplenic candidiases is now quite rare, given the widespread use of fluconazole prophylaxis in patients with prolonged neutropenia. Certain species such as *Streptococcus milleri* or *Staphylococcus aureus* likely indicate a primary bacteremia and warrant a search for the source of this, depending on the typical ecologic niche of the organism isolated. Amebic abscesses should be considered in the context of host epidemiology: those with a low to medium pretest probability based on travel history, who also have a negative amebic serology, are effectively ruled out for disease, without needing to sample the abscess percutaneously. Fever is the most common presenting sign of liver abscess. Only 50% of patients with liver abscess have right upper quadrant pain, hepatomegaly, or jaundice. Therefore, half of patients may have no signs localizing to the liver. An elevated alkaline phosphatase level is the most sensitive laboratory finding in liver abscess, present in ~70% of cases. Other liver function abnormalities are less common.

IV-90. The answer is D. *(Chap. 196)* All patients with *Candida* fungemia should be treated with systemic antifungals. Terbinafine is an agent used for dermatophyte infection of the foot. Fluconazole has been shown to be an effective agent for candidemia with equivalence to amphotericin products and caspofungin. For example, *Candida glabrata* is typically resistant to fluconazole. Voriconazole is also active against *Candida albicans* but has many drug interactions that make it less desirable against this pathogen. Azoles such as fluconazole and voriconazole are often less active against *C. glabrata* and *C. krusei*. Many practitioners therefore prefer to initiate treatment with caspofungin or amphotericin products in a patient with candidemia until the yeast isolate is definitively identified as *C. albicans*. Caspofungin and other echinocandins are gaining popularity due to their broad efficacy against most yeast isolates and benign side-effect profile. Amphotericin B is effective in fungemia but frequently causes rigors, electrolyte wasting, and renal insufficiency. Newer lipid formulations mitigate these effects to varying extents.

I-91. The answer is C. *(Chap. 182)* Immune reconstitution syndrome (IRIS) is commonly seen after the initiation of antiretroviral therapy (ART) in patients with AIDS and a concomitant opportunistic infection (OI). It is a syndrome where either a previously recognized OI worsens after ART despite an initial period of improvement after standard therapy for that particular infection, or when an OI that was not previously recognized is unmasked after ART therapy. The latter scenario occurs presumably as immune cells become reactivated and recognize the presence of a pathogen that disseminated in the absence of adequate T cell response with the patient remaining subclinical prior to ART. Many opportunistic pathogens are known to behave this way but *Cryptococcus*, *Mycobacterium tuberculosis*, and *Mycobacterium avium* complex (MAI/MAC) are the most likely to be associated with IRIS. Risk factors for IRIS are low CD4+ lymphocyte count at ART initiation, initiation of ART within 2 months of treatment initiation for the OI, adequate virologic response to ART, and increase in CD4+ lymphocyte count as a result of ART. IRIS can be diagnostically challenging and is very diverse in terms of clinical presentation and severity. Depending on the organ system and pathogen involved, drug-resistant OI and new OI must be considered, sometimes necessitating invasive biopsies and cultures. In this case, the overlap of organ system with the original presentation, low likelihood of MAI drug resistance, and timing of the syndrome favor IRIS. Therapy is with nonsteroidal anti-inflammatory drugs and sometimes glucocorticoids. OI treatment is continued, and all efforts are made to continue ART as well, except under the most dire of clinical circumstances.

IV-92. **The answer is E.** *(Chap. 179)* Human respiratory syncytial virus (HRSV), previously known as RSV, is an RNA paramyxovirus. HRSV is the major respiratory pathogen in children, the foremost cause of lower respiratory illness in infants, and a cause of a common cold–like syndrome. It is a common and important nosocomial pathogen. RSV Ig, also known as *palivizumab*, has been approved as a monthly injection for children <2 years old who have congenital heart or lung disease or who were born prematurely as a means of preventing RSV infection. It has not been shown to be beneficial in HRSV pneumonia. Barrier precautions should be used, especially in locations where there are high transmission rates; however, with the advent of RSV Ig this is not the only means of prevention. An inactivated, whole-virus RSV vaccine trial found that patients receiving the vaccine appeared more likely to acquire RSV infection. An adequate vaccine has not been developed to date.

IV-93. **The answer is C.** *(Chap. 121)* Primary bacterial peritonitis is a complication of ascites associated with cirrhosis. Clinical presentation can be misleading as only 80% of patients have fever, and abdominal symptoms are only variably present. Therefore, when patients with known cirrhosis develop worsening encephalopathy, fever, and/or malaise, the diagnosis should strongly be considered and ruled out. In this case, a peritoneal polymorphonuclear leukocyte count of >250/μL would be diagnostic of bacterial peritonitis even if Gram's stain were negative. The paracentesis also might provide microbiologic confirmation. CT of the head would be useful for the diagnosis of cerebral edema associated with severe hepatic encephalopathy or in the presence of focal neurologic findings suggesting an epidural bleed. Cirrhotic patients are at great risk of gastrointestinal (GI) bleeding and it may worsen hepatic encephalopathy by increasing the protein load in the colon. Esophagastroduodenoscopy would be a reasonable course of action, particularly if stools were guaiac positive or there was gross evidence of hematemesis or melena. In this case, there is no evidence of GI bleeding and there is mild hemoconcentration, possibly from peritonitis. Lactulose, and possibly neomycin or rifaximin, is a logical therapeutic trial in this patient if peritonitis is not present. Serum ammonia level may suggest hepatic encephalopathy, if elevated, but does not have sufficient predictive value on its own to rule in or rule out this diagnosis.

IV-94. **The answer is B.** *(Chap. 189)* Since its introduction to the United States in 1999, West Nile virus (WNV) causes ~1000–3000 cases of encephalitis with 300 deaths annually. It is a flavivirus of the same family as the causative agents of St. Louis and Japanese encephalitis. Cases typically occur in the summer, often in community outbreaks, associated with dead crows. It is estimated that 1% of infections cause encephalitis, with the remainder being subclinical or having self-limited West Nile fever. The elderly, diabetics, and patients with prior central nervous system (CNS) disease are at greater risk of encephalitis. WNV cannot be cultured, and there is not yet a polymerase chain reaction test. IgM antibodies normally do not cross the blood-brain barrier, and so their presence in the CSF is due to intrathecal production during acute infection with WNV. MRI is abnormal in only 30% of cases of WNV, significantly less often than is the case in herpes simplex virus encephalitis. Stool culture may be useful in the diagnostic evaluation of enteroviral meningitis or encephalitis but not in cases of WNV.

IV-95. **The answer is B.** *(Chap. 180)* Myositis and subsequent rhabdomyolysis and myoglobinuria represent a rare but severe complication of influenza infection. Renal failure may occur. Myalgias are a prominent symptom of influenza infection, but myositis characterized by elevated creatine phosphokinase and marked tenderness of the muscles is very infrequent. The pathogenesis of this complication is unknown. Other extrapulmonary complications of influenza including encephalitis, transverse myelitis, and Guillain-Barré syndrome have been reported, although the etiologic relationship to influenza virus infection is uncertain. Myocarditis and pericarditis were reported during the 1918–1919 influenza pandemic. The most serious complication of influenza is secondary bacterial pneumonia, such as caused by *Staphylococcus aureus*. Arthritis, conjunctivitis, and eczematous rashes have not been described as complications of influenza infection.

IV-96. **The answer is C.** *(Chap. 193)* *Coccidioides immitis* is a mold that is found in the soil in the southwestern United States and Mexico. Case clusters of primary disease may appear 10–14 days after exposure, and the activities with the highest risk include archaeologic excavation, rock hunting, military maneuvers, and construction work. Only 40% of primary pulmonary infections are symptomatic. Symptoms may include those of a hypersensitivity reaction such as erythema nodosum, erythema multiforme, arthritis, or conjunctivitis. Diagnosis can be made by culture of sputum; however, when this organism is suspected, the laboratory needs to be notified as it is a biohazard level 3 fungus. Serologic tests of blood may also be helpful; however, seroconversion of primary disease may take up to 8 weeks. Skin testing is useful only for epidemiologic studies and is not done in clinical practice.

IV-97. **The answer is C.** *(Chap. 167)* Only two rickettsial infections, *R. prowazekii* and *C. burnetii*, have a recrudescent or chronic stage. This patient has louse-borne (epidemic) typhus caused by *R. prowazekii*. Louse-borne typhus occurs most commonly in outbreaks in overcrowded, poorly hygienic areas such as refugee camps. There was an outbreak of ~100,000 people living in refugee camps in Burundi in 1997. It is the second most severe form of rickettsial disease and can recur years after acute infection, as in this patient. This is thought to occur as a result of waning immunity. Rocky Mountain spotted fever would be consistent with this patient's presentation but he has no epidemiologic risk factors apparent for this disease. African tick-borne fever is considerably less severe and is often associated with a black eschar at the site of a tick bite. Murine typhus is usually less severe and does not exist in a recrudescent form. Q fever can cause chronic disease but this is almost always in the form of endocarditis.

IV-98. **The answer is C.** *(Chap. 122)* The patient most likely has food poisoning because of contamination of the fried rice with *Bacillus cereus*. This toxin-mediated disease occurs when heat-resistant spores germinate after boiling. Frying before serving may not destroy the preformed toxin. The emetic form of illness occurs within 6 h of eating and is self-limited. No therapy is necessary unless the patient develops severe dehydration. This patient currently has no symptoms consistent with volume depletion; therefore, she does not need IV fluids at present. Sarcoidosis does not predispose patients to infectious diseases.

IV-99. **The answer is A.** *(Chap. 166)* Lyme serology tests should be done only in patients with an intermediate pretest probability of having Lyme disease. The presence of erythema migrans in both patient B and patient E is diagnostic of Lyme disease in the correct epidemiologic context. The diagnosis is entirely clinical. Patient C's clinical course sounds more consistent with systemic lupus erythematosus, and initial laboratory evaluation should focus on this diagnosis. Patients with chronic fatigue, myalgias, and cognitive change are occasionally concerned about Lyme disease as a potential etiology for their symptoms. However, the pretest probability of Lyme is low in these patients, assuming the absence of antecedent erythema migrans, and a positive serology is unlikely to be a true positive test. Lyme arthritis typically occurs months after the initial infection and occurs in ~60% of untreated patients. The typical attack is large joint, oligoarticular, and intermittent, lasting weeks at a time. Oligoarticular arthritis carries a broad differential diagnosis including sarcoidosis, spondyloarthropathy, rheumatoid arthritis, psoriatic arthritis, and Lyme disease. Lyme serology is appropriate in this situation. Patients with Lyme arthritis usually have the highest IgG antibody responses seen in the infection.

IV-100. **The answer is C.** *(Chap. 120)* This patient has at minimum severe sepsis and has a very high pretest probability of an epidural abscess compressing his spinal cord, based on the development of weakness and upper motor neuron signs. Both represent true emergencies. From a sepsis standpoint, the most likely organisms are gram-positive skin flora with methicillin-resistant or sensitive *Staphylococcus aureus* representing a distinct possibility. Vancomycin given intravenously is therefore imperative. However, other gram-negative organisms such as *Pseudomonas* and the HACEK organisms are sometimes causes of bacteremia and endocarditis in injection drug users. Given this patient's unstable hemodynamic state, it would be sensible to empirically cover gram-negative rods as well with cefepime. As the infection is life threatening, it would not be prudent to await operative culture data prior to starting broad-spectrum antibiotics. An epidural abscess needs to be diagnosed and surgically decompressed as rapidly as possible to prevent permanent loss of neurologic function.

IV-101. **The answer is A.** *(Chap. 195)* Cryptococcal meningoencephalitis presents with early manifestations of headache, nausea, gait disturbance, confusion, and visual changes. Fever and nuchal rigidity are often mild or absent. Papilledema is present in ~30% of cases. Asymmetric cranial nerve palsies occur in 25% of cases. Neuroimaging is often normal. If there are focal neurologic findings, an MRI may be used to diagnose cryptococcomas in the basal ganglia or caudate nucleus, although they are more common in immunocompetent patients with *C. neoformans* var. *gattii*. Imaging does not make the diagnosis. The definitive diagnosis remains CSF culture. However, capsular antigen testing in both the serum and the CSF is very sensitive and can provide a presumptive diagnosis. Approximately 90% of patients, including all with a positive CSF smear, and the majority of AIDS patients have detectable cryptococcal antigen. The result is often negative in patients with pulmonary disease. However, because of a very small false-positive rate in antigen testing, CSF culture remains the definitive diagnostic test. In this condition *C. neoformans* often can also be cultured from the urine; however, other testing methods are more rapid and useful.

IV-102. **The answer is C.** *(Chap. 124)* Acute epididymitis almost always causes unilateral painful swelling of the epididymis. In young men, epididymitis is usually an extension of a primary sexually transmitted infection, and urethral discharge is therefore very suggestive of the diagnosis. The differential diagnosis includes testicular torsion, which is a surgical emergency. An elevated testicle and lack of blood flow on Doppler study suggest this diagnosis. Testicular cancer, unlike epididymitis, does not usually cause tenderness and pain. This is an important consideration in any male with a testicular mass. Response to cefpodoxime and doxycycline should suggest bacterial epididymitis, rather than rule it out.

IV-103. **The answer is E.** *(Chap. 116)* In recent years, rabies virus has been most frequently transmitted by bats in the United States. Usually a bite is noted, but not always. Therefore, patients who have unexpected, unmonitored (i.e., while they are asleep) close contact with bats should be told to seek medical attention and likely vaccination. A bite is a clear indication for the most effective immunization strategy involving both active (inactivated virus vaccine) and passive (human rabies immunoglobulins) immune activation, unless the offending bat is captured and found to be rabies negative with further testing. The vaccination schedule for nonimmunes is intensive, with doses at 0, 3, 7, 14, and 28 days. While there has been at least one report of successful antiviral treatment of rabies, there is no indication for prophylactic antiviral therapy.

IV-104. **The answer is A.** *(Chap. 162)* This patient has syphilis of <1 year duration (early latent). HIV counseling and testing are important for all patients diagnosed with syphilis, given the shared high-risk behaviors associated with transmission of both infections as well as the increased risk of neurosyphilis in co-infected patients. Pregnancy status is important to know as congenital syphilis is a concern. All recent sexual contacts should be screened and treated empirically for syphilis, regardless of serologic or clinical status, as the latency period between exposure and primary syphilis can last as long as 3 months. Individuals with syphilis are at high risk of other STDs such as chlamydia and gonorrhea. Syphilitic aortitis is not a concern in a patient with early latent syphilis.

IV-105. **The answer is E.** *(Chap. 182)* The biologic determinants of HIV transmission and acquisition are complex and have been difficult to study. However, several key factors are now known to increase the per-coital rate of HIV transmission, at least for heterosexual couples. In discordant couples there is a dose-dependent relationship between serum viral load and HIV transmission. In fact, in carefully done studies there was virtually no transmission between discordant couples when serum viral load was low (<400/mL). It is likely that this is due to a fairly tight correlation between serum and genital viral load. A corollary is that during acute HIV or AIDS, the viral load and, therefore, transmissibility are high. There are strong clinical data from randomized trials that circumcised men are less likely to acquire HIV because the interior surface of the foreskin is replete with cellular targets for HIV infection. Nonulcerative sexually transmitted infections cause mucosal breakdown that has been shown to allow for greater acquisition of HIV infection. HSV-2 carriage (not necessarily requiring active genital ulcer disease) leads to increases in HIV genital shedding as well as HIV-1 target cell migration to the genital mucosa, making both transmission and acquisition of HIV higher in HSV-2-positive persons.

IV-106. **The answer is E.** *(Chap. 124)* Pelvic inflammatory disease refers to an ascending infection from the vagina/cervix to the endometrium and/or the fallopian tubes. Infectious complications include peritonitis, perihepatitis, perisplenitis, or pelvic abscess. It is an important cause of infertility. *Neisseria gonorrhoeae* and *Chlamydia trachomatis* are the microbes most commonly implicated in PID. *Mycoplasma genitalium*, anaerobes, and facultative organisms have also been isolated in the peritoneal fluid or fallopian tubes of women with PID. Bacterial vaginosis, a history of salpingitis, the presence of an intrauterine device, or recent exposure to a male partner with urethritis are risk factors for the development of PID. PID is more likely to develop during or soon after a menstrual period, suggesting that menstruation is a risk for ascending infection from the cervix or vagina.

IV-107. **The answer is B.** *(Chap. 182)* CDC guidelines now state that all adults should receive HIV testing, with the availability of a patient opt-out mechanism rather than informed consent. The basis for this is that ~25% of the 1 million Americans infected with HIV are unaware of their status, there is good available treatment for HIV that serves to extend the lifespan and decrease HIV transmission, and HIV testing is shown to correlate with a decrease in risk-taking behaviors. Cost-benefit analysis has suggested this approach has advantages to current approaches focusing on screening high-risk populations. Pretest counseling is desirable but not always built into the testing process so physicians should provide some degree of preparation for a positive test. If the diagnosis is made, support systems should be activated that may include trained nurses, social workers, or community support centers.

IV-108. **The answer is B.** *(Chap. 132)* *Listeria* bacteremia in pregnancy is a relatively rare but serious infection both for mother and fetus. Vertical transmission may occur, with 70–90% of fetuses developing infection from the mother. Preterm labor is common. Prepartum treatment of the mother increases the chances of a healthy delivery. Mortality among fetuses approaches 50% and is much lower in neonates receiving appropriate antibiotics. First-line therapy is with ampicillin, with gentamicin often added for synergy. This recommendation is the same for mother and child. In patients with true penicillin allergy, the therapy of choice is trimethoprim-sulfamethoxazole. Quinolones have shown animal model and in vitro efficacy against *Listeria*, but there is not enough clinical evidence to recommend these agents as first-line therapy.

IV-109. **The answer is A.** *(Chap. 113)* The role of immune modulators in serious infections has received increased attention in recent years as understanding of the cytokine and inflammatory systems have evolved. In several models of disease, an aggressive host anti-inflammatory response may increase organ damage. Steroids are useful adjuncts for several infections as antibiotics alone can increase inflammation and cytokine release due to lysis of intact organism and release of pro-inflammatory intracellular content. However, mold infections, such as *Aspergillus*, are apt to worsen in the setting of glucocorticoids.

IV-110. **The answer is D.** *(Chap. 188)* The patient has been bitten by a member of a species known to carry rabies in an area in which rabies is endemic. Based on the animal vector and the facts that the skin was broken and that saliva possibly containing the rabies virus was present, postexposure rabies prophylaxis should be administered. If an animal involved in an unprovoked bite can be captured, it should be killed humanely and the head should be sent immediately to an appropriate laboratory for rabies examination by the technique of fluorescent antibody staining for viral antigen. If a healthy dog or cat bites a person in an endemic area, the animal should be captured, confined, and observed for 10 days. If the animal remains healthy for this period, the bite is highly unlikely to have transmitted rabies. Postexposure prophylactic therapy includes vigorous cleaning of the wound with a 20% soap solution to remove any virus particles that may be present. Tetanus toxoid and antibiotics should also be administered. Passive immunization with antirabies antiserum in the form of human rabies immune globulin (rather than the corresponding equine antiserum because of the risk of serum sickness) is indicated at a dose of 10 units/kg into the wound and 10 units/kg IM into the gluteal region. Second, one should actively immunize with an antirabies vaccine [either human diploid cell vaccine or rabies vaccine absorbed (RVA)] in five 1-mL doses given IM, preferably in the deltoid or anterior lateral thigh area. The five doses are given over a 28-day period. The administration of either passive or active immunization without the other modality results in a higher failure rate than does the combination therapy.

IV-111. **The answer is D.** *(Chap. 115)* Traumatic splenectomy does not necessarily result in loss of splenic function as functioning splenules can implant within the peritoneum in the setting of trauma. A peripheral smear showing Howell-Jolly bodies implies loss of splenic function. This is important as asplenic patients are at considerably higher risk of overwhelming sepsis and warrant vaccination against encapsulated pathogens.

IV-112. **The answer is A.** *(Chap. 118)* Patients with infective endocarditis on antibiotic therapy can be expected to demonstrate clinical improvement within 5–7 days. Blood cultures will frequently remain positive for 3–5 days for *Staphylococcus aureus* treated with β-lactam antibiotics and 7–9 days with vancomycin. Neither rifampin nor gentamicin has been shown to provide clinical benefit in the scenario described above. Vancomycin peak and trough levels have not been shown to improve drug efficacy in infective endocarditis. It is too early in therapy to consider this case representative of vancomycin failure. The efficacy of daptomycin or linezolid as an alternative to vancomycin for left-sided MRSA endocarditis has not been established.

IV-113. **The answer is B.** *(Chap. 171)* Foscarnet is a potent agent used for drug-resistant CMV, herpes simplex virus (HSV) and varicella-zoster virus (VZV), or for patients who are intolerant of first-line agents. It may cause acute renal failure. It also binds divalent metals, commonly causing hypokalemia, hypocalcemia, hypophosphatemia, and hyperphosphatemia. It is often poorly tolerated as a result of nausea and malaise as well. Ganciclovir commonly causes bone marrow suppression and potential significant neutropenia when used for CMV infections, necessitating a switch to foscarnet. Foscarnet commonly causes renal failure. Acyclovir (used for HSV and VZV) is generally very well tolerated but may cause lethargy and tremors. Aerosolized ribavirin is used to treat respiratory syncytial virus infection in infants. It is a mutagen and teratogen and is embryotoxic.

IV-114. **The answer is A.** *(Chap. 182)* This patient most likely has HIV encephalopathy of moderate severity. Other neurologic conditions associated with HIV may be considered with a broad initial workup, but her reasonably high CD4+ count, lack of focal deficits and lack of mass lesions on high-resolution brain imaging makes toxoplasmosis, central nervous system (CNS) tuberculoma, progressive multifocal leukoencephalopathy (PML), or CNS lymphoma all less unlikely. Immediate highly active antiretroviral therapy is the treatment of choice for HIV encephalopathy, and she warrants this despite her CD4+ lymphocyte count placing her in a gray zone according to current guidelines in regards to starting therapy. A lumbar puncture looking for VDRL is unnecessary as a serum RPR test is a very good screening test for any type of syphilis; JC virus detected in the CSF would suggest PML, but her pretest probability for this is low because it usually affects patients with a low CD4+ T cell count. Serum cryptococcal antigen has excellent performance characteristics, but there is little reason to suspect cryptococcal meningitis in the absence of headache or elevated intracerebral pressure.

IV-115. **The answer is C.** *(Chap. 196)* *Candidemia* may lead to seeding of other organs. Among nonneutropenic patients up to 10% develop retinal lesions; therefore, it is very important to perform thorough funduscopy. Focal seeding can occur within 2 weeks of the onset of candidemia and may occur even if the patient is afebrile or the infection clears. The lesions may be unilateral or bilateral and are typically small white retinal exudates. However, retinal infection may progress to retinal detachment, vitreous abscess, or extension into the anterior chamber of the eye. Patients may be asymptomatic initially but may also report blurring, ocular pain, or scotoma. Abdominal abscess are possible but usually occur in patients recovering from profound neutropenia. Fungal endocarditis is also possible but is more common in patients who use IV drugs and may have a murmur on cardiac examination. Fungal pneumonia and pulmonary abscesses are very rare and are not likely in this patient.

IV-116. **The answer is C.** *(Chap. 162)* This patient has failed therapy for syphilis as his RPR titer has not decreased fourfold over the course of a year. The FTA-ABS may remain positive even after effective treatment. There is no indication for penicillin desensitization. A lumbar puncture is indicated when there is not a fourfold decrease in RPR titre 6–12 months after appropriate therapy, particularly in patients with HIV. A lumbar puncture showing pleocytosis, elevated protein, and/or a positive VDRL will confirm the diagnosis and the need for 10–14 days of IV penicillin. If the CSF is negative, re-treatment with three doses of IM penicillin for late latent syphilis is adequate. There is no reason to begin treatment for neurosyphilis until the diagnosis is made. Doxycycline, 100 mg PO bid for 30 days, is an alternative treatment for syphilis of unknown duration or >1 year duration, but not for neurosyphilis.

IV-117. **The answer is C.** *(Chap. 153)* Although the patient's gardening puts her at risk for *Sporothrix* infection, this infection typically causes a more localized streaking nodular lymphadenitis affecting the forearm. The differential diagnosis for nodular adenitis includes *Sporothrix schenckii*, *Nocardia brasiliensis*, *Mycobacterium marinum*, *Leishmania braziliensis*, and *Francisella tularensis* and is based on direct inoculation of organism due to contact from the soil, marine environment, insect bite, or animal bite. This patient has regional lymphadenitis involving larger lymph nodes that drain the site of inoculation. Most likely in her case is cat scratch disease due to *Bartonella henselae*, based on the kittens in her home, but lymphoma and staphylococcal infection must also be considered and oftentimes a lymph node biopsy is required to make this distinction. Most cases of cat scratch disease resolve without therapy. In immunocompetent patients, antibiotic therapy has minimal benefit but may expedite resolution of lymphadenopathy. Antimicrobial therapy, usually with azithromycin, is indicated in immunosuppressed patients.

IV-118. **The answer is B.** *(Chap. 212)* *Schistosoma mansoni* infection of the liver causes cirrhosis from vascular obstruction resulting from periportal fibrosis but relatively little hepatocellular injury. Hepatosplenomegaly, hypersplenism, and esophageal varices develop quite commonly, and schistosomiasis is usually associated with eosinophilia. Spider nevi, gynecomastia, jaundice, and ascites are observed less commonly than they are in alcoholic and postnecrotic fibrosis.

IV-119. **The answer is A.** *(Chap. 148)* Campylobacters are motile, curved gram-negative rods. The principal diarrheal pathogen is *C. jejuni*. This organism is found in the gastrointestinal tract of many animals used for food production and is usually transmitted to humans in raw or undercooked food products or through direct contact with infected animals. Over half the cases are due to insufficiently cooked contaminated poultry. *Campylobacter* is a common cause of diarrheal disease in the United States. The illness usually occurs within 2–4 days after exposure to the organism in food or water. Biopsy of an affected patient's jejunum, ileum, or colon reveals findings indistinguishable from those of Crohn's disease and ulcerative colitis. Although the diarrheal illness is usually self-limited, it may be associated with constitutional symptoms, lasts more than 1 week, and recurs in 5–10% of untreated patients. Complications include pancreatitis, cystitis, arthritis, meningitis, and Guillain-Barré syndrome. The symptoms of *Campylobacter* enteritis are similar to those resulting from infection with *Salmonella*, *Shigella*, and *Yersinia*; all these agents cause fever and the presence of fecal leukocytes. The diagnosis is made by isolating *Campylobacter* from the stool, which requires selective media. *E. coli* (enterotoxigenic) generally is not associated with the finding of fecal leukocytes; nor is the Norwalk agent.

Campylobacter is a far more common cause of a recurrent relapsing diarrheal illness that could be pathologically confused with inflammatory bowel disease than are *Yersinia, Salmonella, Shigella,* and enteropathogenic *E. coli*.

IV-120. **The answer is E.** *(Chap. 113)* Deficiencies in the complement system predispose patients to a variety of infections. Most of these deficits are congenital. Patients with sickle cell disease have acquired functional defects in the alternative complement pathway. They are at risk of infection from *S. pneumoniae* and *Salmonella* spp. Patients with liver disease, nephrotic syndrome, and systemic lupus erythematosus may have defects in C3. They are at particular risk for infections with *Staphylococcus aureus, S. pneumoniae, Pseudomonas* spp, and *Proteus* spp. Patients with congenital or acquired (usually systemic lupus erythematosus) deficiencies in the terminal complement cascade (C5-8) are at particular risk of infection from *Neisseria* spp such as *N. meningitis* or *N. gonorrhoeae*.

IV-121. **The answer is D.** *(Chap. 166)* This patient's rash is a classic erythema migrans lesion and is diagnostic for Lyme disease in her geographic region. In the United States, Lyme disease is due to *Borrelia burgdorferi*. Partial central clearing, a bright red border, and a target center are very suggestive of this lesion. The fact that multiple lesions exist implies disseminated infection, rather than a primary tick bite inoculation where only one lesion is present. Potential complications of secondary Lyme disease in the United States include migratory arthritis, meningitis, cranial neuritis, mononeuritis multiplex, myelitis, varying degrees of atrioventricular block, and, less commonly myopericarditis, splenomegaly, and hepatitis. Third-degree or persistent Lyme disease is associated with oligoarticular arthritis of large joints and subtle encephalopathy but not frank dementia. *Borrelia garinii* infection is seen only in Europe and can cause a more pronounced encephalomyelitis.

IV-122. **The answer is D.** *(Chap. 166)* As shown in Figure IV-121 (Color Atlas), acute Lyme disease involving the skin and/or joints is treated with oral doxycycline unless the patient is pregnant or <9 years old. Amoxicillin and macrolides (azithromycin) are less effective therapies. Ceftriaxone is indicated for acute disease in the presence of nervous system involvement (meningitis, facial palsy, encephalopathy, radiculoneuritis) or third-degree heart block. It may also be used for treatment of patients with arthritis who do not respond to oral therapy. First-generation cephalosporins are not active against *B. burgdorferi*. While the rash of erythema migrans may look like cellulitis due to staphylococci or streptococci, there is no proven efficacy of vancomycin for Lyme disease.

IV-123. **The answer is D.** *(Chap. 118)* Culture-proven fungal (particularly mold) endocarditis and sinus of Valsalva abscess represent situations where strong evidence supports cardiac surgery; a ruptured sinus of Valsalva abscess represents a surgical emergency, while fungal endocarditis is usually considered more of an elective case, with earlier surgical management preferred. Acute aortic regurgitation plus preclosure of the mitral valve is also an indication for immediate surgery. Septic pulmonary emboli alone do not necessitate surgery; however, if a 10-mm vegetation is also seen this would best be treated surgically. Staphylococcal prosthetic valve endocarditis (PVE) or PVE within 2 months of surgery is an example of reasonable indications for surgical management. In contrast to fungal endocarditis, there are no particular species of bacteria that merit surgical treatment, independent of other factors.

IV-124. **The answer is E.** *(Chaps. 126 and 207)* T. gondii commonly achieves latency in cysts during acute infection. Reactivation in the central nervous system in AIDS patients is well known. However, *Toxoplasma* cysts also reside in the heart. Thus, transplanting a *Toxoplasma*-positive heart into a negative recipient may cause reactivation in the months after transplant. Serologic screening of cardiac donors and recipients for *T. gondii* is important. To account for this possibility, prophylactic doses of trimethoprim-sulfamethoxazole, which is also effective prophylaxis against *Pneumocystis* and *Nocardia*, is standard after cardiac transplantation. Cardiac transplant recipients, similar to all other solid organ transplant recipients, are at risk of developing infections related to impaired cellular immunity, particularly >1 month to 1 year posttransplant. Wound infections or mediastinitis from skin organisms may complicate the early transplant (<1 month) period.

IV-125. **The answer is B.** *(Chap. 123)* Severe *C. difficile*–associated disease may mimic a surgical abdomen and patients may not have diarrhea. The lack of diarrhea should not overshadow the other signs and risk factors that are suggestive of *C. difficile*–associated disease, including significant leukocytosis, long hospitalization, prior antibiotics, and probable enteral tube feeds while on the ventilator. Adynamic ileus is a serious and well-known complication of *C. difficile*–associated disease. All potentially serious manifestations that could be *C. difficile*–associated disease should be empirically treated as such until stool antigen tests are negative and an alternative clinical explanation is found. Intravenous metronidazole may be less optimal then oral vancomycin for severe cases, and this patient may fail therapy. However, oral medicines are less likely to reach the target organ in the presence of an adynamic ileus, necessitating IV metronidazole. Some advocate combining administration of oral vancomycin by NG tube with IV metronidazole. All potentially offending antibiotics should be stopped (if possible, as is the case here with the patient having recovered from her pneumonia) rather than continued. Surgical colectomy may be necessary in fulminant cases when there is no response to medical therapy. Intravenous immunoglobulins, which may provide antibodies to *C. difficile* toxin, are reserved for severe or multiple recurrent cases of *C. difficile*–associated disease.

IV-126. **The answer is B.** *(Chaps. 143 and 282)* *E. coli* is the etiologic agent in 85–95% of uncomplicated urinary tract infections (UTIs) that occur in premenopausal women. Uncomplicated cystitis is the most common UTI syndrome. 20% of women will develop a recurrence in 1 year after their initial UTI. Pregnant women are at high risk of cystitis developing into pyelonephritis. *Proteus* represents only 1–2% of uncomplicated UTI. *Proteus* causes 20–45% of UTIs in patients with long-term bladder catheterization. *Klebsiella* also accounts for only 1–2% of uncomplicated UTIs; however, it is responsible for 5–17% of complicated UTIs. *Enterobacter* is a rare cause of infection outside of the hospital. *Candida* is most often a genitourinary colonizer in healthy patients and is rarely the cause of infection.

IV-127. **The answer is D.** *(Chap. 129)* This patient has infectious pyomyositis, a disease of the tropics and of immunocompromised hosts such as patients with poorly controlled diabetes mellitus or AIDS. The pathogen is usually *S. aureus*. Management includes aggressive debridement, antibiotics, and attempts to reverse the patient's immunocompromised status. *C. perfringens* may cause gas gangrene, particularly in devitalized tissues. Streptococcal infections may cause cellulitis or an aggressive fasciitis, but the presence of abscesses in a patient with poorly controlled diabetes makes staphylococcal infection more likely. Polymicrobial infections are common in diabetic ulcers, but in this case the imaging and physical examination show intramuscular abscesses.

IV-128. **The answer is C.** *(Chap. 180)* Avian influenza epidemics occur when human influenza A undergoes an antigenic exchange with influenza found in poultry. Recent outbreaks have not been associated with effective human-to-human spread; nearly all patients reported exposure to infected poultry. Past influenza pandemics, including the 1918–1919 pandemic, appear to have originated from antigenic exchange between human and avian influenza viruses. Antigenic shifts are defined as major changes in the hemagglutinin (H) and neuraminidase (N) antigens and occur only with influenza A. Minor antigenic changes are known as antigenic drift and can occur with hemagglutinin alone or with both hemagglutinin (H) and neuraminidase (N). While influenza A and B are genetically and morphologically similar, the latter virus' inability to undergo antigenic shifts lessens its virulence and involvement in pandemic flu. Influenza C is a rare cause of disease in humans and is typically a clinically mild, self-limited infection.

IV-129. **The answer is E.** *(Chap. 193)* There is no *Coccidioides* in Northern Arizona (i.e., the Grand Canyon region). The organism can be cultured from dry top soil in the high desert of Southern Arizona surrounding Phoenix and Tucson. Eosinophilia is a common laboratory finding in acute coccidioidomycosis and erythema nodosum is a common cutaneous clinical feature. Mediastinal lymphadenopathy is more commonly seen on radiographs for all acute pneumonias due to endemic mycoses, including *Coccidioides*, rather than due to bacterial pneumonia. A positive complement fixation test is one method to definitively diagnose acute infection.

IV-130. **The answer is E.** *(Chap. 166)* Post-Lyme syndrome is an uncommon but debilitating syndrome similar to fibromyalgia and chronic fatigue syndrome and sometimes occurs after appropriate treatment for Lyme disease. Its etiology is not well understood, but it does not appear to be due to ongoing replication or presence of *Borrelia burgdorferi* at sites of patient discomfort. Clinical trials have compared long courses of IV ceftriaxone followed by oral doxycycline with placebo and found no differences in patient outcome. Prednisone would be indicated only in the presence of documented inflammatory arthritis, a condition that is not evident in this patient. The patient has already received adequate treatment for Lyme disease, and a positive IgG serology would either indicate past infection or serofast state. In either case, the test is not indicated because this information would not be helpful in the current situation and could be misleading to the patient.

IV-131. **The answer is A.** *(Chaps. 145)* *B. cepacia* is an opportunistic pathogen that has been responsible for nosocomial outbreaks. It also colonizes and infects the lower respiratory tract of patients with cystic fibrosis, chronic granulomatous disease, and sickle cell disease. In patients with cystic fibrosis it portends a rapid decline in pulmonary function and a poor clinical prognosis. It also may cause a resistant necrotizing pneumonia. *B. cepacia* is often intrinsically resistant to a variety of antimicrobials, including many β-lactams and aminoglycosides. Trimethoprim-sulfamethoxazole (TMP/SMX) is usually the first-line treatment. *P. aeruginosa* and *S. aureus* are common colonizers and pathogens in patients with cystic fibrosis. *Stenotrophomonas maltophilia* is the pathogen, particularly in patients with cancer, transplants, and critical illness. *S. maltophilia* is a cause of pneumonia, urinary tract infection, wound infection, and bacteremia. TMP/SMX is usually the treatment of choice for *Stenotrophomonas* infections.

IV-132. **The answer is D.** *(Chap. 121)* CAPD-associated peritonitis is different from primary and secondary peritonitis in that most infections are caused by skin flora rather than gut pathogens. Therefore, antibiotics should usually ultimately be directed towards *Staphylococcus* species, especially *S. aureus*. These species, including coagulase-negative staphylococci, account for 40–50% of cases. Recently, *S. aureus* has increased in frequency. Typical signs include diffuse pain and peritoneal signs. Peritoneal fluid will be cloudy with >100 WBCs/μL with >50% neutrophils. Vancomycin is necessary in areas where methicillin-resistant *S. aureus* is common. Intraperitoneal loading doses of this drug are typically given. Though gram-negative and *Candida* infections do occur and should be covered prior to the return of culture data, they are less common. The presence of more than one species in culture should prompt an evaluation for secondary peritonitis. Once definitive culture data are returned, then antibiotics can be narrowed towards only the offending pathogen. If there is no symptomatic improvement within 48 h or the patient appears septic, then catheter removal is standard. These infections are in many ways similar to vascular catheter infections, and their management therefore has many parallels.

IV-133. **The answer is D.** *(Chap. 182)* Indinavir is the only agent to cause nephrolithiasis. Nucleoside reverse transcriptase inhibitors, particularly stavudine and didanosine (d4T and ddI), are associated with mitochondrial toxicity and pancreatitis. Nevirapine can cause hepatic necrosis in women, particularly with a CD4+ lymphocyte count >350/μL. Efavirenz, a very commonly used agent, causes dream disturbances that usually, but not always, subside after the first month of therapy. Both indinavir and atazanavir cause a benign indirect hyperbilirubinemia reminiscent of Gilbert's syndrome.

IV-134. **The answer is E.** *(Chap. 203)* Thick and thin smears are a critical part of the evaluation of fever in a person with recent time spent in a *Plasmodium*-endemic region. Thick smears take a longer time to process but increase sensitivity in the setting of low parasitemia. Thin smears are more likely to allow for precise morphologic evaluation to differentiate between the four different types of *Plasmodium* infection and also allow for prognostic calculation of parasitemia. If clinical suspicion is high, repeat smears should be performed if initially negative. If personnel are not available to rapidly interpret a smear, empirical therapy should be strongly considered to ward off the most severe manifestation of *P. falciparum* infection. Antibody-based diagnostic tests that are sensitive and specific for *P. falciparum* infection have been introduced. They will remain positive for weeks after infection and do not allow quantification of parasitemia.

IV-135.   The answer is B. *(Chap. 134).*   This patient most likely has wound botulism. The use of "black-tar" heroin has been identified as a risk factor for this form of botulism. Typically the wound appears benign, and unlike in other forms of botulism, gastrointestinal symptoms are absent. Symmetric *descending* paralysis suggests botulism, as does cranial nerve involvement. This patient's ptosis, diplopia, dysarthria, dysphagia, lack of fevers, normal reflexes, and lack of sensory deficits are all suggestive. Botulism can be easily confused with Guillain-Barré syndrome (GBS), which is often characterized by an antecedent infection and rapid, symmetric *ascending* paralysis and treated with plasmapheresis. The Miller Fischer variant of GBS is known for cranial nerve involvement with ophthalmoplegia, ataxia, and areflexia being the most prominent features. Elevated protein in the cerebrospinal fluid also favors GBS over botulism. Both botulism and GBS can progress to respiratory failure, so making a diagnosis by physical examination is critical. Other diagnostic modalities that may be helpful are wound culture, serum assay for toxin, and examination for decreased compound muscle action potentials on routine nerve stimulation studies. Patients with botulism are at risk of respiratory failure due to respiratory muscle weakness or aspiration. They should be followed closely with oxygen saturation monitoring and serial measurement of forced vital capacity.

IV-136.   The answer is D. *(Chap. 182)*   *Isospora* and *Cryptosporidium* cause very similar clinical disease in AIDS patients that ranges from intermittent, self-resolved watery diarrhea with abdominal cramping and sometimes nausea, to a potentially fatal cholera-like presentation in the most immunocompromised hosts. *Cryptosporidium* may cause biliary disease and can lead to cholangitis. *Isospora* is limited to the gut lumen. *Cryptosporidium* is not always an opportunistic infection and has led to widespread community outbreaks. *Isospora* is not seen in immunocompetent hosts. Finally, treatment for *Isospora* is usually successful. In fact, this infection is rarely seen in the developed world because trimethoprim/sulfamethoxazole, which is commonly used for *Pneumocystis* prophylaxis, tends to eradicate *Isospora*. Cryptosporidiosis, on the other hand, is very difficult to cure and interventions are controversial. Some clinicians favor nitazoxanone, but cure rates are mediocre and immune reconstitution with antiretroviral therapy is ultimately critical to cure the gastrointestinal disease.

IV-137.   The answer is F. *(Chap. 182)*   Patients with HIV and a CD4+ lymphocyte count <200 μ/L are given the diagnosis of AIDS as this is a rough threshold for an increased risk for several life-threatening opportunistic infections. Different opportunistic infections and HIV-related complications are seen most frequently below certain serum CD4+ lymphocyte count thresholds: disseminated CMV / MAI (<50 μ/L), cryptococcosis (<100 μ/L) and *Pneumocystis* (<200 μ/L). These are all considered AIDS-defining complications. Certain diagnoses, such as active tuberculosis and Kaposi's sarcoma, are considered AIDS-defining even though they may present with higher CD4+ lymphocyte counts because they are historically linked with high mortality rates. Multidermatomal zoster starts to occur with more frequency when CD4+ lymphocyte count descends below 500 μ/L and is not considered AIDS-defining. If multidermatomal zoster occurs in a previously healthy person, it should raise the suspicion of new HIV infection.

IV-138.   The answer is D. *(Chap. 182)*   Acute HIV should be suspected in any at-risk person who presents with a mono-like illness: it is diagnosed by positive plasma RNA PCR. Patients typically have not developed sufficient antibodies to the virus yet to develop a positive EIA, and the diagnosis of HIV is usually missed if this test is sent within the first 2 months of HIV acquisition. It is tempting for clinicians to send an ultrasensitive PCR, but this only decreases specificity (false-positive tests with detection of very low levels of HIV are possible due to cross contamination in the laboratory) with no other benefit. There is typically a massive amount of HIV virus in the plasma during acute infection, and the ultrasensitive assay is never required for detection at this stage of disease. Ultrasensitive assays are helpful in the context of therapy to ensure that there is not persistence of low-level viremia. CD4+ lymphocyte count decreases during many acute infections, including HIV, and is therefore not diagnostically appropriate. CD4+ lymphocyte counts are useful to risk stratify for opportunistic infection in stable patients with known HIV infection. Resistance tests are sent only when the diagnosis is confirmed.

IV-139. **The answer is D.** *(Chap. 160)* Congenital infection from maternal transmission can lead to severe consequences for the neonate; thus, prenatal care and screening for infection are very important. *C. trachomatis* is associated with up to 25% of exposed neonates who develop inclusion conjunctivitis. It can also be associated with pneumonia and otitis media in the newborn. Pneumonia in the newborn has been associated with later development of bronchitis and asthma. Hydrocephalus can be associated with toxoplasmosis. Hutchinson triad, which is Hutchinson teeth (blunted upper incisors), interstitial keratitis, and eighth nerve deafness, is due to congenital syphilis. Sensorineural deafness can be associated with congenital rubella exposure. Treatment of *C. trachomatis* in the infant consists of oral erythromycin.

IV-140. **The answer is B.** *(Chap. 182)* Suppression of HIV replication with combination ART is the cornerstone of management of patients with HIV infection. There are several possible starting regimens for HIV therapy. Tenofovir, emtricitabine, and efavirenz is a popular combination as it is potent, reasonably free of side effects in the long term, and is available in a single pill called Atripla. The combination of stavudine and didanosine (choice A) is now strictly contraindicated as there is a synergistic effect of mitochondrial toxicity resulting in cases of pancreatitis, neuropathy, and lactic acidosis. Indinavir, an older protease inhibitor, has an unacceptably high toxicity (nephrolithiasis) and too frequent dosing (3 times per day) for the current standard of care for an initial regimen. Choice D contains two protease inhibitors (lopinavir/ritonavir, atazanavir), which is atypical and would not be first-line therapy. Choice E (AZT, 3TC, ABC) is available in a combination taken twice a day called Trizivir. It consists of three nucleoside analogues and has been associated with unacceptably high levels of treatment failure in clinical trials comparing it to current standard regimens.

IV-141. **The answer is B.** *(Chap. 176)* Molluscum contagiosum is a cutaneous poxvirus infection with a distinctive cutaneous appearance. The rash typically consists of collections of 2- to 5-mm umbilicated papules that can occur anywhere on the body *except* the palms and soles. It can be accompanied by an eczematous reaction. Molluscum contagiosum is transmitted through close contact including sexual contact, which will cause genital involvement. Unlike other poxvirus lesions, molluscum contagiosum is not associated with inflammation or necrosis. In immunocompetent patients, the disease is usually self-limited; rash will subside within several months time. Systemic involvement does not occur.

IV-142. **The answer is E.** *(Chap. 182)* *P. jiroveci* lung infection is known to worsen after initiation of treatment, likely due to lysis of organism and immune response to its intracellular contents. It is thought that adjunct administration of glucocorticoids may reduce inflammation and subsequent lung injury in patients with moderate to severe pneumonia due to *P. jiroveci*. Adjunct administration of glucocorticoids in patients with moderate to severe disease as determined by a room air Pa_{O_2} <70 mmHg or an A – a gradient >35 mmHg decrease mortality. Glucocorticoids should be given for a total duration of 3 weeks. Patients often do not improve until many days into therapy and often initially worsen; steroids should be used as soon as hypoxemia develops rather than wait for lack of improvement. Pneumothoraces and adult respiratory distress syndrome (ARDS) are common feared complications of *Pneumocystis* infection. If patients present with ARDS due to *Pneumocystis* pneumonia, they would meet the criterion for adjunct glucocorticoids due to the severe nature of disease.

IV-143. **The answer is A.** *(Chap. 191)* Caspofungin and the other echinocandins (anidulafungin, micafungin) inhibit fungal synthesis of B-1,3-glucan synthase, a necessary enzyme for fungal cell wall synthesis that does not have a human correlate. These agents are available only parentally, not orally. They are fungicidal for *Candida* species and fungistatic against

Aspergillus species. Caspofungin is as at least equivalently effective as amphotericin B for disseminated candidiasis and is as effective as fluconazole for candidal esophagitis. It is not a first-line therapy for *Aspergillus* infection but may be used as salvage therapy. The echinocandins, including caspofungin, have an extremely high safety profile. They do not have activity against mucormycosis, paracoccidiomycosis, or histoplasmosis.

IV-144. The answer is D or F. *(Chap. 208)* Giardiasis is diagnosed by detection of parasite antigens, cysts, or trophozoites in feces. There is no reliable serum test for this disease. As a wide variety of pathogens are responsible for diarrheal illness, some degree of diagnostic testing beyond the history and physical examination is required for definitive diagnosis. Colonoscopy does not have a role in diagnosing *Giardia*. Giardiasis can persist in symptomatic patients and should be treated. Cure rates with 5 days of oral metronidazole tid are >90%. A single oral dose of tinidazole is reportedly at least as effective as metronidazole. Paromomycin, an oral poorly absorbed aminoglycoside, can be used for symptomatic patients during pregnancy, but its efficacy for eradicating infection is not known. Clindamycin and albendazole do not have a role in treatment of giardiasis. Refractory disease can be treated with longer duration of metronidazole.

IV-145. The answer is B. *(Chap. 160)* Nontuberculous mycobacteria, such as *M. avium* complex, may cause chronic pulmonary infections in normal hosts and those with underlying pulmonary disease immunosuppression. In immunocompetent patients without underlying disease, treatment of pulmonary infection with *M. avium* complex is considered on an individual basis based on symptoms, radiographic findings, and bacteriology. Treatment should be initiated in the presence of progressive pulmonary disease or symptoms. In patients without any prior lung disease and who do not demonstrate progressive clinical decline, *M. avium* pulmonary infection can be managed conservatively. Patients with underlying lung disease, such as chronic obstructive pulmonary disease or cystic fibrosis, or those with a history of pulmonary tuberculosis should receive antibiotics. In the vignette above, the patient has both clinical and historic reasons for antibiotic treatment. The appropriate regimen in this case is clarithromycin and ethambutol. The combination of pyrazinamide, isoniazid, rifampin, and ethambutol is effective treatment for *M. tuberculosis* infection, which is not present here. Quinolones have shown promise in the treatment of mycobacterial infections but are not first-line therapy in this case. Rifampin has no role in treating *M. avium* infection.

IV-146. The answer is A. *(Chap. 191)* The definitive diagnosis of an invasive fungal infection generally requires histologic demonstration of fungus invading tissue along with an inflammatory response. However, coccidioides serum complement fixation, cryptococcal serum and cerebrospinal fluid antigen, and urine/serum histoplasma antigen are all tests with good performance characteristics, occasionally allowing for presumptive diagnoses before pathologic tissue sections can be examined or cultures of blood or tissue turn positive. There is no such widely used serologic test for blastomycosis. Serum testing for galactomannan is approved for the diagnosis of *Aspergillus* infection. However, false negatives may occur, and further studies of the validity are necessary.

IV-147. The answer is B. *(Chap. 171)* Oral ribavirin combined with pegylated interferon appears to be the most effective regimen for treating hepatitis C. Ribavirin does not exert antiviral effect but may be an immune modulator in combination with the interferon. Hemolytic anemia occurs in nearly 25% of patients receiving this therapy. Common approaches to this problem are dose reduction, cessation of ribavirin therapy, or use of red cell growth factors. Rash can occur but is less common. Interferon has common side effects as well, including flulike symptoms, depression, sleep disturbances, personality change, leukopenia, and thrombocytopenia.

IV-148. The answer is C. *(Chap. 116)* Hepatitis B is efficiently spread as a bloodborne pathogen. In approximately one-third of needle stick cases where the victim is not immunized (either by vaccine or prior clearance of infection), hepatitis B transmission will occur. This is in comparison to 3% for hepatitis C and 0.3% for HIV-1 infections. Moreover, hepatitis B, because it is a DNA virus, can survive for prolonged amount of times on unsterilized surfaces. This speaks to the goal of 100% vaccination against hepatitis B for all health care workers. Rapid administration of both hepatitis B vaccine and immunoglobulins are the most effective way to prevent transmission if a high-risk stick occurs to a nonimmune health care worker. No data exist to support the use of antiviral therapy for hepatitis B needle sticks, though this strategy has proven effective for HIV-1 associated needle sticks.

IV-149. **The answer is C.** *(Chap. 203)* Appropriately and promptly treated, *P. falciparum* malaria without complications has a mortality rate of ~0.1%. The presence or development of organ dysfunction elevates mortality risk significantly. Hypoglycemia is associated with a poor prognosis and is most common in children and pregnant women. It is caused by a failure of hepatic gluconeogenesis and increased glucose consumption by the host. Quinine and quinidine may also increase pancreatic insulin secretion. Obtundation and coma are worrisome in that they often represent cerebral edema, a feared complication of cerebral malaria. The mortality of cerebral malaria is 15–20%. Acute renal failure and profound hemolytic anemia often accompany severe infection and are also poor prognostic features. Their presence may necessitate hemodialysis and exchange transfusion. Though liver enzyme elevations and hemolytic jaundice are common in malaria, hepatic necrosis is not. When severe liver dysfunction occurs, it is usually in the context of multi-organ failure.

IV-150. **The answer is C.** *(Chap. 378)* Prions are infectious proteins that lack nucleic acids and cause neurodegenerative diseases. The most common prion disease in humans is sporadic Creutzfeldt-Jakob disease (s-CJD). Others include familial CJD, fatal familial insomnia, kuru, and iatrogenic CJD. Prions result when an abnormal prion protein binds to a normal isoform of the prion protein, stimulating its conversion into the abnormal isoform. Abnormal prion isoforms have a greater proportion of β-structure and less α-helix than do normal isoforms. The α-to-β structural transition underlies the etiology of the central nervous system degeneration. The patient described has a typical presentation of s-CJD with sleep disturbance, fatigue, and defects in higher cortical functions. CJD progresses quickly to dementia. Over 90% of patients with CJD exhibit myoclonus during the illness. Typically the myoclonus is provoked by startle, loud noises, or bright lights and will occur even during sleep. The diagnosis requires an appropriate clinical presentation and no other etiologies on CSF examination. There is no widely available laboratory test for diagnosis. Brain biopsy may demonstrate spongiform degeneration and the presence of prion proteins.

IV-151. **The answer is D.** *(Chap. 168)* *Mycoplasma pneumoniae* is a common cause of pneumonia that is often underdiagnosed based on difficult and time-consuming culture techniques, it likely causes mild respiratory symptoms, and because it is adequately treated with standard antibiotic regimens for community-acquired pneumonia. It is spread easily person-to-person, and outbreaks in crowded conditions are common. Most patients develop a cough without radiographic abnormalities. Pharyngitis, rhinitis, and ear pain are also common. *M. pneumoniae* commonly induces the production of cold agglutinins, which in turn can cause an IgM- and complement-mediated intravascular hemolytic anemia. The presence of cold agglutinins is specific for *M. pneumoniae* infection only in the context of a consistent clinical picture for infection, as in this patient. Cold agglutinins are more common in children. Blood smear shows no abnormality, which is in contrast to IgG or warm-type hemolytic anemia where spherocytes are seen. Since there is no easy diagnostic test, empirical therapy is often administered.

IV-152. **The answer is B.** *(Chap. 120)* The most common overall cause of acute bacterial osteomyelitis of the spine is *S. aureus*, accounting for ~50% of cases due to a single organism, introduced via the bloodstream in patients at risk for bloodstream infections (injecting drug users, hemodialysis patients, open postoperative wounds). However, in older male patients with lumbar osteomyelitis, genitourinary or enteric pathogens, such as *E. coli*, are common, particularly after recent urinary tract infections and/or urologic surgeries, accounting for up to 25% of cases of vertebral osteomyelitis. Pathogenesis may occur via retrograde introduction of organism into the spine via the spinal venous plexus. Polymicrobial osteomyelitis is most often due to contiguous infection, such as a decubitus ulcer or diabetic foot infection, rather than bloodstream introductions that are more typical in the spine. Tuberculosis (Pott's disease) is always a consideration for osteomyelitis of the spine. However, this patient's presentation is likely too acute for tuberculosis, and the thoracic spine is a slightly more typical location than the lumbar spine. Brucellosis commonly involves the spine, but this patient's potential exposure to *Brucella* spp. is dated and the course of the infection is too acute for brucellosis. Hypothetically each of the listed infections is possible, highlighting the importance of holding antibiotics before culturing the epidural space, provided that the patient does not have sepsis on original presentation.

IV-153. **The answer is A.** *(Chap. 167)* Human granulocytotropic anaplasmosis occurs mostly in the northeastern and upper midwestern United States. It shares the *Ixodes* tick vector with Lyme disease. It is typically a disease of older males (median age 51 years). Because seroprevalence rates are high in endemic areas, subclinical infection is likely common. The disease typically presents with fever (>90% of cases), myalgias, headache, and malaise. Thrombocytopenia, leukopenia, and elevated aminotransferase activity is common. Adult respiratory distress syndrome, toxic shock–like syndrome, and opportunistic infections may occur, particularly in the elderly. Human granulocytotropic anaplasmosis should be considered on the differential of a flulike illness during May through December in endemic regions. Morulae, intracytoplasmic inclusions, are seen in the neutrophils of up to 80% of cases of human granulocytotropic anaplasmosis on peripheral blood smear and are diagnostic in the appropriate clinical context. This patient has high epidemiologic risk based on his long periods of time outside in an endemic region. Human monocytotropic ehrlichiosis, which can be a more severe illness, has morulae in mononuclear cells (not neutrophils) in a minority of cases. Lyme disease, which may be difficult to distinguish from human granulocytotropic anaplasmosis or human monocytotropic ehrlichiosis, will not cause morulae. Treatment of human granulocytotropic anaplasmosis is with doxycycline.

IV-154. **The answer is E.** *(Chap. 197)* Allergic bronchopulmonary aspergillosis (ABPA) is not a true infection but rather a hypersensitivity immune response to colonizing *Aspergillus* species. It occurs in ~1% of patients with asthma and in up to 15% of patients with cystic fibrosis. Patients typically have wheezing that is difficult to control with usual agents, infiltrates on chest radiographs due to mucus plugging of airways, a productive cough often with mucus casts, and bronchiectasis. Eosinophilia is common if glucocorticoids have not been administered. The total IgE is of value if >1000 IU/mL in that it represents a significant allergic response and is very suggestive of ABPA. In the proper clinical context, a positive skin test for *Aspergillus* antigen or detection of serum *Aspergillus*-specific IgG or IgE precipitating antibodies are supportive of the diagnosis. Galactomannan EIA is useful for invasive aspergillosis but has not been validated for ABPA. There is no need to try to culture an organism via BAL to make the diagnosis of ABPA. Chest CT, which may reveal bronchiectasis, or pulmonary function testing, which will reveal an obstructive defect, will not be diagnostic.

IV-155. **The answer is B.** *(Chap. 118)* Prosthetic cardiac valves are at high risk of developing endocarditis after bacteremia. Patients who develop endocarditis within 2 months of valve surgery most likely have acquired their infection nosocomially as a result of intraoperative contamination of the prosthesis or of a bacteremic postoperative event. Coagulase-negative staphylococci are the most common (33%) nosocomial pathogens during this time frame, followed by *Staphylococcus aureus* (22%), facultative gram-negative bacilli (13%), enterococci (8%), diphtheroids (6%), and fungi (6%) (see Table IV-155). The modes of infection and typical organisms causing prosthetic valve endocarditis >12 months after surgery are similar to those in community-acquired endocarditis. Both sets of pathogens must be considered in the intermediate 2–12 months after surgery.

TABLE IV-155 Organisms Causing Major Clinical Forms of Endocarditis

	Percent of Cases							
	Native Valve Endocarditis		Prosthetic Valve Endocarditis at Indicated Time of Onset (Months) after Valve Surgery			Endocarditis in Injection Drug Users		
Organism	Community-Acquired (n = 683)	Health Care–Associated (n = 128)	< 2 (n = 144)	2–12 (n = 31)	> 12 (n = 194)	Right-Sided (n = 346)	Left-Sided (n = 204)	Total (n = 675)[a]
Streptococci[b]	32	8	1	9	31	5	15	12
Pneumococci	1	—	—	—	—	—	—	—
Enterococci	8	16	8	12	11	2	24	9
Staphylococcus aureus	35	44[c]	22	12	18	77	23	57
Coagulase-negative staphylococci	4	15	33	32	11	—	—	—
Fastidious gram-negative coccobacilli (HACEK group)[d]	3	—	—	—	6	—	—	—
Gram-negative bacilli	3	5	13	3	6	5	13	7
Candida spp.	1	6	8	12	1	—	12	4
Polymicrobial/miscellaneous	6	1	3	6	5	8	10	7
Diphtheroids	—	—	6	—	3	—	—	0.1
Culture-negative	5	5	5	6	8	3	3	3

[a]The total number of cases is larger than the sum of right- and left-sided cases because the location of infection was not specified in some cases.
[b]Includes viridans streptococci; *Streptococcus bovis*; other non–group A, groupable streptococci; and *Abiotrophia* spp. (nutritionally variant, pyridoxal-requiring streptococci).
[c]Methicillin resistance is common among these *S. aureus* strains.
[d]Includes *Haemophilus* spp., *Actinobacillus actinomycetemcomitans*, *Cardiobacterium hominis*, *Eikenella* spp., and *Kingella* spp.
Note: Data are compiled from multiple studies.

IV-156. The answer is C. *(Chap. 182)* Clindamycin plus primaquine is a therapeutic, not prophylactic, regimen for mild to moderate disease due to *Pneumocystis* infection. Trimethoprim/sulfamethoxazole is usually given as a first-line agent but carries a significant side-effect profile including hyperkalemia, renal insufficiency, elevation of serum creatinine, granulocytopenia, hemolysis in persons with G6PD insufficiency, and frequent allergic reactions, particularly in those with severe T cell deficiency. Atovaquone is a common alternative that is given at the same dose for *Pneumocystis* prophylaxis as for therapy. Gastrointestinal symptoms are common with atovaquone. Aerosolized pentamidine can be given on a monthly basis with a risk of bronchospasm and pancreatitis. Patients who develop *Pneumocystis* pneumonia while receiving aerosolized pentamidine often have upper lobe–predominant disease. Dapsone is commonly used for *Pneumocystis* prophylaxis; however, the physician must be aware of the possibility of methemoglobinemia, G6PD-mediated hemolysis, rare hepatotoxicity, and rare hypersensitivity reaction when using this medicine.

IV-157. The answer is E. *(Chap. 124)* All of the listed bacterial STIs have had an impressive resurgence among homosexual men in North America and Europe since 1996. This is in part due to the phenomena of serosorting, an imperfect process among many homosexual men who seek sexual partners of the same HIV serostatus. This method allows for no protection against other STIs, and in fact may allow for concentration of these infections among high-risk networks of men. HIV prevalence has unfortunately also increased among homosexual men. Lymphogranuloma venereum, an uncommon chlamydial infection that had virtually disappeared prior to the AIDS era, has been reported in outbreaks amongst homosexual men.

IV-158. The answer is B. *(Chap. 182)* Oral hairy leukoplakia is due to severe overgrowth of Epstein-Barr virus infection in T cell–deficient patients. It is not premalignant, is often unrecognized by the patient, but is sometimes a cosmetic, symptomatic, and therapeutic nuisance. The white thickened folds on the side of the tongue can be pruritic or painful and sometimes resolve with acyclovir derivatives or topical podophyllin resin. Ultimate resolution occurs after immune reconstitution with antiretroviral therapy. Oral candidiasis or thrush is a very common, relatively easy-to-treat condition in HIV patients and takes on an appearance of white plaques on the tongue, palate, and buccal mucosa that bleed with blunt removal. Herpes simplex virus (HSV) recurrences or aphthous ulcers present as painful ulcerating lesions. The latter should be considered when oral ulcers persist, do not respond to acyclovir, and do not culture HSV. Kaposi's sarcoma is uncommon in the oropharynx and takes on a violet hue, suggesting its highly vascularized content.

IV-159.   The answer is A. *(Chap. 160)* Nontuberculous mycobacteria (NTM) were originally classified into "fast-growers" and "slow-growers" based on the length of time they took to grow in culture. While more sophisticated tests have been developed, this classification scheme is still used and is of some benefit to the clinician. Fast-growing NTM include *M. abscessus*, *M. fortuitum*, and *M. chelonae*. They will typically take 7 days or less to grow on standard media, allowing relatively fast identification and drug-resistance testing. Slow-growing NTM include *M. avium*, *M. marinum*, *M. ulcerans*, and *M. kansasii*. They often require special growth media and therefore a high pretest suspicion. The patient described above likely has a cutaneous infection from one of the "fast-growing" NTM, which could be diagnosed with tissue biopsy, Gram stain, and culture.

IV-160.   The answer is D. *(Chap. 205)* This patient comes from an area endemic for visceral leishmaniasis that includes Bangladesh, India, Nepal, Sudan, and Brazil. Although many species can cause cutaneous or mucosal disease, the *L. donovani* complex generally is associated with visceral leishmaniasis. The organism is transmitted by the bite of the sandfly in the majority of cases. Although many patients remain asymptomatic, malnourished persons are at particular risk for progression to symptomatic disease or kala azar, the life-threatening form. The presentation of this disease generally includes fever, cachexia, and splenomegaly. Hepatomegaly is rare compared with other tropical diseases associated with organomegaly, such as malaria, miliary tuberculosis, and schistosomiasis. Pancytopenia is associated with severe disease, as are hypergammaglobulinemia and hypoalbuminemia. Although active investigation is under way to determine a means of diagnosing leishmaniasis by molecular techniques, the current standard remains demonstration of the organism on a stained slide or in tissue culture of a biopsy specimen. Splenic aspiration has the highest yield, with reported sensitivity of 98%. In light of the high mortality associated with this disease, treatment should not be delayed. The mainstay of therapy is a pentavalent antimonial, but newer therapies including amphotericin and pentamidine can be indicated in certain situations. In this case it would be prudent to rule out malaria with a thick and a thin smear. Rarely, the intracellular amastigote forms of *Leishmania* spp. can be seen on a peripheral smear.

IV-161.   The answer is C. *(Chap. 182)* HIV resistance testing is recommended in selecting initial ART where the prevalence of resistance is high (such as in the United States or Europe) and in determining new therapy for patients with virologic failure while on ART. In the United States, the predominant virus in up to 12% of new cases has one major genotypic resistance mutation (patient A). In the patient failing ART, a resistance genotype should be performed while the patient is on therapy. In the absence of ART, the majority of virus reverts to wild type and the genotype appears normal (genotypes only sample the dominant viral form, though many exist); however, archived viruses in latent pools that are not accessible with current commercially available assays may in fact harbor resistance. Therefore a genotype for patient C is likely to be of little value. Following the initiation of therapy the patient should have a 1 log (tenfold) reduction in plasma HIV RNA levels within 1–2 months. Failure to achieve this response (patient B) may warrant a change in therapy. Patient D has breakthrough failure after a period of intermittent compliance. To determine if she has developed a new resistance pattern, she should have a genotype performed while on therapy to allow for adequate selection pressure from the antiviral agents to select the resistant virus leading to failure as the dominant strain.

IV-162. **The answer is C.** *(Chap. 121)* It is important to distinguish between primary (spontaneous) and secondary peritonitis. Primary peritonitis is a result of longstanding ascites, usually as a result of cirrhosis. The pathogenesis is poorly understood but may involve bacteremic spread or translocation across the gut wall of usually only a single species of pathogenic bacteria. Secondary peritonitis is due to rupture of a hollow viscous or irritation of the peritoneum due to a contiguous abscess or pyogenic infection. It typically presents with peritoneal signs and in most cases represents a surgical emergency. Secondary peritonitis in a cirrhotic patient is difficult to distinguish on clinical grounds from primary (spontaneous) peritonitis. It is often overlooked because classic peritoneal signs are almost always lacking, and it is uniformly fatal in the absence of surgery. Suspicion for this diagnosis should occur when ascites shows a protein >1g/dL, LDH greater than serum LDH, glucose <50 mg/dL, and/or a polymicrobial Gram stain. Once this diagnosis is suspected, an abdominal film is indicated to rule out free air, and prompt surgical consultation is warranted. Unlike with primary (spontaneous) bacterial peritonitis, in cases of secondary peritonitis antibiotics should include anaerobic coverage and often antifungal agents. This patient requires IV fluid as he has hypotension and tachycardia due to sepsis. Drotrecogin alfa has been shown to reduce mortality in patients with sepsis; however, patients with thrombocytopenia, cirrhosis, and ascites were excluded from inclusion in phase III trials of this agent.

IV-163. **The answer is B.** *(Chap. 197)* The primary risk factor for developing invasive *Aspergillus* infection is neutropenia and glucocorticoid use. Risk is proportional to the degree and length of neutropenia and the dose of glucocorticoid. HIV patients rarely develop invasive aspergillosis, and if they do, it is in the context of prolonged neutropenia and/or advanced disease. Patients with graft-vs-host disease and uncontrolled leukemia are at particularly elevated risk. The infection is seen in solid organ transplant patients, particularly those requiring high cumulative doses of glucocorticoids for graft rejection.

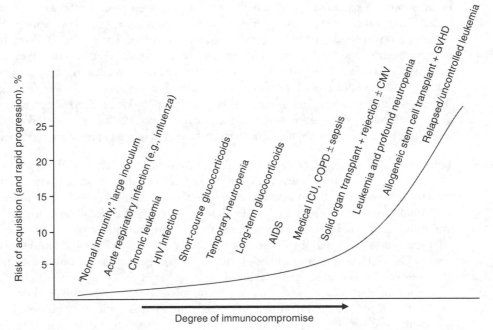

FIGURE IV-163 Invasive aspergillosis: conditions placing patients at elevated risk of acquisition and relatively rapid progression. ICU, intensive care unit; COPD, chronic obstructive pulmonary disease; CMV, cytomegalovirus; GVHD, graft-vs-host disease.

IV-164. **The answer is E.** *(Chaps. 34 and 128)* The PORT score is a system used to classify community-acquired pneumonia (CAP) from mild to severe. The score assigns points to 20 items associated with mortality, including age, nursing home residence, coexisting illness (neoplastic disease, liver disease, congestive heart failure, cerebrovascular disease, renal disease), physical examination findings (mental status, respiratory rate, blood pressure, temperature, pulse rate), and laboratory/radiographic findings (pH, blood urea nitrogen, sodium, glucose, hematocrit, Pa_{O_2}, pleural effusion). The resulting scores are used to define five classes with progressively increasing mortality. These classes correlate with mortality and have been used to derive suggested management and site of treatment (home versus hospital) criteria. Cigarette smoking is a risk factor for the development of pneumonia but is not used in the prognostic scoring system.

IV-165. **The answer is A.** *(Chap. 161)* Rifampin is considered the most potent and important antituberculosis drug. It is also active against other organisms, including some gram-positive and gram-negative organisms, as well as against *Legionella* spp, *Mycobacterium marinum*, and *M. kansasii*. It is notable for turning body fluids a red-orange color. Its use should be avoided or carefully monitored in patients with severe hepatic disease, but it does not need to be dose-adjusted in renal failure. Rifampin is a potent P450 CY3PA inducer and may lower the half-life and therefore effective levels of many important drugs, including anticonvulsants, cyclosporine, hormonal contraceptives, protease inhibitors, narcotics, tricyclic antidepressants, azole antifungals, beta blockers, and many antibiotics. Patients need to be monitored for the effects of subtherapeutic levels whether by directly measuring drug levels (anticonvulsants, cyclosporine), direct effects of the drug (warfarin), or with clinical adjustment (contraceptives, protease inhibitors). While not studied extensively, rifabutin has a similar, although likely lesser, effect on the same medications as rifampin. Amiodarone is not metabolized by CY3PA.

IV-166. **The answer is A.** *(Chap. 145)* Ecthyma gangrenosum is a disseminated collection of geographic, painful, reddish, maculopapular lesions that rapidly progress from pink to purple and finally to a black, dry necrosis. They are teeming with causative bacteria. In reviews on ecthyma, *Pseudomonas aeruginosa* is the most common isolate from blood and skin lesions. However, many organisms can cause this foreboding rash. Neutropenic patients and AIDS patients are at highest risk, but diabetics and intensive care unit (ICU) patients are also affected. Pseudomonal sepsis is severe with a high mortality. Its presentation is otherwise difficult to discern from other severe sepsis syndromes, with hypothermia, fever, hypotension, organ damage, encephalopathy, bandemia, and shock being common findings. Though antibiotic use, severe burns, and long ICU stays increase the risk for *Pseudomonas* infection, these exposures are also risk factors for other bacterial infections, many of which also carry daunting resistant profiles. Because of *P. aeruginosa*'s propensity for multidrug resistance, two agents (usually an anti-pseudomonal β-lactam plus an aminoglycoside or ciprofloxacin) are warranted until culture data return confirming sensitivity to one or both agents. At this point the choice to narrow to one antibiotic or not is still debated and is largely physician preference.

IV-167. **The answer is C.** *(Chaps. 126 and 173)* Reactivation zoster is almost a predictable event after stem cell transplant, occurring in 40% of allogeneic transplants and in 25% of autologous transplants. Patients can develop zoster immediately, but the highest risk period is several months after transplant. Usually just a very painful local infection in the immunocompetent host, transplant recipients' zoster can disseminate systemically from local disease and cause multiorgan disease with effects on the lungs, liver, and central nervous system. Therefore, acyclovir or ganciclovir prophylaxis is the standard of care at most transplant centers. Some data suggest that low doses of acyclovir for a year posttransplant is effective and may eliminate most cases of posttransplant zoster. Acyclovir is still extremely reliable for prophylaxis and treatment of varicella zoster virus, with resistance being a very rare event. Foscarnet would be the drug of choice under these very rare circumstances.

IV-168. **The answer is C.** *(Chap. 158)* Tuberculosis is most commonly transmitted from person to person by airborne droplets. Factors that affect likelihood of developing tuberculosis infection include the probability of contact with an infectious person, the intimacy and duration of contact, the degree of infectiousness of the contact, and the environment in which the contact takes place. The most infectious patients are those with cavitary pulmonary or laryngeal tuberculosis with about 10^5–10^7 tuberculous bacteria per milliliter of sputum. Individuals who have a negative AFB smear with a positive culture for tuberculosis are less infectious but may transmit the disease. However, individuals with only extrapulmonary (e.g., renal, skeletal) tuberculosis are considered noninfectious.

IV-169. **The answer is C.** *(Chap. 158)* While all the patients listed have an increased risk of developing reactivation tuberculosis, the greatest risk factor for development of active tuberculosis is HIV positivity. The risk of developing active infection is greatest in those with the lowest CD4 counts; however, having a CD4 count above a threshold value does not negate the risk of developing an active infection. The reported incidence of developing active tuberculosis in HIV-positive individuals with a positive PPD is 10% per year, compared to a lifetime risk of 10% in immunocompetent individuals. The relative risk of developing active tuberculosis in an HIV-positive individual is 100 times that of an immunocompetent individual. All of the individuals listed as choices have risk factors for developing active tuberculosis. Malnutrition and severe underweight confers a twofold greater risk of developing active tuberculosis, whereas IV drug use increases the risk 10–30 times. Silicosis also increases the risk of developing active tuberculosis 30 times. While the risk of developing active tuberculosis is greatest in the first year after exposure, the risk also increases in the elderly.

IV-170. **The answer is A.** *(Chap. 158)* The CT scan shows a large cavitary lesion in the right upper lobe of the lung. In this man from an endemic area for tuberculosis, this finding should be treated as active pulmonary tuberculosis until proven otherwise. In addition, this patient's symptoms suggest a chronic illness with low-grade fevers, weight loss, and temporal wasting that would be consistent with active pulmonary tuberculosis. If a patient is suspected of having active pulmonary tuberculosis, the initial management should include documentation of disease while protecting health care workers and the population in general. This patient should be hospitalized in a negative-pressure room on airborne isolation until three expectorated sputum samples have been demonstrated to be negative. The samples should preferably be collected in the early morning as the burden of organisms is expected to be higher on a more concentrated sputum. The sensitivity of a single sputum for the detection of tuberculosis in confirmed cases is only 40–60%. Thus, a single sputum sample is inadequate to determine infectivity and the presence of active pulmonary tuberculosis. Skin testing with a PPD of the tuberculosis mycobacterium is used to detect latent infection with tuberculosis and has no role in determining whether active disease is present.

The cavitary lung lesion shown on the CT imaging of the chest could represent malignancy or a bacterial lung abscess, but given that the patient is from a high-risk area for tuberculosis, tuberculosis would be considered the most likely diagnosis until ruled out by sputum testing.

IV-171. **The answer is A.** *(Chap. 158; CA Benson et al: MMWR 53:1, 2004)* Initial treatment of active tuberculosis associated with HIV disease does not differ from that of a non-HIV infected person. The standard treatment regimen includes four drugs: isoniazid, rifampin, pyrazinamide, and ethambutol (RIPE). These drugs are given for a total of 2 months in combination with pyridoxine (vitamin B_6) to prevent neurotoxicity from isoniazid. Following the initial 2 months, patients continue on isoniazid and rifampin to complete a total of 6 months of therapy. These recommendations are the same as those of non-HIV infected individuals. If the sputum culture remains positive for tuberculosis after 2 months, the total course of antimycobacterial therapy is increased from 6 to 9 months. If an individual is already on antiretroviral therapy (ART) at the time of diagnosis of tuberculosis, it may be continued, but often rifabutin is substituted for rifampin because of drug interactions between rifampin and protease inhibitors. In individuals not on ART at the time of diagnosis of tuberculosis, it is not recommended to start ART concurrently because of the risk of immune reconstitution inflammatory syndrome (IRIS) and an increased risk of medication side effects. IRIS occurs as the immune system improves with ART and causes an intense inflammatory reaction directed against the infecting organism(s). There have been fatal cases of IRIS in association with tuberculosis and initiation of ART. In addition, both ART and antituberculosis drugs have many side effects. It can be difficult for a clinician to decide which medication is the cause of the side effects and may lead unnecessarily to alterations in the antituberculosis regimen. For these reasons, it is recommended by the Centers for Disease Control and Prevention to await a response to treatment for tuberculosis prior to initiating ART. Three-drug regimens are associated with a higher relapse rate if used as a standard 6-month course of therapy and, if used, require a total of 9 months of therapy. Situations in which three-drug therapy may be used are pregnancy, intolerance to a specific drug, and in the setting of resistance. A five-drug regimen using RIPE plus streptomycin is recommended as the standard re-treatment regimen. Streptomycin and pyrazinamide are discontinued after 2 months if susceptibility testing is unavailable. If susceptibility testing is available, the treatment should be based upon the susceptibility pattern. In no instance is it appropriate to withhold treatment in the setting of active tuberculosis to await susceptibility testing.

IV-172.   The answer is B. *(Chap. 158)*   The aim of treatment of latent tuberculosis is to prevent development of active disease, and the tuberculin skin test (PPD) is the most common means of identifying cases of latent tuberculosis in high-risk groups. To perform a tuberculin skin test, 5 tuberculin units of PPD are placed subcutaneously in the forearm. The degree of induration is determined after 48–72 h. Erythema only does not count as a positive reaction to the PPD. The size of the reaction to the tuberculin skin test determines whether individuals should receive treatment for latent tuberculosis. In general, individuals in low-risk groups should not be tested. However, if tested, a reaction >15 mm is required to be considered as positive. School teachers are considered low-risk individuals. Thus, the reaction of 7 mm is not a positive result, and treatment is not required.

A size of ≥10 mm is considered positive in individuals who have been infected within 2 years or those with high-risk medical conditions. The individual working in an area where tuberculosis is endemic has tested newly positive by skin testing and should be treated as a newly infected individual. High-risk medical conditions for which treatment of latent tuberculosis is recommended include diabetes mellitus, injection drug use, end-stage renal disease, rapid weight loss, and hematologic disorders.

PPD reactions ≥5 mm are considered positive for latent tuberculosis in individuals with fibrotic lesions on chest radiograph, those with close contact with an infected person, and those with HIV or who are otherwise immunosuppressed.

There are two situations in which treatment for latent tuberculosis is recommended regardless of the results on skin testing. First, infants and children who have had close contact with an actively infected person should be treated. After 2 months of therapy, a skin test should be performed. Treatment can be discontinued if the skin test remains negative at that time. Also, individuals who are HIV positive and have had close contact with an infected person should be treated regardless of skin test results.

IV-173.   The answer is B. *(Chap. 199)*   Tinea versicolor is the most common superficial skin infection. It is caused by lipophilic yeasts of the genus *Malassezia*, most commonly *M. furfur*. In tropical areas, the prevalence of tinea versicolor is 40–60%, whereas in temperate areas it is about 1%. In general, most individuals seek evaluation for cosmetic reasons as the lesions in tinea versicolor are asymptomatic or only mildly pruritic. The lesions typically appear as patches of pink or coppery-brown skin, but the areas may be hypopigmented in dark-skinned individuals. Diagnosis can be made by demonstrating the organism on potassium hydroxide preparation where a typical "spaghetti and meatballs" appearance may be seen. This is due to the presence of both spore forms and hyphal forms within the skin. Under long-wave UVA light (Wood's lamp), the affected areas fluoresce to yellow-green. The organism is sensitive to a variety of antifungals. Selenium sulfide shampoo, topical azoles, terbinafine, and ciclopirox have all been used with success. A 2-week treatment regimen typically shows good results, but the infection typically recurs within 2 years of initial treatment.

IV-174.   Answer is D. *(Chap. 199)*   *Sporothrix schenkii* is a thermally dimorphic fungus found in soil, plants, and moss and occurs most commonly in gardeners, farmers, florists, and forestry workers. Sporotrichosis develops after inoculation of the organism into the skin with a contaminated puncture or scratch. The disease typically presents as a fixed cutaneous lesion or with lymphocutaneous spread. The initial lesion typically ulcerates and become verrucous in appearance. The draining lymphatic channels become affected in up to 80% of cases. This presents as painless nodules along the lymphatic channel, which ulcerate. A definitive diagnosis is made by culturing the organism. A biopsy of the lesion may show ovoid or cigar-shaped yeast forms. Treatment for sporotrichosis is systemic therapy. Options include oral itraconazole, saturated solution of potassium iodide, and terbinafine. However, terbinafine has not been approved for this indication in the United States. Topical antifungals are not effective. In cases of serious system disease such as pulmonary sporotrichosis, amphotericin B is the treatment of choice. Caspofungin is not effective against *S. schenkii*.

IV-175. **The answer is D.** *(Chap. 139)* Generally thought of as a disease of children, epiglottitis is increasingly becoming a disease of adults since the wide use of *Haemophilus influenzae* type B vaccination. Epiglottitis can cause life-threatening airway obstruction due to cellulitis of the epiglottis and supraglottic tissues, classically due to *H. influenzae* type B infection. However, other organisms are also common causes including nontypeable *H. influenzae*, *Streptococcus pneumoniae*, *H. parainfluenzae*, *Staphylococcus aureus*, and viral infection. The initial evaluation and treatment for epiglottitis in adults includes airway management and intravenous antibiotics. The patient presented here is demonstrating signs of impending airway obstruction with stridor, inability to swallow secretions, and use of accessory muscles of inspiration. A lateral neck x-ray shows the typical thumb sign indicative of a swollen epiglottis. In addition, the patient has evidence of hypoventilation with carbon dioxide retention. Thus, in addition to antibiotics, this patient should also be intubated and mechanically ventilated electively under a controlled setting as he is at high risk for mechanical airway obstruction. Antibiotic therapy should cover the typical organisms outlined above and include coverage for oral anaerobes.

In adults presenting without overt impending airway obstruction, laryngoscopy would be indicated to assess airway patency. Endotracheal intubation would be recommended for those with >50% airway obstruction. In children, endotracheal intubation is often recommended as laryngoscopy in children has provoked airway obstruction to a much greater degree than adults, and increased risk of mortality has been demonstrated in some series in children when the airway is managed expectantly.

IV-176. **The answer is E.** *(Chap. 151)* The most likely infecting organism in this patient is *Francisella tularensis*. Gentamicin is the antibiotic of choice for the treatment of tularemia. Fluoroquinolones have shown in vitro activity against *F. tularensis* and have successfully been used in a few cases of tularemia. Currently, however, it cannot be recommended as first-line therapy as data are limited in regards to its efficacy relative to gentamicin, but can be considered if an individual is unable to tolerate gentamicin. To date, there have been no clinical trials of fluoroquinolones to definitively demonstrate equivalency with gentamicin. Third-generation cephalosporins have in vitro activity against *F. tularensis*. However, use of ceftriaxone in children with tularemia resulted in almost universal failure. Likewise, tetracycline and chloramphenicol also have limited usefulness with a higher relapse rate (up to 20%) when compared to gentamicin. *F. tularensis* is a small gram-negative, pleomorphic bacillus that is found both intra- and extracellularly. It is found in mud, water, and decaying animal carcasses, and ticks and wild rabbits are the source for most human infections in the southeast United States and Rocky Mountains. In western states, tabanid flies are the most common vectors. The organisms usually enter the skin through the bite of a tick or through an abrasion. On further questioning, the patient above reported that during the camping trip he was primarily responsible for skinning the animals and preparing dinner. He did suffer a small cut on his right hand at the site where the ulceration is apparent. The most common clinical manifestations of *F. tularensis* are ulceroglandular and glandular disease, accounting for 75–85% of cases. The ulcer appears at the site of entry of the bacteria and lasts for 1–3 weeks and may develop a black eschar at the base. The draining lymph nodes become enlarged and fluctuant. They may drain spontaneously. In a small percentage of patients, the disease becomes systemically spread, as is apparent in this case, with pneumonia, fevers, and sepsis syndrome. When this occurs, the mortality rate approaches 30% if untreated. However, with appropriate antibiotic therapy the prognosis is very good. Diagnosis requires a high clinical suspicion as demonstration of the organism is difficult. It rarely seen on Gram's stain because the organisms stain weakly and are so small that they are difficult to distinguish from background material. On polychromatically stained tissue, they may be seen both intra- and extracellularly, singly or in clumps. Moreover, *F. tularensis* is a difficult organism to culture and requires cysteine-glucose–blood agar. However, most labs do not attempt to culture the organism because of the risk of infection in laboratory workers, requiring biosafety level 2 practices. Usually the diagnosis is confirmed by agglutination testing with titers >1:160 confirming diagnosis.

IV-177.   **The answer is A.** *(Chap. 154)* Donovanosis is caused by the intracellular organism *Calymmatobacterium granulomatis* and most often presents as a painless erythematous genital ulceration after a 1–4 week incubation period. However, incubation periods can be as long as 1 year. The infection is predominantly sexually transmitted, and autoinoculation can lead to formation of new lesions by contact with adjacent infected skin. Typically the lesion is painless but bleeds easily. Complications include phimosis in men and pseudo-elephantiasis of the labia in women. If the infection is untreated, it can lead to progressive destruction of the penis or other organs. Diagnosis is made by demonstration of *Donovan bodies* within large mononuclear cells on smears from the lesion. Donovan bodies refers to the appearance of multiple intracellular organisms within the cytoplasm of mononuclear cells. These organisms are bipolar and have an appearance similar to a safety pin. On histologic examination, there is an increase in the number of plasma cells with few neutrophils; additionally, epithelial hyperplasia is present and can resemble neoplasia. A variety of antibiotics can be used to treat donovanosis including macrolides, tetracyclines, trimethoprim-sulfamethoxazole, and chloramphenicol. Treatment should be continued until the lesion has healed, often requiring ≥5 weeks of treatment.

All of the choices listed in the question above are in the differential diagnosis of penile ulcerations. Lymphogranuloma venereum is endemic in the Caribbean. The ulcer of primary infection heals spontaneously, and the second phase of the infection results in markedly enlarged inguinal lymphadenopathy, which may drain spontaneously. *H. ducreyi* results in painful genital ulcerations, and the organism can be cultured from the lesion. The painless ulcerations of cutaneous leishmaniasis can appear similarly to those of donovanosis but usually occur on exposed skin. Histologic determination of intracellular parasites can distinguish leishmaniasis definitively from donovanosis. Finally, it is unlikely that the patient has syphilis in the setting of a negative rapid plasma reagin test, and the histology is inconsistent with this diagnosis.

IV-178.   **The answer is C.** *(Chap. 140)* This patient has subacute bacterial endocarditis due to infection with one of the HACEK organisms. The HACEK organisms (*Haemophilus, Actinobacillus, Cardiobacterium, Eikenella,* and *Kingella*) are gram-negative rods that reside in the oral cavity. They are responsible for about 3% of cases of infective endocarditis in most series. They are the most common cause of gram-negative endocarditis in non-drug abusers. Most patients have a history of poor dentition or recent dental procedure. Often, patients are initially diagnosed with culture-negative endocarditis, as these organisms may be slow growing and fastidious. Cultures must be specified for prolonged culture of fastidious organisms. HACEK endocarditis is typically subacute, and the risk of embolic phenomena to the bone, skin, kidneys, and vasculature is high. Vegetations are seen on ~85% of transthoracic echocardiograms. Cure rates are excellent with antibiotics alone; native valves require 4 weeks and prosthetic valves require 6 weeks of treatment. Ceftriaxone is the treatment of choice, with ampicillin/gentamicin as an alternative. Sensitivities may be delayed due to the organism's slow growth.

IV-179.   **The answer is B.** *(Chap. 140)* *Capnocytophaga canimorsus* is the most likely organism to have caused fulminant disease in this alcoholic patient following a dog bite. *Eikenella* and *Haemophilus* are common mouth flora in humans but not in dogs. *Staphylococcus* can cause sepsis but is less likely in this scenario.

IV-180. **The answer is A.** *(Chap. 117)* Influenza occurs year round in the tropics and is the most common vaccine-preventable infection in travelers. Documentation of vaccination against yellow fever is required in many countries. Measles is prevalent in much of the developing world, and all travelers should have documented vaccination. Tetanus should be up to date for international travelers, and rabies vaccination should be discussed with patients.

IV-181. **The answer is B.** *(Chap. 117)* Malaria prophylaxis recommendations vary by region. Currently the recommended malaria prophylaxis for Central America is chloroquine. In contrast, due to chloroquine resistance of falciparum malaria, prophylaxis in India and most areas in Africa is with atovaquone/proguanil, doxycycline, or mefloquine. The following table represents the chemoprophylaxis regimens for malaria arranged by country as currently recommended by the Centers for Disease Control and Prevention.

TABLE IV-181   Malaria Chemosuppressive Regimens According to Geographic Area[a]

Geographic Area	Drug of Choice	Alternatives
Central America (north of Panama), Haiti, Dominican Republic, Iraq, Egypt, Turkey, northern Argentina, and Paraguay	Chloroquine	Mefloquine Doxycycline Atovaquone/ proguanil
South America including Panama (except northern Argentina and Paraguay); Asia (including Southeast Asia); Africa; and Oceania	Mefloquine Doxycycline Atovaquone-proguanil (Malarone)	Primaquine
Thai-Myanmar and Thai-Cambodian borders	Doxycycline Atovaquone-proguanil (Malarone)	

[a]See CDC's *Health Information for International Travel 2005–2006.*
Note: See also Chap. 203.

IV-182. **The answer is A.** *(Chap. 117)* The causes of fever in travelers vary by geography. In general, all febrile travelers returning from malaria-endemic regions should be assumed to have malaria until ruled out or another diagnosis established, since falciparum malaria may be life-threatening and effective therapy is available. Dengue is particularly common in Southeast Asia. Most cases are self-limited and require supportive therapy. A small proportion, however, can develop hemorrhagic fever or a shock syndrome. The table below lists the most common causes of febrile illness in returning travelers by country.

TABLE IV-182   Etiology and Geographic Distribution (Percent) of Systemic Febrile Illness in Returned Travelers (N = 3907)

Etiology	Carib	CAm	SAm	SSA	SCA	SEA
Malaria	<1	13	13	**62**	14	13
Dengue	**23**	12	14	<1	14	**32**
Mononucleosis	7	7	8	1	2	3
Rickettsia	0	0	0	6	1	2
Salmonella	2	3	2	<1	14	3

Note: Carib, Caribbean; CAm, Central America; SAm, South America; SSA, Sub-Saharan Africa; SCA, South Central Asia; SEA, Southeast Asia. Bold type is for emphasis only.
Source: Revised from Table 2 in Freedman et al, 2006. Used with permission from the Massachusetts Medical Society.

IV-183. **The answer is D.** *(Chap. 119)* Erysipelas is a soft tissue infection caused by *Streptococcus pyogenes* that occurs most frequently on the face or extremities. The infection is marked by abrupt onset of fiery-red swelling with intense pain. The infection progresses rapidly and is marked by well-defined and indurated margins. Flaccid bullae may develop on the second or third day. Only rarely does the infection involve the deeper soft tissues.

Penicillin is the treatment of choice. However, swelling may progress despite appropriate treatment with desquamation of the affected area.

IV-184. **The answer is C.** *(Chap. 119)* This patient is presenting with septic shock secondary to necrotizing fasciitis with group A streptococcus. Necrotizing fasciitis presents with fever and pain of the affected area that progresses rapidly to severe systemic symptoms. Swelling and brawny edema may be present early in the disease, progressing rapidly to dark-red induration with bullae filled with bluish to purple fluid. Pathologically, the underlying dermis shows extensive thrombosis of vessels in the dermis. Necrotizing fasciitis is commonly caused by group A streptococcus, specifically *S. pyogenes*, or mixed aerobic-anaerobic infections. In this patient, the presence of gram-positive cocci in chains suggests *S. pyogenes* as the underlying cause. The initial treatment of patients with necrotizing fasciitis is surgical debridement of the affected area. The area of debridement is frequently very large. During surgery, all necrotic tissue should be removed and any increased compartment pressure should be relieved. In addition, appropriate antibiotics should be initiated. For group A streptococcus, the combination of clindamycin and penicillin should be used. Penicillin is bacteriocidal for streptococcus as is clindamycin. Clindamycin also neutralizes the toxins produced by group A streptococcus. Antibiotic therapy alone should not be used as necrotizing fasciitis is rapidly fatal without surgical intervention. Vancomycin is not a first-line antibiotic in necrotizing fasciitis and should be considered only for those with penicillin allergy.

IV-185. **The answer is C.** *(Chap. 198)* This patient has signs and symptoms of mucormycosis. Although mucormycosis is a relatively uncommon invasive fungal infection, patients with poorly controlled diabetes, patients receiving glucocorticoids, immunocompromised patients, or patients with iron overload syndromes receiving desferrioxamine have an enhanced susceptibility to this devastating infection. The "gold standard" diagnosis is tissue culture, but a common hallmark is the black eschar noted on the palate, which represents invasion of the fungus into tissue, with necrosis. The black eschar in this scenario should prompt the clinician to do more than prescribe treatment for sinusitis. Black eschars on the extremities can be found with anthrax infection or spider bites. Given the mortality associated with this infection and the rapidity with which it progresses, it is not prudent to wait for an ENT consultation after a course of antibiotics. The infection is usually fatal. Successful therapy requires reversal of the underlying predisposition (glucose control in this case), aggressive surgical debridement, and early initiation of antifungal therapy. Voriconazole is not thought to be effective in the treatment of mucormycosis. Posaconazole, an experimental azole antifungal, has been shown to be effective in mouse models of the disease and has been used in patients unable to tolerate amphotericin.

IV-186. **The answer is A.** *(Chap. 194)* Although spontaneous cures of pulmonary infection with *Blastomyces dermatitidis* have been well documented, almost all patients with blastomycosis should be treated since there is no way to distinguish which patients will progress or disseminate. Extrapulmonary disease should always be treated, especially if the patient is immunocompromised. Itraconazole is indicated for non-central nervous system extrapulmonary disease in mild to moderate cases. Otherwise, amphotericin B is the treatment of choice, especially if there has been treatment failure with itraconazole. The echinocandins have variable activity against *B. dermatitidis* and are not recommended for blastomycosis. The triazole antifungals have not been studied extensively in human cases of blastomycosis. Fluoroquinolones have activity against many mycobacterial species, but do not have activity against fungi, including *B. dermatitidis*.

V. DISORDERS OF THE CARDIOVASCULAR SYSTEM

QUESTIONS

DIRECTIONS: Choose the **one best** response to each question.

V-1. A 46-year-old white female presents to your office with concerns about her diagnosis of hypertension 1 month previously. She asks you about her likelihood of developing complications of hypertension, including renal failure and stroke. She denies any past medical history other than hypertension and has no symptoms that suggest secondary causes. She currently is taking hydrochlorothiazide 25 mg/d. She smokes half a pack of cigarettes daily and drinks alcohol no more than once per week. Her family history is significant for hypertension in both parents. Her mother died of a cerebrovascular accident. Her father is alive but has coronary artery disease and is on hemodialysis. Her blood pressure is 138/90. Body mass index is 23. She has no retinal exudates or other signs of hypertensive retinopathy. Her point of maximal cardiac impulse is not displaced but is sustained. Her rate and rhythm are regular and without gallops. She has good peripheral pulses. An electrocardiogram reveals an axis of −30 degrees with borderline voltage criteria for left ventricular hypertrophy. Creatinine is 1.0 mg/dL. Which of the following items in her history and physical examination is a risk factor for a poor prognosis in a patient with hypertension?

A. Family history of renal failure and cerebrovascular disease
B. Persistent elevation in blood pressure after the initiation of therapy
C. Ongoing tobacco use
D. Ongoing use of alcohol
E. Presence of left ventricular hypertrophy on ECG

V-2. A 68-year-old male presents to your office for routine follow-up care. He reports that he is feeling well and has no complaints. His past medical history is significant for hypertension and hypercholesterolemia. He continues to smoke a pack of cigarettes daily. He is taking chlorthalidone 25 mg daily, atenolol 25 mg daily, and pravastatin 40 mg nightly. Blood pressure is 133/85, and heart rate is 66. Cardiac and pulmonary examinations are unremarkable. A pulsatile abdominal mass is felt just to the left of the umbilicus and measures approximately 4 cm. You confirm the diagnosis of abdominal aortic aneurysm by CT imag-

V-2. *(Continued)*
ing. It is located infrarenally and measures 4.5 cm. All the following are true about the patient's diagnosis *except*

A. The 5-year risk of rupture of an aneurysm of this size is 1 to 2%.
B. Surgical or endovascular intervention is warranted because of the size of the aneurysm.
C. Infrarenal endovascular stent placement is an option if the aneurysm experiences continued growth in light of the location of the aneurysm infrarenally.
D. Surgical or endovascular intervention is warranted if the patient develops symptoms of recurrent abdominal or back pain.
E. Surgical or endovascular intervention is warranted if the aneurysm expands beyond 5.5 cm.

V-3. A 45-year-old woman presents to the emergency room complaining of progressive dyspnea on exertion and abrupt onset of painful ulcerations on her toes. She has noted the symptoms for the past 3 months. The dyspnea has progressed such that she is only able to walk about 1 block without stopping. Over this same time, she has noticed a cough that occasionally produces thin, pink-tinged sputum. She also has reports that her breathing is worse at night. She sleeps on three pillows but awakens with dyspnea once or twice nightly. Over the past 2 days, she has developed painful ulcerations on toes 1 and 4 on her left foot. She reports that the areas started as reddish painful discoloration that ulcerated over the ensuing days. She denies fevers, chills, or weight loss. She has no history of chest pain, heart disease, or heart murmurs. She has been in good health until the past 3 months. She takes no medications. Her last dental visit was ~8 months ago. On physical examination, she appears in no distress. Vital signs: blood pressure of 145/92 mmHg, heart rate of 95 beats/min, respiratory rate of 24 breaths/min, temperature is 37.7°C, and Sa_{O_2} is 95% on room air. The cardiovascular examination reveals a regular rate and rhythm. There is a III/VI mid-diastolic murmur with an occasional low-pitched mid-diastolic sound that occurs when the patient is in the upright position. The jugular venous

V-3. (Continued)

pressure is measured at 10 cm above the sternal angle. A few bibasilar crackles are noted. There is 1+ pitting edema bilaterally to the knees. On her left great toe, there is an area of erythema with central ulceration covered by a black eschar. A similar area is present on her left fourth toe. The peripheral pulses are full and 2+. The patient undergoes an echocardiogram, shown in the figure. What is the most appropriate plan of care for this patient?

V-3. (Continued)

A. Consult cardiac surgery for definitive therapy.
B. Initiate therapy with IV penicillin and gentamicin.
C. Obtain blood cultures and initiate therapy based upon results.
D. Obtain a positron emission tomographic scan to assess for primary malignancy.
E. Perform left heart catheterization and consider surgery based upon results.

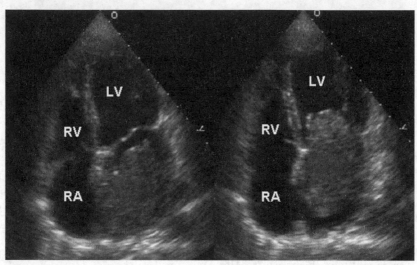

FIGURE V-3

V-4. Your 57-year-old clinic patient is seeing you in follow-up for chronic stable angina. He is a former heavy tobacco smoker who maintained an unhealthy diet and exercise routine until recently. Since initiating a healthy diet and commencing an exercise regimen, he has lost weight and improved his blood pressure control. A cardiac catheterization 1 month ago showed two nonobstructive coronary lesions in the left circumflex artery. He still has angina, which is reproducible with moderate exercise that is fully relieved by one sublingual nitroglycerin. Which of the following factors is least likely to be contributing to his angina?

A. Epicardial coronary artery resistance
B. Heart rate
C. Hemoglobin concentration
D. Diffusion capacity of the lung

V-5. In the tracing below, what type of conduction abnormality is present and where in the conduction pathway is the block usually found?

A. First-degree AV block; intranodal
B. Second-degree AV block type 1; intranodal
C. Second-degree AV block type 2; infranodal
D. Second-degree AV block type 2; intranodal

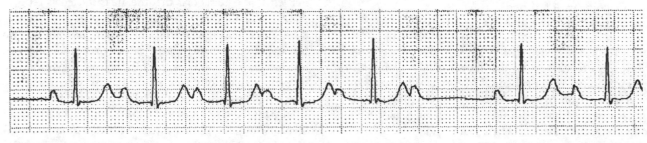

FIGURE V-5

V-6. A 62-year-old male loses consciousness in the street, and resuscitative efforts are undertaken. In the emergency room an electrocardiogram is obtained, part of which is shown below. Which of the following disorders could account for this man's presentation?

V-6. *(Continued)*

A. Hypokalemia
B. Hyperkalemia
C. Intracerebral hemorrhage
D. Digitalis toxicity
E. Hypocalcemic tetany

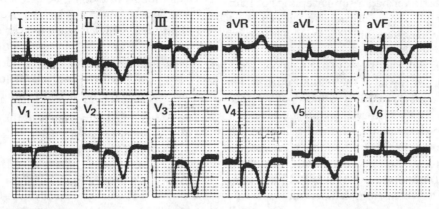

FIGURE V-6

V-7. You are seeing an 86-year-old male patient with severe aortic stenosis in follow-up. He has had severe aortic stenosis for 4 years without symptoms. Recently, he has scaled back his activities due to light-headedness with exertion. His wife reports one episode a week ago when he passed out briefly while trying to do his gardening. On examination, his blood pressure is 150/85 mmHg, heart rate is 76 beats/min. He has a grade III/VI systolic ejection murmur that extends to S_2 with radiation to the carotids. S_2 is barely audible, consistent with his prior examinations. Carotid pulses are delayed as they have been in the past. He has femoral and abdominal aortic bruits. Peripheral pulses are 2+ bilaterally. Laboratory data show a creatinine of 0.9 mg/dL, low-density lipoprotein cholesterol of 75 mg/dL, high-density lipoprotein of 50 mg/dL. What is the next appropriate step in this patient's management?

A. Aortic valve surgery
B. Cardiac rehabilitation
C. End-of-life arrangements with hospice
D. Improved blood pressure control
E. Transthoracic echocardiogram

V-8. A 35-year-old man is evaluated for dyspnea. He first noticed shortness of breath with exertion about 12 months ago. It has become progressively worse such that he is only able to walk about 20 ft without stopping. In general, he rates his health as good, although he recalls being told when he was younger that he had a heart murmur. He has not seen a physician in 15 years. On examination, he is noted to be hypoxic with an Sa_{O_2} of 85% on room air. His cardiac examination reveals a harsh machinery-like murmur that is continuous throughout systole and diastole with a palpable thrill. There is late systolic accentuation of the murmur at the upper left ster-

nal angle. He is noted to have cyanosis and clubbing of his toes but not his fingers. What is the most likely cause of the patient's murmur?

A. Anomalous pulmonary venous return
B. Coarctation of the aorta
C. Patent ductus arteriosus
D. Tetralogy of Fallot
E. Ventricular septal defect

V-9. In the cardiac care unit, you are caring for a 69-year-old man with an inferior ST-segment elevation myocardial infarction (MI). He has undergone successful urgent percutaneous coronary intervention and is recovering. Later that day, he complains of shortness of breath and orthopnea. His vital signs show blood pressure of 118/74 mmHg, heart rate of 63 beats/min, respiratory rate of 20 breaths/min, and oxygen saturation of 91% on room air. Lung examination shows crackles bilaterally. On cardiac examination, the jugular venous pressure is elevated. There is a grade III/VI musical systolic murmur heard at the base of the heart with a crescendo-decrescendo pattern. The intensity of the murmur does not change with respiration. The murmur does not radiate to the axilla. A two-dimensional echocardiogram is requested. Which of the following echocardiographic findings is most likely?

A. Eccentric mitral regurgitant jet
B. High-frequency fluttering of the anterior mitral leaflet
C. Respiratory variation in velocity across the mitral valve
D. Systolic anterior motion of the aortic (anterior) mitral valve
E. Ventricular septal defect

V-10. A 44-year-old man with a history of hypertension that is poorly controlled presents to the emergency room complaining of severe chest pain. The pain began abruptly this afternoon while at rest. He describes the pain as tearing and radiates to the back. He also is complaining of feeling lightheaded but does not have nausea or vomiting. He has never had a similar episode of pain and is usually able to exercise at the gym without chest pain. In addition to hypertension, he also has a history of hypercholesterolemia. He has been prescribed felodipine, 10 mg once daily, and rosuvastatin, 10 mg once daily, but says that he only takes them intermittently. He smokes 1 pack of cigarettes daily and has done so since the age of 20. His family history is significant for coronary artery disease in his father, who had a heart attack at the age of 60. On physical examination, the patient appears uncomfortable and diaphoretic. Vital signs: blood pressure is 190/110 mmHg, heart rate is 112 beats/min, respiratory rate is 26 breaths/min, temperature is 36.3°C, and Sa_{O_2} is 98% on room air. His carotid pulses are full and bounding. His cardiac examination reveals a hyperdynamic precordium. The rhythm is tachycardic but regular. An S_4 is present. There is a II/VI diastolic murmur heard at the lower left sternal border. An electrocardiogram (ECG) shows 1 mm of ST elevation in leads II, III, and aV_F. A contrast-enhanced chest CT shows a dissection of the ascending aorta with a small amount of pericardial fluid. What is the most appropriate management of the patient?

A. Emergent cardiac catheterization
B. Emergent cardiac surgery
C. Intravenous nitroprusside and esmolol alone

V-10. *(Continued)*

D. Intravenous nitroprusside and esmolol and cardiac surgery emergently
E. Thrombolysis with tenecteplase

V-11. A 42-year-old male from El Salvador complains of several months of dyspnea on exertion. Physical examination reveals an elevated jugular venous pressure, clear lungs, a third heart sound, a pulsatile liver, ascites, and dependent edema. Chest radiography reveals no cardiomegaly and clear lung fields. An echocardiogram demonstrates normal to mildly decreased left ventricular systolic function. The initial diagnostic workup should include all the following *except*

A. computed tomography of the chest
B. coronary angiogram
C. fat pad biopsy
D. iron studies
E. tuberculin skin test

V-12. A 29-year-old woman is in the intensive care unit with rhabdomyolysis due to compartment syndrome of the lower extremities after a car accident. Her clinical course has been complicated by acute renal failure and severe pain. She has undergone fasciotomies and is admitted to the intensive care unit. An electrocardiogram (ECG) is obtained (shown below). What is the most appropriate course of action at this point?

A. 18-lead ECG
B. Coronary catheterization
C. Hemodialysis
D. Intravenous fluids and a loop diuretic
E. Ventilation/perfusion imaging

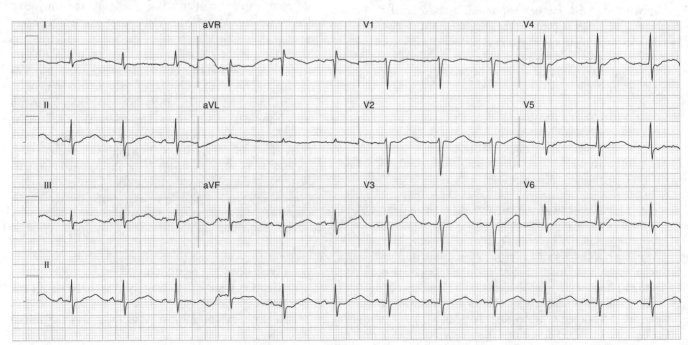

FIGURE V-12

V-13. A 54-year-old male with type 2 diabetes mellitus reports 3 months of exertional chest pain. His physical examination is notable for obesity with a body mass index (BMI) of 32 kg/m^2, blood pressure of 150/90, an S_4, no cardiac murmurs, and no peripheral edema. Fasting glucose is 130 mg/dL, and serum triglycerides are 200 mg/dL. Which of the following is most likely in this patient?

A. Elevated high-density lipoprotein (HDL) cholesterol
B. Insulin resistance
C. Larger than normal LDL particles
D. Reduced serum endothelin level
E. Reduced serum homocysteine level

V-14. A 45-year-old man is admitted to the intensive care unit with symptoms of congestive heart failure. He is addicted to heroin and cocaine and uses both drugs daily via injection. His blood cultures have yielded methicillin-sensitive *Staphylococcus aureus* in four of four bottles within 12 h. His vital signs show a blood pressure of 110/40 mmHg and a heart rate of 132 beats/min. There is a IV/VI diastolic murmur heard along the left sternal border. A schematic representation of the carotid pulsation is shown in the figure below. What is the most likely cause of the patient's murmur?

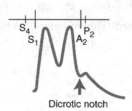

FIGURE V-14

A. Aortic regurgitation
B. Aortic stenosis
C. Mitral stenosis
D. Mitral regurgitation
E. Tricuspid regurgitation

V-15. A 30-year-old male is transported to the emergency room after a motor vehicle accident. He is complaining of moderate chest pain. He becomes hypotensive, and his blood pressure pattern reveals a pulsus paradoxus. The heart sounds appear distant. An examination of the neck veins fails to reveal a Kussmaul's sign. An electrocardiogram is unremarkable, and a chest x-ray reveals an enlarged cardiac silhouette. A right heart catheter is placed. Which of the following values is consistent with this patient's diagnosis?

	Pressure, RA mmHg	Pressure, PA mmHg	Pressure, PCW mmHg
A	16	75/30	11
B	16	34/16	16
C	16	100/30	28
D	16	45/22	20
E	16	22/12	10
Normal values	0–5	12–28/3–13	3–11

Note: RA, atrial pressure; PA, pulmonary arterial; PCW, pulmonary capillary wedge

V-16. You are treating a patient with stable angina pectoris. She is a postmenopausal woman with refractory angina despite therapy with metoprolol and isosorbide dinitrate, as well as her other anti-ischemic medications. Past medical history is significant for coronary artery bypass grafting (CABG), chronic obstructive pulmonary disease, first-degree atrioventricular block, left bundle branch block, and dyslipidemia. A recent cardiac catheterization showed coronary artery disease not amenable to percutaneous intervention, and the patient is not interested in redo of the CABG. Renal function is normal. Her left ventricular ejection fraction is 15%, and she has New York Heart Association class II heart failure symptoms. Blood pressure and pulse allow for the addition of a calcium channel blocker to her regimen. Which calcium channel–blocking medication is appropriate for this patient?

A. Amlodipine
B. Diltiazem
C. Immediate-release nifedipine
D. Verapamil

V-17. A 30-year-old female is seen in the clinic before undergoing an esophageal dilation for a stricture. Her past medical history is notable for mitral valve prolapse with mild regurgitation. She takes no medications and is allergic to penicillin. Her physician should recommend which of the following?

A. Clarithromycin 500 mg PO 1 h before the procedure
B. Clindamycin 450 mg PO 1 h before the procedure
C. Vancomycin 1 g intravenously before the procedure
D. The procedure is low-risk, and therefore no prophylaxis is indicated.
E. Her valvular lesion is low-risk, and therefore no prophylaxis is indicated.

V-18. A 78-year-old male presents to the clinic complaining that every time he shaves with a straight razor, he passes out. His symptoms have been occurring for the last 2 months. Occasionally, when he puts on a tight collar, he passes out as well. The loss of consciousness is brief, he has no associated prodrome, and he feels well afterward. His past medical history is notable for hypertension and hypercholesterolemia. His only medication is hydrochlorothiazide. On physical exam his vital signs are normal, and his cardiac exam is normal with the exception of a fourth heart sound. Which of the following is the most appropriate next diagnostic test?

A. Stress echocardiography
B. Adenosine thallium scan
C. Computed tomogram of the neck
D. Carotid sinus massage
E. Tilt table test

V-19. You are called to the bedside to see a patient with Prinzmetal's angina who is having chest pain. The patient had cardiac catheterization 2 days prior showing a 60%

V-19. *(Continued)*

stenosis of the right coronary artery with associated spasm during coronary angiogram. At the patient's bedside, which finding is consistent with the diagnosis of Prinzmetal's angina?

- A. Chest pain reproduced by palpation of the chest wall
- B. Nonspecific ST-T-wave abnormalities
- C. Relief of pain with drinking cold water
- D. ST-segment elevation in II, III, and aV_F
- E. ST-segment depression in I, aV_L, and V_6

V-20. A 32-year-old female is seen in the emergency department for acute shortness of breath. A helical CT shows no evidence of pulmonary embolus, but incidental note is made of dilatation of the ascending aorta to 4.3 cm. All the following are associated with this finding *except*

- A. syphilis
- B. Takayasu's arteritis
- C. giant cell arteritis
- D. rheumatoid arthritis
- E. systemic lupus erythematosus

V-21. A 38-year-old Bolivian man is admitted to the cardiac intensive care unit with decompensated heart failure. He has no known past medical history and takes no medications. He emigrated from Mexico 10 years ago and currently works in a retail store. On physical examination, he has signs of congestion and poor perfusion. An electrocardiogram shows first-degree atrioventricular block and right bundle branch block. An echocardiogram shows dilated and thinned ventricles. He has an apical aneurysm in the left ventricle with thrombus formation. You treat his heart failure symptomatically and begin anticoagulation. A cardiac catheterization shows normal coronaries without atherosclerosis. Which statement is true regarding this patient's prognosis?

- A. Aggressive lipid lowering (low-density lipoprotein <70 mg/dL) has been shown to be beneficial in this condition.
- B. Calcium channel blockers will prevent progression of his disease.
- C. Cardiac transplantation offers the only cure for this condition.
- D. His cardiac function will improve over time.
- E. Nifurtimox offers a reasonable chance for cure.

V-22. You are evaluating a 43-year-old woman who complains of dyspnea on exertion. She was well until 2 months ago when she noticed decreasing exercise tolerance and fatigue. She denies chest pain but does have New York Heart Association class II symptoms. She has no orthopnea or paroxysmal nocturnal dyspnea. She has noticed bilateral ankle swelling that improves with recumbency. She has one child and has no other past medical history. On cardiac examination, the jugular venous pressure is slightly elevated. There is a prominent *a* wave. There is a right-ventricular

V-22. *(Continued)*

tap felt along the left sternal border. S_1 is prominent and P_2 is accentuated. There is a sharp opening sound heard best during expiration just medial to the cardiac apex, which occurs shortly after S_2. A diastolic rumble is heard at the apex with the patient in the left lateral decubitus position. Hepatomegaly and ankle edema are present. The pulse is regular and blood pressure is 108/60 mmHg. This patient is at high risk for developing which of the following?

- A. Atrial fibrillation
- B. Left-ventricular dysfunction
- C. Multifocal atrial tachycardia
- D. Right bundle branch block
- E. Right-ventricular outflow tract tachycardia

V-23. Which of the following conditions is not associated with sinus bradycardia?

- A. Brucellosis
- B. Leptospirosis
- C. Hypothyroidism
- D. Advanced liver disease
- E. Typhoid fever

V-24. All of the following are common consequences of congenital heart disease in the adult *except*

- A. Eisenmenger syndrome
- B. erythrocytosis
- C. infective endocarditis
- D. pulmonary hypertension
- E. stroke

V-25. Acute hyperkalemia is associated with which of the following electrocardiographic changes?

- A. QRS widening
- B. Prolongation of the ST segment
- C. A decrease in the PR interval
- D. Prominent U waves
- E. T-wave flattening

V-26. All of the following clinical findings are consistent with severe mitral stenosis *except*

- A. atrial fibrillation
- B. opening snap late after S_2
- C. pulmonary vascular congestion
- D. pulsatile liver
- E. right-ventricular heave

V-27. All the following patients should be evaluated for secondary causes of hypertension *except*

- A. a 37-year-old male with strong family history of hypertension and renal failure who presents to your office with a blood pressure of 152/98
- B. a 26-year-old female with hematuria and a family history of early renal failure who has a blood pressure of 160/88

V-27. *(Continued)*

C. a 63-year-old male with no past history with a blood pressure of 162/90

D. a 58-year-old male with a history of hypertension since age 45 whose blood pressure has become increasingly difficult to control on four antihypertensive agents

E. a 31-year-old female with complaints of severe headaches, weight gain, and new-onset diabetes mellitus with a blood pressure of 142/89

V-28. You are seeing a 71-year-old patient with tachycardia-bradycardia syndrome in follow-up. She had a single-lead ventricular pacemaker implanted 2 years ago and has no new complaints. Past medical history also includes an old stroke with mild residual left hand weakness and diabetes. Her last transthoracic echocardiogram showed a left ventricular ejection fraction of 35–40% but no valvular abnormalities. The left atrium is mildly enlarged. Her medical regimen includes aspirin, metformin, metoprolol, lisinopril, lasix, and dipyridamole. What intervention, if any, should be considered for this patient at this time?

A. Anticoagulation

B. Cardiac catheterization

C. Discontinuation of dipyridamole

D. None, as she has no new complaints

V-29. A 64-year-old woman with known stage IV breast cancer presents to the emergency room with severe dyspnea and hypotension. Her blood pressure is 92/50 mmHg, and heart rate is 112 beats/min. She has distended neck veins that do not collapse with inspiration. Heart sounds are muffled. The systolic blood pressure drops to 70 with inspiration. An echocardiogram shows a large pericardial effusion with right ventricular diastolic collapse consistent with pericardial tamponade. Which of the following values most accurately demonstrate the expected values on right heart catheterization?

	Right-atrial pressure, mmHg	Right-ventricular pressure, mmHg	Pulmonary artery pressure, mmHg	Pulmonary capillary wedge pressure, mmHg
A.	5	20/5	25/10	12
B.	8	20/10	30/12	20
C.	17	40/17	45/17	17
D.	18	40/20	45/25	10

V-30. The ECG most likely was obtained from which of the following patients?

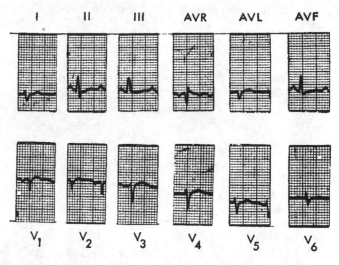

FIGURE V-30

A. A 33-year-old female with acute-onset severe headache, disorientation, and intraventricular blood on head CT scan

B. A 42-year-old male with sudden-onset chest pain while playing tennis

C. A 54-year-old female with a long history of smoking and 2 days of increasing shortness of breath and wheezing

D. A 64-year-old female with end-stage renal insufficiency who missed dialysis for the last 4 days

E. A 78-year-old male with syncope, delayed carotid upstrokes, and a harsh systolic murmur in the right second intercostal space

V-31. You are evaluating a new patient in your clinic who brings in this electrocardiogram (ECG) to the visit. The ECG was performed on the patient 2 weeks ago. What complaint do you expect to elicit from the patient?

V-31. *(Continued)*
A.   Angina
B.   Hemoptysis
C.   Paroxysmal nocturnal dyspnea
D.   Tachypalpitations

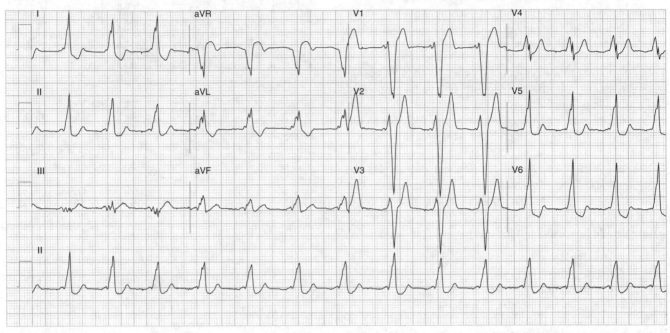

FIGURE V-31

V-32. A patient is found to have a holosystolic murmur on physical examination. With deep inspiration, the intensity of the murmur increases. This is consistent with which of the following?

A.   Atrial-septal defect
B.   Austin Flint murmur
C.   Carvallo's sign
D.   Chronic mitral regurgitation
E.   Gallavardin effect

V-33. A 37-year-old male with Wolff-Parkinson-White syndrome develops a broad-complex irregular tachycardia at a rate of 200 beats per minute. He appears comfortable and has little hemodynamic impairment. Useful treatment at this point might include

A.   Digoxin
B.   Amiodarone
C.   Propranolol
D.   Verapamil
E.   Direct-current cardioversion

V-34. A 72-year-old man seeks evaluation for leg pain with ambulation. He describes the pain as an aching to crampy pain in the muscles of his thighs. The pain subsides within minutes of resting. On rare occasions, he has noted numbness of his right foot at rest and pain in his right leg has woken him at night. He has a history of hypertension and cerebrovascular disease. He previously had a transient ischemic attack and underwent right carotid endarterectomy 4 years previously. He currently takes aspirin, irbesartan, hydrochlorothiazide, and atenolol on a daily basis. On examination, he is noted to have diminished dorsalis pedis and posterior tibial pulses bilaterally. The right dorsal pedis pulse is faint. There is loss of hair in the distal extremities. Capillary refill is approximately 5 s in the right foot and 3 s in the left foot. Which of the following findings would be suggestive of critical ischemia of the right foot?

A.   Ankle-brachial index <0.3
B.   Ankle-brachial index <0.9
C.   Ankle-brachial index >1.2
D.   Lack of palpable dorsalis pedis pulse
E.   Presence of pitting edema of the extremities

V-35. A 24-year-old male seeks medical attention for the recent onset of headaches. The headaches are described as "pounding" and occur during the day and night. He has had minimal relief with acetaminophen. Physical examination is notable for a blood pressure of 185/115 mmHg in the right arm, a heart rate of 70/min, arterioventricular (AV) nicking on funduscopic examination, normal jugular veins and carotid arteries, a pressure-loaded PMI with an apical S_4, no abdominal bruits, and reduced pulses in both lower extremities. Review of symptoms is positive only for leg fatigue with exertion. Additional measurement of blood pressure reveals the following:

Right arm	185/115
Left arm	188/113
Right thigh	100/60
Left thigh	102/58

Which of the following diagnostic studies is most likely to demonstrate the cause of the headaches?

A.   MRI of the head
B.   MRI of the kidney
C.   MRI of the thorax
D.   24-h urinary 5-HIAA
E.   24-h urinary free cortisol

V-36. The patient described in Question V-35 is most likely to have which of the following associated cardiac abnormalities?

A.   Bicuspid aortic valve
B.   Mitral stenosis
C.   Preexcitation syndrome
D.   Right bundle branch block
E.   Tricuspid atresia

V-37. A 30-year-old female with a history of irritable bowel syndrome presents with complaints of palpitations. On further questioning, the symptoms occur randomly throughout the day, perhaps more frequently after caffeine. The primary sensation is of her heart "flip-flopping" in her chest. The patient has never had syncope. Her vital signs and exam are normal. An electrocardiogram is ob-

V-37. *(Continued)*
tained, and it shows normal sinus rhythm with no other abnormality. A Holter monitor is obtained and shows premature ventricular contractions occurring approximately six times per minute. The next most appropriate step in her management is

A.   referral to a cardiologist for electrophysiologic study
B.   beta blocker administration
C.   amiodarone administration
D.   reassurance that this is not pathologic
E.   verapamil administration

V-38. All the following ECG findings are suggestive of left ventricular hypertrophy *except*

A.   (S in V_1 + R in V_5 or V_6) >35 mm
B.   R in aVL >11 mm
C.   R in aVF >20 mm
D.   (R in I + S in III) >25 mm
E.   R in aVR >8 mm

V-39. A 27-year-old woman is hospitalized in the intensive care unit (ICU) for Lyme disease. Complete heart block is noted and a single-lead pacemaker is implanted. She is discharged on a long course of antibiotics with a permanent pacemaker. She returns to see you in clinic complaining of inability to concentrate, fatigue, palpitations, and cough. On examination, her blood pressure is 121/72 mmHg; heart rate 60 beats per minute, respiratory rate 18 breaths per minute. She has an elevated jugular venous pressure with cannon *a* waves. She has rales on lung auscultation and an S_3 on cardiac auscultation but no peripheral edema. Electrocardiogram (ECG) shows a ventricular paced rate at 60/min with repolarization abnormalities. These findings are most consistent with

A.   acute myocardial infarction
B.   ICU psychosis syndrome
C.   Kearne-Sayer syndrome
D.   pacemaker syndrome
E.   pacemaker twiddler's syndrome

V-40. You are evaluating a new patient in clinic. He is a 72-year-old man who had a myocardial infarction (MI) and a stroke 3 years ago. He comes to your office to establish a primary care physician and because he ran out of medications (metoprolol, aspirin, lovastatin, lisinopril) 1 week ago. He brings in with him an electrocardiogram (ECG) performed 1 year ago (below). You obtain another tracing and it is not significantly changed. Other than occasional weakness in his right upper extremity, he has no com-

V-40. *(Continued)*
plaint. He has not had any medications for 2 weeks. Which is the next most appropriate step?

A. Obtain chest radiograph in clinic today
B. Obtain a transthoracic echocardiogram
C. Refill medications and ask him to return to clinic in 6 months
D. Transfer him to the hospital for thrombolytic therapy
E. Transfer him to the hospital for cardiac catheterization

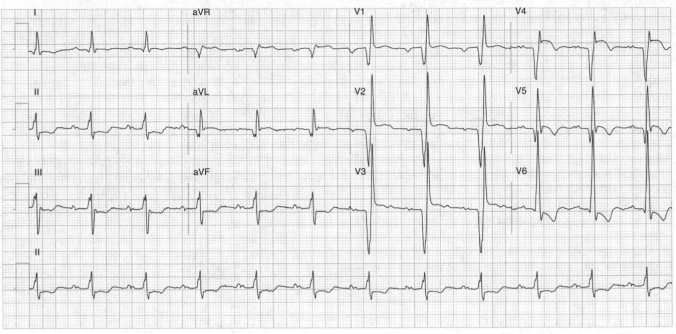

FIGURE V-40

V-41. All the following disorders may be associated with thoracic aortic aneurysm *except*

A. osteogenesis imperfecta
B. Takayasu's arteritis
C. Ehlers-Danlos syndrome
D. ankylosing spondylitis
E. Klinefelter's syndrome

V-42. All the following may cause elevation of serum troponin *except*

A. congestive heart failure
B. myocarditis
C. myocardial infarction
D. pneumonia
E. pulmonary embolism

V-43. What is the correct interpretation of this electrocardiogram (ECG) tracing?

A. Atrial fibrillation
B. Complete heart block with junctional escape rhythm

V-43. *(Continued)*
C. Idioventricular sinus arrhythmia
D. Mobitz Type 2 AV Block
E. Respiratory sinus arrhythmia

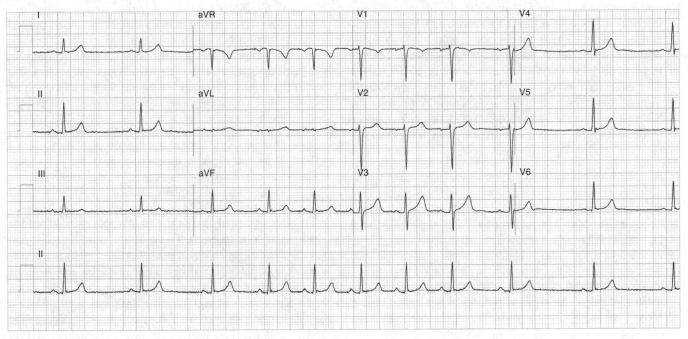

FIGURE V-43

V-44. A 44-year-old man with history of HIV infection is brought to the Emergency Department by friends because of an altered mental status. They note that he has been coughing with worsening shortness of breath for the past 2–3 weeks. His antiretroviral therapy includes a protease inhibitor. In triage, his blood pressure is 110/74 mmHg; heart rate 31 beats per minute, respiratory rate 32, temperature 38.7°C, and oxygen saturation 74% on room air. He appears well perfused. Chest radiograph shows bilateral fluffy infiltrates. An electrocardiogram shows sinus bradycardia without ST changes. A chest CT scan shows no pulmonary embolus. After initiating oxygen and establishing an airway, you direct your attention to his bradycardia. Which is the most appropriate step at this time?

A. Correct the oxygen deficit, check an arterial blood gas, and monitor closely
B. Glucagon to reverse the effects of protease inhibitors
C. Temporary transvenous pacemaker
D. Urgent cardiac catheterization for percutaneous coronary intervention

V-45. A 55-year-old woman is undergoing evaluation of dyspnea on exertion. She has a history of hypertension since age 32 and is also obese with a body mass index (BMI) of 44 kg/m². Her pulmonary function tests show mild restrictive lung disease. An echocardiogram shows a thickened left-ventricular wall, left-ventricular ejection

fraction of 70%, and findings suggestive of pulmonary hypertension with an estimated right-ventricular systolic pressure of 55 mmHg, but the echocardiogram is technically difficult and of poor quality. She undergoes a right heart catheterization that shows the following results:

Mean arterial pressure	110 mmHg
Left-ventricular end-diastolic pressure	25 mmHg
Pulmonary artery (PA) systolic pressure	48 mmHg
PA diastolic pressure	20 mmHg
PA mean pressure	34 mmHg
Cardiac output	5.9 L/min

What is the most likely cause of the patient's dyspnea?

A. Chronic thromboembolic disease
B. Diastolic heart failure
C. Obstructive sleep apnea
D. Pulmonary arterial hypertension
E. Systolic heart failure

V-46. Which of the following congenital cardiac disorders will lead to a left-to-right shunt, generally with cyanosis?

A. Anomalous origin of the left coronary artery from the pulmonary trunk
B. Patent ductus arteriosus without pulmonary hypertension
C. Total anomalous pulmonary venous connection
D. Ventricular septal defect
E. Sinus venosus atrial septal defect

V-47. You are evaluating a new patient in clinic. On cardiac auscultation, there is a high-pitched, blowing, decrescendo diastolic murmur heard best in the third intercostal space along the left sternal border. A second murmur is heard at the apex, which is a low-pitched rumbling mid-diastolic murmur. Sustained hand-grip increases the intensity of the murmurs. The murmurs are heard best at end-expiration. There are also an S_3 and a systolic ejection murmur. The left ventricular impulse is displaced to the left and inferiorly. Radial pulses are brisk with a prominent systolic component. Blood pressure is 170/70 mmHg, heart rate is 98 beats/min, respiratory rate 18 breaths/min. An electrocardiogram (ECG) is obtained in clinic. Which of the following findings do you expect on the ECG tracing for this patient?

A. Diffuse ST-segment elevation and PR-segment depression
B. Inferior Q-waves
C. Left-ventricular hypertrophy
D. Low voltage
E. Right-atrial enlargement

V-48. A 65-year-old male is seen in the emergency department with palpitations. His symptoms began 30 min before arrival. He has not had any dizziness, light-headedness, or chest pain. His past medical history is notable for a myocardial infarct 2 years ago, chronic atrial fibrillation, and a three-vessel coronary artery bypass graft surgery 1 year ago. Medications include aspirin, metoprolol, warfarin, and lisinopril. An electrocardiogram shows wide complex tachycardia at a rate of 170. Which of the following will prove definitively that his rhythm is ventricular tachycardia?

A. Hypotension
B. Cannon *a* waves
C. An odd electrocardiogram with similar QRS morphology
D. Irregular rhythm
E. Syncope

V-49. You have referred your patient for an exercise-electrocardiography stress test. The report indicates that he walked for 7 min of the Bruce protocol and had no chest pain during or after the test. During the exercise, he had multiple premature ventricular complexes and reached 90% of maximum predicted heart rate. He had 2-mm upsloping ST-segment response during exercise. At the end of the protocol and during recovery, he had 1-mm ST-segment depressions, which lasted for 6 min. Blood pressure rose from 127/78 to 167/102 mmHg at maximal exertion. Which feature of this report is most suggestive of severe ischemic heart disease and a high risk of future events?

A. Diastolic pressure >100 mmHg
B. Not achieving 95% of maximum predicted heart rate
C. Persistent ST-segment depressions into recovery
D. Upsloping ST-segments during exercise
E. Ventricular ectopy during exercise

V-50. A 45-year-old female who immigrated to the United States 10 years ago from Peru presents with dyspnea on exertion for the last 4 months. She denies chest pain but has noted significant accumulation of fluid in her abdomen and lower extremity edema. She has a history of tuberculosis, which was treated with a four-drug regimen when she was a child. Electrocardiography shows normal sinus rhythm but no other abnormality. A CT of the chest is obtained and shows pericardial calcifications. In addition to an elevated jugular venous pressure and a third heart sound, which of the following is likely to be found on physical exam?

A. Rapid *y* descent in jugular venous pulsations
B. Double systolic apical impulse on palpation
C. Loud, fixed split P_2 on auscultation
D. Cannon *a* wave in jugular venous pulsations
E. An opening snap on auscultation

V-51. During a yearly physical, a 55-year-old man is found to have a systolic murmur. The murmur is mid-systolic and begins shortly after S_1 and peaks in mid-systole. It is a low-pitched, rough murmur heard best at the base of the heart in the right second intercostal space. There is radiation to the carotids bilaterally. The rest of his physical examination is unremarkable, and you make a presumptive diagnosis of aortic stenosis. Laboratory data show a hemoglobin A1C of 7.2%, high-density lipoprotein cholesterol 45 mg/dL, low-density lipoprotein cholesterol 144 mg/dL, and creatinine 1.2 mg/dL. Blood pressure is 159/85 mmHg, heart rate is 75 beats/min. Body mass index is 33 kg/m². What is the most likely etiology of this patient's aortic stenosis?

A. Age-related degeneration
B. Dyslipidemia
C. Glucose intolerance
D. Hypertension
E. Obesity

V-52. All the following are associated with a high risk of stroke in patients with atrial fibrillation *except*

A. diabetes mellitus
B. hypercholesterolemia
C. congestive heart failure
D. hypertension
E. age over 65

V-53. You are asked to evaluate a 66-year-old male for preoperative cardiovascular risk before the surgical removal of a 2-cm sigmoid colon cancer. The patient has an 80-pack-year history of cigarette use but quit 6 months before this presentation. His past medical history is also significant for hypertension and hypercholesterolemia. He has no past cardiac history and has never received cardiac imaging or stress testing. He currently is taking lisinopril 20 mg/d, hydrochlorothiazide 25 mg/d, and pravastatin 20 mg/d. He has not tolerated atenolol in the past because of fatigue and decreased libido. Functionally, the patient is quite healthy and

V-53. *(Continued)*

continues to play golf weekly while carrying his own golf bag. He lives on the fourth floor of an apartment complex and prefers climbing the stairs to using the elevator. He has no limiting dyspnea or chest pain. On physical examination the patient appears his stated age and has a blood pressure of 136/88. Heart rate is 90. Cardiovascular and pulmonary examinations are normal. The patient has good peripheral pulses and no carotid bruits. His electrocardiogram reveals no evidence of prior ischemia or left ventricular hypertrophy, but he does have a right bundle branch block. What do you advise the patient and his surgeon about his operative risk?

A. He should undergo cardiac stress testing with imaging before surgery to rule out silent ischemia in the setting of a right bundle branch block.
B. His hypertension, hypercholesterolemia, and tobacco use place him in a high-risk surgical category, and he should undergo immediate cardiac catheterization before abdominal surgery.
C. Functional status is such that the patient can perform to greater than four metabolic equivalents, and the patient has only one risk factor for predicting cardiovascular events. Thus, he can proceed to surgery without further investigation.
D. The patient should not receive preoperative metoprolol because he had a bad reaction to it in the past.
E. Because of his smoking history, the patient's pulmonary risk outweighs his cardiovascular risk.

V-54. A 54-year-old man with hypercholesterolemia and poorly controlled hypertension is admitted to the coronary care unit after coming to the emergency room with sudden chest pain. A coronary catheterization is performed, and complete occlusion of the posterior descending artery is identified. Percutaneous intervention fails and the patient is medically managed. Two days later he appears to be acutely ill. Physical examination reveals a new murmur. Which of the following would account for an early decrescendo systolic murmur in this case?

A. Acute mitral regurgitation
B. Hypertrophic cardiomyopathy
C. Chronic mitral regurgitation
D. Severe aortic stenosis
E. Ventricular septal rupture

V-55. A 73-year-old female develops substernal chest pain, severe nausea, and vomiting while mowing the lawn. In the emergency department she has cool extremities, right arm and left arm blood pressure of 85/70 mmHg, heart rate of 65/min, clear lungs, and no murmurs. She has no urine output. A Swan-Ganz catheter is placed and reveals cardiac index of 1.1 L/min per mm^2, PA pressure of 20/14 mmHg, PCW pressure of 6 mmHg, and RA pressure of 24 mmHg. The patient most likely has

A. gram-negative sepsis
B. occlusion of the left main coronary artery

V-55. *(Continued)*

C. occlusion of the right coronary artery
D. perforated duodenal ulcer
E. ruptured aortic aneurysm

V-56. Which of the following patients with echocardiographic evidence of significant mitral regurgitation has the best indication for surgery with the most favorable likelihood of a positive outcome?

A. A 52-year-old man with an ejection fraction of 25%, NYHA class III symptoms, and a left-ventricular end-systolic dimension of 60 mm
B. A 54-year-old man with an ejection fraction of 30%, NYHA class II symptoms, and pulmonary hypertension
C. A 63-year-old man in sinus rhythm without symptoms, an ejection fraction of 65%, and a normal right heart catheterization
D. A 66-year-old man without symptoms, an ejection fraction of 50%, and left-ventricular end-systolic dimension of 45 mm
E. A 72-year-old asymptomatic woman with newly discovered atrial fibrillation, ejection fraction of 60%, and end-systolic dimension of 35 mm

V-57. Which of the following patients meets criteria for the diagnosis of the metabolic syndrome?

A. A man with waist circumference of 110 cm, well-controlled diabetes mellitus with fasting plasma glucose of 98 mg/dL, and blood pressure of 140/75 mmHg
B. A woman with triglycerides of 180 mg/dL, waist circumference of 75 cm, and polycystic ovary syndrome
C. A man with nonalcoholic liver disease, obstructive sleep apnea, and blood pressure of 135/90 mmHg
D. A woman with high-density lipoprotein (HDL) of 54 mg/dL, blood pressure of 125/80 mmHg, and fasting plasma glucose of 85 mg/dL

V-58. In the maternity ward, 2 days after assisted vaginal delivery of a healthy boy, a 31-year-old African-American woman has developed shortness of breath and wheezing. On examination, blood pressure is 113/78 mmHg, heart rate is 102, and regular and jugular venous pressures are elevated. Chest auscultation shows rales 2/3 bilaterally without evidence of consolidation. Cardiac examination reveals an S$_3$. An echocardiogram shows a dilated left ventricle with an ejection fraction of 30%. A diagnosis of peripartum cardiomyopathy is made and she improves with treatment. Which of the following factors is predictive of her risk for developing peripartum cardiomyopathy or mortality with subsequent pregnancies?

A. Age >30 years
B. African ancestry
C. Interpartum left ventricular function
D. Male child
E. Nadir ejection fraction

V-59. A 55-year-old man complains of 6 months of shortness of breath. He has new dyspnea on exertion and three-pillow orthopnea. Lung auscultation reveals rales 2/3 bilaterally. He has 2+ pitting lower extremity edema. Jugular venous pressure is estimated to be 14 cmH$_2$0 measured at a 45° angle. Chest radiograph reveals pulmonary infiltrates and an enlarged cardiac silhouette. Electrocardiography shows low-voltage in the precordial and limb leads. An echocardiogram shows a dilated left ventricle, ejection fraction of 20%, mild mitral regurgitation, and a small pericardial effusion. Which finding on cardiac examination would be consistent with this patient's diagnosis?

A.   Absent S$_2$
B.   Narrow pulse pressure
C.   Paradoxical splitting of S$_2$ with inspiration
D.   Pulsus bisferiens

V-60. A 49-year-old male is found to have persistently elevated total cholesterol and low-density lipoprotein (LDL) despite lifestyle modification. You prescribe an HMG-CoA reductase inhibitor to reduce the risk of coronary events. This medication will exert all the following beneficial effects *except*

A.   direct action on atheroma progression
B.   improvement in endothelial-dependent vasomotion
C.   long-term reduction of serum LDL
D.   regression of existing coronary stenosis
E.   stabilization of existing atherosclerotic lesions

V-61. Dipyridamole is often used during nuclear cardiac stress tests. Based on the pathophysiology of myocardial ischemia and the mechanism of action of dipyridamole, in which circumstance might the stress test underestimate the degree of ischemic tissue?

A.   Three-vessel high-grade obstruction
B.   Bradycardia
C.   Left bundle branch block
D.   Osteoarthritis
E.   Right coronary artery 99% occlusion

V-62. A 62-year-old female with a history of chronic left bundle branch block is admitted to the coronary care unit with 4 hours of substernal chest pain and shortness of breath. She has elevation of serum troponin-T. She receives urgent catheterization with angioplasty and stent placement of a left anterior descending (LAD) artery lesion. Three days after admission she develops recurrent chest pain. Which of the following studies is most useful for detecting new myocardial damage since the initial infarction?

A.   Echocardiogram
B.   Electrocardiogram
C.   Serum myoglobin
D.   Serum troponin-I
E.   Serum troponin-T

V-63. A 38-year-old woman presents with complaints of fevers and chest pain. She is noted to have a widened mediastinum on chest radiograph, and a diastolic murmur is present at the lower left sternal border. She is hypertensive, with a blood pressure of 180/72 mmHg. All blood cultures are negative on three occasions from separate anatomic sites drawn 6 h apart. Further evaluation of the murmur demonstrates a dilation of the aortic root to 4 cm with subsequent aortic regurgitation. She is diagnosed with aortitis. Which of the following is the *least* likely cause of aortitis in this patient?

A.   Ankylosing spondylitis
B.   Giant cell arteritis
C.   Rheumatoid arthritis
D.   Syphilis
E.   Takayasu's arteritis

V-64. Echocardiogram of a patient with this electrocardiogram (ECG) tracing is likely to show which of the following?

A.   Catheter in the right ventricle
B.   Focal hypokinesis
C.   Global hypokinesis
D.   Small pericardial effusion
E.   Thickened left ventricle

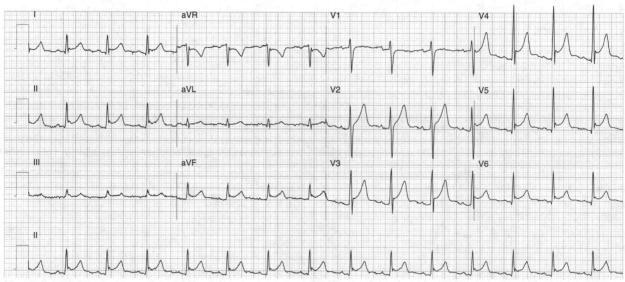

FIGURE V-64

V-65. A 54-year-old male is brought to the emergency department with 1 hour of substernal crushing chest pain, nausea, and vomiting. He developed the pain while playing squash. The pain was improved with the administration of sublingual nitroglycerine in the field. His ECG is shown below. Emergent cardiac catheterization is most likely to show acute thrombus in which of the following vessels?

V-65. *(Continued)*
A. Left anterior descending coronary artery
B. Left circumflex coronary artery
C. Left main coronary artery
D. Obtuse marginal coronary artery
E. Right main coronary artery

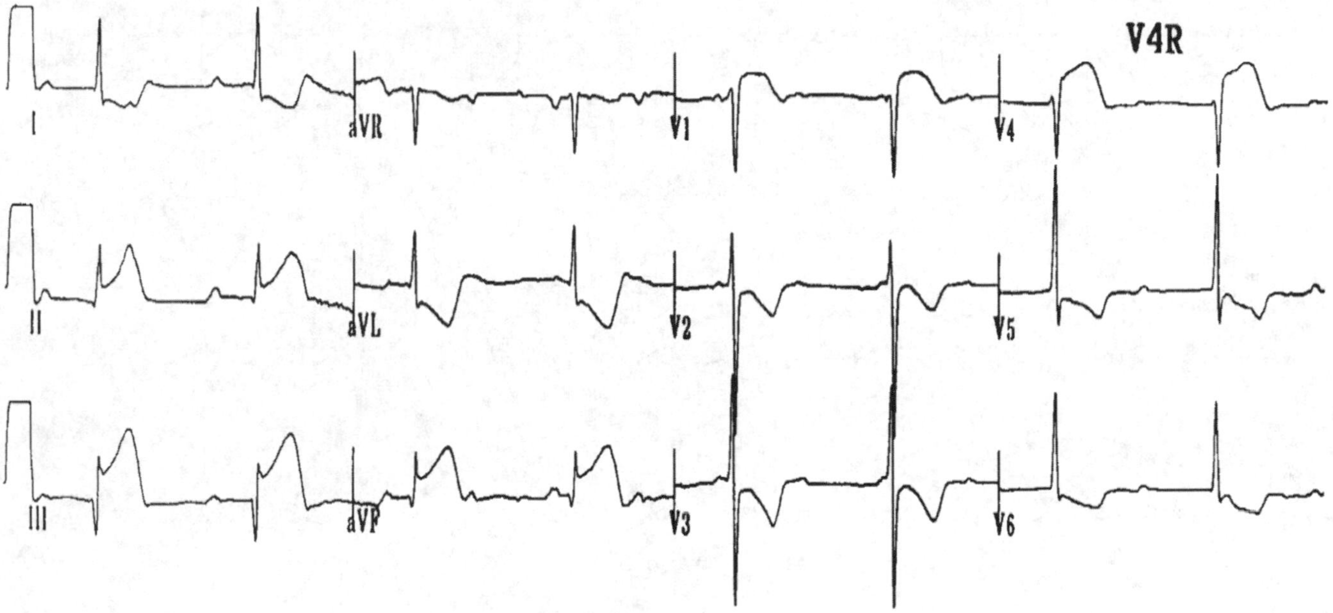

FIGURE V-65

V-66. A 54-year-old man presents to the emergency department with chest pain. He has had three episodes of chest pain in the past 24 h with exertion. Each has lasted 20–30 min and resolved with rest. His past medical history is significant for hypertension, hyperlipidemia, asthma, and chronic obstructive pulmonary disease. He currently smokes one pack/day of cigarettes. His family history is remarkable for early coronary artery disease in a sibling. Home medications include chlorthalidone, simvastatin, aspirin, albuterol, and home oxygen. In the emergency department, he becomes chest pain–free after receiving three sublingual nitroglycerin tablets and IV heparin. ECG shows 0.8-mm ST-segment depression in V_5, V_6, lead I and aV_L. Cardiac biomarkers are negative. An exercise stress test shows inducible ischemia. Which aspects of this patient's history add to the likelihood that he might have death, myocardial infarction (MI), or urgent revascularization in the next 14 days?

A. Age
B. Aspirin usage
C. Beta-agonist usage
D. Diuretic usage

V-67. A 62-year-old woman presents to your office with dyspnea of 4 months duration. She has a history of monoclonal gammopathy of unclear significance (MGUS) and has been lost to follow-up for the past 5 years. She is able to do only minimal activity before she has to rest but has no symptoms at rest. She has developed orthopnea but denies paroxysmal nocturnal dyspnea. She complains of fatigue, light headedness, and lower extremity swelling. On examination, blood pressure is 110/90 mmHg and heart rate 94. Jugular venous pressure is elevated, and the jugular venous wave does not fall with inspiration. An S_3 and S_4 are present, as well as a mitral regurgitation murmur. The point of maximal impulse is not displaced. Abdominal examination is significant for ascites and a large, tender, pulsatile liver. Chest radiograph shows bilateral pulmonary edema. An electrocardiogram shows an old left bundle branch block. Which clinical features differentiate constrictive pericarditis from restrictive cardiomyopathy?

A. Elevated jugular venous pressure
B. Kussmaul's sign
C. Narrow pulse pressure
D. Pulsatile liver
E. None of the above

V-68. This electrocardiogram (ECG) is obtained from a 47-year-old man after an exercise stress test. Which of the following additional tests would be important to obtain at this point?

V-68. *(Continued)*

A. 18-lead ECG
B. Chest CT scan with IV contrast
C. Chest radiograph
D. Erythrocyte sedimentation rate
E. Rhythm strip analysis

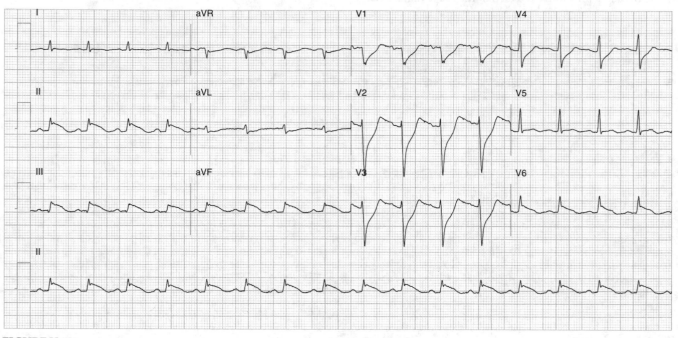

FIGURE V-68

V-69. All of the following are potential causes of tricuspid regurgitation *except*

A. congenital heart disease
B. infective endocarditis
C. inferior wall myocardial infarction
D. pulmonary arterial hypertension
E. rheumatic heart disease
F. all will cause tricuspid regurgitation

V-70. A 45-year-old man is evaluated following an episode of syncope. He has had occasional chest pain with exertion. Today, while he was climbing a flight of stairs in his home, he abruptly lost consciousness and fell two steps. His wife was home with him and heard the fall. He regained consciousness rapidly prior to arrival of emergency medical services but has no memory of the event. He is being treated for a broken radius that occurred during the fall. He has no history of childhood illnesses or previous history of heart murmur. His physical activity has not been limited until recently, because of anginal symptoms for which he has not sought evaluation. He has no history of hypertension or hypercholesterolemia and does not smoke. He last saw a physician about 8 years ago for a job-related physical examination and was told his health was good. You are asked to evaluate for a possible cardiac cause of syncope. On physical examination, his blood pressure is 160/90 mmHg and heart rate is 88 beats/min. He has a IV/VI harsh crescendo-decrescendo midsystolic murmur. His carotid upstroke is delayed. His electrocardiogram shows left-ventricular hypertrophy with a strain pattern. You suspect aortic stenosis. What is the most likely cause of aortic stenosis in this individual?

A. Bicuspid aortic valve
B. Calcification of the aortic valve
C. Congenital aortic stenosis
D. Rheumatic fever

V-71. All of the following statements regarding cardiac transplantation are true *except*

A. Most transplant programs routinely perform endomyocardial biopsies on a routine schedule for 5 years to detect acute transplant rejection.
B. Patients requiring inotropic support with a pulmonary artery catheter or mechanical circulatory support (left- or right-ventricular assist device) are given highest priority for transplantation.
C. The average posttransplant "half-life" for a transplanted heart is 9.3 years.
D. The most common cause of late mortality (>1 year) following cardiac transplantation is coronary artery disease.
E. While the survival following heart transplantation is 76% at 3 years, most patients are unable to return to unrestricted functional status after heart transplant.

V-72. You are managing a patient with the metabolic syndrome. She is an obese woman with poorly controlled diabetes and dyslipidemia. Her HbA1C is 8.8% and fasting plasma glucose is 195 mg/dL. Low-density lipoprotein (LDL) cholesterol is 98 mg/dL and triglycerides are 276 mg/dL. Her medications include insulin, atorvastatin, hydrochlorothiazide, and aspirin. What is the best option for a medication to treat this patient's hypertriglyceridemia?

A. Cholestyramine
B. Colestipol
C. Ezetimibe
D. Fenofibrate
E. Nicotinic acid

V-73. All of the following statements regarding percutaneous coronary interventions (PCI) accompanied by stenting for ischemic heart disease are true *except*

A. Coronary artery bypass grafting (CABG) is preferred over PCI in patients with isolated left main artery disease.

V-73. *(Continued)*

B. Compared to balloon angioplasty, PCI with stenting has higher target vessel patency rates at 6 months.
C. Drug-eluting stents delay endothelial healing and expose the patient to an increased risk of subacute stent thrombosis compared to bare metal stents.
D. PCI with stenting reduces the occurrence of coronary death and myocardial infarction (MI) in patients with symptomatic ischemic heart disease.

V-74. You are evaluating a new patient with chronic pain syndrome. This electrocardiogram (ECG) is obtained in clinic. What medication is contraindicated in this patient?

A. Codeine
B. Fentanyl
C. Gabapentin
D. Methadone

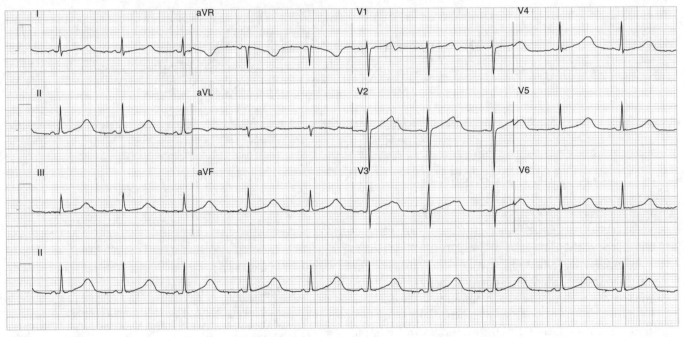

FIGURE V-74

V-75. When treating a patient with a non-ST-segment elevation myocardial infarction (NSTEMI), risk stratification and timely administration of anti-ischemic and antithrombotic therapies are paramount. For a patient with unstable angina with negative biomarkers, which medication regimen is most appropriate as initial treatment?

A. Aspirin, beta blocker, spironolactone, HMG-CoA reductase inhibitor (statin)
B. Aspirin, clopidogrel, nitroglycerin, beta blocker, heparin
C. Aspirin, nitroglycerin, beta blocker, heparin, glycoprotein IIB/IIIa inhibitor
D. Aspirin, morphine, oxygen, nitrates

V-76. All the following are true about cardiac valve replacement *except*

A. Bioprosthetic valve replacement is preferred to mechanical valve replacement in younger patients because of the superior durability of the valve.
B. Bioprosthetic valves have a low incidence of thromboembolic complications.
C. The risk of thrombosis with mechanical valve replacement is higher in the mitral position than in the aortic position.
D. Mechanical valves are relatively contraindicated in patients who wish to become pregnant.

V-76. *(Continued)*

    E.   Double-disk tilting mechanical prosthetic valves offer superior hemodynamic characteristics over single-disk tilting valves.

V-77. A 35-year-old female undergoes a physical examination while obtaining new insurance coverage. She reports 1 year of slowly progressive dyspnea on exertion and a change in skin color. Her physical examination is notable for the presence of cyanosis, an elevated jugular venous pulse, a fixed split loud second heart sound, and peripheral edema. Arterial oxygen saturation is 84%. Chest radiography shows an enlarged heart and normal lung parenchyma. Ten years ago, at her last insurance physical examination, her physical examination, oxygen saturation, and chest radiogram were normal. Echocardiography most likely will reveal

    A.   atrial septal defect

    B.   Ebstein's anomaly

V-77. *(Continued)*

    C.   tetralogy of Fallot

    D.   truncus arteriosus

    E.   ventricular septal defect

V-78. A 66-year-old man has a history of ischemic cardiomyopathy. He undergoes right and left heart catheterization for evaluation of unexplained dyspnea on exertion and an equivocal result on noninvasive cardiac stress testing. Sample tracings from his right and left heart catheterization at rest and during exercise are shown. What abnormality is demonstrated in the pulmonary capillary wedge tracing?

    A.   Aortic stenosis

    B.   Congestive heart failure

    C.   Mitral regurgitation

    D.   Mitral stenosis

    E.   Pulmonary arterial hypertension

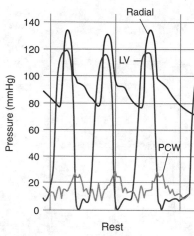 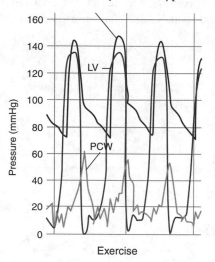

FIGURE V-78

V-79. A 28-year-old female has hypertension that is difficult to control. She was diagnosed at age 26. Since that time she has been on increasing amounts of medication. Her current regimen consists of labetalol 1000 mg bid, lisinopril 40 mg qd, clonidine 0.1 mg bid, and amlodipine 5 mg qd. On physical examination she appears to be without distress. Blood pressure is 168/100, and heart rate is 84 beats per minute. Cardiac examination is unremarkable, without rubs, gallops, or murmurs. She has good peripheral pulses and has no edema. Her physical appearance does not reveal any hirsutism, fat maldistribution, or abnormalities of genitalia. Laboratory studies reveal a potassium of 2.8 mEq/dL and a serum bicarbonate of 32 mEq/dL. Fasting blood glucose is 114 mg/dL. What is the likely diagnosis?

    A.   Congenital adrenal hyperplasia

    B.   Fibromuscular dysplasia

    C.   Cushing's syndrome

    D.   Conn's syndrome

    E.   Pheochromocytoma

V-80. What is the best way to diagnose this disease?

    A.   Renal vein renin levels

    B.   24-h urine collection for metanephrines

    C.   Magnetic resonance imaging of the renal arteries

    D.   24-h urine collection for cortisol

    E.   Plasma aldosterone/renin ratio

V-81. You are evaluating a new patient in clinic. The 25-year-old patient was diagnosed with "heart failure" in another state and has since relocated. He has New York Heart Association class II symptoms and denies angina. He presents for evaluation and management. On review of systems, the patient has been wheel-chair bound for many years and has severe scoliosis. He has no family history of hyperlipidemia. His physical examination is notable for bilateral lung crackles, an S_3, and no cyanosis. An electrocardiogram (ECG) is obtained in clinic and shows tall R waves in V_1 and V_2 with deep Qs in V_5 and V_6. An echocardiogram reports severe global left ventricular dysfunction with reduced ejection fraction. What is the most likely diagnosis?

V-81. (Continued)

A. Amyotrophic lateral sclerosis
B. Atrial septal defect
C. Chronic thromboembolic disease
D. Duchenne's muscular dystrophy
E. Ischemic cardiomyopathy

V-82. Which of the following congenital heart defects causes fixed splitting of the second heart sound?

A. Atrial septal defect
B. Epstein's anomaly
C. Patent foramen ovale
D. Tetralogy of Fallot
E. Ventricular septal defect

V-83. In chronic severe aortic regurgitation, the left ventricle adapts to maintain cardiac output. Left-ventricular hypertrophy occurs over time and maintains cardiac output in the face of increased preload. All of the following are adverse effects of left ventricular hypertrophy *except*

A. decreased coronary blood flow
B. equalization of aortic and left-ventricular pressures in end-diastole
C. increased myocardial oxygen consumption
D. increased wall stress

V-84. A 41-year-old patient is referred to you for evaluation of a cardiac murmur. The patient has a diastolic murmur with a rumbling quality, with an opening snap heard best at the left-ventricular apex. An electrocardiogram shows the patient to be in sinus rhythm with evidence of left atrial enlargement. A two-dimensional echocardiogram shows mitral stenosis with an estimated valve area of 1.7 cm^2 indicative of mild mitral stenosis. When deciding on whether or not to correct this patient's valvular heart disease, which of the following tests is indicated?

A. Coronary arteriogram
B. Coronary CT angiogram
C. Exercise stress test
D. Right heart catheterization
E. 24-h Holter monitor

V-85. A 35-year-old woman comes in for a routine visit. Her past medical history is significant for poorly controlled type 2 diabetes mellitus (HbA1C of 8.4%), obstructive sleep apnea, hypertension, and dyslipidemia. Her body mass index is 42 kg/m². Blood pressure in clinic is 154/87 mmHg and fasting plasma glucose is 130 mg/dL. Her medications include metformin, insulin, ramipril, hydrochlorothiazide, and atorvastatin. You have diagnosed her with the metabolic syndrome. Based on our current understanding of the metabolic syndrome, treating which of the following underlying conditions is the primary approach to treating this disorder?

A. Hyperglycemia
B. Hypercholesterolemia

V-85. (Continued)

C. Hypertension
D. Inflammatory cytokines
E. Obesity

V-86. A 24-year-old man is referred to cardiology after an episode of syncope while playing basketball. He has no recollection of the event, but he was told that he collapsed while running. He awakened lying on the ground and suffered multiple contusions as a result of the fall. He has always been an active individual but recently has developed some chest pain with exertion that has caused him to restrict his activity. His father died at age 44 while rock climbing. He believes his father's cause of death was sudden cardiac death and recalls being told his father had an enlarged heart. On examination, the patient has a III/VI mid-systolic crescendo-decrescendo murmur. His electrocardiogram shows evidence of left ventricular hypertrophy. You suspect hypertrophic cardiomyopathy as the cause of the patient's heart disease. Which of the following maneuvers would be expected to cause an increase in the loudness of the murmur?

A. Handgrip exercise
B. Squatting
C. Standing
D. Valsalva maneuver
E. A and B
F. C and D

V-87. A patient is noted to have a crescendo-decrescendo mid-systolic murmur on examination. The murmur is loudest at the left sternal border. The patient is asked to squat, and the murmur decreases in intensity. The patient stands and the murmur increases. Finally, the patient is asked to perform a Valsalva maneuver and the murmur increases in intensity. Which of the following is most likely to be the cause of this murmur?

A. Aortic stenosis
B. Chronic mitral regurgitation
C. Hypertrophic cardiomyopathy (HOCM)
D. Mitral valve prolapse
E. Pulmonic stenosis

V-88. You are asked to give medical clearance for a 75-year-old male before an elective carotid endarterectomy. His past medical history is significant for hypercholesteremia and hypertension. He also has diet-control diabetes mellitus. Current medications include simvastatin and hydrochlorothiazide. He denies any current or prior cardiac symptoms and has never had a myocardial infarction. Physical examination is unrevealing with the exception of a right carotid bruit. An electrocardiogram is unremarkable with the exception of premature ventricular contractions (PVCs) at a rate of two to three per minute. Laboratory analysis is unremarkable, including normal renal function and liver function tests. Oxygen satura-

V-88. *(Continued)*

tions are also normal. What would be the expected serious complication rate (perioperative MI, pulmonary edema, or ventricular tachycardia) in this patient?

A. <0.1%
B. 0.1–1.0%
C. 1.0–3.0%
D. 3.0–10%
E. 10%

V-89. Which of the following disorders is not associated with ventricular tachycardia as a cause of syncope?

A. Hypertrophic obstructive cardiomyopathy
B. Prior myocardial infarction
C. Atrial myxoma
D. Aortic valvular stenosis
E. Congenital long QT syndrome

V-90. A 20-year-old female is seen in the emergency department with symptoms of severe periodic headaches, sweating, and nausea with vomiting. She also complains of feeling light-headed with standing. Her blood pressure on presentation is 240/136, with a heart rate of 92. On standing, the patient has a blood pressure of 204/98, with a heart rate of 136. On ophthalmologic examination the patient has mild blurring of the optic discs without hemorrhage. The examination is otherwise normal. What is the best medication for the management of this patient's hypertension?

A. Phentolamine
B. Fenoldopam
C. Esmolol
D. Nicardipine
E. Diazoxide

V-91. What test would best determine the patient's diagnosis?

V-91. *(Continued)*

A. Plasma catecholamines
B. 24-h urine collection for 5-hydroxy-indoleacetic acid
C. Abdominal CT scan
D. 24-h urine collection for metanephrines and vanillylmandelic acid
E. Adrenal vein sampling for renin levels

V-92. Which of the following statements about cardiovascular disease in the United States is correct?

A. Death secondary to cardiovascular disease remains higher in men compared to women.
B. Dysfunction of the coronary microcirculation is more common in men than women.
C. The prevalence of cardiovascular disease is ~25% in individuals >75 years.
D. While age-adjusted cardiovascular deaths are declining in the United States, hospital admissions for cardiovascular disease and congestive heart failure continue to rise.
E. Women are more likely than men to present with symptoms of chest pain with nausea, vomiting, and diaphoresis.

V-93. A 40-year-old male with diabetes and schizophrenia is started on antibiotic therapy for chronic osteomyelitis in the hospital. His osteomyelitis has developed just underlying an ulcer where he has been injecting heroin. He is found unresponsive by the nursing staff suddenly. His electrocardiogram is shown here. The most likely cause of this rhythm is which of the following substances?

A. Furosemide
B. Metronidazole
C. Droperidol
D. Metformin
E. Heroin

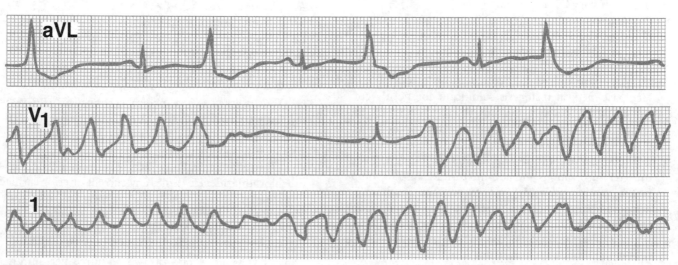

FIGURE V-93

V-94. Normal sinus rhythm is restored with electrical cardioversion. A 12-lead electrocardiogram is notable for a prolonged QT interval. Besides stopping the offending drug, the most appropriate management for this rhythm disturbance should include intravenous administration of which of the following?

A. Amiodarone
B. Lidocaine
C. Magnesium
D. Metoprolol
E. Potassium

V-95. A 52-year-old man with a history of stable angina presents to the hospital with 30 min of chest pain. He reports that over the past 2 weeks, he has developed his typical anginal symptoms of chest pressure radiating to his jaw and left arm with progressively less exertion. He has been using sublingual nitroglycerin more frequently. His other medication includes a beta blocker, aspirin, and lovastatin. On the day of admission, he developed pain at rest that was not relieved with three nitroglycerin tablets. On examination, he is anxious and short of breath. His vital signs are notable for a blood pressure of 140/88 mmHg; a heart rate of 110/min, and a respiratory rate of 25/min. He has bilateral crackles halfway up both lung fields and has a 3/6 systolic murmur that radiates to his axilla. His electrocardiogram shows 3-mm ST-segment depression in leads V_3–V_5. In addition to his outpatient medications, all of the following additional therapies are indicated *except*

A. cardiac catheterization
B. clopidogrel

V-95. (*Continued*)
C. enoxaparin
D. eptifibatide
E. tissue plasminogen activator

V-96. Which of the following patients with aortic dissection can be managed without surgical or endovascular intervention?

A. A 72-year-old male with a dissection of the descending aorta that begins just distal to the left subclavian artery and extends to below the left renal artery and with a baseline creatinine of 1.8 mg/dL that is not increasing
B. A 41-year-old male with an ascending aortic dissection that extends past the left common carotid artery after an automobile accident
C. A 42-year-old male with Marfan's syndrome with a distal aortic dissection beginning just below the left subclavian artery and an aortic root of 53 mm
D. A 72-year-old male with a chronic type B dissection with a CT that shows advancement of the dissection at 6 months
E. A 56-year-old male with a descending aortic dissection that encompasses the origin of the renal and iliac arteries with rest claudication

V-97. Based on the electrocardiogram below, treating which condition might specifically improve this patient's tachycardia?

A. Anemia
B. Chronic obstructive pulmonary disease (COPD)
C. Myocardial ischemia
D. Pain

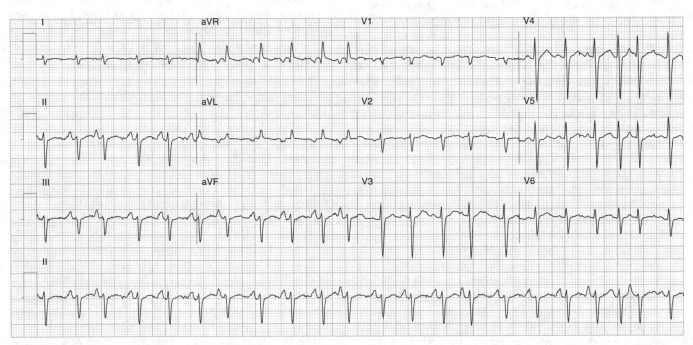

FIGURE V-97

V-98. Each of these patients is alert and oriented and has a blood pressure of 110/60. In which patient would adenosine constitute appropriate initial therapy?

A.   A 65-year-old male with no ischemic heart disease and wide complex tachycardia

B.   A 65-year-old female with known ischemic disease and narrow complex tachycardia

C.   A 25-year-old female with known preexcitation syndrome and narrow complex tachycardia

D.   A 28-year-old male with known preexcitation syndrome and wide complex tachycardia

E.   A 44-year-old male with atrial fibrillation without a prior history of heart disease

V-99. A 68-year-old man with a history of coronary artery disease is seen in his primary care clinic for complaint of cough with sputum production. His care provider is concerned about pneumonia, so a chest radiograph is ordered. On the chest radiograph, the aorta appears tortuous with a widened mediastinum. A contrast-enhanced CT of the chest confirms the presence of a descending thoracic aortic aneurysm measuring 4 cm with no evidence of dissection. What is the most appropriate management of this patient?

A.   Consult interventional radiology for placement of an endovascular stent.

B.   Consult thoracic surgery for repair.

C.   No further evaluation is needed.

D.   Perform yearly contrast-enhanced chest CT and refer for surgical repair when the aneurysm size is >4.5 cm.

E.   Treat with beta blockers, perform yearly contrast-enhanced chest CT, and refer for surgical repair if the aneurysm grows more than 1 cm/year.

V-100. A 55-year-old male presents with severe substernal chest pain for the last hour. It began at rest and is associated with dyspnea and nausea. The electrocardiogram shows bradycardia with a Mobitz type II second-degree block. Chest plain film is normal. Which of the following is likely to be found in addition on the electrocardiogram?

A.   ST elevation V_1–V_3

B.   Wellen's T waves

C.   ST elevation II, III, and aVF

D.   ST depression in I and aVL

E.   No other abnormality

V-101. A 44-year-old woman presents to the emergency room complaining of acute onset of chest pain. She describes the chest pain as 10/10 in intensity, with a sharp stabbing quality. The chest pain is worse when lying flat and better when sitting upright. The pain came on suddenly, awakening the patient from sleep. There is no radiation of the pain and no nausea, vomiting, or lightheadedness. She has no other complaints. She has no history of hypertension, hypercholesterol-

V-101. *(Continued)*
emia, or diabetes mellitus. She does not smoke. On physical examination, she appears in distress moving in bed frequently. Her vital signs are: temperature 38.3°C, blood pressure 112/62 mmHg, heart rate 102 beats/min, respiratory rate 18 breaths/min, and Sa_{O_2} 100% on room air. She has a regular tachycardia. There are no murmurs, rubs, or gallops. There is no pulsus paradoxus. The pulmonary, abdominal, extremity, and neurologic examinations are normal. An echocardiogram demonstrates a normal ejection fraction without an effusion. Initial troponin I level is 0.26 ng/mL (normal values <0.06–0.50 ng/mL). What is the most appropriate treatment for this patient? (See also Figure V-64.)

A.   Anticoagulation with heparin and serial troponin measurements

B.   Immediate cardiac catheterization with angioplasty and stent

C.   Indomethacin, 50 mg three times daily

D.   Reassurance only

E.   Reteplase, 10 units IV now, followed by an additional dose in 30 min

V-102. A 22-year-old man collapses immediately after being hit in the chest with a ball while playing lacrosse. Emergency medical personnel were present during the game and noted the initial rhythm to be ventricular fibrillation. The patient underwent prompt defibrillation within 3 min, and normal sinus rhythm was restored. The patient has been transported to the emergency room and is stable with a blood pressure of 128/76 mmHg and heart rate of 112 beats/min. He has no prior history of syncope and no family history of sudden cardiac death. His electrocardiogram (ECG) is normal. There is no evidence of broken ribs or sternum by x-ray. What is the most likely diagnosis?

A.   Brugada syndrome

B.   Cardiac contusion

C.   Commotio cordis

D.   Hypertrophic cardiomyopathy

E.   Right ventricular dysplasia

V-103. You are examining a new patient in clinic. On cardiac auscultation you palpate a double apical impulse. There is a III/VI harsh crescendo "diamond-shaped" murmur that begins well after the first heart sound. The murmur is best heard at the lower left sternal border as well as at the apex. The murmur does not radiate to the neck. There is no respiratory variation. S_1 and S_2 are normal. With passive elevation of the legs, the murmur decreases in intensity. During the strain phase of the Valsalva maneuver, the murmur increases in intensity. With inhalation of amyl nitrate, the murmur increases in intensity. What is the etiology of this patient's murmur?

V-103. (Continued)

- A. Aortic sclerosis
- B. Aortic stenosis
- C. Hypertrophic cardiomyopathy
- D. Mitral regurgitation
- E. Tricuspid regurgitation

V-104. Insulin resistance and fasting hyperglycemia are important when creating a treatment program for the metabolic syndrome. Often, lifestyle modifications will occur at the same time medications are prescribed. In addressing the treatment of insulin resistance and fasting hyperglycemia, which of the following statements is true?

- A. Metformin is more effective than the combination of weight reduction, dietary fat restriction, and increased physical activity for the prevention of diabetes mellitus.
- B. Metformin is superior to other drug classes for increasing insulin sensitivity.
- C. Thiazolidinediones, but not metformin, improve insulin-mediated glucose uptake in muscle.
- D. Lifestyle interventions alone are not effective in reducing the incidence of diabetes mellitus.

V-105. A 63-year-old male with end-stage ischemic cardiomyopathy is offered a heart transplant from a 20-year-old female with brain death after a skiing accident. Which of the following is not a risk that the patient should be advised about if he decides to accept the heart?

- A. Increased risk of malignancy
- B. Risk of rejection of transplanted organ
- C. Coronary artery disease
- D. Increased risk of infections
- E. Increased risk of bradyarrhythmias

V-106. A 38-year-old man presents to the emergency department with chest pain. He has had chest pressure for the past 2 days. He has never had this pain before. At baseline, his exercise tolerance is normal, but he has limited his activity in the past few days due to fear of exacerbating the chest pain. The pain has been present for most of the past 48 h. In the emergency department, he has a normal blood pressure, heart rate is 104 beats per minute, respiratory rate 22 breaths per minute; oxygen saturation 91% on room air. Lung auscultation is clear bilaterally. Cardiac examination reveals tachycardia but no other significant findings. Laboratory data show a white blood cell count of 9000/μL, CK is 190 U/L; CK-MB 8 μg/L; and troponin 0.7 ng/mL. Electrocardiogram (ECG) shows tachycardia, a rightward axis, left ventricular hypertrophy, and T-wave inversions in V_2 and V_3. An old ECG is not available for comparison. What is the most likely diagnosis?

- A. Esophageal spasm
- B. Myocarditis
- C. Non-ST-segment elevation myocardial infarction

V-106. (Continued)

- D. Pulmonary embolism
- E. Unstable angina

V-107. All the following interventions have demonstrated a decrease in macrovascular complications (coronary artery disease, stroke) in patients with diabetes and dyslipidemia except

- A. ACE inhibitors
- B. gemfibrozil therapy
- C. goal blood pressure below 130/85
- D. HMG-CoA reductase therapy
- E. tight glycemic control

V-108. Pulsus paradoxus can be described by which of the following statements?

- A. Pulsus paradoxus can be seen in patients with acute asthma exacerbations in which the negative intrathoracic pressure decreases afterload of the heart with a resultant increase in systolic pressure during inspiration.
- B. Pulsus paradoxus has not been described in patients with superior vena cava syndrome.
- C. Pulsus paradoxus describes the finding of diminished pulses during inspiration, when the peripheral pulse is normally augmented during inspiration.
- D. A drop in systolic pressure during inspiration of more than 5 mmHg indicates the presence of pulsus paradoxus.
- E. Pulsus paradoxus occurs during cardiac tamponade when there is an exaggeration of the normal decrease in the systolic blood pressure during inspiration.

V-109. A 35-year-old woman is admitted to the hospital with malaise, weight gain, increasing abdominal girth, and edema. The symptoms began about 3 months ago and gradually progressed. The patient reports an increase in waist size of ~15 cm. The swelling in her legs has gotten increasingly worse such that she now feels her thighs are swollen as well. She has dyspnea on exertion and two-pillow orthopnea. She has a past history of Hodgkin's disease diagnosed at age 18. She was treated at that time with chemotherapy and mediastinal irradiation. On physical examination, she has temporal wasting and appears chronically ill. Her current weight is 96 kg, an increase of 11 kg over the past 3 months. Her vital signs are normal. Her jugular venous pressure is ~16 cm, and the neck veins do not collapse on inspiration. Heart sounds are distant. There is a third heart sound heard shortly after aortic valve closure. The sound is short and abrupt and is heard best at the apex. The liver is enlarged and pulsatile. Ascites is present. There is pitting edema extending throughout the lower extremities and onto the abdominal wall. Echocardiogram shows pericardial thickening, dilatation of the inferior vena cava and hepatic veins, and abrupt cessation of ventricular filling in early diastole. Ejection

V-109. *(Continued)*

fraction is 65%. What is the best approach for treatment of this patient?

A. Aggressive diuresis only
B. Cardiac transplantation
C. Mitral valve replacement
D. Pericardial resection
E. Pericardiocentesis

V-110. A 52-year-old man is brought to the emergency room complaining of shortness of breath, chest pain, and dizziness. The chest pain began acutely about 90 min ago. He had been working in the yard at that time and thought he might have strained a muscle in his chest. He took an aspirin and lay down, but the symptoms worsened. He soon developed dizziness and shortness of breath. He called 911, and upon arrival to the emergency room, he was found to be hypotensive and tachycardic. His vital signs on presentation were: blood pressure 75/44 mmHg, heart rate 132 beats/min, respiratory rate 24 breaths/min, and Sa_{O_2} 88% on room air. On physical examination, he appears in distress and is diaphoretic. He is unable to speak in full sentences. His neck veins appear distended. There are crackles throughout both lung fields. The heart sounds are regular and tachycardic. There is no edema. The extremities are cool, and the pulses are thready. An electrocardiogram shows ST elevations in lead V2–V6. Chest radiograph shows diffuse pulmonary edema. Emergency cardiac catheterization is scheduled, and it is estimated that the catheterization laboratory will be available in ~45 min. The patient remains hypotensive with a blood pressure that is now 68/38 mmHg, and the oxygen saturation has fallen to 82% on room air. What is the best management for the patient's hypotension?

A. Aortic counterpulsation
B. Dobutamine, 2.5 μg/kg per min IV
C. Furosemide, 40 mg IV
D. Metoprolol, 5 mg IV
E. Norepinephrine, 4 μg/min IV

V-111. A 64-year-old woman is admitted to the emergency room with hypotension and chest pain. Her symptoms began 30 min ago, awakening the patient from sleep. She vomited twice and has felt dizzy and lightheaded. Upon arrival in the emergency room, her blood pressure was 80/40 mmHg, with a heart rate of 64 beats/min. She appears in distress and has another episode of emesis in the emergency room. The lungs are clear to auscultation. Pulses are thready. An electrocardiogram demonstrates elevations in leads II, III, and aV_F. There are ST depressions in V_1 and V_2. The rhythm is sinus with occasional premature ventricular contractions. A chest radiograph is clear. An echocardiogram shows normal left ventricular function and right ventricular dilatation. What is the best immediate treatment for this patient's hypotension?

V-111. *(Continued)*

A. Aortic counterpulsation
B. Dobutamine, 5 μg/kg per min
C. Dopamine, 5 μg/kg per min
D. Normal saline bolus, 500 mL
E. Transvenous pacemaker placement

V-112. All of the following statements regarding sudden cardiac death in the United States are true *except*

A. A strong parental history of sudden cardiac death as a presenting history of coronary artery disease increases the likelihood of a similar presentation in an offspring.
B. An estimated 50% of all cardiac deaths are sudden and unexpected.
C. As many as 70–75% of men who die of sudden cardiac death have evidence of acute myocardial infarction (MI), while only 20–30% have preexisting healed MIs.
D. By 5 min after sudden cardiac arrest, the estimated survival rates are no better than 25–30% in the out-of-hospital setting.

V-113. A 64-year-old man suddenly collapses while playing the sousaphone with his alumni band during halftime of a football game. Emergency medical services with training in advanced cardiac life support are present within 2 min of collapse. Initial rhythm on cardiac monitor is ventricular fibrillation. What is the first step in the treatment of this patient?

A. Continue cardiopulmonary resuscitation (CPR) for a full 5 min prior to attempting defibrillation
B. Endotracheal intubation followed by rapid defibrillation
C. Immediate defibrillation at 300–360 J once, followed by CPR for 60–90 s before additional defibrillation
D. Obtain IV access and administer amiodarone, 150 mg
E. Obtain IV access and administer epinephrine, 1 mg

V-114. Which of the following therapies has been demonstrated to improve survival to hospital discharge with favorable neurologic outcome in out-of-hospital cardiac arrest?

A. Amiodarone
B. Epinephrine
C. Hypothermia
D. Time to initial defibrillation <10 min
E. Vasopressin

V-115. A 65-year-old man is evaluated for chest pain. Given the characteristics of his chest pain, it is decided that he should undergo cardiac stress testing. He has a history of myocardial infarction involving the left anterior descending artery 2 years ago, for which he received reteplase with restoration of coronary flow. His adenosine technetium

V-115. *(Continued)*

99m nuclear stress test is shown in Figure V-115 (Color Atlas). What abnormality is indicated by the arrows?

A. Apical aneurysm
B. Fixed defect of the anteroapical wall
C. Reversible ischemia of the anteroapical wall
D. Tissue attenuation due to obesity

V-116. A 54-year-old man presents to the emergency department with chest pain. He has had three episodes of chest pain in the past 24 h with exertion. Each has lasted 20–30 min and resolved with rest. His past medical history is significant for hypertension, hyperlipidemia, asthma, and chronic obstructive pulmonary disease. He currently smokes one pack/day of cigarettes. His family history is remarkable for early coronary artery disease in a sibling. Home medications include chlorthalidone, simvastatin, aspirin, albuterol, and home oxygen. In the emergency department, he becomes free of chest pain after receiving three sublingual nitroglycerin tablets and IV heparin. Electrocardiogram shows 0.8mm ST-segment depression in leads V_5, V_6, I, and aV_L. Cardiac biomarkers are negative. An exercise stress test shows inducible ischemia. Which aspects of this patient's history add to the likelihood that he might have death, myocardial infarction (MI) or urgent revascularization in the next 14 days?

A. Age
B. Aspirin use
C. Beta-agonist use
D. Diuretic use

V-117. A 38-year-old man presents to the emergency department with chest pain. He has had substernal chest pressure for the past 2 days. He has never had this pain before. At baseline, his exercise tolerance is normal, but he has limited his activity in the past few days due to fear of exacerbating the chest pain. The pain has been present for most of the past 48 h. In the emergency department, he has a normal blood pressure; heart rate is 104 beats/min, respiratory rate 22 breaths/min, oxygen saturation 91% on room air. Lung auscultation is clear bilaterally. Cardiac examination reveals tachycardia but no other significant findings. Laboratory data show a white blood cell count of 9000/μl, CK is 190, CK-MB 8 μg/mL, troponin 0.9 μg/mL. Electrocardiogram (ECG) shows tachycardia, a rightward axis, left ventricular hypertrophy, and T-wave inversions in V_2 and V_3. An old ECG is not available for comparison. What is the most likely diagnosis?

A. Esophageal spasm
B. Myocarditis
C. Non-ST-elevation myocardial infarction
D. Pulmonary embolism
E. Unstable angina

V-118. You are called to the bedside to see a patient with Prinzmetal's angina who is having chest pain. The patient had a cardiac catheterization 2 days prior showing a 60% stenosis of the right coronary artery with associated spasm during coronary angiogram. The spasm was relieved with nitroglycerin infusion. Which of the following additional disorders is the patient most likely to have?

A. Migraine
B. Peptic ulcer disease
C. Peripheral vascular disease
D. Reactive arthritis
E. Rheumatoid arthritis

V-119. A 56-year-old man is admitted to the hospital for newly diagnosed heart failure. On cardiac examination his pulse is irregular, he has an S_3, and a laterally displaced point of maximal impulse. There is a high-pitched holosystolic murmur beginning with the first heart sound and extending to the second heart sound heard best in the axilla. Neurologic examination shows decreased sensation to pin prick in a stocking-glove distribution. Electrocardiogram (ECG) shows atrial fibrillation, low voltage in the limb leads, and first-degree atrioventricular block without evidence of prior myocardial infarction. Chest radiograph shows cardiomegaly. Blood chemistries show potassium 4.1 meq/L, magnesium 1.6 mg/dL, creatinine 0.8 mg/dL, calcium 11.4 mg/dL, albumin 3.7 mg/dL, total protein 8.4 mg/dL, AST 27 U/L, ALT 17 U/L, alkaline phosphatase 76 U/L. An echocardiogram is performed. Which finding on echocardiogram is most likely?

A. Akinesis of the inferior wall
B. Aortic stenosis
C. Protrusion of the left ventricular apex with hypercontractility of the base
D. Systolic anterior motion of the mitral valve
E. Thickened interatrial septum

V-120. A cardiac biopsy is obtained from a 24-year-old man with new-onset heart failure during a right heart catheterization. Congo red staining shows positive birefringence characteristic of amyloid. Immunohistochemical staining of the biopsy reveals an abundance of the transthyretin protein. What is the next step in the management of this type of amyloidosis?

A. Bone marrow biopsy
B. Evaluation for underlying inflammatory disease
C. Family pedigree analysis
D. Neurocognitive testing
E. Urine for Bence-Jones protein

V-121. You are caring for a patient with heart rate-related angina. With minor elevations in heart rate, the patient has anginal symptoms that impact his quality of life. On review of a 24-h Holter monitor, it appears that the pa-

V-121. *(Continued)*

tient has sinus tachycardia at the time of his symptoms. What is the mechanism for this patient's arrhythmia?

- A. Delayed afterdepolarizations
- B. Early afterdepolarizations
- C. Increased automaticity
- D. Reentry pathway

V-122. Where are the most common drivers of atrial fibrillation anatomically located?

- A. Left atrial appendage
- B. Mitral annulus
- C. Pulmonary vein orifice
- D. Sinus venosus
- E. Sinus node

V-123. Symptoms of atrial fibrillation vary dramatically from patient to patient. A patient with which of the following clinical conditions will likely be the *most* symptomatic (e.g., short of breath) if they develop atrial fibrillation?

- A. Acute alcohol intoxication
- B. Hypertrophic cardiomyopathy
- C. Hyperthyroidism
- D. Hypothermia
- E. Postoperative after thoracotomy

V-124. When deciding whether to initiate anticoagulation for a patient with atrial fibrillation, which of the following factors is *least* important?

- A. Age
- B. History of diabetes
- C. Mitral stenosis
- D. Use of antiarrhythmic medications
- E. Hypertension

V-125. Which of the following electrocardiographic findings suggests a focal atrial tachycardia as opposed to an automatic atrial tachycardia (e.g., sinus tachycardia)?

- A. Initiation of tachycardia with programmed stimulation
- B. One P-wave morphology
- C. Slow-onset and termination phase
- D. Slowing of the rate with adenosine infusion

V-126. You are seeing a return patient in clinic. The patient is a 76-year-old man with a history of hypertension, remote cerebrovascular accident, diet-controlled diabetes, and congestive heart failure with left ventricular systolic dysfunction (ejection fraction = 30%). The patient reports no new complaints and feels well. On physical examination, you palpate an irregular pulse, and an electrocardiogram verifies atrial fibrillation. The patient does not have a history of atrial fibrillation. You and the patient are interested in a trial of direct current cardioversion (DCCV). What is the appropriate management of anticoagulation for this patient?

V-126. *(Continued)*

- A. Initiate warfarin (with goal INR 2.0–3.0) following DCCV only if cardioversion is unsuccessful.
- B. Give full-dose aspirin (325 mg daily) 3 weeks prior to DCCV, perform transesophageal echocardiogram (TEE) and DCCV (if not contraindicated), then discontinue aspirin if DCCV is successful.
- C. Initiate IV heparin and warfarin, perform transesophageal echocardiogram (TEE) and DCCV (if not contraindicated), then discontinue warfarin if DCCV is successful.
- D. Initiate IV heparin, perform TEE and DCCV (if not contraindicated), then continue warfarin for at least 1 month.

V-127. You are evaluating a patient with a wide-complex tachycardia. The patient has a history of Wolff-Parkinson-White (WPW) syndrome. Which medication is the most effective for treating this patient's tachycardia?

- A. Adenosine
- B. Digoxin
- C. Diltiazem
- D. Procainamide
- E. Verapamil

V-128. All of the following are electrocardiographic clues supporting the diagnosis of ventricular tachycardia *except*

- A. capture beats
- B. concordance of QRS complex in all precordial leads
- C. fusion beats
- D. QRS duration during tachycardia shorter than during sinus rhythm
- E. RSR' pattern in V_1

V-129. A 68-year-old man with a history of myocardial infarction and congestive heart failure is comfortable at rest. However, when walking to his car, he develops dyspnea, fatigue, and sometimes palpitations. He must rest for several minutes before these symptoms resolve. His New York Heart Association classification is which of the following?

- A. Class I
- B. Class II
- C. Class III
- D. Class IV

V-130. The husband of a 68-year-old woman with congestive heart failure is concerned because his wife appears to stop breathing for periods of time when she sleeps. He has noticed that she stops breathing for ~10 s and then follows this with a similar period of hyperventilation. This does not wake her from sleep. She does not snore. She feels well rested in the morning but is very dyspneic with even mild activity. What is your next step in management?

- A. Electroencephalography
- B. Maximize heart failure management

V-130. *(Continued)*

   C. Nasal continuous positive airway pressure (CPAP) during sleep

   D. Obtain a sleep study

   E. Prescribe bronchodilators

V-131. A 28-year-old man with long-standing cardiomyopathy presents with worsening dyspnea. Physical examination reveals a blood pressure of 85/50 mmHg, heat rate of 112 beats/min, elevated jugular venous pressure, positive hepatojugular reflex, quiet S_1/S_2, apical S_3, no pulmonary rales, and 3+ lower extremity edema. Chest radiograph shows no pulmonary edema and a small left-sided pleural effusion. What information does the patient's pulmonary examination give you in regards to his likely pulmonary capillary wedge pressure?

   A. It is likely to be elevated.

   B. It is likely to be normal.

   C. It is likely to be decreased.

   D. No information.

V-132. All of the following findings on echocardiographic assessment of patients with congestive heart failure with preserved ejection fraction are relevant *except*

   A. atrial fibrillation

   B. left atrial dilatation

   C. left ventricular wall thickness

   D. left ventricular diastolic filling as measured by tissue Doppler

   E. systolic anterior motion of the mitral valve

V-133. All of the following medications have been shown to worsen heart failure in patients with left ventricular systolic dysfunction *except*

V-133. *(Continued)*

   A. angiotensin receptor blockers

   B. calcium channel antagonists

   C. nonsteroidal anti-inflammatory drugs (NSAIDs)

   D. sotalol

   E. thiazolidinediones

V-134. Which of the following is true regarding dose escalation of angiotensin-converting enzyme (ACE) inhibitors and beta blockers in patients newly diagnosed with congestive heart failure?

   A. ACE inhibitors should be escalated on a daily basis to maximal tolerated doses, while beta blockers should be gently increased in dose over weeks, as tolerated.

   B. Beta blockers should be escalated on a daily basis to maximal tolerated doses, while ACE inhibitors should be gently increased in dose over weeks, as tolerated.

   C. Both should be escalated rapidly to maximally tolerated doses.

   D. Both should be escalated slowly to maximally tolerated doses.

   E. Both should be initiated at full doses.

V-135. In African Americans with New York Heart Association class II heart failure, which of the following drug combinations should be added to an angiotensin-converting enzyme inhibitor and beta blocker?

   A. Hydralazine/angiotensin receptor blockers

   B. Hydrazaline/digoxin

   C. Isosorbide dinitrate/angiotensin receptor blockers

   D. Isosorbide dinitrate/digoxin

   E. Isosorbide dinitrate/hydralazine

V. DISORDERS OF THE CARDIOVASCULAR SYSTEM

ANSWERS

V-1. The answer is C. *(Chap. 241)* Several factors have been shown to confer an increased risk of complications from hypertension. In the patient described here there is only one: ongoing tobacco use. Epidemiologic factors that have poorer prognosis include African-American race, male sex, and onset of hypertension in youth. In addition, comorbid factors that independently increase the risk of atherosclerosis worsen the prognosis in patients with hypertension. These factors include hypercholesterolemia, obesity, diabetes mellitus, and tobacco use. Physical and laboratory examination showing evidence of end organ damage also may portend a poorer prognosis. This includes evidence of retinal damage or hypertensive heart disease with cardiac enlargement or congestive heart failure. Furthermore, electrocardiographic evidence of ischemia or left ventricular strain but not left ventricular hypertrophy alone may predict worse outcomes. A family history of hypertensive complications does not worsen the prognosis if diastolic blood pressure is maintained at less than 110 mmHg.

V-2. The answer is B. *(Chap. 242)* Abdominal aortic aneurysms (AAAs) affect 1 to 2% of men older than age 50. Most AAAs are asymptomatic and are found incidentally on physical examination. The predisposing factors for AAA are the same as those for other cardiovascular disease, with over 90% being associated with atherosclerotic disease. Most AAAs are located infrarenally, and recent data suggest that an uncomplicated infrarenal AAA may be treated with endovascular stenting instead of the usual surgical grafting. Indications for proceeding to surgery include any patient with symptoms or an aneurysm that is growing rapidly. Serial ultrasonography or CT imaging is imperative, and all aneurysms larger than 5.5 cm warrant intervention because of the high mortality associated with repair of ruptured aortic aneurysms. The rupture rate of an AAA is directly related to size, with the 5-year risk of rupture being 1 to 2% with aneurysms less than 5 cm and 20 to 40% with aneurysms more than 5 cm. Mortality of patients undergoing elective repair is 1 to 2% and is greater than 50% for emergent treatment of a ruptured AAA. Preoperative cardiac evaluation before elective repair is imperative as coexisting coronary artery disease is common.

V-3. The answer is A. *(Chap. 233)* This patient is presenting with symptoms of congestive heart failure with evidence of systemic embolization. The physical examination suggests mitral valve stenosis with a positional low-pitched sound heard when the patient is in the upright position. This is characteristic of a "tumor plop," which should alert the physician to the possibility of a cardiac tumor. This is confirmed by the echocardiogram revealing a large left atrium tumor, which is most likely an atrial myxoma. Myxomas are the most common type of benign primary cardiac tumors, accounting for over three-quarters of surgically resected cardiac tumors. Myxomas generally present in between ages 20 and 50 and are seen more commonly in women. The clinical presentation of myxomas resembles that of valvular heart disease due either to obstruction of flow from the tumor obscuring valvular flow or to regurgitation due to abnormal valve closure. The tumor plop is heard in mid-diastole and results from the impact of the tumor against the valve or ventricular wall. Most tumors are solid masses located in the atria and measure 4–8 cm. They usually arise from the interatrial septum near the fossa ovalis. Histologically, they appear as gelatinous structures with scattered myxoma cells embedded in a glycosaminoglycan stromal matrix. They may embolize and can be mistaken for endocarditis, particularly as systemic symptoms, including fevers and weight loss, may be seen. Echocardiogram is useful to document tumor size and site of attachment. MRI or CT scanning may also be utilized for preoperative planning. However, cardiac catheterization is no longer considered mandatory prior to tumor resection, especially as catheterization of the chamber containing the tumor increases the likelihood of embolization. Primary surgical excision is the treatment of choice and should be performed regardless of tumor size as even small tumors can cause embolization or valvular obstruction. Surgical resection is generally curative with only a 1–2% recurrence rate in sporadic cases. Tumors metastatic to the heart are more common than primary cardiac tumors and occur with the highest incidence in metastatic melanoma. However, by absolute numbers of cases, breast and lung cancer account for the largest number of cases. Cardiac metastases usually occur in patients with known malignancies, are usually not the cause of presentation, and are found incidentally. Only 10% are clinically apparent at the time of presentation, and most are found at autopsy.

V-4. **The answer is A.** *(Chap. 237)* Myocardial ischemia is determined by the balance between myocardial oxygen supply and demand. Myocardial oxygen demand $(M\dot{V}O_2)$ is determined by heart rate, myocardial contractility, and myocardial wall tension. A normal oxygen supply to the myocardium requires adequate inspired oxygen, intact lung function (including diffusion capacity, which is abnormal in emphysema), normal hemoglobin concentration and function, and normal coronary blood flow. The resistance to coronary blood flow is determined by three vascular regions: large epicardial arteries, pre-arteriolar vessels, and arteriolar and intramyocardial capillaries. In the absence of significant flow-limiting atherosclerosis, the resistance in the epicardial arteries is negligible. The major determinant of coronary-resistance is due to the pre-arteriolar, arteriolar, and intramyocardial capillary vessels.

V-5. **The answer is B.** *(Chap. 225)* Second-degree AV block type 1 (Mobitz type 1) is characterized by a progressive lengthening of the PR interval preceding a pause. The pause in this tracing is between the third and fourth QRS complex. First-degree AV block is a slowing of conduction through the AV junction and is diagnosed when the PR interval >200 ms. Type 2 second-degree AV block is characterized by intermittent failure of conduction of the P wave without changes in the preceeding PR or RR intervals. Second-degree AV block type 2 usually occurs in the distal or infra-His conduction systems.

V-6. **The answer is C.** *(Chap. 221)* The electrocardiographic T wave represents myocardial repolarization, and its configuration can be altered nonspecifically by metabolic abnormalities, drugs, neural activity, and ischemia through a dispersion effect on the activation or repolarization of action potentials. Although myocardial ischemia and subendocardial infarction can produce deep, symmetric T-wave inversions which would result in tachyarrhythmias and syncope, noncardiac phenomena such as intracerebral hemorrhage can similarly affect ventricular repolarization. Hyperkalemia is manifested by tall peaked T waves, not inverted ones. Hypocalcemia is manifested by prolonged QT intervals.

V-7. **The answer is A.** *(Chap. 230)* Aortic stenosis (AS) may remain asymptomatic for many years. However, once symptoms develop, surgery is indicated owing to the increased mortality associated with symptomatic AS. The average time to death after onset of symptoms is as follows: angina pectoris, 3 years; syncope, 3 years; dyspnea, 2 years; congestive heart failure, 1.5–2 years. In addition, surgery is advocated when the ejection fraction falls below 50% or when severe calcification, rapid progression, or expected delays in surgery are present. There is no specific age cut-off or degree of left-ventricular function that precludes surgical correction. This is, in part, due to the fact that there are no good medical therapies to treat aortic stenosis. Percutaneous balloon valvuloplasty has been used as a bridge to surgery and in patients with severe left-ventricular dysfunction or who are otherwise too ill to tolerate surgery. Improving blood pressure will not improve this patient's symptomatic AS, and vasodilation to an excessive degree can precipitate syncope in these patients due to having a fixed cardiac output. Further characterization of the patient's AS will not alter management. An exercise regimen is likely to result in more episodes of syncope.

V-8. **The answer is C.** *(Chap. 229)* The ductus arteriosus is an embryonic vessel connecting the pulmonary artery to the aorta just distal to the left subclavian artery, shunting blood from the fluid-filled lungs of the fetus. After birth, the ductus arteriosus closes as blood now circulates through the low-resistance pulmonary vascular bed. If the ductus arteriosus fails to close after birth, a left-to-right shunt develops between the aorta and the pulmonary vasculature. Because the pressure in the aorta is greater than that of the pulmonary artery through all portions of the cardiac cycle, the murmur of a patent ductus arteriosus is a continuous murmur. There is late systolic accentuation of the murmur at the upper left sternal angle. The murmur is described as "machinery"-like, and often a palpable thrill is present. If Eisenmenger syndrome occurs, as in this patient, the shunt changes directional flow and becomes a right-to-left shunt as a result of pulmonary hypertension. That is when patients will become cyanotic. Because of the anatomic location of the ductus arteriosus below the level of the left subclavian artery, a characteristic of Eisenmenger syndrome in those with patent ductus arteriosus is cyanosis and clubbing of the toes but not the fingers. Total anomalous pulmonary venous return occurs when all four pulmonary veins drain into the systemic venous circulation. This condition is fatal soon after birth if there is not also an atrial or ventricular septal defect or a patent foramen ovale. Most patients with this condition are identified shortly after birth because of cyanosis. Coarctation of the aorta is a relatively common congenital abnormality that is associated with a stricture of the aorta near the insertion site of the ligamentum arteriosus (the remnant of the ductus arteriosus). A patient with coarctation of the aorta frequently presents with headache. Upper extremity hypertension is present in association with low blood pressures in the lower extremities. Patients may also complain of claudication in the lower extremities. Tetralogy of Fallot is a congenital heart disease syndrome with ventricular septal defect, right-ventricular outflow obstruction, aortic override of the ventricular septal defect, and right-ventricular hypertrophy. This defect is almost always identified and corrected during childhood. Ventricular septal defect results in left-to-right shunt and a holosystolic murmur rather than a continuous murmur.

V-9. **The answer is A.** *(Chap. 230)* In the post-MI setting, posterior (mural) mitral valve chordae rupture is more common than aortic (anterior) mitral valve rupture due to its singular blood supply. In contrast to functional mitral regurgitation, the regurgitant jet of valvular mitral regurgitation (MR) is eccentric and directed towards one wall of the atrium. The musical quality of the murmur has been described when the cause is a flail leaflet. Systolic anterior motion (SAM) of the mitral valve is a finding on echocardiogram when MR is associated with hypertrophic cardiomyopathy. Acute ventricular septal defect can be seen within the first few days of an MI. These patients usually have hypotension and rapidly develop pulmonary hypertension and signs of cardiogenic shock. In the post-MI setting, ventricular free wall rupture into the pericardium is a catastrophic event that can cause tamponade and shock. Respiratory variation in mitral inflow velocity is an echocardiographic sign of tamponade physiology. High-frequency fluttering of the anterior mitral leaflet is the characteristic echocardiographic finding of acute aortic regurgitation, seen most commonly in primary aortic valvular disease, aortic dissection, infective endocarditis, or chest trauma.

V-10. **The answer is D.** *(Chap. 242)* This patient presents with severe chest pain that is tearing in quality and associated with hypertension. These symptoms should raise the concern for aortic dissection as the cause of the chest pain, and prompt evaluation and treatment are essential to decrease mortality from this often fatal condition. In the presence of an aortic regurgitation murmur and ECG changes consistent with myocardial injury, an ascending aortic dissection should be considered with dissection of the right coronary artery. Aortic dissections are classified by either the DeBakey or Stanford classifications. The DeBakey system classifies aortic dissections into three types. Type I is caused by an intimal tear in the ascending aorta and has propagated to include the descending aorta. A type II dissection involves only the ascending aorta, and a type III dissection involves only the descending aorta. The Stanford classification has only two categories: type A, which involves the ascending aorta, and type B, which involves only the descending aorta. Risk factors for developing an aortic dissection include systemic hypertension (70%), Marfan syndrome, inflammatory aortitis, congenital valve abnormalities, coarctation of the aorta, and trauma. Aortic dissections are a medical emergency with a high in-hospital mortality due to aortic rupture, pericardial tamponade, or visceral ischemia. Ascending aortic dissections have the highest mortality, and studies have demonstrated that medical management alone in an ascending aortic dissection has a mortality rate of >50% (*PG Hagan et al, JAMA 283:897, 2000*). The greatest mortality occurs early after presentation with the mortality reported at 1–2% per hour initially after symptoms onset (*CA Nienaber, KA Eagle, Circulation 108:628, 2003*). Because of the high associated mortality, it is imperative to evaluate and treat aggressively with early surgical intervention. Transesophageal echocardiography has 80% sensitivity for diagnosing ascending aortic dissections and will also provide information regarding valvular function and presence of pericardial tamponade. CT angiography and MRI both have sensitivities for diagnosing aortic dissection of >90%. The decision regarding which test to perform should be based on the rapid availability of testing and clinical stability of the patient. Management of an aortic dissection initially begins with medical therapy to stabilize the patient and decrease blood pressure. This should be occurring concurrently with surgical consultation to plan definitive operative repair on an emergent basis. Medical therapy should consist of antihypertensive therapy to rapidly reduce the systolic blood pressure to 100–120 mmHg. Most often this is accomplished with nitroprusside. In addition, use of a beta blocker to reduce cardiac contractility and heart rate is recommended. Surgery involves excision of the intimal flap, removal of the intramural hematoma, and placement of a graft. In some cases, replacement of the entire aortic root and aortic valve is necessary when the aortic valve is involved. With coronary artery involvement, coronary artery bypass may also be required. With prompt surgical intervention, mortality from ascending aortic dissection is ~15–25%.

V-11. The answer is B. *(Chaps. 231 and 244)* This patient presents with classic findings of right-sided heart failure. The differential diagnosis includes pulmonary vascular disease, restrictive cardiomyopathy, constrictive pericarditis, cor pulmonale, and any cause of longstanding left-sided heart failure. A CT or MRI of the chest would assess for pericardial calcifications or parenchymal lung disease not visualized on radiography. Iron studies are a component of the evaluation for hemochromatosis, and fat pad biopsy is a component of the evaluation for amyloidosis, both of which may cause restrictive cardiomyopathy. The tuberculin test is useful for ascertaining the presence of prior infection with *Mycobacterium tuberculosis*, which is associated with the development of constrictive pericarditis. A coronary angiogram would not be helpful in a young patient with no physical signs or echocardiographic findings of left-sided heart failure.

V-12. The answer is D. *(Chaps. 221 and e19)* This ECG shows a short ST segment that is most prominent in V_2, V_3, V_4, and V_5. Hypercalcemia, by shortening the duration of repolarization, abbreviates the total time from depolarization through repolarization. This is manifested on the surface ECG by a short QT interval. In this scenario, the hypercalcemia is due to the rhabdomyolysis and renal failure. Fluids and a loop diuretic are an appropriate therapy for hypercalcemia. Hemodialysis is seldom indicated. Hemodialysis is indicated for significant hyperkalemia, which may also develop after rhabdomyolysis, manifest by "tenting" of the T waves or widening of the QRS. Classic ECG manifestations of a pulmonary embolus (S_1, Q_3, T_3 pattern) are infrequent in patients with pulmonary embolism (PE), though the changes may be seen with massive PE. There are no signs of myocardial ischemia on this ECG, which would make coronary catheterization and 18-lead ECG interpretation of low yield.

V-13. The answer is B. *(Chaps. 235 and 350)* This patient meets the criteria for the metabolic syndrome. These patients with type 2 diabetes and an abnormal lipid profile have insulin resistance and a marked increase in cardiovascular risk. The LDL in these patients may not be markedly elevated, but the particles are smaller and denser. These small LDL particles are thought to be more atherogenic than are normal LDL particles. Patients with the metabolic syndrome have reduced HDL levels. Elevated serum endothelin levels may contribute to hypertension, and elevated homocysteine levels have been suggested as a cardiovascular risk factor.

Clinical Identification of the Metabolic Syndrome—Any Three Risk Factors	
Risk Factor	Defining Level
Abdominal obesity[a]	
Men (waist circumference)[b]	>102 cm (>40 in.)
Women	>88 cm (>35 in.)
Triglycerides	>1.7 mmol/L (>150 mg/dL)
HDL cholesterol	
Men	<1.0 mmol/L (<40 mg/dL)
Women	<1.3 mmol/L (<50 mg/dL)
Blood pressure	≥130/≥85 mmHg
Fasting glucose	>6.1 mmol/L (>110 mg/dL)

[a]Overweight and obesity are associated with insulin resistance and the metabolic syndrome. However, the presence of abdominal obesity is more highly correlated with the metabolic risk factors than is an elevated body-mass index (BMI). Therefore, the simple measure of waist circumference is recommended to identify the BMI component of the metabolic syndrome.

[b]Some male patients can develop multiple metabolic risk factors when the waist circumference is only marginally increased, e.g., 94–102 cm (37–39 in.). Such patients may have a strong genetic contribution to insulin resistance. They should benefit from life-style changes, similarly to with categorical increases in waist circumference.

V-14.   The answer is A. *(Chap. 220)*   The presentation of this patient is consistent with the diagnosis of acute valvular dysfunction due to infective endocarditis. The presence of a widened pulse pressure and diastolic murmur heard best along the lower sternal border suggests aortic regurgitation. The figure shown below in panel *C* shows a typical bisferiens pulse that is characteristic of aortic regurgitation. With a bisferiens pulse, there are two distinct pulsations that can be palpated with systole. The initial pulse represents an exaggerated percussion wave reflecting the increased stroke volume that occurs in aortic regurgitation, with the second peak reflecting the tidal, or anacrotic, wave.

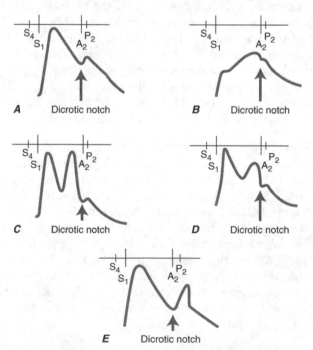

FIGURE V-14   Schematic diagrams of the configurational changes in carotid pulse and their differential diagnoses. Heart sounds are also illustrated. *A.* Normal. A$_2$, aortic component of the second heart sound; S$_1$, first heart sound; S$_4$, atrial sound. *B.* Anacrotic pulse with a slow initial upstroke. The peak is close to S$_2$. These features suggest fixed left ventricular outflow obstruction, such as occurs with valvular aortic stenosis. *C.* Pulsus bisferiens with both percussion and tidal waves occurring during systole. This type of carotid pulse contour is most frequently observed in patients with hemodynamically significant aortic regurgitation or combined aortic stenosis and regurgitation with dominant regurgitation. It is rarely appreciated at the bedside by palpation. *D.* In hypertrophic obstructive cardiomyopathy, the pulse wave upstroke rises rapidly and the trough is followed by a smaller slowly rising positive pulse. *E.* A dicrotic pulse results from an accentuated dicrotic wave and tends to occur in patients with sepsis, severe heart failure, hypovolemic shock, cardiac tamponade, and aortic valve replacement. *[From K Chatterjee: Bedside evaluation of the heart: The physical examination, in Cardiology: An Illustrated Text/Reference, K Chatterjee, W Parmley (eds). Philadelphia, JB Lippincott, 1991.]*

Infective endocarditis causes loss of valvular integrity and acutely causes valvular regurgitation. Of the other options, both mitral regurgitation and tricuspid regurgitation (choice E) would cause systolic and not diastolic murmurs. A hyperkinetic pulse may occur in these conditions, particularly if associated with fever or sepsis. With a hyperkinetic pulse the usual dichrotic notch is more pronounced as seen in panel *E* of the figure. Mitral stenosis causes a diastolic murmur but is not a common lesion associated with infective endocarditis, unless underlying valvular stenosis was present prior to acquiring the infection. It is not associated with a bisferiens pulse. Aortic stenosis is associated with pulsus parvus et tardus, with a delayed and prolonged carotid upstroke as shown here in panel *B* of the figure. Aortic stenosis has an associated harsh crescendo-decrescendo systolic murmur.

V-15. **The answer is B.** *(Chap. 232)* This patient presents with pericardial tamponade. These patients often have distant heart sounds and on examination typically have pulsus paradoxus. Jugular veins are distended and typically show a prominent *x* descent and an absent *y* descent, as opposed to patients with constrictive pericarditis. In addition, Kussmaul's sign is absent in tamponade but present in constrictive pericarditis. The electrocardiogram is normal or shows low voltage. Rarely, electrical alternans may be present. Echocardiographic findings typically reveal right atrial collapse and right ventricular diastolic collapse. Cardiac catheterization will reveal equalization of diastolic pressures across the cardiac chambers. Therefore, the pulmonary capillary wedge pressure will be equal to the diastolic pulmonary arterial pressure, and this will be equal to the right atrial pressure. These catheterization findings are also present in a patient with constrictive pericarditis.

V-16. **The answer is A.** *(Chap. 237)* Calcium channel blockers are potent coronary vasodilators, which also reduce myocardial oxygen demand, contractility, and arterial pressure. When beta blockers are ineffective or poorly tolerated, calcium channel blockers are indicated for the treatment of stable angina. Adverse effects of the calcium channel blockers include hypotension, conduction disturbances, and the propensity to exacerbate heart failure due to the negative inotropic effects. In general, verapamil should not be used in conjunction with beta blockers because of the combined effect on heart rate and contractility. Diltiazem should not be used in patients taking beta blockers with conduction disturbances and a low ejection fraction. Immediate-release nifedipine and other short-acting dihydropyridines should be avoided due to the increased risk of precipitating myocardial infarction. Amlodipine and other second-generation dihydropyridines dilate coronary arteries and decrease blood pressure. In conjunction with beta blockers, which slow heart rate and decrease contractility, amlodipine has a favorable effect in the treatment of angina.

V-17. **The answer is A.** *(Chaps. 118 and 230)* Indications for endocarditis prophylaxis with procedures are assessed by taking into account the nature of the cardiac lesion and the risk posed by the procedure. High-risk cardiac lesions include prosthetic heart valves, a history of bacterial endocarditis, complex cyanotic congenital heart disease, patent ductus arteriosus, coarctation of the aorta, and surgically constructed systemic portal shunts. Moderate-risk patients include those with congenital cardiac malformations other than high-risk or low-risk lesions, acquired aortic or mitral valve dysfunction, hypertrophic cardiomyopathy with asymmetric septal hypertrophy, and mitral valve prolapse with valve thickening or regurgitation. Low-risk lesions include isolated secundum atrial septal defect (ASD), a surgically repaired ASD, ventricular septal defect (VSD), patent ductus arteriosis (PDA), prior coronary bypass graft, mitral valve prolapse without regurgitation or thickened valves, a history of rheumatic fever without valvular dysfunction, and cardiac pacemakers or implantable defibrillators. This patient falls into the moderate-risk category. Her procedure is an esophageal dilation, which, like dental procedures, calls for prophylaxis in the moderate- to high-risk groups. Amoxicillin 2 g PO 1 h before the procedure is the standard recommendation, but this patient may be penicillin-allergic. Acceptable alternatives include clarithromycin 500 mg PO 1 h before the procedure, clindamycin 600 mg PO 1 h before, or cephalexin 2 g PO 1 h before if the patient is able to tolerate cephalosporins.

V-18. **The answer is D.** *(Chap. 22)* The patient presents with carotid hypersensitivity syndrome in which pressure on the carotid sinus baroreceptors results in activation of the sympathetic nervous system with subsequent bradycardia caused by sinus arrest or atrioventricular block, vasodilation, or both. Generally, men older than 50 are at risk for this condition, and it classically presents with syncope in the setting of shaving, wearing a tight collar, or turning the head to one side. Diagnosis is suggested by carotid sinus massage with prolonged (more than 3 s) asystole.

V-19. **The answer is D.** *(Chap. 238)* Prinzmetal and colleagues described a syndrome of angina that occurs at rest but not usually with exertion associated with transient ST-segment elevation. The pathophysiology is due to coronary artery vasospasm. Proximal nonobstructive coronary plaques are usually present. The vasospasm usually occurs within 1 cm of a coronary plaque and is associated with ST-segment elevations on the 12-lead surface electrocardiogram. Due to further vasospasm, cold water ingestion may exacerbate the patient's symptoms. Costochondritis or muscular strain can reproduce the patient's pain. By definition, Prinzmetal's angina is associated with ST-segment elevation, not depression, during the anginal episode.

V-20. **The answer is E.** *(Chap. 242)* Aortitis and ascending aortic aneurysms are commonly caused by cystic medial necrosis and mesoaortitis that result in damage to the elastic fibers of the aortic wall with thinning and weakening. Many infectious, inflammatory, and inherited conditions have been associated with this finding, including syphilis, tuberculosis, mycotic aneurysm, Takayasu's arteritis, giant cell arteritis, rheumatoid arthritis, and the spondyloarthropathies (ankylosing spondylitis, psoriatic arthritis, Reiter's syndrome, Behçet's disease). In addition, it can be seen with the genetic disorders Marfan's syndrome and Ehlers-Danlos syndrome.

V-21. **The answer is C.** *(Chap. 206)* This patient presents with the classic findings of chronic Chagas' disease with cardiomyopathy. Chagas' disease, or American trypanosomiasis, is due to infection with *Trypanosoma cruzi* and only occurs in the Americas. Acute Chagas' disease is usually a mild illness. A minority of chronically infected patients develop serious cardiac or gastrointestinal disease (megaesophagus or megacolon). This diagnosis should be considered in a person from Central or South America presenting with this degree of cardiomyopathy with conduction delays (most commonly right bundle branch block) and normal angiogram. Apical aneurysm and thrombus formation are common and may lead to systemic embolization, including stroke. Although medical therapy for acute Chagas' improves mortality, the role in chronic Chagas' has not been proven. Treatment for coronary vasospasm and aggressive lipid lowering therapy do not have an established role in the treatment of Chagas' disease. Since the cardiomyopathy is considered irreversible, cardiac transplantation is the only viable option to improve function. The prognosis after cardiac transplantation tends to be favorable since this form of chronic Chagas' disease is usually limited to the heart. Many forms of acute viral myocarditis or stress cardiomyopathy are expected to improve with time.

V-22. **The answer is A.** *(Chap. 230)* This patient has the opening snap, diastolic rumble, and signs of pulmonary hypertension indicative of mitral stenosis (MS). The most common cause is sequelae of rheumatic carditis, and symptoms of stenosis usually develop two decades after the onset of carditis. MS can remain asymptomatic for many years but be exaggerated when there is tachycardia, increased left-ventricular filling pressure, or reduced cardiac output (e.g., fever, excitement, anemia, atrial fibrillation, pregnancy, or thyrotoxicosis). Due to elevated left atrial pressure and concomitant left atrial dilation, these patients are at high risk for developing atrial fibrillation, pulmonary hypertension, and right-ventricular failure. Multifocal atrial tachycardia is commonly due to diseases of the lung parenchyma. Right-ventricular outflow tract tachycardia is unrelated to valvular pathology and is common in the young and women. Patients with MS do not develop primary left-ventricular dysfunction because the left ventricle is protected from the pressure and volume load by the diseased mitral valve. Patients with MS can develop right-ventricular hypertrophy and right-ventricular failure. Right bundle branch block is usually unrelated to MS.

V-23. **The answer is B.** *(Chap. 225)* Although sinoatrial node dysfunction is seen most commonly in the elderly with no specific etiology identified, certain disease states are associated with sinoatrial dysfunction, including infiltrative diseases such as amyloid and sarcoidosis. Additionally, multiple systemic disorders are associated with sinus bradycardia, for instance, hypothyroidism, advanced liver disease, hypoxemia, hypercapnia, acidemia, and acute hypertension. Finally, several infectious diseases are classically associated with sinus bradycardia, notably typhoid fever and brucellosis. Leptospirosis is not associated with sinus bradycardia.

V-24. **The answer is E.** *(Chap. 229)* Congenital heart disease (CHD) affects about 1% of all live births, and >85% of affected individuals survive until adulthood. Currently, there are more adults than children living with CHD in the United States, and many of these individuals are unaware of the presence of CHD until other complications develop. Pulmonary hypertension may develop in individuals with a significant left-to-right shunt such as an undiagnosed atrial septal defect. Pulmonary hypertension is the result of increased blood flow across the pulmonary vascular bed, leading to obliteration of the vascular bed. With the development of significant pulmonary hypertension, Eisenmenger syndrome may develop. This occurs when a right-to-left shunt develops as a result of pulmonary hypertension. Patients will have cyanosis. Erythrocytosis due to chronic hypoxemia is a common feature of cyanotic congenital heart disease with a hematocrit of up to 65–70% commonly seen. However, symptoms of hyperviscosity rarely develop, and phlebotomy is not frequently required. The risk of infective endocarditis is increased in those with CHD, and prophylactic antibiotics are recommended for all individuals with CHD undergoing invasive procedures. Stroke is greatest in children <4 years of age but is not increased in adults unless there is inappropriate use of anticoagulants, concomitant atrial fibrillation, or infective endocarditis.

V-25. **The answer is A.** *(Chap. 221)* Hyperkalemia leads to partial depolarization of cardiac cells. As a result, there is slowing of the upstroke of the action potential as well as reduced duration of repolarization. The T wave becomes peaked, the RS complex widens and may merge with the T wave (giving a sine-wave appearance), and the P wave becomes shallow or disappears. Prominent U waves are associated with hypokalemia; ST-segment prolongation is associated with hypocalcemia.

V-26. **The answer is B.** *(Chap. 230)* The time interval between closure of the aortic valve (A_2) and the opening snap of mitral stenosis is inversely related to the severity of mitral stenosis. In severe mitral stenosis, the left atrial pressure is high. In a patient with elevated left atrial pressures, the mitral valve opens quickly after closure of the aortic valve (A_2) due to the relatively low pressure gradient across the mitral valve in early diastole. If the left atrial pressure were lower, it would take longer for the pressure gradient across the mitral valve to cause mitral valve opening. A short interval between A_2 and the opening snap indicates very elevated left atrial pressures. Atrial fibrillation, pulmonary vascular congestion, pulmonary hypertension, and right-ventricular failure (elevated jugular pressure, pulsatile liver, peripheral edema) are all potential sequelae of severe mitral stenosis.

V-27. **The answer is A.** *(Chaps. 219 and 241)* Essential hypertension causes 92 to 94% of cases of hypertension in the general population, and screening for secondary causes of hypertension is not cost-effective in most instances. The abrupt onset of severe hypertension or the onset of any hypertension before the age of 35 or after age 55 should prompt evaluation for renovascular hypertension. In addition, patients should be evaluated for secondary causes if previously well-controlled blood pressure suddenly becomes increasingly difficult to control as this may indicate the development of renovascular disease. Any symptoms or physical findings of concern should be investigated further as well. In the scenarios presented in Question 27, (B) should signal concern for adult-onset polycystic kidney disease and (E) describes a woman with possible Cushing's disease. Other causes of secondary hypertension include pheochromocytoma, primary hyperaldosteronism, medication-induced, and vasculitis.

V-28. **The answer is A.** *(Chap. 225)* One-third of patients with sinoatrial node dysfunction will develop supraventricular tachycardia, usually atrial fibrillation or atrial flutter. Patients with the tachycardia-bradycardia variant of sick sinus syndrome are at risk for thromboembolism. Those at greatest risk include age >65 years, prior history of stroke, valvular heart disease, left ventricular dysfunction, or atrial enlargement. These patients should be treated with anticoagulants. There is no reason to discontinue dypyridamole at this time as she is complaining of no side effects, and the absence of angina argues against the need for cardiac catheterization.

V-29. **The answer is C.** *(Chap. 232)* Cardiac tamponade occurs with accumulation of fluid in the pericardial space such that the resulting pericardial pressure obstructs venous inflow and subsequently cardiac output. The most common causes of cardiac tamponade are neoplasm, renal failure, and idiopathic acute pericarditis. The amount of fluid required to cause cardiac tamponade varies widely, depending upon the acuity with which the effusion develops. Rapid accumulation of pericardial fluid will result in tamponade with as little as 200 mL of fluid, whereas a slow accumulation of pericardial fluid may result in a pericardial effusion of ≥2000 mL. Cardiac tamponade can be rapidly fatal if not recognized and treated quickly with pericardiocentesis. Clinical features of pericardial tamponade are hypotension, muffled heart sounds, and jugular venous distention, with a rapid *x* descent but without a *y* descent. These symptoms collectively are known as Beck's triad. In more slowly accumulating effusions, symptoms may be those of heart failure, with dyspnea and orthopnea common. An elevated pulsus paradoxus is also present in cardiac tamponade. Normally, blood pressure falls during inspiration, due to an increase in blood flow into the right ventricle with displacement of the interventricular septum to the left, decreasing left-ventricular filling and cardiac output. This fall in blood pressure results in a fall in systolic blood pressure of ≤10 mmHg in normal individuals but is exaggerated in cardiac tamponade. On electrocardiogram, electrical alternans may be seen. Echocardiogram is frequently diagnostic, showing a large pericardial effusion with collapse of the right ventricle during diastole. A right heart catheterization demonstrates equalization of pressures in all chambers of the heart. This is exemplified in option C where the right-atrial pressure, right-ventricular diastolic pressure, pulmonary artery diastolic pressure, and pulmonary capillary wedge pressure are equal. Option A are normal values on right heart catheterization. Option B would be seen in congestive heart failure, and option D is seen in pulmonary arterial hypertension.

V-30. **The answer is C.** *(Chaps. 221 and 231)* The ECG shows slight right axis deviation and low voltage. These changes are typical of emphysema when the thorax is hyperinflated with air and the flattened diaphragm pulls the heart inferiorly and vertically. An acute central nervous system (CNS) event such as a subarachnoid hemorrhage may cause QT prolongation with deep, wide inverted T waves. Hyperkalemia will cause peaked narrowed T waves or a wide QRS complex. Patients with hypertrophic cardiomyopathy will have left ventricular hypertrophy and widespread deep, broad Q waves.

V-31. **The answer is D.** *(Chaps. 221 and e21)* This ECG tracing shows the triad of a short PR interval, wide QRS, and delta waves (seen best in leads I, II, and V$_5$), consistent with Wolff-Parkinson-White (WPW) syndrome. Patients with WPW syndrome are commonly diagnosed asymptomatically when an ECG is performed showing the classic findings. Symptoms are due to conduction via an accessory pathway and include tachypalpitations, light headedness, syncope, cardiopulmonary collapse, and sudden cardiac death. Life-threatening presentations are usually due the development of atrial fibrillation or atrial flutter with 1:1 conduction, which can both precipitate ventricular fibrillation.

V-32. **The answer is C.** *(Chap. e8)* Causes of holosystolic murmurs include mitral regurgitation, tricuspid regurgitation, and ventricular septal defects. Carvallo's sign describes the increase in intensity of a tricuspid regurgitation murmur with inspiration. This occurs due to the increase in venous return during inspiration with falling pleural pressure. The Gallavardin effect occurs when the murmur of aortic stenosis is transmitted to the apex (and becomes higher pitched), approximating the murmur heard in mitral regurgitation. The Austin Flint murmur is a late diastolic murmur heard at the apex in aortic regurgitation. The murmur of chronic mitral regurgitation does not worsen with inspiration. Atrial septal defects cause a mid-systolic murmur at the mid to upper left sternal border, with fixed splitting of S_2. There is no change with respiration.

V-33. The answer is E. *(Chap. 226)* Persons who have Wolff-Parkinson-White syndrome are predisposed to develop two major types of atrial tachyarrhythmias. The first, which resembles paroxysmal supraventricular tachycardia (SVT) with reentry, involves the atrioventricular node in anterograde conduction and the bypass tract in retrograde conduction. This tachycardia typically has a narrow QRS complex and can be treated similarly to other forms of SVT. The other, more dangerous tachyarrhythmia (present in the patient described in this question) is atrial fibrillation, which usually is conducted anterograde down the bypass tract and has a wide QRS configuration. The ventricular rate in this situation is quite rapid, and cardiovascular collapse or ventricular fibrillation may result. The usual treatment is direct-current cardioversion, though quinidine may slow conduction through the bypass tract. Verapamil and propranolol have little effect on the bypass tract and may further depress ventricular function, which already is compromised by the rapid rate. Digoxin may accelerate conduction down the bypass tract and lead to ventricular fibrillation.

V-34. The answer is A. *(Chap. 220)* Peripheral arterial disease (PAD) affects 5–8% of Americans with increasing incidence with age. Over the age of 65, the incidence of PAD rises to between 12 and 20%. The primary symptom of PAD is claudication. As this patient describes, claudication occurs with ambulation and is often described as a crampy to aching pain that is relieved with rest. On physical examination, those with PAD often have diminished peripheral pulses, delayed capillary refill, and hair loss in the distal extremities. The skin is often cool to touch with a thin, shiny appearance. In severe PAD, pain in the extremities occurs at rest. Diagnosis of PAD can be suggested by these findings and should be documented by determination of the ankle-brachial index (ABI), as physical examination alone is insufficient to diagnose PAD. Although lack of a palpable pulse suggests critical ischemia, it is not diagnostic. To perform an ABI, blood pressures are determined in the arm and the lower extremities. Either the dorsalis pedis or posterior tibial pulses can be used. The ABI is calculated by dividing the ankle systolic pressure by the brachial systolic pressure. A resting ABI < 0.9 is abnormal, but critical ischemia with rest pain does not occur until the ABI is < 0.3. In individuals with heavily calcified blood vessels, the ABI can be abnormally elevated (ABI > 1.2) when PAD is present. In this situation, toe pressures to determine ABI or employing imaging techniques such as MRI or arteriography should be considered. Lower extremity edema is suggestive of congestive heart failure, not PAD.

V-35 and V-36. The answers are C and A. *(Chap. 229)* This patient has a coarctation of the aorta presenting with marked hypertension proximal to the lesion. The narrowing most commonly occurs distal to the origin of the left subclavian artery, explaining the equal pressure in the arms and reduced pressure in the legs. Coarctations account for approximately 7% of congenital cardiac abnormalities, occur more frequently (2×) in men than in women, and are associated with gonadal dysgenesis and bicuspid aortic valves. Adults will present with hypertension, manifestations of hypertension in the upper body (headache, epistaxis), or leg claudication. Physical examination reveals diminished and/or delayed lower extremity pulses, enlarged collateral vessels in the upper body, or reduced development of the lower extremities. Cardiac examination may reveal findings consistent with left ventricular (LV) hypertrophy. There may be no murmur, a midsytolic murmur over the anterior chest and back, or an aortic murmur with a bicuspid valve. Transthoracic (suprasternal/parasternal) or transesophageal echocardiography, contrast CT or MRI of the thorax, or cardiac catheterization can be diagnostic. MRI of the head would not be useful diagnostically. The clinical picture is not consistent with renal artery stenosis, pheochromocytoma, carcinoid, or Cushing's syndrome.

V-37. The answer is D. *(Chap. 226)* The patient is a young woman with no cardiac disease. In this population asymptomatic premature ventricular contractions (PVCs) require no specific therapy as they are not associated with increased mortality. In patients with symptoms such as palpitations, the primary therapy should be patient reassurance. If this is unsuccessful, beta blockers can be helpful, especially in patients whose symptoms are more prominent during stressful situations and patients with hyperthyroidism. Even in patients with myocardial infarction and PVCs there is no benefit to administering antiarrhythmic therapy with the goal of decreasing the PVC rate. Trials such as CAST comparing ectopy suppression by encainide, flecainide, moricizine, or placebo showed that mortality was increased in all the drug groups compared with placebo at 2 years. Thus, it has become clear that PVC reduction cannot be used as a surrogate endpoint for reduction of risk from sudden cardiac death.

V-38. The answer is E. *(Chap. 221)* The limb lead aVR generally has a negative deflection as the primary vector for ventricular depolarization is directed down and away from this lead. Therefore, in the case of left ventricular hypertrophy the negative deflection, or S wave, would be expected to be larger without an effect on the R wave. There are multiple criteria for diagnosing left ventricular hypertrophy on ECG.

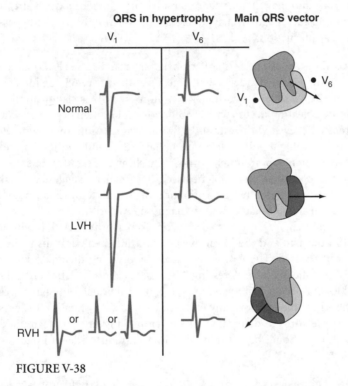

FIGURE V-38

V-39. The answer is D. *(Chap. 225)* Pacemaker syndrome occurs as a result of disrupted AV synchrony. The symptoms are similar to those in this scenario but can also include neck pulsation, confusion, exertional dyspnea, dizziness, and syncope. Signs on examination may suggest cardiac congestive failure. The management involves changing the pacing mode to restore AV synchrony. Lyme disease does not increase the risk of coronary artery diseases. The ECG shows only changes consistent with ventricular pacing, and there is no suggestion of ischemia. ICU psychosis is a cause of delirium among patients with prolonged stays in intensive care settings. Pacemaker twiddler's syndrome occurs when the pulse generator of the pacemaker rotates in its subcutaneous pocket, leading to lead dislodgement and failure to sense or pace. In this case, the stable paced rhythm at 60/min makes this unlikely. Kearne-Sayer syndrome is a rare syndrome caused by abnormal mitochondrial DNA in muscle, which can manifest as cardiac conduction delays.

V-40. The answer is B. *(Chaps. 221 and e19)* This ECG shows findings consistent with an old anterolateral MI. Given the patient's history and that the ST-segment elevations in aV$_L$ and V$_2$–V$_4$ are unchanged from prior; this ECG is consistent with a left ventricular aneurysm. A transthoracic echocardiogram should be obtained to assess for severity as well as the presence of ventricular thrombus. Presence of left ventricular thrombus would warrant discussion of arrhythmogenic and embolic complications. Chest radiography may show an enlarged cardiac silhouette but will not be specific for the patient's pathology. As the patient's symptoms may be indicative of a more serious problem (i.e., left ventricular thrombus), it is not appropriate to schedule follow-up months from now. Without symptoms of chest pain and a stable electrocardiogram, neither cardiac catheterization nor thrombolysis is indicated.

V-41. **The answer is E.** *(Chaps. 230 and 242)* Aortic aneurysm results from numerous mechanisms. The vast majority are associated with atherosclerosis. The risk factors for atherosclerosis (hypertension, hypercholesterolemia, etc.) are also risk factors for aneurysm formation. It is unclear if atherosclerosis is the primary cause or a result of the same pathophysiologic mechanisms that lead to dilatation. Other etiologies include congenital causes. Marfan's syndrome and Ehlers-Danlos syndrome are the most frequently noted. However, there is also an association with osteogenesis imperfecta. Turner's syndrome is associated with coarctation of the aorta. Repair of coarctation may predispose to later dilation and aneurysm formation. Klinefelter's syndrome, however, is not associated with aneurysm formation. Chronic infectious causes include syphilis and mycotic aneurysm from bacterial endocarditis. Chronic inflammatory states such as Takayasu's arteritis, giant cell arteritis, and seronegative spondyloarthropathies such as Reiter's syndrome and ankylosing spondylitis are also associated with aneurysms.

V-42. **The answer is D.** *(Chap. 238)* Although troponin is a commonly used biomarker for myocardial necrosis in the setting of acute myocardial infarction, it is also associated with and caused by a number of other clinical entities, including pulmonary embolism, myocarditis, and congestive heart failure. Troponin elevations are not known to be caused by pneumonia in the absence of myocardial necrosis.

V-43. **The answer is E.** *(Chaps. 221 and e21)* This ECG tracing shows a normal physiologic finding of respiratory sinus arrhythmia. The sinus pacemaker is slow at the beginning of the tracing, accelerates during inspiration in the middle of the tracing, and then slows again during expiration. In atrial fibrillation there are no discernable conducting P waves and the rate is irregularly irregular. In complete heart block, the QRS complexes are usually wider than normal and the R-R interval is regular; variability in the R-R interval rules out complete heart block. There are no nonconducted P waves in this tracing to suggest type 2 AV block. In a ventriculophasic sinus arrhythmia or idioventricular sinus arrhythmia, there is 2:1 AV block with two distinct P-P intervals, which appear to alternate with the QRS complexes.

V-44. **The answer is A.** *(Chap. 225)* This patient's bradycardia may be symptomatic in that he has altered mental status, but he is also severely hypoxic with an active pulmonary infection. Correction of reversible etiologies is indicated since he is still able to generate enough pulse pressure to perfuse his vital organs. Although myocardial infarction due to right coronary artery disease can cause sinus bradycardia, there is no indication that this patient has any disease process other than his pulmonary infection. Glucagon can reverse the bradycardic effects of beta blockers. Temporary transvenous pacing is not indicated since the patient is well-perfused and reversible etiologies are yet to be corrected.

V-45. **The answer is B.** *(Chap. 223)* In the diagnostic algorithm for pulmonary hypertension, the right heart catheterization is important to document the presence and degree of pulmonary hypertension. The right-ventricular systolic pressure (RVSP) on echocardiography provides an estimate of pulmonary arterial pressures, but accurate determination of the RVSP relies upon the presence of triscupid regurgitation and good quality echocardiography. In this patient, her body habitus is prohibitive in obtaining good windows for echocardiography. Thus, a right heart catheterization is imperative for documenting pulmonary hypertension as well as for determining the cause. The right heart catheterization demonstrates an elevated mean arterial pressure, elevated left-ventricular end-diastolic pressure (pulmonary capillary wedge pressure), and elevated mean pulmonary artery pressure. In the presence of a normal cardiac output and an elevated left-ventricular ejection fraction, this is consistent with the diagnosis of diastolic heart failure. Systolic heart failure is associated with similar indices on right heart catheterization, but left-ventricular function is depressed in systolic heart failure. The other causes listed as options are known causes of pulmonary hypertension but would not be expected to cause an increase in the left-ventricular end-diastolic pressure. Obstructive sleep apnea is usually associated only with mild elevations in pulmonary artery pressure. This patient's BMI puts her at risk for obstructive sleep apnea but would not be responsible for these right heart catheterization values. Both chronic thromboembolic disease and pulmonary arterial hypertension can cause severe elevations in the pulmonary arterial pressure but have a normal left atrial pressure.

V-46. **The answer is C.** *(Chap. 229; Brickner et al, 2000.)* Left-to-right shunts occur in all types of atrial and ventricular septal defects but generally do not result in cyanosis, whereas large right-to-left shunts frequently do. The magnitude of the shunt depends on the size of the defect, the diastolic properties of both ventricles, and the relative impedance of the pulmonary and systemic circulations. Defects of the sinus venosus type occur high in the atrial septum near the entry of the superior vena cava or lower near the orifice of the inferior vena cava and may be associated with anomalous connection of the right inferior pulmonary vein to the right atrium. In the case of anomalous origin of the left coronary artery from the pulmonary artery, as pulmonary vascular resistance declines immediately after birth, perfusion of the left coronary artery from the pulmonary trunk ceases and the direction of flow in the anomalous vessel reverses. Twenty percent of patients with this defect can survive to adulthood because of myocardial blood supply flowing totally through the right coronary artery. In the absence of pulmonary hypertension blood will flow from the aorta to the pulmonary artery throughout the cardiac cycle, resulting in a "continuous" murmur at the left sternal border. In total anomalous pulmonary venous connection all the venous blood returns to the right atrium; therefore, an interatrial communication is required and right-to-left shunts with cyanosis are common.

V-47. **The answer is C.** *(Chap. 230)* This patient's murmur is consistent with chronic aortic regurgitation. The high-pitched blowing murmur in the left third intercostal space is commonly present, whereas the second diastolic murmur at the apex, resembling mitral stenosis (Austin Flint murmur), is not always present. Peripheral signs of chronic aortic regurgitation are manifestations of a widened pulse pressure and equalization of aortic and ventricular end-diastolic pressures. As pressure increases in the left ventricle, hypertrophy develops as a compensatory mechanism. Left atrial, but not right atrial, enlargement may be apparent on the ECG if there is concomitant mitral regurgitation. Inferior Q waves may be seen if there has been a myocardial infarction. ST-segment depressions may be seen in the lateral leads when there is significant left-ventricular hypertrophy. Low voltage on the ECG can be seen in obstructive lung diseases, pericardial effusions, and infiltrative diseases of the myocardium. Diffuse ST-segment elevation and PR-segment depression are seen in pericarditis.

V-48. **The answer is B.** *(Chap. 226)* The differentiation of ventricular tachycardia from supraventricular tachycardia with an aberration of intraventricuar conduction can be challenging and has important implications for management. By definition, however, ventricular tachycardia is associated with atrioventricular (AV) dissociation. Cannon *a* waves are found in the jugular venous pulsations when the atria are contracting against a closed tricuspid valve. This can occur only with AV dissociation, thus proving ventricular tachycardia. Hypotension, irregular rhythm, and syncope can all be seen in both ventricular tachycardia and supraventricuar tachycardia with aberrancy.

V-49. **The answer is C.** *(Chap. 237)* The ischemic ST-segment response during exercise is characterized by flat or downsloping ST-segment depression of at least 1 mm lasting for >0.08 s. Upsloping ST segments, ventricular arrhythmias, T-wave abnormalities, and conduction disturbances that develop during exercise should be noted, but are not diagnostic.

A decrease in blood pressure or a failure to increase blood pressure with signs of ischemia on the stress test may be indicative of global dyskinesis and severe ischemic heart disease. The normal response to the graded exercise protocol is a gradual increase in blood pressure. Isolated hypertension during a stress test, despite its severity, is not indicative of myocardial ischemia. Developing angina at a low work-load (i.e., before completion of stage II of a Bruce protocol) or persistent ST-segment depressions lasting >5 min into recovery increase the specificity of the test and indicate a high risk of future events. The target heart rate for exercise stress tests is ≥85% of maximal predicted heart rate for age and sex.

V-50. **The answer is A.** *(Chap. 220)* The patient presents with signs and symptoms consistent with congestive heart failure. Her history of tuberculosis puts her at risk for constrictive pericarditis, and indeed, chest CT shows the classic pericardial calcifications of this disorder. As she is relatively young and does not have enlarged chambers or ischemic changes on the electrocardiogram, dilated or ischemic cardiomyopathy is unlikely. Constrictive pericarditis has certain suggestive physical findings, notably the prominent and rapid *y* descent in the jugular venous pulsations that represents early and rapid filling of the right ventricle during early diastole. Other findings that have been associated include rapid *x* descent, pericardial knock that is similar to a third heart sound, and impressive ascites, edema, and occasionally Kussmaul's sign (lack of inspiratory decline in jugular venous pressure). A double systolic apical impulse has been described in patients with hypertrophic cardiomyopathy. A loud and fixed split P_2 suggests pulmonary hypertension. Cannon *a* waves are most commonly seen in arrhythmias that cause atrioventricular dissociation. Finally, opening snaps are brief, high-pitched diastolic sounds that usually are due to mitral stenosis.

V-51. **The answer is A.** *(Chap. 230)* Aortic stenosis in adults may be due to congenital degenerative calcification of the aortic cusps. Age-related degenerative calification is the most common cause of aortic stenosis (so-called senile aortic stenosis). Approximately 30% of persons over age 65 have evidence of aortic valve sclerosis. Many have a murmur without obstruction, while 2% exhibit stenosis. The risk factors for developing aortic stenosis (dyslipidemia, chronic kidney disease, diabetes, etc.) are similar to those for developing atherosclerotic coronary artery disease. Pathology of the affected valves will show evidence of vascular inflammation, lipid deposition, and calcification. However, treating risk factors such as dyslipidemia has not been shown to improve severe aortic stenosis. There is no effective medical therapy for aortic stenosis. In younger patients presenting with aortic stenosis, the aortic valve apparatus is commonly bicuspid.

V-52. **The answer is B.** *(Chap. 226)* Atrial fibrillation is characterized by disorganized atrial activity with an irregular ventricular response to atrial activity. This lack of organization results in stasis of blood in the atria and puts the patient at risk for cardioembolic stroke. Several factors associated with increased stroke risk have been identified, including diabetes mellitus, hypertension, age over 65, rheumatic heart disease, a prior stroke or transient ischemic attack, congestive heart failure, and a transesophageal echocardiogram showing spontaneous echo contrast in the left atrium, left atrial atheroma, or left atrial appendage velocity <20 cm/s. Hypercholesterolemia is not associated with an increased risk of stroke in patients with atrial fibrillation.

V-53. **The answer is C.** *(Chap. 8)* Cardiac complications are the most important cause of perioperative morbidity and mortality, and primary care physicians are frequently asked to assess a patient's perioperative risk for cardiac events before cardiac procedures. Multiple clinical risk scores have been developed by various professional organizations, such as the American College of Physicians and the American Heart Association. Patients deemed to be at low risk may proceed to surgery without further intervention. The patient described above has only one major risk—intraperitoneal surgery—on the six-point revised cardiac risk index (see Table V-53). This puts the patient into an intermediate-risk classication by this scale; however, further testing is indicated only if the patient is undergoing vascular surgery. In addition, the patient has excellent functional status and can achieve greater than four metabolic equivalents with ease. Examples of activities that consume four metabolic equivalents are climbing one flight of stairs and walking two blocks on level ground. The risk of postoperative cardiovascular complications does not appear to be influenced by stable hypertension, elevated cholesterol, obesity, cigarette smoking, or bundle branch block. Perioperative beta blockade has been shown to decrease rates of postoperative myocardial infarction and cardiac death by at least 50% and is recommended for any patient who has cardiac risk factors or is at intermediate risk of cardiovascular complications after surgery. The patient's prior adverse reaction to beta blockade should not preclude its use in the perioperative period, as it consisted of only mild fatigue and decreased sexual functioning. Finally, the patient's pulmonary risk is likely to be low as he quit smoking more than 8 weeks before surgery and has good functional status without dyspnea.

TABLE V-53   The Revised Cardiac Risk Index

Factor	Adjusted Odds Ratio (OR) for Cardiac Complications in Derivation Cohort
1. High-risk surgery	2.8
2. Ischemic heart disease	2.4
3. History of congestive heart failure	1.9
4. History of cerebrovascular disease	3.2
5. Insulin therapy for diabetes mellitus	3.0
6. Preoperative serum creatinine >2.0 mg/dL	3.0

Class	Number of Factors	Cardiac Complication Rates, %	
		Derivation Cohort	Validation Cohort
I	0	0.5	0.4
II	1	1.3	0.9
III	2	3.6	6.6
IV	3–6	9.1	11.0

Source: Adapted from TH Lee et al. Circulation 100:1043, 1999; with permission.

V-54.   The answer is A. *(Chap. e8)* This patient most likely experienced papillary muscle rupture, which led to acute mitral regurgitation. Other settings where acute mitral regurgitation may occur include rupture of chordae tendineae in the setting of myxomatous mitral valve disease, infective endocarditis, or chest wall trauma. The regurgitation into a normal-sized noncompliant left atrium results in an early systolic descrescendo murmur heard best near the apical impulse. The decrescendo nature contrasts with chronic mitral regurgitation due to the rapid pressure rise in the left atrium during systole. Chronic mitral regurgitation causes a holosystolic murmur. Ventricular septal rupture also causes a holosystolic murmur and is associated with a systolic thrill at the left sternal border. Severe aortic stenosis and hypertrophic cardiomyopathy both present with a mid-systolic murmur.

V-55.   The answer is C. *(Chaps. 239 and 264)* This patient has a right ventricular infarction. The combination of findings consistent with bradycardia, cardiogenic shock, low normal left ventricular and PA pressures, and markedly elevated right atrial pressure is consistent with acute right ventricular (RV) failure. An acute pulmonary embolus may also cause acute RV failure, but the PA pressure is usually elevated. RV infarction is usually due to occlusion of the right coronary artery; the bradycardia is due to sinus or AV node ischemia. Right-sided precordial ECG will show ST-segment elevation. Occlusion of the left main artery will cause cardiogenic shock, but the PCW pressure will be elevated. Perforated duodenal ulcer and ruptured aortic aneurysm will cause hypovolemic shock with low RA and PCW pressures. Gram-negative sepsis will generally have a normal or increased cardiac index with normal filling pressures and low blood pressure.

V-56.   The answer is D. *(Chap. 230)* Indications for surgical repair of mitral regurgitation are dependent on left-ventricular function, ventricular size, and the presence of sequelae of chronic mitral regurgitation. The experience of the surgeon and the likelihood of successful mitral valve repair are also an important consideration. The management strategy for chronic severe mitral regurgitation depends on the presence of symptoms, left-ventricular function, left-ventricular dimensions, and the presence of complicating factors such as pulmonary hypertension and atrial fibrillation. With very depressed left-ventricular function (<30% or end-systolic dimension > 55 mm), the risk of surgery increases, left-ventricular recovery is often incomplete, and long-term survival is reduced. However, since medical therapy offers little for these patients, surgical repair should be considered if there is a high likelihood of success (>90%). When ejection fraction is between 30 and 60% and end-systolic dimension rises above 40 mm, surgical repair is indicated even in the absence of symptoms, owing to the excellent long-term results achieved in this group. Waiting for worsening left-ventricular function leads to irreversible left-ventricular remodeling. Pulmonary hypertension and atrial fibrillation are important to consider as markers for worsening regurgitation. For asymptomatic patients with normal left-ventricular function and dimensions, the presence of new pulmonary hypertension or atrial fibrillation in patients with normal ejection fraction and end-systolic dimensions are class IIa indications for mitral valve repair.

V-57.   **The answer is A.** *(Chap. 236)* The metabolic syndrome (according to the NCET:ATP III guidelines) is defined by three or more of the following: central obesity (men >102 cm; women >88 cm), hypertriglyceridemia (≥150 mg/dL or on specific medication), low HDL cholesterol (men <40 mg/dL; women <50 mg/dL), hypertension (systolic ≥130 mmHg or diastolic ≥85 mmHg, or on specific medication), and hyperglycemia (fasting plasma glucose ≥100 mg/dL, or previous diagnosis of diabetes mellitus, or on specific medication). The International Diabetes Foundation also has criteria that further subdivide the cut-offs of waist circumference based on ethnicity. Patients with the metabolic syndrome are at greater risk than patients without the syndrome for developing conditions such as atherosclerotic cardiovascular disease, type 2 diabetes mellitus, peripheral vascular disease, sleep apnea, and polycystic ovary syndrome. The presence of one of the criteria should prompt the clinician to search for other criteria and treat the conditions as necessary.

V-58.   **The answer is C.** *(Chap. 231)* Peripartum cardiomyopathy can develop in the last trimester of pregnancy or within 6 months of delivery. The cause is unknown and mortality is high (25–50%). Risk factors for developing the disease are African ancestry, age >30 years, and multiparity. Counseling patients with peripartum cardiomyopathy who are considering becoming pregnant in the future is important as it directly impacts maternal and fetal mortality. Some of these patients may become pregnant again; however, women whose ventricular function has not returned to normal usually are advised against pregnancy since the mortality can be as high as 50% during subsequent pregnancies in this population. Among all-comers, there is a 25–67% chance of having another bout of peripartum cardiomyopathy during future pregnancies. Sex of the child during the incident episode of peripartum cardiomyopathy, maternal age, or nadir ejection fraction is not known to be associated with future events. African ancestry is a risk for developing peripartum cardiomyopathy but subsequent risk of mortality depends on the resolution of the first episode.

V-59.   **The answer is B.** *(Chap. 231)* Varying degrees of cardiac enlargement and findings of congestion can be found in patients with dilated cardiomyopathies, depending on the chronicity of the illness. In severe left ventricular dilatation, the jugular venous pressure is elevated, murmurs of mitral and tricuspid regurgitation are common, and third or fourth heart sounds may be heard. Owing to the depressed cardiac output, systemic vascular resistance increases, and with it, diastolic blood pressure. Systolic blood pressure may decrease as a result of decreased cardiac output leading to a narrow pulse pressure. Conditions in which S_2 becomes absent include severe aortic stenosis and severe aortic insufficiency when the insufficiency murmur is louder than S_2. Paradoxical splitting occurs when P_2 and A_2 become closer during inspiration and can be seen in patients with left bundle branch block. Pulsus bisferiens (double-impulse pulse) is classically detected when aortic insufficiency exists in association with aortic stenosis, but it may also be found in isolated but severe aortic insufficiency and hypertrophic obstructive cardiomyopathy.

V-60.   **The answer is D.** *(Chap. 235)* HMG-CoA reductase inhibitors ("statins") clearly reduce cardiovascular events in patients with atherosclerosis. The mechanism appears to be more complex than simply the reduction of serum LDL. Lipid-lowering drugs do not appear to cause significant regression of fixed coronary lesions. The benefit of statins appears to be related to stabilization of plaques, long-term egress of lipids, and/or improved vasodilatory tone. The improved vasodilatory tone appears to be mediated by modulation of endothelial-dependent vasodilators such as nitric oxide. Thus, the beneficial effect of the statins probably consists of an early effect on vasomotion (or other mechanisms) and a long-term effect on serum and plaque lipids.

V-61.   The answer is A. *(Chap. 237)*   Dipyridamole inhibits the activity of adenosine deaminase and phosphodiesterase, which cause an accumulation of adenosine and coronary artery vasodilation. Where there is significant obstructive coronary disease, there is a pressure gradient between prestenotic and poststenotic segments, and the poststenotic vascular bed dilates to allow for preserved coronary blood flow. Higher degrees of obstruction cause maximal poststenotic vasodilation. In nonaffected regions of myocardium, there is no distal vasodilation. Dipyridamole, by disproportionately dilating nonobstructed areas of myocardium, is useful as a pharmacologic agent to differentiate ischemic from nonischemic tissue. Where there is high-grade, three-vessel disease, the usefulness of dipyridamole or adenosine infusion is limited by (1) baseline maximal vasodilation, and (2) lack of ability to differentiate affected from nonaffected regions of myocardium. Dipyridamole testing is helpful in identifying ischemic tissue in a single-vessel territory. Intraventricular conduction abnormalities limit the use of electrocardiography or echocardiography as a stress-imaging technique. Dipyridamole, as a pharmacologic stressor, is not affected by heart rate and may be particularly useful for patients who are unable to exercise.

V-62.   The answer is C. *(Chap. 239)*   Myoglobin is released from ischemic myocardial cells and appears in serum within hours. It has a very short half-life in serum as it is excreted rapidly in the urine. Serum myoglobin returns to normal within 24 h after an infarction. Therefore, in this patient a new elevation of myoglobin would be helpful in distinguishing new myocardial necrosis. Troponin-I and troponin-T are more specific markers of myocardial necrosis but have a long half-life in the circulation. They may remain elevated for over a week after an acute MI. Therefore, they are not as useful for detecting new or recurrent injury. In the presence of a preexisting left bundle branch ECG is of limited utility in detecting new ischemia. Serial echocardiograms may detect new wall motion abnormalities that suggest new ischemia or infarction, but in the absence of a prior study a single echocardiogram would have limited utility in this patient.

V-63.   The answer is B. *(Chap. 242)*   Aortitis is an uncommon cause of an ascending aortic aneurysm and commonly presents with fevers and chest pain. Malaise and weight loss may also occur in association with underlying rheumatic disease. Physical examination frequently reveals evidence of aortic regurgitation. All of the listed choices can cause aortitis. However, giant cell arteritis almost never occurs in individuals <50 years of age (*SM Levine, DB Hellmann: Curr Opin Rheumatol 14:3, 2002*).

V-64.   The answer is D. *(Chaps. 221 and e19)*   This ECG shows ST-segment elevation in all leads except for aV_L, aV_R and V_1. There is PR depression in the inferior leads and PR elevation in aV_R, consistent with acute pericarditis. Acute pericarditis can be due to infectious, neoplastic, autoimmune, cardiac, metabolic, or pharmacologic events. Most often, a causal factor is not identified. The ECG in acute pericarditis evolves through four stages. In stage 1 (hours to days), there are diffuse ST-segment elevations and PR-segment depressions. Stage 2 is characterized by normalization of the ST and PR segments. In stage 3, there are diffuse T-wave inversions. In stage 4, the tracing may become normal or the T-wave inversions may persist. Proximal main coronary artery occlusion can manifest as diffuse ST-segment elevations; however, PR-segment depression is highly specific for acute pericarditis. The echocardiogram will show a small to moderate amount of pericardial effusion with normal left ventricular function. Focal ST-segment elevations consistent with acute myocardial infarction would correlate with focal hypokinesis on echocardiography. This ECG does not meet any criteria for left ventricular hypertrophy. There are no pacemaker lead depolarizations or right bundle branch block, which might suggest a catheter irritating the right ventricular myocardium.

V-65.   The answer is E. *(Chap. 221)*   The ECG shows a junctional rhythm with an atrioventricular (AV) block and ST-segment elevation in leads II, III, and aVF. There are also reciprocal changes in I and aVL. These changes are consistent with an acute inferior wall myocardial infarction. The ECG is more useful in localizing regions of ischemia in ST elevation than in non-ST elevation MI. Anteroseptal ischemia causes changes in V_1–V_3 and apical/lateral ischemia in V_4–V_6. The right coronary artery (RCA) generally supplies blood flow to the right ventricle and the AV node. The inferior-posterior region of the left ventricle is supplied by the right coronary artery or the left circumflex coronary artery. In approximately 60 to 70% of people it is supplied by the RCA (right dominant). In this case the presence of AV nodal dysfunction and inferior ischemia makes disease of the RCA most likely.

V-66.   The answer is B. *(Chap. 238)*   Patients with unstable angina/non-ST-segment elevation myocardial infarction (UA/NSTEMI) exhibit a wide spectrum of risk of death, MI, or urgent revascularization. Risk stratification tools such as the TIMI risk score are useful for identifying patients who benefit from an early invasive strategy and those who are best suited for a more conservative approach. The TIMI risk score is composed of seven independent risk factors: Age ≥65, three or more cardiovascular risk factors, prior stenosis >50%, ST-segment deviation ≥0.5mm, two or more anginal events in <24 h, aspirin usage in the past 7 days, and elevated cardiac markers. Aspirin resistance can occur in 5–10% of patients and is more common among those taking lower doses of aspirin. Having unstable angina despite aspirin usage suggests aspirin resistance. Use of a beta-agonist and a diuretic do not confer an independent risk for death, MI, or need for urgent revascularization.

V-67.   The answer is E. *(Chap. 231)*   A common diagnostic dilemma is differentiating constrictive pericarditis from a restrictive cardiomyopathy. Elevated jugular venous pressure is almost universally present in both. Kussmaul's sign (increase in or no change in jugular venous pressure with inspiration) can be seen in both conditions. Other signs of heart failure do not reliably distinguish the two conditions. In restrictive cardiomyopathy, the apical impulse is usually easier to palpate than in constrictive pericarditis and mitral regurgitation is more common. These clinical signs, however, are not reliable to differentiate the two entities. In conjunction with clinical information and additional imaging studies of the left ventricle and pericardium, certain pathognomic findings increase diagnostic certainty. A thickened or calcified pericardium increases the likelihood of constrictive pericarditis. Conduction abnormalities are more common in infiltrating diseases of the myocardium. In constrictive pericarditis, measurements of diastolic pressures will show equilibrium between the ventricles, while unequal pressures and/or isolated elevated left ventricular pressures are more consistent with restrictive cardiomyopathy. The classic "square root sign" during right heart catheterization (deep, sharp drop in right ventricular pressure in early diastole, followed by a plateau during which there is no further increase in right ventricular pressure) can be seen in both restrictive cardiomyopathy and constrictive pericarditis. The presence of a paraprotein abnormality (MGUS, myeloma, amyloid) makes restrictive cardiomyopathy more common.

V-68.   The answer is A. *(Chaps. 221 and e19)*   This ECG demonstrates marked ST-segment elevations in the inferior leads (II, III, aV_F) and laterally (V_6) as well as prominent ST-segment depressions with upright T waves in V_1–V_4 consistent with an acute posterior and anterolateral myocardial infarction (MI). The 12-lead ECG is most useful for detecting infarctions in the inferior, lateral, and anterior walls of the left ventricle. As 40% of patients with inferior wall infarctions have right ventricular or posterior wall involvement, additional testing is recommended in the acute care of patients with inferior MIs. The addition of right ventricular leads (V_4R, V_5R, V_6R) and posterior leads (V_7, V_8, V_9) improves both sensitivity and specificity for detecting infarctions in these territories. Although posterior infarctions predispose a patient to high-grade AV block, a specific rhythm strip analysis is not indicated. These patients should be monitored on telemetry. Chest radiography and CT scanning are not routinely obtained when a patient has an acute MI. Unnecessary testing will delay the time to reperfusion therapy, which has a direct impact on mortality and morbidity. Pericarditis may cause diffuse ST-segment elevation but not focal changes as described above.

V-69.   The answer is F. *(Chap. 230)* Tricuspid regurgitation is most commonly caused by dilation of the tricuspid annulus due to right-ventricular enlargement of any cause. Any cause of left-ventricular failure that results in right-ventricular failure may lead to tricuspid regurgitation. Congenital heart diseases or pulmonary arterial hypertension leading to right-ventricular failure will dilate the tricuspid annulus. Inferior wall infarction may involve the right ventricle. Rheumatic heart disease may involve the tricuspid valve, although less commonly than the mitral valve. Infective endocarditis, particularly in IV drug users, will infect the tricuspid valve, causing vegetations and regurgitation. Other causes of tricuspid regurgitation include carcinoid heart disease, endomyocardial fibrosis, congenital defects of the atrioventricular canal, and right-ventricular pacemakers.

V-70.   The answer is A. *(Chap. 229)* Given the young age of this patient, bicuspid aortic valve is the most likely cause of aortic stenosis. Bicuspid aortic valve is one of the most common abnormalities of the circulatory system, affecting 1–2% of the population. For unknown reasons, males are twice as likely as females to have a bicuspid aortic valve. Bicuspid aortic valves often are undetected until symptomatic aortic stenosis develops. This most commonly occurs between the fourth and fifth decades of life. Congenital aortic stenosis would be expected to present earlier in life. A murmur is often present from birth and requires valvular replacement before adulthood. Calcific aortic stenosis is the most common cause of aortic stenosis and most commonly presents in the seventh or eighth decade. Rheumatic heart disease as a result of rheumatic fever is also commonly associated with aortic valve disease. The age of presentation of rheumatic heart disease falls between that of bicuspid aortic valve and calcific aortic stenosis, usually around the sixth or seventh decade.

V-71.   The answer is E. *(Chap. 228)* Cardiac transplantation was first performed in 1967 and since the 1990s, about 4000 cardiac transplants are performed yearly worldwide. Approximately 2200 of these are performed in the United States. Severe heart failure with refractory symptoms is the main indication for cardiac transplantation and may be caused by a variety of underlying diseases. In general, cardiac transplantation is reserved for younger individuals without significant comorbidities. The patients given highest priority for transplant are those requiring vasopressor support with concomitant use of a pulmonary artery catheter or those requiring mechanical circulatory support. Individuals requiring vasopressor support managed without pulmonary artery catheter are given second highest priority. All other transplants are determined by a variety of factors including time on waiting list, immune sensitization, and ABO blood type. Following transplantation, individuals largely have good outcomes. One-year survival is 83%, and 76% survive >3 years. The average "half-life" of a cardiac transplant is 9.3 years. More than 90% of individuals return to good functional status. Acute rejection and infection are the commonest causes of early transplant failure and death. Most programs perform routine endomyocardial biopsies to detect rejection for a period of 5 years after transplant. Mortality that occurs >1 year after transplant is most likely related to coronary artery disease, which is accelerated posttransplant due to immunosuppression.

V-72.   The answer is D. *(Chap. 236)* According to the NCEP:ATP III guidelines, treating the dyslipidemia of the metabolic syndrome should first be directed towards LDL cholesterol goals (usually <100 mg/dL, depending on the presence of risk factors). If triglyceride levels are ≥200 mg/dL after the LDL goal is reached, the clinician should set a secondary goal for non-high-density lipoprotein cholesterol 30 points higher than the LDL goal. When triglyceride levels are between 200 and 499 mg/dL, options include nicotinic acid, a fibrate, or intensifying therapy with an HMG-CoA reductase inhibitor (statin). Average efficacy of these drug classes are as follows: nicotinic acid, 20–40%; fibrate, 35–50%; statin, 7–30%). Cholestyramine and colestipole are bile acid sequestrants. They lower cholesterol but often increase triglyceride levels and should not be used in patients with triglycerides >200 mg/dL. The effects of ezetimibe on hypertriglyceridemia are not well established. Nicotinic acid is effective for treating hypertriglyceridemia but may worsen glucose control and therefore should be used cautiously in patients with the metabolic syndrome. Gemfibrozil is more likely to worsen statin myopathy than fenofibrate.

V-73. **The answer is D.** *(Chap. 237)* The use of PCI with stenting relieves angina better than best medical therapy, but the salutary effects on coronary death or MI are not well established. In a recent large clinical trial (COURAGE trial) of patients with stable coronary artery disease, death rates with medical therapy were equivalent to death rates with PCI at 4 years of follow-up. Balloon angioplasty reocclusion rates are up to two times higher compared to restenosis with stenting. This type of restenosis is mediated by hyperproliferation of smooth muscle cells into the intima as they react to the vascular injury induced by the balloon angioplasty. However, due to the delayed endothelial healing that is achieved with drug-eluting stents, the patient is exposed to a higher risk of subacute in-stent restenosis. This type of restenosis is mediated by thrombus formation as the denuded endothelium is exposed to the circulation. Patients with left-main coronary occlusion, three-vessel disease, two-vessel disease including the left main, impaired left ventricular function, or diabetes should be considered for CABG.

V-74. **The answer is D.** *(Chaps. 221 and e21)* This ECG shows an example of the hereditary long-QT syndrome. There is a wide range of abnormal rate-corrected QT interval values, ranging from 400–640 ms. A $QT_c \geq 600$ ms is associated with greater risk for cardiac events, but only a minority of patients have this degree of QT prolongation. T-wave notching, or "humps," may be common in asymptomatic patients and are of prognostic importance. Avoiding life-threatening drug interactions is important when managing a patient with hereditary long-QT syndrome. Of the choices above, only methadone is known to prolong the QT interval, and it should be avoided in patients with hereditary long-QT syndrome.

V-75. **The answer is B.** *(Chap. 238)* Unstable angina is defined as angina or ischemic discomfort with at least one of three factors: pain at rest lasting >10 min, severe recent pain (within 4–6 weeks), or crescendo angina. NSTEMI is diagnosed when a patient with unstable angina has positive cardiac biomarkers. Anti-ischemic therapy (nitrates, beta blockers) is important for symptom relief and to prevent recurrence of chest pain. Antithrombotic therapy is directed against the platelet aggregation at the site of the ruptured plaque. Initially, this therapy should consist of aspirin. Addition of clopidogrel confers an additional 20% risk reduction in both low- and high-risk NSTEMI patients, as demonstrated in the CURE trial. Continuation of treatment for up to 12 months confers additional benefit in patients treated conservatively and among those who underwent percutaneous coronary intervention. The glycoprotein IIb/IIIa inhibitors are usually reserved for high-risk (i.e., troponin-positive) patients and may not be beneficial for patients treated conservatively. Statin therapy is important for secondary prevention; however, spironolactone is not a first-line therapy for NSTEMI.

V-76. **The answer is A.** *(Chap. 230)* Bioprosthetic valves are made from human, porcine, or bovine tissue. The major advantage of a bioprosthetic valve is the low incidence of thromboembolic phenomena, particularly 3 months after implantation. Although in the immediate postoperative period some anticoagulation may occur, after 3 months there is no further need for anticoagulation or monitoring. The downside is the natural history and longevity of the bioprosthetic valve. Bioprosthetic valves tend to degenerate mechanically. Approximately 50% will need replacement at 15 years. Therefore, these valves are useful in patients with contraindications to anticoagulation, such as elderly patients with comorbidities and younger patients who desire to become pregnant. Elderly people may also be spared the need for repeat surgery as their life span may be shorter than the natural history of the bioprosthesis. Mechanical valves offer superior durability. Hemodynamic parameters are improved with double-disk valves compared with single-disk or ball-and-chain valves. However, thrombogenicity is high and chronic anticoagulation is mandatory. Younger patients with no contraindications to anticoagulation may be better served by mechanical valve replacement.

V-77. **The answer is A.** *(Chap. 229)* This patient is presenting with Eisenmenger's syndrome. This designation is applied to patients with communications between the right and left circulations, pulmonary hypertension, and a predominantly right-to-left shunt. Eisenmenger's syndrome can develop in patients with communication at the atrial, ventricular, or aortopulmonary level. These shunts are initially left to right and therefore do not present with cyanosis. Pulmonary hypertension develops over years as a result of increased pulmonary flow, increased vascular tone, and erythrocytosis. Cyanosis develops when the pulmonary hypertension becomes so severe that it reverses the shunt. Atrial septal defects are most common in adults presenting with Eisenmenger's syndrome. This patient had no evidence of pulmonary hypertension or cyanosis 10 years ago. Ebstein's anomaly, tetralogy of Fallot, and truncus arteriosis all cause cyanosis.

V-78.   The answer is C. *(Chap. 223)*   The pulmonary capillary wedge tracing shows a large *v* wave at rest that substantially increases during exercise. This is a finding seen with mitral regurgitation. In this patient, the mitral regurgitation worsened during exercise and was due to occult coronary artery disease. The patient's dyspnea improved with following angioplasty and stenting of the left circumflex artery. The pulmonary capillary wedge pressure reflects the left-ventricular end-diastolic pressure in the absence of mitral stenosis or pulmonary venous hypertension. In mitral stenosis, there is a significant drop between left-atrial and left-ventricular diastolic pressures and elevation of the pulmonary capillary wedge pressure. Pulmonary arterial hypertension would have a normal pulmonary capillary wedge pressure but an elevated pulmonary artery mean pressure, which is not shown in these tracings. In aortic stenosis, the pulmonary capillary wedge pressure may be elevated if heart failure is present, but no abnormal wave forms would be expected. Congestive heart failure causes an elevated pulmonary capillary wedge pressure, which is not present here. The large *v* waves of mitral regurgitation should not be read as the pulmonary capillary wedge pressure.

V-79 and V-80.   The answers are D and E. *(Chap. 241)*   This patient presents at a young age with hypertension that is difficult to control, raising the question of secondary causes of hypertension. The most likely diagnosis in this patient is primary hyperaldosteronism, also known as Conn's syndrome. The patient has no physical features that suggest congenital adrenal hyperplasia or Cushing's syndrome. In addition, there is no glucose intolerance as is commonly seen in Cushing's syndrome. The lack of episodic symptoms and the labile hypertension make pheochromocytoma unlikely. The findings of hypokalemia and metabolic alkalosis in the presence of difficult to control hypertension yield the likely diagnosis of Conn's syndrome. Diagnosis of the disease can be difficult, but the preferred test is the plasma aldosterone/renin ratio. This test should be performed at 8 A.M., and a ratio above 30 to 50 is diagnostic of primary hyperaldosteronism. Caution should be made in interpreting this test while the patient is on ACE inhibitor therapy as ACE inhibitors can falsely elevate plasma renin activity. However, a plasma renin level that is undetectable or an elevated aldosterone/renin ratio in the presence of an ACE inhibitor therapy is highly suggestive of primary hyperaldosteronism. Selective adrenal vein renin sampling may be performed after the diagnosis to help determine if the process is unilateral or bilateral. Although fibromuscular dysplasia is a common secondary cause of hypertension in young females, the presence of hypokalemia and metabolic alkalosis should suggest Conn's syndrome. Thus, magnetic resonance imaging of the renal arteries is unnecessary in this case. Measurement of 24-h urine collection for potassium wasting and aldosterone secretion can be useful in the diagnosis of Conn's syndrome. The measurement of metanephrines or cortisol is not indicated.

V-81.   The answer is D. *(Chap. 231)*   Cardiac involvement is common in many of the neuromuscular diseases. The ECG pattern of Duchenne's muscular dystrophy is unique and consists of tall R waves in the right precordial leads with an R/S ratio >1.0, often with deep Q waves in the limb and precordial leads. These patients often have a variety of supraventricular and ventricular arrhythmias and are at risk for sudden death due to the intrinsic cardiomyopathy as well as the low ejection fraction. Implantable cardioverter defibrillators should be considered in the appropriate patient. Global left ventricular dysfunction is a common finding in dilated cardiomyopathies, whereas focal wall motion abnormalities and angina are more common if there is ischemic myocardium. This patient is at risk for venous thromboembolism; however, chronic thromboembolism would not account for the severity of the left heart failure and would present with findings consistent with pulmonary hypertension. Amyotrophic lateral sclerosis is a disease of motor neurons and does not involve the heart. This patient would be young for that diagnosis. An advanced atrial septal defect would present with cyanosis and heart failure (Eisenmenger's physiology).

V-82. **The answer is A.** *(Chap. 220)* Splitting of the second heart sound normally occurs during inspiration when there is increased venous return to the right ventricle that increases its stroke volume and delays closure of the pulmonic valve. During inspiration, it is normal to hear the closing of the aortic valve (A_2) before the closing of the pulmonic valve (P_2). A fixed split of the second heart sound occurs in the setting of an atrial septal defect. With this congenital heart defect, the volume of blood that is shunted from the left atrium to the right atrium results in a stable right-ventricular stroke volume. Thus, there is no difference between inspiration and expiration, resulting in a fixed split of the second heart sound.

V-83. **The answer is D.** *(Chap. 230)* As described by LaPlace's law ($S = Pr/h$; where $S =$ wall stress, $P =$ pressure, $r =$ radius, $h =$ wall thickness), the initial effect of left-ventricular hypertrophy is to reduce or maintain wall stress as the intraventricular pressures increase. Initially, the hypertrophy is adaptive, but eventually the ventricle fails. Reasons for this failure are multifactorial. Thickened myocardium increases back pressure in the coronary circulation thereby reducing coronary perfusion, leading to ischemia. In addition, diastolic pressures are lower when there is severe aortic regurgitation, which further decreases coronary perfusion. Myocardial oxygen consumption increases when there is ventricular hypertrophy as a result of increased mass and contractility. In chronic aortic regurgitation, the equilibration of end-diastolic left-ventricular and aortic pressures exacerbates left-ventricular remodeling and will cause premature closure of the mitral valve or functional mitral regurgitation.

V-84. **The answer is D.** *(Chap. 230)* Mild mitral stenosis may be followed yearly unless there has been systemic embolization or severe pulmonary hypertension has developed (pulmonary arterial pressure >50 mmHg at rest or >60 mmHg with exercise). Diagnosing paroxysmal atrial fibrillation with a 24-h monitor is an option if there is no evidence of pulmonary hypertension. There is no evidence that percutaneous or surgical repair of mitral stenosis is beneficial for slight or no functional impairment. Coronary assessment with CT, stress test, or arteriogram is not usually necessary in males <45 years or females <55 years without a significant risk factor profile or unless symptoms are suggestive of coronary artery disease.

V-85. **The answer is E.** *(Chap. 236)* The most accepted hypothesis to describe the pathophysiology of the metabolic syndrome involves an overabundance of free fatty acids and ensuing insulin resistance. Insulin resistance is thought to be a mediator of many of the other aspects of the metabolic syndrome, including hypertension and hyperglycemia. Free fatty acids are derived mainly from adipose tissue. Increases in visceral obesity are thought to be more harmful than subcutaneous stores because of the direct effect of free fatty acids on the liver from the visceral stores. The inflammatory milieu of the metabolic syndrome is enhanced by the overproduction of the proinflammatory cytokines by the expanded adipose tissue. Treating hypertension, hyperglycemia, dyslipidemia, and the oxidative stress of the proinflammatory state is important when treating metabolic syndrome. However, adipose tissue loss is the primary approach to treating the underlying cause of the disorder.

V-86. **The answer is F.** *(Chap. 220)* When a murmur of uncertain cause is identified on physical examination, a variety of physiologic maneuvers can be used to assist in the elucidation of the cause. Commonly used physiologic maneuvers include change with respiration, Valsalva maneuver, position, and exercise. In hypertrophic cardiomyopathy, there is asymmetric hypertrophy of the interventricular septum, which creates a dynamic outflow obstruction. Maneuvers that decrease left-ventricular filling will cause an increase in the intensity of the murmur, whereas those that increase left-ventricular filling will cause a decrease in the murmur. Of the interventions listed, both standing and a Valsalva maneuver will decrease venous return and subsequently decrease left ventricular filling, resulting in an increase in the loudness of the murmur of hypertrophic cardiomyopathy. Alternatively, squatting increases venous return and thus decreases the murmur. Maximum handgrip exercise also results in a decreased loudness of the murmur.

V-87.   The answer is C. *(Chap. e8)* Causes of mid-systolic murmurs include aortic stenosis, aortic sclerosis, hypertrophic cardiomyopathy (HOCM), coarctation of the aorta, and pulmonary valve stenosis. In the obstructive form of HOCM, maneuvers that increase the amount of outflow obstruction will increase the intensity of the murmur. Outflow obstruction is increased by decreasing preload, which occurs in standing, performing a Valsalva maneuver, or with the administration of vasodilators. Increasing preload by squatting or passive leg raise will lead to reduction of outflow tract obstruction and a diminished murmur. The murmur of HOCM will also decrease with increasing afterload (vasopressors) or decreasing contractility (beta blockers). The murmur of aortic stenosis is typically in the right second intercostal space and radiates to the carotids. Valsalva maneuver will classically lead to a decreased aortic stenosis murmur. The murmur of congenital pulmonic stenosis is in the right second intercostal space. There is often a parasternal lift. Mitral valve prolapse causes a late systolic murmur usually introduced by an ejection click. It does not cause a crescendo-decrescendo murmur. Chronic mitral regurgitation causes a holosystolic murmur that radiates to the apex.

V-88.   The answer is B. *(Chap. 219)* Cardiovascular disease is the leading cause of death in the United States. Many patients have undiagnosed cardiovascular disease and therefore are at unsuspected risk for perioperative cardiac morbidity, defined as perioperative MI, pulmonary edema, or ventricular tachycardia. Multivariable analysis first proposed by Goldman and colleagues identified several risk factors, including age over 70 years, an MI within the last 6 months, evidence of aortic stenosis or pulmonary edema on exam, and abnormalities within the electrocardiogram or laboratory analysis, as well as the type of surgical procedure being performed, with an emergency surgery being more highly associated with complication risk. In this patient the only risk is age over 70 years. The presence of two to three PVCs per minute is within the normal range. His hypertension, hypercholesterolemia, and diabetes mellitus, although significant, were not identified as independent risk factors. Therefore, this patient's risk of serious complication is ~0.6%.

V-89.   The answer is C. *(Chap. 22)* Although ventricular tachycardia is classically associated with ischemic heart disease, in which scarred myocardium provides a substrate for reentrant tachyarrhythmias, other cardiac lesions put a patient at risk for ventricular tachycardia. Notably, hypertrophic obstructive cardiomyopathy, aortic stenosis, and long QT syndrome carry an increased risk for ventricular tachycardia. Atrial myxoma, which can cause syncope by obstructing blood flow with resultant decreased cardiac output, is not associated with ventricular tachycardia.

V-90 and V-91.   The answers are A and D. *(Chaps. 335 and 337)* The scenario describes a young patient with severe hypertension and should prompt consideration of secondary causes of hypertension. The episodic symptoms and orthostasis despite marked hypertension are suggestive of pheochromocytoma. Thus, the most appropriate management of this patient should include an α-adrenergic receptor blocker. Phentolamine and nitroprusside are two agents that can be used intravenously in the setting of hypertensive crises. This patient should be managed as such as she has evidence of increased intracranial pressure on ophthalmologic examination. An oral α-adrenergic blocker is available in the form of phenoxybenzamine. The diagnosis of pheochromocytoma is best made by 24-h urine collection for metanephrines and vanillylmandelic acid. Plasma catecholamines are elevated in patients with pheochromocytoma, but the routine measurement of these levels for diagnosis is confounded by the wide variation in levels associated with various stressors. If plasma catecholamines are to be used, the levels must be drawn with the patient at rest for at least 30 minutes and drawn through an indwelling intravenous catheter. False-positive results are common. Abdominal CT imaging can also be adjunctive to assess for an adrenal or periaortic mass associated with pheochromocytoma but is not diagnostic without concurrent demonstration of elevated catecholamines. Measurement of 5-HIAA and renin levels is done for diagnosis of carcinoid syndrome and primary hyperaldosteronism, respectively.

V-92. **The answer is D.** *(Chap. 219)* Cardiovascular disease remains the top cause of death in the United States and is responsible for 40% of all deaths. Cardiovascular disease is more prevalent with age, affecting only 5% at age 20 with a rise to 75% at age >75 years. Although age-adjusted death rates for cardiovascular disease have declined by two-thirds since 1965, the actual number of hospitalizations for cardiovascular disease and congestive heart failure are increasing as more individuals are surviving an initial heart attack to live with chronic cardiovascular disease and heart failure. The absolute number of deaths in men due to cardiovascular disease is falling. However, in women, this number continues to rise. In 2002, it was estimated by the American Heart Association that 32 million women and 30 million men had cardiovascular disease. Heart disease is responsible for 43% of deaths in females and 37% of deaths in males. Cardiovascular disease in women is more likely to present atypically without chest pain and is also more likely to be due to dysfunction of the microcirculation and thus less amenable to current interventional therapies.

V-93 and V-94. **The answers are C and C.** *(Chap. 226)* The patient's rhythm is torsade de pointes, with polymorphic ventricular tachycardia and QRS complexes with variations in amplitude and cycle length giving the appearance of oscillation about an axis. Torsades de pointes is associated with a prolonged QT interval; thus, anything that is associated with a prolonged QT can potentially cause torsade. Most commonly, electrolyte disturbances such as hypokalemia and hypomagnesemia, phenothiazines, fluoroquinolones, antiarrhythmic drugs, tricyclic antidepressants, intracranial events, and bradyarrhythmias are associated with this malignant arrhythmia. Management, besides stabilization, which may require electrical cardioversion, consists of removing the offending agent. In addition, success in rhythm termination or prevention has been reported with the administration of magnesium as well as overdrive atrial or ventricular pacing, which will shorten the QT interval. Beta blockers are indicated for patients with congenital long QT syndrome but are not indicated in this patient.

V-95. **The answer is E.** *(Chap. 238)* Standard therapy for a patient with unstable angina or non-ST-segment elevation myocardial infarction (NSTEMI) includes aspirin and clopidogrel. If an anticoagulant is added, enoxaparin has been shown to be superior to unfractionated heparin in reducing recurrent cardiac events. Glycoprotein IIb/IIIa inhibitors have also been shown to be beneficial in treating unstable angina/NSTEMI. Eptifibatide, tirofiban, and abciximab are beneficial for patients likely to receive percutaneous intervention. Clinical trials have shown benefit of early invasive strategy in the presence of high-risk factors such as recurrent rest angina, elevated troponin, new ST-segment depression, congestive heart failure symptoms, rales, mitral regurgitation, positive stress test, ejection fraction < 0.40, decreased blood pressure, sustained ventricular tachycardia, or recent coronary intervention. The presence of ST depressions, rales, and mitral regurgitation puts this patient at high risk. Tissue plasminogen factor is beneficial in ST-segment elevation myocardial infarction, not NSTEMI.

V-96. **The answer is A.** *(Chap. 242)* Ascending aortic dissections require surgical intervention, whereas descending aortic dissections that are uncomplicated may be managed medically. Indications for intervention for descending dissections acutely include occlusion of a major aortic branch with symptoms. For example, paralysis may occur with occlusion of the spinal artery or worsening renal failure may occur in the case of dissection that involves the renal arteries. Once a descending dissection has been found, intensive medical management of blood pressure is imperative and should include agents that decrease cardiac contractility and aortic shear force. Follow-up with CT or MRI imaging every 6 to 12 months is recommended, and surgical intervention should be considered if there is continued advancement despite medical therapy. Finally, patients with Marfan's syndrome have increased complications with descending dissections and should be considered for surgical repair, especially if there is concomitant disease in the ascending aorta as demonstrated by aortic root dilation to greater than 50 mm.

V-97. **The answer is B.** *(Chaps. 221 and e21)* This ECG tracing shows multifocal atrial tachycardia (MAT), right atrial overload, a superior axis, and poor R-wave progression in the precordial leads. There are varying P-wave morphologies (more than three morphologies) and P-P intervals. MAT is most commonly caused by COPD, but other conditions associated with this arrhythmia include coronary artery disease, congestive heart failure, valvular heart disease, diabetes mellitus, hypokalemia, hypomagnesemia, azotemia, postoperative state, and pulmonary embolism. Anemia, pain, and myocardial ischemia are also causes of tachycardia that should be considered when managing a new tachycardia. These states are usually associated with sinus tachycardia.

V-98. **The answer is B.** *(Chap. 226; Camm and Garratt, 1991.)* Adenosine is currently approved for the termination of paroxysmal supraventricular tachycardias at a dose of 6 mg or, if 6 mg fails, 12 mg. The primary mechanism of adenosine is to decrease conduction velocity through the atrioventricular (AV) node. Thus, it is an ideal drug for acute termination of regular reentrant supraventricular tachycardia involving the AV node. Side effects may include chest discomfort and transient hypotension. The half-life is extremely short, and the side effects tend to be brief. Patients with wide complex tachycardia suggestive of ventricular tachycardia or known preexcitation syndrome should be treated with agents that decrease automaticity, such as quinidine and procainamide. However, in patients with apparent ventricular tachycardia who have neither a history of ischemic heart disease nor preexcitation syndrome, adenosine may be a useful diagnostic agent to determine whether a patient has a reentrant tachycardia, in which case the drug may terminate it; an atrial tachycardia, in which case the atrial activity may be unmasked; or a true, preexcited tachycardia, in which case adenosine will have no effect. Although adenosine is not the recommended primary therapy for patients with wide complex tachyarrhythmia, patients with junctional tachycardia who have evidence of poor ventricular function or concomitant β-adrenergic blockade may be reasonable candidates for its use.

V-99. **The answer is E.** *(Chap. 242)* Descending aortic aneurysms are most commonly associated with atherosclerosis. The average growth rate is ~0.1–0.2 cm yearly. The risk of rupture and subsequent management are related to the size of the aneurysm as well as symptoms related to the aneurysm. However, most thoracic aortic aneurysms are asymptomatic. When symptoms do occur, they are frequently related to mechanical complications of the aneurysm causing compression of adjacent structures. This includes the trachea and esophagus, and symptoms can include cough, chest pain, hoarseness, and dysphagia. The risk of rupture is ~2–3% yearly for aneurysms <4 cm and rises to 7% per year once the size is greater than >6 cm. Management of descending aortic aneurysms includes blood pressure control. Beta blockers are recommended because they decrease contractility of the heart and thus decrease aortic wall stress, potentially slowing aneurysmal growth. Individuals with thoracic aortic aneurysms should be monitored with chest imaging at least yearly, or sooner if new symptoms develop. This can include CT angiography, MRI, or transesophageal echocardiography. Operative repair is indicated if the aneurysm expands by >1 cm in a year or reaches a diameter of >5.5–6.0 cm. Endovascular stenting for the treatment of thoracic aortic aneurysms is a relatively new procedure with limited long-term results available. The largest study to date included >400 patients with a variety of indications for thoracic endovascular stents. In 249 patients, the indication for stent was thoracic aortic aneurysm. This study showed an initial success rate of 87.1%, with a 30-day mortality rate of 10%. However, if the procedure was done emergently, the mortality rate at 30 days was 28%. At 1 year, data were available on only 96 of the original 249 patients with degenerative thoracic aneurysms. In these individuals, 80% continued to have satisfactory outcomes with stenting and 14% showed growth of the aneurysm *(LJ Leurs, J Vasc Surg 40:670, 2004)*. Ongoing studies with long-term follow-up are needed before endovascular stenting can be recommended for the treatment of thoracic aortic aneurysms, although in individuals who are not candidates for surgery, stenting should be considered.

V-100. **The answer is C.** *(Chap. 225)* The atrioventricular node is supplied by the posterior descending coronary artery in 90% of the population. Furthermore, this artery in the majority of the population arises from the right coronary artery. Thus, a patient who presents as this one does with symptoms consistent with an acute coronary syndrome and who has a Mobitz type II second-degree block probably has significant ischemia in the right coronary artery. Right coronary artery transmural infarct is manifest most commonly by ST elevation in II, III, and aVF. Wellen's T waves are deep symmetric T-wave inversions that are seen in either significant left main coronary artery stenosis or proximal left anterior descending artery stenosis.

V-101. **The answer is C.** *(Chap. 232)* The presentation of this patient is one of acute pericarditis. Acute pericarditis is the most common disease of the pericardium and typically presents as a sharp, intense anterior chest pain. It may be referred to the neck, arms, or left shoulder and may be pleuritic in nature. The positional nature of the pain is characteristic in acute pericarditis. The pain is worse with lying supine and improved with sitting up and leaning forward. A pericardial friction rub is present in 85% of cases of acute pericarditis. A pericardial friction rub is described as high-pitched, grating, or scratching and is heard throughout the cardiac cycle. The ECG, shown here, classically shows elevation of the ST segment in the limb leads and V_2–V_6 with reciprocal depression of the ST segment in aV_R and sometimes V_1. In addition, the PR segment is depressed in all leads except aV_R and V_1, where it may be elevated. Mild elevations in cardiac enzymes may be seen. An echocardiogram should be performed if there is suspicion of a possible effusion. Treatment of acute pericarditis involves rest and anti-inflammatory treatment. Aspirin or nonsteroidal anti-inflammatory drugs in high doses are most commonly used. Alternative treatments include colchicine, glucocorticoids, and intravenous immunoglobulin (IVIg). IVIg is indicated for pericarditis due to cytomegalovirus, adenovirus, or parvovirus. As this patient is in severe pain, reassurance only is not the best option but would be a possible treatment if panic attack were suspected. The other choices are utilized in the case of unstable angina and acute myocardial infarction and should not be utilized in this patient. Both heparin and reteplase would increase the risk of developing a hemorrhagic pericardial effusion. Cardiac catheterization is an unnecessary procedure.

V-102. **The answer is C.** *(Chap. 223)* Commotio cordis occurs due to a blunt force injury to the chest wall that results in an often fatal arrhythmia, most frequently ventricular fibrillation. While all of the diagnoses listed are causes of sudden cardiac death in young individuals, commotio cordis is the likely diagnosis because of the occurrence of the injury in relation to blunt trauma to the chest wall. In contrast to cardiac contusion (contusion cordis), the force of the injury is insufficient to cause cardiac contusion or injury to the ribs or chest wall. All of the other choices would result in abnormalities in the ECG, and a family history of sudden cardiac death is frequent.

In animal studies, commotio cordis has been found to occur when the blunt force is applied at 20–50 mph and only during specific timing within the cardiac cycle (*C Madias et al: J Cardiovasc Electrophysiol 18:115, 2007; MS Link et al: N Engl J Med 338:1805, 1998*). If the force were delivered during the upstroke of the T wave (10–30 msec before the peak), ventricular fibrillation would frequently result. If the force were applied during the QRS (depolarization), transient complete heart block might occur (*MS Link et al: N Engl J Med 338:1805, 1998*). In reported case series, the survival of commotio cordis is only 15%. Defibrillation is most successful if applied within 3 min.

V-103. **The answer is C.** *(Chap. 231)* This patient's murmur is due to hypertrophic cardiomyopathy (HCM). A normal S_2, the location of the murmur, the absence of radiation to the neck, and being loudest at the lower left sternal border make aortic sclerosis or aortic stenosis less likely. These murmurs are usually heard best in the second right intercostal space. Maneuvers such as going from standing to squatting and passively raising the legs decrease the gradient across the outflow tract and intensity of the murmur due to increased preload. Amyl nitrate causes a decrease in systemic vascular resistance and arterial pressure. The murmur of HCM increases in intensity while there is less regurgitation across the mitral valve and the murmur of mitral regurgitation gets softer. Right-sided murmurs, except for the pulmonic ejection "click" of pulmonary stenosis, usually increase in intensity during inspiration.

V-104. **The answer is C.** *(Chap. 236)* Reversing insulin resistance and hyperglycemia can be achieved by lifestyle modifications, metformin or other biguanide medications, and/or thiazolidinedione medications. Of the medications, only the thiazolidinediones improve insulin-mediated glucose uptake in the muscle and adipose tissue. The mechanism of action of metformin is uncertain, but it appears to work by reducing hepatic gluconeogenesis and intestinal absorption of glucose. In a large trial of lifestyle modifications and metformin in the prevention of diabetes (Diabetes Prevention Program), subjects in the lifestyle arm of the trial had a more significant reduction in the incidence of diabetes than those assigned to metformin. In resource-poor settings and the developing world, lifestyle modifications have also been shown to be more cost-effective than metformin for preventing diabetes.

V-105. **The answer is E.** *(Chap. 228)* Approximately 3000 heart transplants are performed each year in the United States. Generally the recipients do well, with survival rates of 76% at 3 years and an average transplant "half-life" of 9.3 years. However, certain complications are common with the necessary immunosuppression, including an increased risk of malignancy and infections. Additionally, patients are at risk of rejection of the transplanted organ that can be acute or chronic. Chronic cardiac transplant rejection manifests as coronary artery disease, with characteristic long, diffuse, and concentric stenosis seen on angiography. It is thought that these changes represent chronic rejection of the transplanted organ. The only definitive therapy is retransplantation. Bradyarrhythmias are not known to occur more frequently in transplant recipients.

V-106. **The answer is C.** *(Chap. 238)* Although this patient has positive cardiac biomarkers that could represent myocardial ischemia, in patients with an unclear history of angina, low levels of these biomarkers may not always indicate an acute coronary syndrome. Common alternative diagnoses in this setting include exacerbations of congestive heart failure, myocarditis, and pulmonary embolism. This patient has atypical features of his chest pain for angina: lasting for more than minutes at a time, nonexertional. In a young host, without other significant risk factors, atherosclerotic coronary artery disease would be less likely, especially if the history is atypical. Myocarditis is a diagnosis of exclusion; however, ST-segment elevations throughout the ECG with PR interval depressions suggest myocarditis. Esophageal spasm may mimic cardiac pain; however, it would not be expected to cause the described ECG abnormalities nor the positive cardiac biomarkers.

V-107. **The answer is E.** *(Chap. 235)* Although tight glycemic control clearly decreases the risk of the microvascular complications of diabetes (renal function, retinopathy), demonstration of a benefit for myocardial infarction or stroke is less compelling. However, other factors in the management of these patients have been shown to decrease risk. These factors include the use of HMG-CoA reductase inhibitors over all ranges of LDL cholesterol; gemfibrazil, particularly in patients with the metabolic syndrome; strict control of hypertension; and the use of an antihypertensive agent that inhibits the actions of angiotensin II, such as an ACE inhibitor or an angiotensin receptor blocker.

V-108. **The answer is E.** *(Chap. 220)* During normal inspiration there is a small, less than 10 mmHg decrease in systolic pressure. In several disease states, notably severe obstructive lung disease, pericardial tamponade, and superior vena cava obstruction, an accentuation of this normal finding can occur. Indeed, in the most pronounced cases the peripheral pulse may not be palpable during inspiration.

V-109. **The answer is D.** *(Chap. 232)* This patient's presentation and physical examination are most consistent with the diagnosis of constrictive pericarditis. The most common cause of constrictive pericarditis worldwide is tuberculosis, but given the low incidence of tuberculosis in the United States, constrictive pericarditis is a rare condition in this country. With the increasing ability to cure Hodgkin's disease with mediastinal irradiation, many cases of constrictive pericarditis in the United States are in patients who received curative radiation therapy 10–20 years prior. These patients are also at risk for premature coronary artery disease. Risks for these complications include dose of radiation and radiation windows that include the heart. Other rare causes of constrictive pericarditis are recurrent acute pericarditis, hemorrhagic pericarditis, prior cardiac surgery, mediastinal irradiation, chronic infection, and neoplastic disease. Physiologically, constrictive pericarditis is characterized by the inability of the ventricles to fill because of the noncompliant pericardium. In early diastole, the ventricles fill rapidly, but filling stops abruptly when the elastic limit of the pericardium is reached. Clinically, patients present with generalized malaise, cachexia, and anasarca. Exertional dyspnea is common, and orthopnea is generally mild. Ascites and hepatomegaly occur because of increased venous pressure. In rare cases, cirrhosis may develop from chronic congestive hepatopathy. The jugular venous pressure is elevated, and the neck veins fail to collapse on inspiration (Kussmaul's sign). Heart sounds may be muffled. A pericardial knock is frequently heard. This is a third heart-sound that occurs 0.09–0.12 s after aortic valve closure at the cardiac apex. Right heart catheterization would show the "square root sign" characterized by an abrupt y descent followed by a gradual rise in ventricular pressure. This finding, however, is not pathognomonic of constrictive pericarditis and can be seen in restrictive cardiomyopathy of any cause. Echocardiogram shows a thickened pericardium, dilatation of the inferior vena cava and hepatic veins, and an abrupt cessation of ventricular filling in early diastole. Pericardial resection is the only definitive treatment of constrictive pericarditis. Diuresis and sodium restriction are useful in managing volume status preoperatively, and paracentesis may be necessary. Operative mortality ranges from 5–10%. Underlying cardiac function is normal; thus, cardiac transplantation is not indicated. Pericardiocentesis is indicated for diagnostic removal of pericardial fluid and cardiac tamponade, which is not present on the patient's echocardiogram. Mitral valve stenosis may present similarly with anasarca, congestive hepatic failure, and ascites. However, pulmonary edema and pleural effusions are also common. Examination would be expected to demonstrate a diastolic murmur, and echocardiogram should show a normal pericardium and a thickened immobile mitral valve. Mitral valve replacement would be indicated if mitral stenosis were the cause of the patient's symptoms.

V-110. **The answer is A.** *(Chap. 266)* This patient is presenting in pulmonary edema and cardiogenic shock due to acute myocardial infarction (MI). Given the distribution of ST-segment elevation, the left anterior descending artery is the most likely artery occluded. Initial management should include high-dose aspirin, heparin, and stabilization of blood pressure. Initial management of acute MI also includes use of nitroglycerin and beta blockers such as metoprolol in most individuals, but are contraindicated in this individuals because of his profound hypotension. In addition, use of furosemide for the treatment of pulmonary edema is also contraindicated because of the degree of hypotension. Intravenous fluids should be used with caution as the patient also has evidence of pulmonary edema. The best choice for treatment of this patient's hypotension is aortic counterpulsation. Aortic counterpulsation requires placement of an intraaortic balloon pump percutaneously into the femoral artery. The sausage-shaped balloon inflates during early diastole, augmenting coronary blood flow, and collapses during early systole, markedly decreasing afterload. In contrast to vasopressors and inotropic agents, aortic counterpulsation decreases myocardial oxygen consumption. Both dobutamine and norepinephrine can increase myocardial oxygen demand and worsen ischemia.

V-111. **The answer is D.** *(Chap. 266)* This patient is presenting with right ventricular (RV) myocardial infarction. The usual clinical features of right ventricular infarction are hypotension, elevated right heart filling pressures, absence of pulmonary congestion, and evidence of RV dilatation and dysfunction. In most cases of RV infarction, the vessel involved is the right coronary artery, which manifests as ST elevation in leads II, III, and aV_F. When RV infarction occurs, ST depression is commonly seen in V_1 and V_2. An electrocardiogram with the precordial leads placed on the right side of the chest demonstrates ST elevation in RV_4. The initial treatment of hypotension of RV infarction is IV fluids to raise the central venous pressure to 10–15 mmHg. If fluid administration fails to alleviate the hypotension, sympathomimetic agents or aortic counterpulsation can be used. However, care must be taken to avoid excess fluid administration, which would shift the interventricle septum to the left and further impede cardiac output. A transvenous pacemaker would be useful if the hypotension were related to heart block or profound bradycardia, which can be associated with right coronary artery ischemia.

V-112.   The answer is C.   *(Chap. 267)*   Sudden cardiac death (SCD) is defined as death due to cardiac causes heralded by the abrupt loss of consciousness within 1 h of onset of acute symptoms. Sudden cardiac death accounts for about 50% of all cardiac deaths, and of these, two-thirds are initial cardiac events or occur in populations with previously known heart disease who are considered to be relatively low risk. The most common electrical mechanism of SCD is ventricular fibrillation, accounting for 50–80% of cardiac arrests. The risk of SCD rises with age and is greater in men and individuals with a history of coronary artery disease. In addition, several inherited conditions increase the risk of SCD, including hypertrophic cardiomyopathy, right ventricular dysplasia, and long-QT syndromes, among others. A strong parental history of sudden cardiac death as a presenting history of coronary artery disease increases the likelihood of a similar presentation in an offspring. Interestingly, 70–80% of men who die from SCD have preexisting healed MIs while only 20–30% have had recent acute MI. On autopsy, individuals who die of SCD most commonly show longstanding atherosclerotic disease as well as evidence of an unstable coronary lesion. When this is considered with the fact that most individuals do not have pathologic evidence of an acute MI by pathology, this suggests that transient ischemia is the mechanism of onset of the fatal arrhythmia. Rapid intervention and restoration of circulation is important for survival in SCD. Within 5 min, the likelihood of surviving SCD is only 25–30% for out-of-hospital arrests.

V-113.   The answer is C.   *(Chap. 267)*   Immediate defibrillation should be the initial choice of action in the treatment of sudden cardiac arrest due to ventricular fibrillation (VF) or ventricular tachycardia (VT). Defibrillation should occur prior to endotracheal intubation or placement of intravenous access. If the time to potential defibrillation is <5 min, the medical team should proceed immediately to defibrillation at 300–360 J if a monophasic defibrillator is used (150 J if a biphasic defibrillator is used). If there is >5-min delay to defibrillation, then brief CPR should be given prior to defibrillation. A single shock should be given with immediate resumption of CPR for 60–90 s before delivering additional shocks. After each shock, CPR should be given without delay. Even if there is return of a perfusable rhythm, there is often a delayed return of pulse because of myocardial stunning. If the patient remains in VF or pulseless VT after initial defibrillation, the patient should be intubated and have IV access attained while CPR is performed. Once IV access is obtained, the initial drug of choice is either epinephrine, 1 mg, or vasopressin, 40 units. Amiodarone is a second-line agent.

V-114.   The answer is C.   *(Chap. 267; J Nolan et al: Circulation 108:118, 2003.)*   In 2002, two studies conducted in Europe and Australia confirmed the benefit of therapeutic hypothermia following out-of-hospital cardiac arrest. In these trials, patients were rapidly cooled to 32–34°C and maintained at these temperatures for the initial 12–24 h. Individuals who received therapeutic hypothermia were 40–85% more likely to have good neurologic outcomes upon hospital discharge. In addition, therapeutic hypothermia also decreased in-hospital morality. Time to initial defibrillation of >5 min is associated with no more than a 25–30% survival rate, and survival continues to decrease linearly from 1 to 10 min. Defibrillation within 5 minutes has the greatest likelihood for good neurologic outcomes. Of the medications used in treatment of cardiac arrest due to ventricular fibrillation or pulseless ventricular tachycardia, none have been demonstrated to have any effects on neurologic outcome.

V-115.   The answer is B.   *(Chap. e20)*   Adenosine technetium99m and thallium201 scans are frequently used for further evaluation of cardiac disease via stress testing. Pharmacologic agents used in cardiac stress testing are either vasodilators (adenosine, dipyridamole) or inotropic agents (dobutamine). When vasodilator agents are used, ischemic myocardium develops as normal coronary artery segments dilate in response to the drug, whereas fixed coronary lesions are unable to fully dilate. This causes a diversion of blood away from areas with fixed coronary lesions, a phenomenon known as *coronary steal*. Alternatively, inotropic agents induce stress by causing increased myocardial oxygen demand, and ischemia is diagnosed by the failure to increase blood flow in response to this stress. Using radionuclide labeled perfusion agents, images of the heart are taken following the stress-inducing agent and with rest. Reversible ischemia, indicative of coronary artery ischemia, is demonstrated by lack of perfusion with stress, but perfusion is present at rest. In the images depicted in the figure, there is no evidence of reperfusion of the affected area upon rest. These images are typical of an old myocardial infarction resulting in scar formation and is described as a *fixed defect*. Tissue attenuation due to obesity or breast tissue is a particular problem, especially with the use of thallium. When tissue attenuation occurs, it typically appears as a reversible defect and is a cause of a false-positive stress test. An apical aneurysm may be difficult to ascertain by thallium images, but typically there should be evidence of ballooning of the cardiac apex outward and distortion of the cardiac silhouette, which is not seen here.

V-116. **The answer is B.** *(Chap. 238)* Patients with unstable angina/non-ST-segment elevation myocardial infarction (UA/NSTEMI) exhibit a wide spectrum of risk of death, MI, or urgent revascularization. Risk stratification tools, such as the TIMI risk score, are useful for identifying patients who benefit from an early invasive strategy and those who are best suited for a more conservative approach. The TIMI risk score is composed of seven independent risk factors: Age ≥65, at least three cardiovascular risk factors, prior stenosis >50%, ST-segment deviation ≥0.5 mm, at least two anginal events in <24 h, aspirin usage in the past 7 days, and elevated cardiac markers. Aspirin resistance can occur in 5–10% of patients and is more common among those taking lower doses of aspirin. Having unstable angina despite aspirin usage suggests aspirin resistance. Use of a beta-agonist and a diuretic do not confer an independent risk for death, MI, or need for urgent revascularization.

V-117. **The answer is D.** *(Chap. 238)* Although this patient has positive cardiac biomarkers that could represent myocardial ischemia, in patients with an unclear history of angina, low levels of these biomarkers may not always indicate an acute coronary syndrome. Common alternative diagnoses in this setting include exacerbations of congestive heart failure, myocarditis, and pulmonary embolism. This patient has atypical features of his chest pain for angina, with it lasting for more than minutes at a time and being nonexertional. In a young host, without other significant risk factors, atherosclerotic coronary artery disease would be less likely, especially if the history is atypical. Myocarditis is a diagnosis of exclusion; however, ST-segment elevations throughout the ECG with PR-interval depressions suggest myocarditis. Esophageal spasm may mimic cardiac pain; however, it would not be expected to cause the described ECG abnormalities nor the positive cardiac biomarkers.

V-118. **The answer is A.** *(Chap. 238)* In 1959, Prinzmetal and colleagues described a syndrome of angina that occurs at rest but not usually with exertion, associated with transient ST-segment elevation. The pathophysiology is due to focal epicardial coronary artery vasospasm. While the exact mechanism is not clear, proximal nonobstructive coronary plaques are usually present. It is associated with other vasospastic disorders such as migraine, Raynaud's phenomenon, and aspirin-induced asthma. Patients typically are younger with less coronary artery disease and peripheral vascular disease than those with typical angina or non-ST-segment elevation myocardial infarction. The coronary vasospasm responds to nitrates or calcium channel blockers. The vasospasm is associated with ST-segment elevations on the 12-lead surface electrocardiogram. Cold water ingestion may exacerbate symptoms by causing further vasospasm. Prinzmetal's angina is not associated with autoimmunity, HLA B27 positivity, or *Helicobacter pylori* infection.

V-119. **The answer is E.** *(Chap. 324)* Amyloidosis is in the differential diagnosis of a patient with newly diagnosed heart failure. The cardiac examination is not specific for cardiac amyloid, but accessory findings such as neurologic involvement, low voltage on the ECG and an elevated globulin fraction (total protein – albumin ≥4 mg/dL) are suggestive of cardiac amyloid. Echocardiographic findings include left ventricular hypertrophy, dilated atria, thickened interatrial septum, and a "starry-sky" appearance of the myocardium. The starry-sky appearance is rarely seen using contemporary ultrasound technology. Focal myocardial wall motion abnormalities (akinesis) are more suggestive of coronary artery disease. Valvular heart disease can cause heart failure if left uncorrected. This patient's murmur is characteristic of mitral regurgitation and is not consistent with aortic stenosis. Protrusion of the left ventricular apex with hypercontractility of the base is characteristic of stress cardiomyopathy, which is usually accompanied by clinical findings suggesting acute heart failure and ECG findings suggesting acute anterior myocardial infarction.

V-120. **The answer is C.** *(Chap. 324)* Amyloidosis is a term for diseases that are due to the extracellular deposition of insoluble protein fibrils. The specific diseases are defined by the biochemical nature of the protein in the fibril deposits. Primary systemic amyloidosis (AL) is amyloid composed of immunoglobulin light chains and is usually due to a plasma cell dyscrasia. Bence-Jones protein is often in the urine of patients with plasma cell dyscrasia. Bone marrow biopsy is indicated when AL is diagnosed. AA (secondary amyloidosis) is due to an accumulation of serum amyloid A protein and occurs in the setting of chronic inflammatory or infectious diseases. Alzheimer's disease is caused by accumulation of Aβ protein. Neurocognitive testing may be helpful in patients diagnosed with early cognitive decline. There is currently no clinically available test for early accumulation of Aβ protein. Mutant transthyretin (prealbumin) is the protein usually found in the fibril deposits of the familial amyloidoses (AF). The disease is transmitted in an autosomal dominant fashion, although sporadic cases occur. Typical symptoms include neuropathy, cardiomyopathy, and autonomic neuropathy. Without intervention, survival is typically 5–15 years. Orthotopic liver transplantation removes the source of variant protein production and provides a source of normal protein production. While neuropathy usually improves, cardiomyopathy may not. Screening family members is important for counseling family members who may also be affected.

V-121. **The answer is C.** *(Chap. 226)* There are three main mechanisms by which arrhythmias are initiated and maintained: automaticity, afterdepolarizations, and reentry. Automaticity, such as seen with sinus tachycardia, atrial premature complexes, and some atrial tachycardias, is due to an increase in the slope of phase 4 of the action potential. The depolarization threshold is reached more quickly and repeatedly. Afterdepolarizations are associated with an increase in cellular calcium accumulation, leading to repeated myocardial depolarization during phase 3 (early) and phase 4 (delayed) of the action potential. Early afterdepolarizations may be related to the initiation of torsades de pointes. Delayed afterdepolarizations are responsible for arrhythmias related to digoxin toxicity and for catecholamine-induced ventricular tachycardia. Reentry is due to inhomogeneities in myocardial conduction and refractory periods. With reentry, conduction is blocked in one pathway, allowing slow conduction in the other. This allows for sufficient delay so that the blocked site has time for reentry and propagation of the tachycardia within the two pathways. Reentry appears to be the mechanism for most supraventricular and ventricular tachycardias.

V-122. **The answer is C.** *(Chap. 226)* The mechanisms for atrial fibrillation initiation and maintenance are still debated; however, there are anatomic structures that play a role in both of these processes. Muscularized tissue at the orifices of the pulmonary vein inlets are the predominant anatomic drivers of atrial fibrillation, although metabolic disturbances (e.g., hyperthyroidism, inflammation, infection) are also very common. Radiofrequency ablation of the tissue in the area of the pulmonary vein inlets can terminate atrial fibrillation; however, recurrences are not uncommon and other anatomic drivers may be present. The left atrial appendage is an important site of thrombus formation in patients with atrial fibrillation. Any focus within the left or right atrium can be a focus of reentry of focal atrial tachycardia, including the mitral annulus or sinus venosus. Increased automaticity of the sinus node is the mechanism for sinus tachycardia.

V-123. **The answer is B.** *(Chap. 226)* Symptoms of atrial fibrillation vary dramatically. The most common symptom is tachypalpitations; however, the hemodynamic effects account for symptoms of impaired left ventricular filling. In atrial fibrillation, there is not an effective atrial contraction to augment late-diastolic left ventricular filling. In patients with impaired ventricular diastolic function, this loss of effective atrial contraction causes impaired left ventricular filling, increased left atrial filling pressures, and pulmonary congestion. These hemodynamic effects are more common in the elderly and in patients with long-standing hypertension, hypertrophic cardiomyopathy, and obstructive aortic valve disease. The tachycardia of atrial fibrillation further compromises left ventricular filling and increases atrial filling pressures. Atrial fibrillation may occur with acute alcohol intoxication, warming of hypothermic patients, and postoperative after thoracic surgery. The magnitude of the hemodynamic effect and symptoms will be related to ventricular rate (slower allows more time for left ventricular filling) and underlying cardiac function.

V-124. **The answer is D.** *(Chap. 226)* A common risk scoring system for anticoagulant use in patients with atrial fibrillation is the CHADS2 scoring system; C = congestive heart failure, H = hypertension, A = age >75 years, D = diabetes, S = history of stroke. The presence of any of these risk factors assigns a score of 1, except for stroke, which is worth 2 points. Low-risk patients (score of 0, stroke risk 0.5%/year without warfarin) can be managed with aspirin alone. High-risk patients (score ≥3, stroke risk ≥5.2%/year without warfarin) should be managed with warfarin. Intermediate-risk patients (score 1 or 2, stroke risk 1.5%–2.5%/year without warfarin) may be managed with aspirin or warfarin, depending upon the clinician's assessment of risk, the ability to monitor the intensity of anticoagulation, the patient's risk of bleeding with anticoagulation, and patient preference. If warfarin is used, the goal INR should be 2–3.

V-125. **The answer is A.** *(Chap. 226)* Focal atrial tachycardias can be divided into two categories based on mechanism: automatic and reentry. Sinus tachycardia is the classic automatic tachycardia in which onset and termination have a "warm-up" and "slow-down" period, respectively. The P-wave morphology, which initiates the tachycardia of automatic tachycardias, is the same as the P wave of the tachycardia, whereas the initiating P wave of focal reentrant atrial tachycardia is usually different from those of the tachycardia. Automatic tachycardias are not reliably initiated by programmed stimulation during an electrophysiologic study, whereas reentrant atrial tachycardias can be initiated by programmed stimulation or premature beats. Adenosine receptors within sinus and atrioventricular nodal tissue are thought to account for the ability of this drug to slow and terminate arrhythmias involving these structures.

V-126. **The answer is D.** *(Chap. 226)* Anticoagulation is of particular importance for patients with atrial fibrillation for whom chemical or electrical cardioversion is considered. If the duration of atrial fibrillation is unknown or >24 h, there is an increased risk of an atrial appendage thrombus and subsequent embolization. When DCCV is being considered, one of two strategies is used most often. Intravenous heparin can be initiated and transesophageal echocardiogram obtained. Once the activated partial thromboplastin time is at a therapeutic level, DCCV can be performed if there is no thrombus visualized on TEE. Alternatively, anticoagulation with warfarin can be initiated immediately and continued for at least 3 weeks. If the INR >1.8 on at least two separate occasions, DCCV can be safely performed. Using either strategy, anticoagulation must be continued for at least 1 month after DCCV if the duration of atrial fibrillation has been prolonged or unknown, due to the increased risk of thrombus formation and embolization after DCCV.

V-127. **The answer is D.** *(Chap. 226)* Tachycardias that involve an accessory pathway, like WPW, are at risk for degeneration into 1:1 atrial:ventricular conduction down the accessory pathway and subsequent ventricular tachycardia or fibrillation. If the circuit can conduct anterogradely (i.e., down the accessory pathway, up the His-Purkinje tract), then atrioventricular (AV) nodal blocking agents can precipitate ventricular tachycardia. With a wide-complex tachycardia, the AV nodal blocking agents (adenosine, digoxin, diltiazem, verapamil) will not be as effective as the class 1a antiarrhythmic agent procainamide. Lidocaine and amiodarone would also be effective agents for treating stable wide-complex tachycardias.

V-128. **The answer is E.** *(Chap. 226)* Diagnosing ventricular tachycardia based on the surface electrocardiogram is challenging. All of the answers above, except for E, are clues supporting ventricular tachycardia. In the presence of any interventricular conduction delay, the sinus rhythm QRS duration may be prolonged while the ventricular tachycardia depolarization pattern may originate from closer to the interventricular septum, resulting in a narrower QRS complex. Other clues supporting ventricular tachycardia include a bizarre QRS pattern that does not mimic typical left bundle branch block (LBBB) or right bundle branch block (RBBB) QRS complexes, delayed activation of the initial phase of the QRS complex, a frontal plane axis between −90° and 180° and a prolonged QRS duration in the presence of an LBBB or RBBB. Fusion beats and atrial capture signify atrioventricular dissociation and are the most specific clues for ventricular tachycardia; however, they are also the least commonly found.

V-129. **The answer is C.** *(Chap. 227)* The NY Heart Association classification is a tool to define criteria that describe the functional ability and clinical manifestations of patients in heart failure. It is also used in patients with pulmonary hypertension. These criteria have been shown to have prognostic value with worsening survival as class increases. They are also useful to clinicians when reading studies to understand the entry and exclusion criteria of large clinical trials. Class I is used for patients with no limiting symptoms; class II for patients with slight or mild limitation; class III implies no symptoms at rest but dyspnea or angina or palpitations with little exertion; patients are moderately limited; class IV is severely limited, so that even minimal activity causes symptoms. Treatment guidelines also frequently base recommendations on these clinical stages. This patient has symptoms with mild exertion but is comfortable at rest; therefore he is NY Heart Association class III.

V-130. **The answer is B.** *(Chap. 227)* Patients with severe congestive heart failure often exhibit Cheyne-Stokes breathing, defined as intercurrent short periods of hypoventilation and hyperventilation. The mechanism is thought to relate to the prolonged circulation time between the lungs and the respiratory control centers in the brain, leading to poor respiratory control of P_{CO_2}. The degree of Cheyne-Stokes breathing is related to the severity of heart failure. This pattern of breathing is different from obstructive sleep apnea, which is notable for periods of loud snoring, apnea, and sudden waking. Patients are also often hypersomnolent during the day. While sleep apnea is managed with weight loss and overnight CPAP, Cheyne-Stokes breathing is difficult to address as it is often a sign of advanced systolic dysfunction and implies a poor prognosis. All efforts to further maximize heart failure management are indicated. A sleep study would demonstrate this pattern of breathing, but this history and clinical presentation is typical. There is no role for bronchodilators or an electroencephalogram.

V-131. **The answer is D.** *(Chaps. 220 and 227)* Patients with chronic congestive heart failure develop substantial lymphatic reserve in their lungs. Consequently, they may not display signs of pulmonary edema on physical examination or chest radiograph, even in the presence of a very elevated left ventricular filling pressure. The lack of these findings carries a very limited predictive value and does not rule out heart failure. This phenomenon also occurs in patients with chronic mitral stenosis so is likely an effect of long-standing elevation of pulmonary venous pressure. Acute heart failure will present with bilateral rales on pulmonary examination. However, noncardiac causes of pulmonary edema will also cause rales, so this finding is nonspecific.

V-132. **The answer is E.** *(Chaps. 222 and 227)* Heart failure with a preserved ejection fraction is very common but can be challenging to evaluate serially. Each of the described parameters gives important adjunct information regarding heart function in this type of patient. Left atrial dilatation often implies a chronic elevation in left ventricular diastolic pressures as the atria is relatively compliant and will dilate in this setting. Atrial fibrillation is easily seen on echocardiography and is problematic in these patients as they are often dependent on their atrial kick to maintain preload and therefore cardiac output. Left ventricular wall thickness and diastolic filling may imply severity and duration of disease. Systolic anterior motion of the mitral valve with asymmetric septal hypertrophy is a characteristic echocardiographic finding in hypertrophic cardiomyopathy.

V-133. **The answer is A.** *(Chap. 227)* Angiotensin receptor blockers (ARBs) are useful in heart failure patients who do not tolerate angiotensin-converting enzyme inhibitors due to cough or other side effects. Inhibition of the renin-angiotensin pathway reduces left ventricular afterload and remodeling. They have been shown to improve symptoms and exercise capacity and to reduce need for hospitalization and mortality in patients with systolic heart failure. Calcium channel blockers, particularly first-generation medications, may worsen function in patients with systolic dysfunction. Thiazolidinediones (rosiglitazone, pioglitazone) are associated with fluid retention and may worsen heart failure. NSAID use in patients with a reduced cardiac output may cause acute renal failure. Sotalol has been shown to increase mortality in patients with left ventricular dysfunction.

V-134. **The answer is A.** *(Chap. 227)* Because beta blockers take longer to achieve a steady state, can decrease inotropic function, and cause bradycardia or heart block, the dose of these medicines should be escalated slowly. ACE inhibitors are typically increased to doses achieved in clinical trials at a more rapid rate with careful monitoring of renal function.

V-135. **The answer is E.** *(Chap. 227; AL Taylor et al: N Eng J Med 351:2049, 2004.)* Isosorbide dinitrate/hydralazine in a fixed combination (BiDil) was shown to decrease mortality and hospitalizations in African Americans with impaired left ventricular function (<35–45%) when added to standard heart failure therapy. The drug was approved by the U.S. Food and Drug Administration in 2005 as the first race-specific drug therapy.

VI. DISORDERS OF THE RESPIRATORY SYSTEM

QUESTIONS

DIRECTIONS: Choose the **one best** response to each question.

VI-1. A patient is evaluated in the emergency department for peripheral cyanosis. Which of the following is not a potential etiology?

A. Cold exposure
B. Deep venous thrombosis
C. Methemoglobinemia
D. Peripheral vascular disease
E. Raynaud's phenomenon

VI-2. Which of the following associations correctly pairs clinical scenarios and community-acquired pneumonia (CAP) pathogens?

A. Aspiration pneumonia: *Streptococcus pyogenes*
B. Heavy alcohol use: atypical pathogens and *Staphylococcus aureus*
C. Poor dental hygiene: *Chlamydia pneumoniae, Klebsiella pneumoniae*
D. Structural lung disease: *Pseudomonas aeruginosa, S. aureus*
E. Travel to southwestern United States: *Aspergillus* spp.

VI-3. A 54-year-old female presents to the hospital because of hemoptysis. She has coughed up approximately 1 teaspoon of blood for the last 4 days. She has a history of cigarette smoking. A chest radiogram shows diffuse bilateral infiltrates predominantly in the lower lobes. The hematocrit is 30%, and the serum creatinine is 4.0 mg/dL. Both were normal previously. Urinalysis shows 2+ protein and red blood cell casts. The presence of autoantibodies directed against which of the following is most likely to yield a definitive diagnosis?

A. Glomerular basement membrane
B. Glutamic acid decarboxylase
C. Phospholipids
D. Smooth muscle
E. U1 ribonucleoprotein (RNP)

VI-4. All the following drugs can cause eosinophilic pneumonia *except*

A. nitrofurantoin
B. sulfonamides

VI-4. *(Continued)*
C. nonsteroidal anti-inflammatory drugs (NSAIDs)
D. isoniazid
E. amiodarone

VI-5. A 26-year-old man presents to the clinic with 3 days of severe sore throat and fever. All of the following support the diagnosis of streptococcal pharyngitis *except*

A. cough
B. fever
C. pharyngeal exudates
D. positive rapid streptococcal throat antigen test
E. tender cervical lymphadenopathy

VI-6. Which of the following has been shown to decrease duration of nonspecific upper respiratory tract symptoms?

A. Azithromycin
B. Echinacea
C. Vitamin C
D. Zinc
E. None of the above
F. All of the above

VI-7. A 24-year-old man presents to the emergency room complaining of shortness of breath and right-sided chest pain. The symptoms began abruptly about 2 hours previously. The pain is worse with inspiration. He denies fevers or chills and has not had any leg swelling. He has no past medical history but smokes 1 pack of cigarettes daily. On physical examination, he is tachypneic with a respiratory rate of 24 breaths/min. His oxygen saturation is 94% on room air. Breath sounds are decreased in the right lung, and there is hyperresonance to percussion. A chest radiograph confirms a 50% pneumothorax of the right lung. What is the best approach for treatment of this patient?

A. Needle aspiration of the pneumothorax
B. Observation and administration of 100% oxygen
C. Placement of a large-bore chest tube
D. Referral for thoracoscopy with stapling of blebs and pleural abrasion

237

VI-8. A 23-year-old female complains of dyspnea and substernal chest pain on exertion. Evaluation for this complaint 6 months ago included arterial blood gas testing, which revealed pH 7.48, P_{O_2} 79 mmHg, and P_{CO_2} 31 mmHg. Electrocardiography then showed a right axis deviation. Chest x-ray now shows enlarged pulmonary arteries but no parenchymal infiltrates, and a lung perfusion scan reveals subsegmental defects that are thought to have a "low probability for pulmonary thromboembolism." Echocardiography demonstrates right heart strain but no evidence of primary cardiac disease. The most appropriate diagnostic test now would be

A. open lung biopsy
B. Holter monitoring
C. right-heart catheterization
D. transbronchial biopsy
E. serum α_1-antitrypsin level

VI-9. A 53-year-old woman presents to the hospital following an episode of syncope, with ongoing lightheadedness and shortness of breath. She had a history of antiphospholipid syndrome with prior pulmonary embolism and has been nonadherent to her anticoagulation recently. She has been prescribed warfarin, 7.5 mg daily, but reports taking it only intermittently. She does not know her most recent INR. On presentation to the emergency room, she appears diaphoretic and tachypneic. Her vital signs are: blood pressure 86/44 mmHg, heart rate 130 beats/min, respiratory rate 30 breaths/min, Sa_{O_2} 85% on room air. Cardiovascular examination shows a regular tachycardia without murmurs, rubs, or gallops. The lungs are clear to auscultation. On extremity examination, there is swelling of her left thigh with a positive Homan's sign. Chest CT angiography confirms a saddle pulmonary embolus with ongoing clot seen in the pelvic veins on the left. Anticoagulation with unfractionated heparin is administered. After a fluid bolus of 1 L, the patient's blood pressure remains low at 88/50 mmHg. Echocardiogram demonstrates hypokinesis of the right ventricle. On 100% non-rebreather mask, the Sa_{O_2} is 92%. What is the next best step in management of this patient?

A. Continue current management.
B. Continue IV fluids at 500 mL/hr for a total of 4 L of fluid resuscitation.
C. Refer for inferior vena cava filter placement and continue current management.
D. Refer for surgical embolectomy.
E. Treat with dopamine and recombinant tissue plasminogen activator, 100 mg IV.

VI-10 to VI-13. Among the following pulmonary function test results, pick those which are the most likely finding in each of the following respiratory disorders:

A. Increased total lung capacity (TLC), decreased vital capacity (VC), decreased FEV_1/FVC ratio

VI-10 to VI-13. *(Continued)*

B. Decreased TLC, decreased VC, decreased residual volume (RV), increased FEV_1/FVC ratio, normal maximum inspiratory pressure (MIP)
C. Decreased TLC, increased RV, normal FEV_1/FVC ratio, decreased MIP
D. Normal TLC, normal RV, normal FEV_1/FVC ratio, normal MIP

VI-10. Myasthenia gravis

VI-11. Idiopathic pulmonary fibrosis

VI-12. Familial pulmonary hypertension

VI-13. Chronic obstructive pulmonary disease

VI-14. A 52-year-old female presents with a community-acquired pneumonia complicated by pleural effusion. A thoracentesis is performed, with the following results:

Appearance	Viscous, cloudy
pH	7.11
Protein	5.8 g/dL
LDH	285 IU/L
Glucose	66 mg/dL
WBC	3800/mm^3
RBC	24,000/mm^3
PMNs	93%
Gram stain	Many PMNs; no organism seen

Bacterial cultures are sent, but the results are not currently available. Which characteristic of the pleural fluid is most suggestive that the patient will require tube thoracostomy?

A. Presence of more than 90% polymorphonucleocytes (PMNs)
B. Glucose less than 100 mg/dL
C. Presence of more than 1000 white blood cells
D. pH less than 7.20
E. Lactate dehydrogenase (LDH) more than two-thirds of the normal upper limit for serum

VI-15. A 63-year-old male with a long history of cigarette smoking comes to see you for a 4-month history of progressive shortness of breath and dyspnea on exertion. The symptoms have been indolent, with no recent worsening. He denies fever, chest pain, or hemoptysis. He has a daily cough of 3 to 6 tablespoons of yellow phlegm. The patient says he has not seen a physician for over 10 years. Physical examination is notable for normal vital signs, a prolonged expiratory phase, scattered rhonchi, elevated jugular venous pulsation, and moderate pedal edema. Hematocrit is 49%. Which of the following therapies is most likely to prolong his survival?

A. Atenolol
B. Enalapril
C. Oxygen
D. Prednisone
E. Theophylline

VI-16. A 23-year-old male is climbing Mount Kilimanjaro. He has no medical problems and takes no medications. Shortly after beginning the climb, he develops severe shortness of breath. Physical examination shows diffuse bilateral inspiratory crackles. Which of the following is the most likely etiology?

A. Acute interstitial pneumonitis
B. Acute respiratory distress syndrome
C. Cardiogenic shock
D. Community-acquired pneumonia
E. High-altitude pulmonary edema

VI-17. Which of the following statements about this condition is true?

A. Acetazolamide is indicated for the treatment of this disorder.
B. Older patients are more at risk for this disorder than are younger patients because hypoxic vasoconstriction is more pronounced as patients age.
C. Oxygen is an ineffective therapy for this disorder.
D. Persons who live at high altitudes are not at risk for this disorder even when they return to a high altitude after time spent at sea level.
E. Prevention can be achieved by means of gradual ascent.

VI-18. Which of the following organisms is unlikely to be found in the sputum of a patient with cystic fibrosis?

A. *Haemophilus influenzae*
B. *Acinetobacter baumannii*
C. *Burkholderia cepacia*
D. *Aspergillus fumigatus*
E. *Staphylococcus aureus*

VI-19. A 63-year-old female is seen in the pulmonary clinic for evaluation of progressive dyspnea. She underwent single-lung transplantation 4 years ago for idiopathic pulmonary fibrosis and did well until the last 6 months, when she noted that her exercise tolerance had decreased as a result of shortness of breath. She denies fevers, chills, weight loss, or medication noncompliance. The patient does have an occasional dry cough. Her current medications include tacrolimus, prednisone, trimethoprim-sulfamethoxazole (TMP-SMX), pantoprazole, diltiazem, and mycophenolate mofetil. She denies any current habits but has a remote history of tobacco use. Physical examination is notable for dry crackles on the side of the native lung and decreased breath sounds on the side of the transplanted lung but no adventitious sounds. Review of pulmonary function testing shows an FEV_1/FVC ratio of 50% of the predicted value and an FEV_1 of 0.91 L. Additionally, FEV_1 has fallen by 30% progressively over the last year. Which of the following can ameliorate the fall in FEV_1 in this patient?

VI-19. *(Continued)*
A. Augmented immunosuppression
B. Reduced immunosuppression
C. Antifungal therapy
D. Antiviral therapy
E. Administration of α_1 antitrypsin
F. None of the above

VI-20. A 60-year-old male is seen in the clinic for counseling about asbestos exposure. He is well and has no symptoms. He also has hypertension, for which he takes hydrochlorothiazide. The patient smokes one pack of cigarettes a day but has no other habits. He is currently retired but worked for 30 years as a pipefitter and says he was around "lots" of asbestos, often without wearing a mask or other protective devices. Physical examination is normal except for nicotine stains on the left second and third fingers. Chest radiography shows pleural plaques but no other changes. Pulmonary function tests, including lung volumes, are normal. Which of the following statements should be made to this patient?

A. He must quit smoking immediately as his risk of emphysema is higher than that of other smokers because of asbestos exposure.
B. He does not have asbestosis.
C. His risk of mesothelioma is higher than that of other patients with asbestos exposure because he has a history of tobacco use.
D. He has no evidence of asbestos exposure on chest radiography.
E. He should undergo biannual chest radiography screening for lung cancer.

VI-21. Which of the following patients with community-acquired pneumonia meet the CURB-65 criteria for hospital admission?

A. A 23-year-old man with normal mental status, blood urea nitrogen (BUN) = 17 mg/dL, respiratory rate 25 breaths/min, and blood pressure 110/70 mmHg
B. A 35-year-old woman with normal mental status, BUN = 13 mg/dL, respiratory rate 35 breaths/min, and systolic blood pressure 140/80 mmHg
C. A 48-year-old man with normal mental status, BUN = 25 mg/dL, respiratory rate 32 breaths/min, blood pressure 110/75 mmHg
D. A 62-year-old woman who is confused, BUN = 15 mg/dL, respiratory rate 25 breaths/min, blood pressure 115/65 mmHg
E. A 73-year-old woman with normal mental status, BUN = 10 mg/dL, respiratory rate 18 breaths/min, blood pressure 145/70 mmHg

VI-22. What mode of ventilation is depicted in the graphic below?

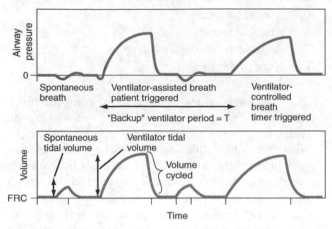

FIGURE VI-22

A. Assist control
B. Continuous positive airway pressure
C. Pressure control
D. Pressure support
E. Synchronized intermittent mandatory ventilation

VI-23. A 67-year-old female is admitted to the hospital with a hip fracture after a fall. Which of the following regimens constitutes appropriate venous thromboembolism prophylaxis for this patient?

A. Intermittent pneumatic compression devices
B. Subcutaneous unfractionated heparin
C. Subcutaneous low-molecular-weight heparin
D. Warfarin, with a target international normalized ratio (INR) of 1.5 to 2.0
E. A and B

VI-24. A 35-year-old male is seen in the clinic for evaluation of infertility. He has never fathered any children, and after 2 years of unprotected intercourse his wife has not achieved pregnancy. Sperm analysis shows a normal number of sperm, but they are immotile. Past medical history is notable for recurrent sinopulmonary infections, and the patient recently was told that he has bronchiectasis. Chest radiography is likely to show which of the following?

A. Bihilar lymphadenopathy
B. Bilateral upper lobe infiltrates
C. Normal findings
D. Situs inversus
E. Water balloon–shaped heart

VI-25. A 78-year-old woman is admitted to the medical intensive care unit with multilobar pneumonia. On initial presentation to the emergency room, her initial oxygen saturation was 60% on room air and only increased to 82% on a non-rebreather face mask. She was in marked respiratory distress and intubated in the emergency

VI-25. (Continued)
room. Upon admission to the intensive care unit, she was sedated and paralyzed. The ventilator is set in the assist-control mode with a respiratory rate of 24, tidal volume of 6 mL/kg, F_{IO_2} of 1.0, and positive end-expiratory pressure of 12 cmH$_2$O. An arterial blood gas measurement is performed on these settings; the results are pH 7.20, Pa_{CO_2} of 32 mmHg, and Pa_{O_2} 54 mmHg. What is the cause of the hypoxemia?

A. Hypoventilation alone
B. Hypoventilation and ventilation-perfusion mismatch
C. Shunt
D. Ventilation-perfusion mismatch

VI-26. A 17-year-old boy is admitted to the intensive care unit with fever, jaundice, renal failure, and respiratory failure. Ten days ago he was part of a community service group from his school that cleaned up a rat-infested alley. Two of his colleagues developed a flulike illness with headache, fever, myalgias, and nausea that has begun to resolve. He developed similar symptoms with the addition of jaundice. On the day of admission he developed shortness of breath. The physical examination is notable for a temperature of 38.4°C (101.1°F), blood pressure of 95/65 mmHg, heart rate of 110/min, respiratory rate of 25/min, and oxygen saturation of 92% on 100% face mask. He has notable jaundice and icterus as well as bilateral conjunctival suffusion. A chest radiogram shows bilateral diffuse infiltrates. Laboratory studies are notable for creatinine 2.5 mg/dL, total bilirubin 12.3 mg/dL, and normal aspartate aminotransferase (AST), alanine aminotransferase (ALT), and prothrombin time. Which of the following antibiotics should be included in his therapy?

A. Cefipime
B. Ciprofloxacin
C. Clindamycin
D. Penicillin
E. Vancomycin

VI-27. A 68-year-old woman presents to the emergency room complaining of dyspnea. She has developed progressive shortness of breath over the past 2 weeks. She has a slight dry cough and a right-sided pleuritic chest pain. There have been no associated fevers or chills. She smokes a pack of cigarettes daily and has done so since the age of 18. On physical examination, she appears dyspneic at rest. Her vital signs are: blood pressure 138/86 mmHg, heart rate 92 beats/min, temperature 37.1°C, respiratory rate 24 breaths/min, and Sa$_{O_2}$ 94% on room air. There is dullness to percussion halfway up her right lung field with decreased tactile fremitus. Breath sounds are decreased without egophony. The examination is otherwise normal. A chest radiograph shows a large free-flowing pleural effusion on the right and also suggests mediastinal lymphadenopathy. The patient undergoes

VI-27. *(Continued)*

thoracentesis, and 1500 mL of bloody-appearing fluid is removed. The results of the pleural fluid are: pH 7.46, red blood cell count too numerous to count, hematocrit 3%, white blood cell count 230/μL (85% lymphocytes, 10% neutrophils, 5% mesothelial cells), protein 4.6 g/dL, lactate dehydrogenase (LDH) 340 U/L, and glucose 35 mg/dL. The corresponding values in the serum are: protein 6.8 g/dL, LDH 360 U/L, and glucose 115 mg/dL. A chest CT performed after the thoracentesis shows residual moderate pleural effusion with collapse of the right lower lobe and enlarged mediastinal lymph nodes. Which of the following tests is most likely to yield the cause of the pleural effusion?

A. Mammography
B. Mediastinoscopy
C. Pleural fluid cytology
D. Pleural fluid culture
E. Thoracoscopic biopsy of the pleura

VI-28. A 36-year-old male comes to his primary care physician complaining of 3 days of worsening headache, left frontal facial pain, and yellow nasal discharge. The patient reports that he has had nasal stuffiness and coryza for about 5 days. Past medical history is notable only for seasonal rhinitis. The physical examination is notable for a temperature of 37.9°C (100.2°F) and tenderness to palpation over the left maxillary sinus. The oropharynx has no exudates, and there is no lymphadenopathy. Which of the following is the most appropriate next intervention?

A. Aspiration of the maxillary sinus
B. Nasal fluticasone
C. Oral amoxicillin
D. Serum antineutrophil cytoplasmic antibodies (ANCA)
E. Sinus CT scan

VI-29. Which of the following conditions would be expected to increase the residual volume of the lung?

A. Bacterial pneumonia
B. Cryptogenic organizing pneumonia
C. Emphysema
D. Idiopathic pulmonary fibrosis
E. Obesity

VI-30. A 24-year-old man from Cincinnati, OH, comes into your clinic requesting treatment for "the flu." He is in your town for a business trip. He reports 1 day of chills, sweats, headaches, myalgias, and a nonproductive cough. He has no known occupational exposures but has just recently finished doing structural repairs on his old house. His blood pressure is 106/72 mmHg, heart rate 98 beats/min, temperature 39.5°C, respiratory rate 24 breaths/min, and Sa$_{O_2}$ is 88% on room air. You obtain a chest ra-

VI-30. *(Continued)*

diograph which shows signs of bilateral pneumonitis and mediastinal lymphadenopathy. An induced sputum silver stain is shown in the figure (see also Figure VI-30, Color Atlas). What is the preferred treatment for this patient?

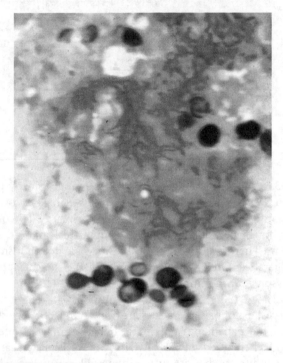

FIGURE VI-30

A. Amphotericin
B. Caspofungin
C. Ciprofloxacin
D. Glucocorticoids
E. Piperacillin/tazobactam

VI-31. Match the following vasopressors with the statement that best describes their action on the cardiovascular system.

1. Dobutamine
2. Low-dose dopamine (2–4 μg/kg per min)
3. Norepinephrine
4. Phenylephrine

A. Acts solely at α-adrenergic receptors to cause vasoconstriction
B. Acts at β$_1$-adrenergic receptors and dopaminergic receptors to increase cardiac contractility and heart rate. It also causes vasodilatation and increased splanchnic and renal blood flow
C. Acts at β$_1$- and, to a lesser extent, β$_2$-adrenergic receptors to increase cardiac contractility, heart rate, and vasodilatation.
D. Acts at α and β$_1$-adrenergic receptors to increase heart rate, cardiac contractility, and vasoconstriction

VI-32. What sleep disorder is depicted in the graphic below (see also Figure VI-32, Color Atlas)?

A.   Cheyne-Stokes respiration

VI-32. *(Continued)*

B.   Central sleep apnea
C.   Obstructive sleep apnea
D.   Periodic limb movement disorder of sleep

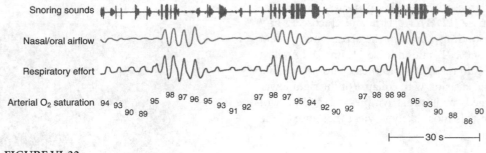

FIGURE VI-32

VI-33. A 42-year-old male presents with progressive dyspnea on exertion, low-grade fevers, and weight loss over 6 months. He also is complaining of a primarily dry cough, although occasionally he coughs up a thick mucoid sputum. There is no past medical history. He does not smoke cigarettes. On physical examination, the patient appears dyspneic with minimal exertion. The patient's temperature is 37.9°C (100.3°F). Oxygen saturation is 91% on room air at rest. Faint basilar crackles are heard. On laboratory studies, the patient has polyclonal hypergammaglobulinemia and a hematocrit of 52%. A CT scan reveals bilateral alveolar infiltrates that are primarily perihilar in nature with a mosaic pattern. The patient undergoes bronchoscopy with bronchoalveolar lavage. The effluent appears milky. The cytopathology shows amorphous debris with periodic acid-Schiff (PAS)-positive macrophages. What is the diagnosis?

A.   Bronchiolitis obliterans organizing pneumonia
B.   Desquamative interstitial pneumonitis
C.   Nocardiosis
D.   *Pneumocystis carinii* pneumonia
E.   Pulmonary alveolar proteinosis

VI-34. What treatment is most appropriate at this time?

A.   Prednisone and cyclophosphamide
B.   Trimethoprim-sulfamethoxazole
C.   Prednisone
D.   Whole-lung saline lavage
E.   Doxycycline

VI-35. An 86-year-old nursing home resident is brought by ambulance to the local emergency room. He was found unresponsive in his bed and 911 was called. Apparently he had been coughing and complaining of chills for the past few days; no further history is available from the nursing home staff. His past medical history is remarkable for Alzheimer's dementia and treated prostate cancer. The emergency responders were able to appreciate a faint pulse and obtained a blood pressure of 91/49 mmHg and a heart rate of 120 beats/min. In the emergency room his pressure is 88/51 mmHg and heart rate is 131 beats/min. He is moan-

ing and obtunded, localizes to pain, and has flat neck veins. Skin tenting is noted. A peripheral IV is placed, specimens for initial laboratory testing sent off, and electrocardiogram and chest x-ray are obtained. Anesthesiology has been called to the bedside and is assessing the patient's airway. What is the best immediate step in management?

A.   Infuse hypertonic saline to increase the rate of vascular filling.
B.   Infuse isotonic crystalloid solution via IV wide open.
C.   Initiate IV pressors starting with levophed.
D.   Infuse a colloidal solution rapidly.
E.   Transfuse packed red blood cells until hemoglobin is >10 g/dL.

VI-36. Which of the following is true regarding hypovolemic shock?

A.   Loss of 20–40% of the blood volume leads to shock physiology.
B.   Loss of <20% of the blood volume will manifest as orthostasis.
C.   Oliguria is a crucial prognostic sign of impending vascular collapse.
D.   Symptoms of hypovolemic shock differ from those of hemorrhagic shock.
E.   The first sign of hypovolemic shock is mental obtundation.

VI-37. A 24-year-old woman is brought to the emergency room after attempting suicide with an overdose of heroin. On arrival at the emergency department in Jacksonville, FL, she is obtunded and has a respiratory rate of 6 breaths/min. She is hypotensive with a blood pressure of 84/60 mmHg and a heart rate of 80 beats/min. The oxygen saturation is 70% on room air. An arterial blood gas is performed showing the following: pH 7.09, Pa_{CO_2} 80 mmHg, Pa_{O_2} 42 mmHg. Which of the following statements is true regarding the patient's arterial blood gas?

A.   The patient is hypoxic due to hypoventilation with an increased A – a (alveolar-arterial) gradient.

VI-37. *(Continued)*

    B. The patient is hypoxic due to hypoventilation with a normal $A - a$ gradient.

    C. The patient is hypoxic due to shunt with an increased $A - a$ gradient.

    D. The patient is hypoxic due to ventilation-perfusion ($\dot{V}/\dot{Q}$) mismatch with an increased $A - a$ gradient.

VI-38. Which of the following statements best describes the functional residual capacity of the lung?

    A. The volume of gas at which the tendency of the lungs to collapse (elastic recoil pressure) and the tendency of the chest wall to expand are equal.

    B. The volume of gas remaining in the lungs at the end of a normal tidal exhalation

    C. The volume of gas remaining in the lungs after a maximal expiratory effort

    D. A and B

    E. A and C

VI-39. A 49-year-old woman is admitted for an evaluation of weakness. She complains of fatigue with repetitive muscle use, with significant fatigue and dysphagia by the end of the day. Her activities have been significantly limited due to her fatigue, and there is significant orthopnea. During her evaluation, laboratory analysis reveals: Sodium 137 meq/L, potassium 3.8 meq/L, chloride 94 meq/L, bicarbonate 31 meq/L. An arterial blood gas shows a pH of 7.33, Pa_{CO_2} 60 mmHg, and Pa_{O_2} 65 mmHg. A chest x-ray is interpreted as "poor inspiratory effort." The oxygen saturation is 92% on room air. A ventilation-perfusion scan has normal perfusion. Which of the following tests will most likely identify the cause of this patient's respiratory acidosis?

    A. CT scan of the brain

    B. Diffusing capacity for carbon monoxide

    C. Esophagoscopy

    D. Forced vital capacity (supine and upright)

    E. Pulmonary angiogram

VI-40. The most common cause of a pleural effusion is

    A. cirrhosis

    B. left ventricular failure

    C. malignancy

    D. pneumonia

    E. pulmonary embolism

VI-41. A 52-year-old man presents with crushing sub-sternal chest pain. He has a history of coronary artery disease and has suffered two non-ST-elevation myocardial infarctions in the past 5 years, both requiring percutaneous intervention and intracoronary stent placement. His electrocardiogram shows ST elevations across the precordial leads, and he is taken emergently to the catheterization laboratory. After angioplasty and stent placement he is transferred to the coronary care unit. His vital signs are

VI-41. *(Continued)*

stable on transfer; however, 20 min after arrival he is found to be unresponsive. His radial pulse is thready, extremities are cool, and blood pressure is difficult to obtain; with a manual cuff it is 65/40 mmHg. The nurse turns to you and asks what you would like to do next. Which of the following accurately represents the physiologic characteristics of this patient's condition?

	Central Venous Pressure	Cardiac Output	Systemic Vascular Resistance
A	↓	↓	↓
B	↓	↑	↓
C	↑	↑	↓
D	↑	↓	↑
E	↓	↓	↑

VI-42. A 19-year-old normal nonsmoking female has a moderately severe pulmonary embolism while on oral contraceptive pills. Which of the following is the most likely predisposing factor?

    A. Abnormal factor V

    B. Abnormal protein C

    C. Diminished protein C level

    D. Diminished protein S level

    E. Diminished antithrombin III level

VI-43. A 22-year-old man has cystic fibrosis. He currently is hospitalized about three times yearly for infectious exacerbations. He is colonized with *Pseudomonas aeruginosa* and *Staphylococcus aureus*, but has never had *Burkholderia cepacia* complex. He remains active and is in college studying architecture. He requires 2 L of oxygen with exertion. The most recent pulmonary function tests demonstrate an FEV_1 that is 28% of the predicted value and an FEV_1/FVC ratio of 44%. Measurement of his arterial blood gas on room air is pH 7.38, Pa_{CO_2} 46 mmHg, and Pa_{O_2} 62 mmHg. Which of these characteristics is an indication for referral for lung transplantation?

    A. Colonization with *Pseudomonas aeruginosa*

    B. FEV_1 <30% predicted

    C. FEV_1/FVC ratio <50%

    D. Pa_{CO_2} >40 mmHg

    E. Use of oxygen with exertion

VI-44. A 42-year-old woman presents to the emergency room with acute onset of shortness of breath. She recently had been to visit her parents out of state and rode in a car for about 9 h each way. Two days ago, she developed a mild calf pain and swelling, but she thought that this was not unusual after having been sitting with her legs dependent for the recent trip. On arrival to the emergency room, she is noted to be tachypneic. The vital signs are: blood pressure 98/60 mmHg, heart rate 114 beats/min, respiratory rate 28 breaths/min, Sa_{O_2} 92% on room air, weight 89 kg. The lungs are clear bilaterally. There is

VI-44. *(Continued)*

pain in the right calf with dorsiflexion of the foot, and the right leg is more swollen when compared to the left. An arterial blood gas measurement shows a pH of 7.22, Pa_{CO_2} 18 mmHg, and Pa_{O_2} 68 mmHg. Kidney and liver function are normal. A helical CT scan is performed using shielding of the uterus and confirms a pulmonary embolus. All of the following agents can be used alone as initial therapy in this patient *except*

A.   enoxaparin, 1 mg/kg SC twice daily
B.   fondaparinux, 7.5 mg SC once daily
C.   tinzaparin, 175 units/kg SC once daily
D.   unfractionated heparin IV adjusted to maintain activated partial thromboplastin time (aPTT) two to three times the upper limit of normal
E.   warfarin, 7.5 mg PO once daily to maintain INR at 2–3

VI-45. Which of the following contacts with a patient infected with tuberculosis is most likely to develop the disease?

A.   The child of a parent with smear-negative, culture-positive pulmonary tuberculosis
B.   The co-worker in a small office of a patient with laryngeal tuberculosis
C.   The HIV-negative partner of an HIV-infected patient with pulmonary tuberculosis
D.   The parent of a young child in diapers with renal tuberculosis
E.   The spouse of a patient with miliary tuberculosis

VI-46. A 32-year-old male is brought to the emergency department after developing sudden-onset shortness of breath and chest pain while coughing. He reports a 3-month history of increasing dyspnea on exertion, nonproductive cough, and anorexia with 15 lb of weight loss. He has no past medical history and takes no medications. The patient smokes one or two packs of cigarettes a day, uses alcohol socially, and has no risk factors for HIV infection. A chest radiogram shows a right 80% pneumothorax, and there are nodular infiltrates in the left base that spare the costophrenic angle. After placement of a chest tube, a chest CT shows bilateral small nodular opacities in the lung bases and multiple small cystic spaces in the lung apex. Which of the following interventions is most likely to improve the symptoms and radiograms?

A.   Intravenous α_1 antitrypsin
B.   Isoniazid, rifampin, ethambutol, and pyrazinamide
C.   Prednisone and cyclophosphamide
D.   Smoking cessation
E.   Trimethoprim-sulfamethoxazole

VI-47. A 68-year-old man presents for evaluation of dyspnea on exertion. He states that he first noticed the symptoms about 3 years ago. At that time, he had to stop walking the golf course and began to use a cart, but he was still able to complete a full 18 holes. Over the past

VI-47. *(Continued)*

year, he has stopped golfing altogether because of breathlessness and states that he has difficulty walking to and from his mailbox, which is about 50 yards (46 m) from his house. He also has a dry cough that occurs on most days. It is not worse at night, and he can identify no triggers. He denies wheezing. He has had no fevers, chills, or weight loss. He denies any joint symptoms. He is a former smoker of about 50 pack-years, but quit 8 years previously after being diagnosed with coronary artery disease. In addition to coronary artery disease, he also has benign prostatic hypertrophy for which he takes tamsulosin. His other medications include aspirin, atenolol, and simvastatin. On physical examination, he appears breathless after walking down the hallway to the examination room, but quickly recovers upon resting. Vital signs are: blood pressure 118/67 mmHg, heart rate 88 beats/min, respiratory rate 20 breaths/min, Sa_{O_2} 94% at rest, decreasing to 86% after ambulating 300 ft (91 m). His lung examination shows normal percussion and expansion. There are Velcro-like crackles at both bases, and they are distributed halfway through both lung fields. No wheezing was noted. Cardiovascular examination is normal. Digital clubbing is present. A chest CT is performed and is shown below. He is referred for surgical lung biopsy. Which statement below is most typical of the pathology seen in this disease?

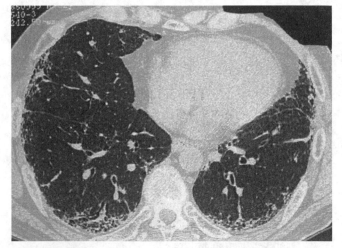

FIGURE VI-47

A.   Dense amorphous fluid within the alveoli diffusely that stains positive with periodic acid–Schiff stain
B.   Destruction of alveoli with resultant emphysematous areas, predominantly in the upper lobes
C.   Diffuse alveolar damage
D.   Formation of noncaseating granulomas
E.   Heterogeneous collagen deposition with fibroblast foci and honeycombing

VI-48. A 68-year-old woman has been receiving mechanical ventilation for 10 days for community-acquired pneu-

VI-48. *(Continued)*
monia. You are attempting to decide whether the patient is appropriate for a spontaneous breathing trial. Which of the following factors would indicate that the patient is not likely to be successfully extubated?

A. Alert mental status
B. Positive end-expiratory pressure (PEEP) of 5 cmH$_2$O
C. pH >7.35
D. Rapid shallow breathing index (respiratory rate/tidal volume) >105
E. Sa$_{O_2}$ >90% on F$_{IO_2}$ <0.5

VI-49. A 34-year-old man presents for evaluation of a cough that has been persistent for the past 3 months. He recalls having an upper respiratory tract infection prior to the onset of cough with complaints of rhinitis, sore throat, and low-grade fever. After these symptoms resolved, he states that "the cold moved to my chest" about 10 days later. He reports severe coughing episodes that have been associated with posttussive emesis in the past, but these are less frequent now. His biggest complaint has been coughing that awakens him from sleep at night and ultimately has resulted in progressive fatigue. He denies wheezing. Specific triggers for his cough include eating cold foods, especially ice cream. He has no history of asthma or prior history of prolonged cough. He denies symptoms of gastroesophageal reflux disease. He breathes easily through his nose and does not have seasonal rhinitis. He has no past medical history. He works as an accountant in a new office building. He does not have any fume exposure. He does not smoke or drink alcohol. He has no pets. He does not recall his vaccination history, but thinks he has not had any vaccinations since graduating from high school. On physical examination, he appears well. He is speaking in full sentences. He is 190 cm tall and weighs 95.5 kg. His temperature is 37.5°C, respiratory rate of 14 breaths/min, heart rate of 64 beats/min, and blood pressure of 112/72 mmHg. His oxygen saturation is 97% on room air at rest. Head, eyes, ears, nose, and throat examination reveals no enlargement of the nasal turbinates, with open nasal passages. The airway is Mallampati class I without cobblestoning or erythema. The lung examination is clear to auscultation. No forced expiratory wheezes are present. The cardiac, gastrointestinal, extremity, and neurologic examinations are normal. His peak expiratory flow rate is 650 L/min. The forced expiratory volume in one second (FEV$_1$) is 4.86 L (96% predicted) and forced vital capacity (FVC) is 6.26 (99% predicted). The FEV$_1$/FVC ratio is 78%. Which test is most likely to establish the diagnosis correctly?

A. 24-h pH probe
B. *Bordetella pertussis* IgG and IgA levels
C. Methacholine challenge testing
D. Peak expiratory flow monitoring in the workplace
E. Skin testing for allergens

VI-50. A 45-year-old male is evaluated in the clinic for asthma. His symptoms began 2 years ago and are characterized by an episodic cough and wheezing that responded initially to inhaled bronchodilators and inhaled corticosteroids but now require nearly constant prednisone tapers. He notes that the symptoms are worst on weekdays but cannot pinpoint specific triggers. His medications are an albuterol MDI, a fluticasone MDI, and prednisone 10 mg PO daily. The patient has no habits and works as a textile worker. Physical examination is notable for mild diffuse polyphonic expiratory wheezing but no other abnormality. Which of the following is the most appropriate next step?

A. Exercise physiology testing
B. Measurement of FEV$_1$ before and after work
C. Methacholine challenge testing
D. Skin testing for allergies
E. Sputum culture for *Aspergillus fumigatus*

VI-51. A 46-year-old man is brought to your office by his wife. He is reluctant to admit that he has any health problems. His wife, on the other hand, is adamant that something be done about his sleepiness. He admits that he is frequently sleepy at work and falls asleep while watching television at night, but he attributes this to stress on the job. She describes loud snoring at night that begins almost immediately when he falls asleep, punctuated by long periods of no breathing at all. She believes that neither of them is getting enough sleep. On examination, he is a pleasant, obese man in no distress. He is 178 cm tall and weighs 111 kg. Blood pressure is elevated at 146/92 mmHg. He has a normal oropharynx and has a short, squat neck. His lung sounds are clear, and he has a protuberant, obese abdomen. Pulses are intact. After completing the physical examination, the patient's wife demands to know what is wrong and what you are going to do about it. What are the next steps in diagnosis and treatment?

A. He and his wife should be reassured that his symptoms will improve as his work stress lessens.
B. He meets clinical criteria for obstructive sleep apnea (OSA) and should be referred for surgery.
C. He should be prescribed a therapeutic trial of modafinil.
D. He should be started on low-dose continuous-positive airway pressure (CPAP) ventilation at home.
E. He should undergo a polysomnogram, potentially followed by a CPAP trial.

VI-52. A 34-year-old female seeks evaluation for a complaint of cough and dyspnea on exertion that has gradually worsened over 3 months. The patient has no past history of pulmonary complaints and has never had asthma. She started working in a pet store approximately 6 months ago. Her duties there include cleaning the reptile and bird cages. She reports occasional low-grade fevers but has had no wheezing. The cough is dry and nonpro-

VI-52. *(Continued)*

ductive. Before 3 months ago the patient had no limitation of exercise tolerance, but now she reports that she gets dyspneic climbing two flights of stairs. On physical examination the patient appears well. She has an oxygen saturation of 95% on room air at rest but desaturates to 91% with ambulation. Temperature is 37.7°C (99.8°F). The pulmonary examination is unremarkable. No clubbing or cyanosis is present. The patient has a normal chest radiogram. A high-resolution chest CT shows diffuse ground-glass infiltrates in the lower lobes with the presence of centrilobular nodules. A transbronchial biopsy shows an interstitial alveolar infiltrate of plasma cells, lymphocytes, and occasional eosinophils. There are also several loose noncaseating granulomas. All cultures are negative for bacterial, viral, and fungal pathogens. What is the diagnosis?

A. Sarcoidosis
B. Psittacosis
C. Hypersensitivity pneumonitis
D. Nonspecific interstitial pneumonitis related to collagen vascular disease
E. Aspergillosis

VI-53. What treatment do you recommend?

A. Glucocorticoids
B. Doxycycline
C. Glucocorticoids plus azathioprine
D. Glucocorticoids plus removal of antigen
E. Amphotericin

VI-54. A 71-year-old man presents with complaints of cough and sputum production. He describes coughing up a small amount of blood occasionally. He states that his symptoms have worsened over a period of years, and he now gets winded going up one flight of stairs. He has a distant history of treated tuberculosis and has been treated for community-acquired pneumonia two-to-three times per year for the past several years. He received a flu vaccination this fall. He has never smoked. On examination, his respirations are 16/min and regular. He has scattered rhonchi and faint expiratory wheezes bilaterally on auscultation. He is not using accessory muscles to breathe. You suspect that this patient may have bronchiectasis to explain his recurrent infections. Which of the following is true regarding making this diagnosis?

A. Bronchiectasis cannot be diagnosed in the setting of an acute pulmonary infection.
B. Bronchoscopy is required to definitively diagnose bronchiectasis.
C. Chest x-ray demonstrating honeycombing pattern will make the diagnosis.
D. High-resolution chest CT scan is the preferred confirmatory test for bronchiectasis.
E. Physical examination is sufficient to diagnose bronchiectasis in a patient with this history.

VI-55. All the following are pulmonary manifestations of systemic lupus erythematosus *except*

A. pleuritis
B. progressive pulmonary fibrosis
C. pulmonary hemorrhage
D. diaphragmatic dysfunction with loss of lung volumes
E. pulmonary vascular disease

VI-56. Which of the following is the most appropriate therapy for a 60-year-old male with 2 weeks of productive cough, fever, shortness of breath, and the chest radiogram as shown in the following figure?

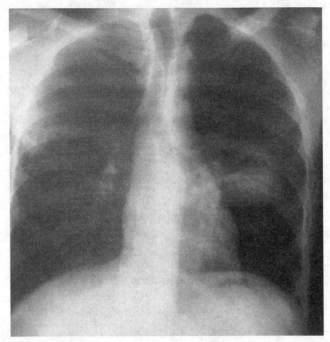

FIGURE VI-56

A. Cephalexin
B. Ciprofloxacin
C. Clindamycin
D. Penicillin
E. Vancomycin

VI-57. A 68-year-old man presents to the emergency room with fever and productive cough. His illness began abruptly 4 days ago. He describes his cough as productive of a rusty-colored sputum. There is associated left-sided pleuritic chest pain. He is a smoker with a 48 pack-year history. On physical examination, there is dullness to percussion over the lower one-third of the left chest. There is decreased tactile fremitus and distant breath sounds. A chest radiograph shows dense consolidation of the left lower lobe and an associated effusion. Which of the following factors would be an indication for tube thoracostomy for treatment of the pleural effusion?

A. Loculated pleural fluid
B. Pleural fluid pH <7.20
C. Pleural fluid glucose <60 mg/dL
D. Positive Gram stain or culture of the pleural fluid
E. All of the above

VI-58. In the first year following lung transplant, which of the following is the most common cause of mortality?

 A. Acute rejection
 B. Bronchiolitis obliterans
 C. Infection
 D. Posttransplant lymphoproliferative disorder
 E. Primary graft failure

VI-59. A 52-year-old alcoholic man presents to a local emergency room with purulent, productive cough, shortness of breath, right-sided chest pain, and fever. He thinks his symptoms started a few days ago. On examination, he has a temperature of 38.8°C, heart rate of 96 beats/min, respirations of 22 breaths/min, oxygen saturation of 85% on room air, and a blood pressure of 115/92 mmHg. He has poor dentition and fetid breath. There is dullness to percussion over the right lower lung field, and rales are auscultated bilaterally. A chest radiograph shows a right-sided opacity in the superior portion of the right lower lobe with an air-fluid level present. There appears to be right-sided parenchymal consolidation as well. Which of the following is the most likely etiologic organism based on this presentation?

 A. *Candida glabrata*
 B. Influenza virus
 C. *Mycobacterium tuberculosis*
 D. *Peptostreptococcus*
 E. *Streptococcus pneumoniae*

VI-60. A 45-year-old woman presents for evaluation of abnormal sensations in her legs that keep her from sleeping at night. She first notices the symptoms around 8 P.M. when she is sitting quietly watching television. She describes the symptoms as "ants crawling in her veins." While the symptoms are not painful, they are very uncomfortable and worsen when she lies down at night. They interfere with her ability to fall asleep about four times weekly. If she gets out of bed to walk or rubs her legs, the symptoms disappear almost immediately only to recur as soon as she is still. She also sometimes takes a very hot bath to alleviate the symptoms. During sleep, her husband complains that she kicks him throughout the night. She has no history of neurologic or renal disease. She currently is perimenopausal and has been experiencing very heavy and prolonged menstrual cycles over the past several months. The physical examination, including thorough neurologic examination, is normal. Her hemoglobin is 9.8 g/dL and hematocrit is 30.1%. The mean corpuscular volume is 68 fL. Serum ferritin is 22 ng/mL. Which is the most appropriate initial therapy for this patient?

 A. Carbidopa/levodopa
 B. Hormone replacement therapy
 C. Iron supplementation
 D. Oxycodone
 E. Pramipexole

VI-61. A 45-year-old female is seen in the clinic for evaluation of a chronic cough. She reports a cough that began in her early twenties that is occasionally productive of yellow or green thick sputum. She has been treated with innumerable courses of antibiotics, all with brief improvements in the symptoms. The patient has been told that she has asthma, and her only medications are fluticasone and albuterol metered-dose inhalers (MDIs). Physical examination is notable for normal vital signs and an oxygen saturation of 92% on room air. The patient's lungs have dullness in the upper lobes bilaterally and diffuse expiratory wheezing. She has mild digital clubbing. The remainder of the physical examination is normal. Pulmonary function testing shows airflow obstruction. Review of the sputum culture data shows that she has had multiple positive cultures for *Pseudomonas aeruginosa* and *Staphylococcus aureus*. Posteroanterior (PA) and lateral chest radiography shows bilateral upper lobe infiltrates. Which of the following tests is the most important first step in diagnosing the underlying disease?

 A. Chest computed tomogram (CT)
 B. Bronchoscopy with transbronchial biopsy
 C. Sweat chloride testing
 D. Blood polymerase chain reaction (PCR) for ΔF508 mutation
 E. Sputum cytology

VI-62. A 23-year-old hospital worker is evaluated for a known contact with a patient with active tuberculosis. One year ago his intermediate-strength PPD had 3 mm of induration; now it has 13 mm of induration at 48 h. He has no significant past medical history and is on no medications. Subsequent management should include

 A. chest radiography
 B. isoniazid 300 mg/d for 3 months
 C. measurement of baseline liver function tests
 D. measurement of liver function tests every 3 months
 E. repeated intermediate-strength PPD testing in 2 weeks

VI-63. A 72-year-old male with a long history of tobacco use is seen in the clinic for 3 weeks of progressive dyspnea on exertion. He has had a mild nonproductive cough and anorexia but denies fevers, chills, or sweats. On physical examination, he has normal vital signs and normal oxygen saturation on room air. Jugular venous pressure is normal, and cardiac examination shows decreased heart sounds but no other abnormality. The trachea is midline, and there is no associated lymphadenopathy. On pulmonary examination, the patient has dullness over the left lower lung field, decreased tactile fremitus, decreased breath sounds, and no voice transmission. The right lung examination is normal. After obtaining chest plain film, appropriate initial management at this point would include which of the following?

 A. Intravenous antibiotics
 B. Thoracentesis

VI-63. (Continued)

   C.   Bronchoscopy
   D.   Deep suctioning
   E.   Bronchodilator therapy

VI-64. Which of the following is specific in differentiating bacterial from viral acute sinusitis?

   A.   Duration of illness >7 days
   B.   Mucosal thickening on CT scan
   C.   Nasal culture
   D.   Purulent nasal discharge
   E.   All of the above
   F.   None of the above

VI-65. Which of the following is the most common underlying medical condition of patients undergoing lung transplantation?

   A.   Chronic obstructive pulmonary disease (COPD)
   B.   Cystic fibrosis
   C.   Idiopathic pulmonary fibrosis (IPF)
   D.   Pulmonary hypertension
   E.   Sarcoidosis

VI-66. A 34-year-old woman complains of cough productive of green sputum, malaise, and headache over the past week. She notes that two of her children recently had colds, and she thought she caught this from one of them. She smokes two packs of cigarettes a day. On examination, she is afebrile, with a heart rate of 125 beats/min and respiratory rate of 32 breaths/min. Oxygen saturation is 94% on room air. She has pronounced use of her accessory respiratory musculature. Physical examination reveals diffuse expiratory wheezing on auscultation of the lungs. There are no areas of bronchophony or egophony. In the proper clinical context, which of the following is necessary to diagnose community-acquired pneumonia?

   A.   Abnormal white blood cell (WBC) count
   B.   Bronchial breath sounds
   C.   Elevated measures of inflammation (erythrocyte sedimentation rate, C-reactive protein)
   D.   Infiltrate on chest radiograph
   E.   Supportive microbiologic data

VI-67. In a patient with severe bullous emphysema, the most appropriate method for measuring lung volumes is

   A.   body plethysmography
   B.   diffusing capacity of carbon monoxide
   C.   spirometry
   D.   helium dilution
   E.   transdiaphragmatic pressure

VI-68. A 50-year-old female receives an uncomplicated double lung transplant for a history of primary pulmonary hypertension. She was cytomegalovirus (CMV)-seropositive and received CMV prophylaxis immediately after the transplant. On postoperative day 7 she developed fever and a new infil-

VI-68. (Continued)

trate in the right lung. Which of the following organisms is most likely to be the causative agent of these findings?

   A.   Cytomegalovirus
   B.   *Listeria monocytogenes*
   C.   *Nocardia asteroides*
   D.   *Pneumocystis carinii*
   E.   *Pseudomonas aeruginosa*

VI-69. A 20-year-old man presents for evaluation of excessive daytime somnolence. He is finding it increasingly difficult to stay awake during his classes. Recently, his grades have fallen because whenever he tries to read he finds himself drifting off. He finds that his alertness is best after exercising or brief naps of 10–30 min. Because of this, he states that he takes 5 or 10 "catnaps" daily. The sleepiness persists despite averaging 9 h of sleep nightly. His Epworth Sleepiness Scale score is 21/24. In addition to excessive somnolence, he reports occasional hallucinations that occur as he is falling asleep. He describes these occurrences as a voice calling his name as he drifts off. Perhaps once weekly, he awakens from sleep but is unable to move for a period of about 30 s. He has never had apparent loss of consciousness but states that whenever he is laughing, he feels a heaviness in his neck and arms. Once he had to lean against a wall to keep from falling down. He undergoes an overnight sleep study and multiple sleep latency test. There is no sleep apnea. His mean sleep latency on five naps is 2.3 min. In three of the five naps, rapid-eye-movement sleep is present. Which of the following findings of this patient is most specific for the diagnosis of narcolepsy?

   A.   Cataplexy
   B.   Excessive daytime somnolence
   C.   Hypnagogic hallucinations
   D.   Rapid-eye-movement sleep in more than two naps on a multiple sleep latency test
   E.   Sleep paralysis

VI-70. Which of the following is the most common sleep disorder in the population?

   A.   Delayed sleep phase syndrome
   B.   Insomnia
   C.   Obstructive sleep apnea
   D.   Narcolepsy
   E.   Restless legs syndrome

VI-71. Patients with chronic hypoventilation disorders often complain of a headache upon wakening. What is the cause of this symptom?

   A.   Arousals from sleep
   B.   Cerebral vasodilation
   C.   Cerebral vasoconstriction
   D.   Polycythemia
   E.   Nocturnal microaspiration and cough

VI-72. From which stage of sleep are the parasomnias somnambulism and night terrors most likely to occur?

A. Stage 1
B. Stage 2
C. Stage 3/4 (Slow-wave sleep)
D. Rapid-eye-movement (REM) sleep

VI-73. Secondhand tobacco smoke has been associated with which of the following?

A. Increased risk of lung cancer
B. Increased prevalence of respiratory illness
C. Excess cardiac mortality
D. A and B
E. All of A, B, and C

VI-74. All of the following are factors that are related to the increased incidence of sepsis in the United States *except*

A. aging of the population
B. increased longevity of individuals with chronic disease
C. increased risk of sepsis in individuals without comorbidities
D. increased risk of sepsis in individuals with AIDS
E. increased use of immunosuppressive drugs

VI-75. A 28-year-old man comes to the emergency department with complaints of 1–2 days of fever, malaise, cough, green sputum production, and dyspnea. He is a cigarette smoker and works in a restaurant. He has no significant past medical history and takes no medications. He is uncomfortable but alert with temperature of 39.2°C, respiratory rate 28 breaths/min, blood pressure 110/70 mmHg, heart rate 105 beats/min, Sa_{O_2} on room air is 94%. His chemistry studies are normal. White blood cell (WBC) count is 15,500/μL. There are bronchial breath sounds in the right lower lobe, and chest radiograph shows consolidation in that area. Which of the following is the most appropriate antibiotic therapy?

A. Azithromycin
B. Ceftriaxone plus clarithromycin
C. Fluconazole
D. Piperacillin/tazobactam
E. Vancomycin

VI-76. A 68-year-old woman comes to the emergency department with complaints of 3 days of fever, malaise, cough with green sputum, dyspnea, and right lower chest pain that is worse on inspiration. She is a 1 pack per day cigarette smoker and works in a retail store. Her only medication is hydrochlorothiazide for hypertension. She is alert but in mild respiratory distress. Her temperature is 39.2°C, respiratory rate 32 breaths/min, blood pressure 110/70 mmHg, heart rate 105 beats/min, Sa_{O_2} on room air is 91%. Her chemistry studies show a serum glucose of 140 mg/dL and a BUN of 32 mg/dL. WBC is 12,500/μL with a left shift. There are bronchial breath sounds in the right lower lobe, and chest radiograph shows consolida-

VI-76. *(Continued)*
tion in the right and left lower lobes. Which of the following is the most appropriate antibiotic therapy?

A. Azithromycin
B. Ceftriaxone plus clarithromycin
C. Fluconazole
D. Piperacillin/tazobactam
E. Vancomycin

VI-77. A 45-year-old woman with HIV is admitted to the intensive care unit with pneumonia secondary to *Pneumocystis jiroveci*. She requires mechanical ventilatory support. The ventilator settings are: PC mode, inspiratory pressure 30 cmH2O, FI_{O_2} 1.0, and PEEP 10 cmH2O. An arterial blood gas measured on these settings shows: pH 7.32, Pa_{CO_2} 46 mmHg, and Pa_{O_2} 62 mmHg. All of the following are important supportive measures for this patient *except*

A. frequent ventilator circuit changes
B. gastric acid suppression
C. nutritional support
D. prophylaxis against deep venous thrombosis
E. sedation and analgesia to maintain patient comfort

VI-78. A 68-year-old woman is brought to the emergency room for fever and lethargy. She first felt ill yesterday and experienced generalized body aches. Overnight, she developed a fever to 39.6°C and had shaking chills. By this morning, she was feeling very fatigued. Her son feels that she has had periods of waxing and waning mental status. She denies cough, nausea, vomiting, diarrhea, or abdominal pain. She has a past medical history of rheumatoid arthritis. She takes prednisone, 5 mg daily, and methotrexate, 15 mg weekly. On examination, she is lethargic but appropriate. Her vital signs are: blood pressure 85/50 mmHg, heart rate 122 beats/min, temperature 39.1°C, respiratory rate 24 breaths/min, Sa_{O_2} 97% on room air. Physical examination shows clear lung fields and a regular tachycardia without murmur. There is no abdominal tenderness or masses. Stool is negative for occult blood. There are no rashes. Hematologic studies show a white blood cell count of 24,200/μL with a differential of 82% PMNs, 8% band forms, 6% lymphocytes, 3% monocytes. Hemoglobin is 8.2 g/dL. A urinalysis has numerous white blood cells with gram-negative bacteria on Gram stain. Chemistries reveal the following: bicarbonate 16 meq/L, BUN 60 mg/dL, and creatinine 2.4 mg/dL. After fluid administration of 2 L, the patient has a blood pressure of 88/54 mmHg and a heart rate of 112 beats/min with a central venous pressure of 18 cmH2O. There is 25 mL of urine output in the first hour. The patient has been initiated on antibiotics with ciprofloxacin. What should be done next for the treatment of this patient's hypotension?

A. Dopamine, 3 μg/kg per minute IV
B. Hydrocortisone, 50 mg IV every 6 h
C. Norepinephrine, 2 μg/min IV

VI-78. *(Continued)*

    D.   Ongoing colloid administration at 500–1000 mL/h

    E.   Transfusion of 2 units packed red blood cells

VI-79. All of the following statements about the epidemiology and pathogenesis of sepsis and septic shock are true *except*

    A.   Blood cultures are positive in only 20–40% of cases of severe sepsis.

    B.   Microbial invasion of the bloodstream is not necessary for the development of severe sepsis.

    C.   The hallmark of septic shock is a marked decrease in peripheral vascular resistance that occurs despite increased plasma levels of catecholamines.

    D.   The incidence and mortality from septic shock have declined over the past 20 years.

    E.   Widespread vascular endothelial injury is present in severe sepsis and is mediated by cytokines and procoagulant factors that stimulate intravascular thrombosis.

VI-80. All of the following statements about the physiology of mechanical ventilation are true *except*

    A.   Application of positive end-expiratory pressure decreases preload and afterload.

    B.   High inspired tidal volumes contribute to the development of acute lung injury due to overdistention of alveoli with resultant alveolar damage.

    C.   Increasing the inspiratory flow rate will increase the ratio of inspiration to expiration (I:E) and allow more time for expiration.

    D.   Mechanical ventilation provides assistance with inspiration and expiration.

    E.   Positive end-expiratory pressure helps prevent alveolar collapse at end-expiration.

VI-81. A 64-year-old man requires endotracheal intubation and mechanical ventilation for chronic obstructive pulmonary disease. He was paralyzed with rocuronium for intubation. His initial ventilator settings were AC mode, respiratory rate 10 breaths/min, $F_{I_{O_2}}$ 1.0, V_t (tidal volume) 550 mL, and PEEP 0 cmH$_2$O. On admission to the intensive care unit, the patient remains paralyzed; arterial blood gas is pH 7.22, Pa$_{CO_2}$ 78 mmHg, and Pa$_{O_2}$ 394 mmHg. The $F_{I_{O_2}}$ is decreased to 0.6. Thirty minutes later, you are called to the bedside to evaluate the patient for hypotension. Current vital signs are: blood pressure 80/40 mmHg, heart rate 133 beats/min, respiratory rate 24 breaths/min, and Sa$_{O_2}$ 92%. Physical examination shows prolonged expiration with wheezing continuing until the initiation of the next breath. Breath sounds are heard in both lung fields. The high-pressure alarm on the ventilator is triggering. What should be done first in treating this patient's hypotension?

    A.   Administer a fluid bolus of 500 mL

    B.   Disconnect the patient from the ventilator

    C.   Initiate a continuous IV infusion of midazolam

    D.   Initiate a continuous IV infusion of norepinephrine

    E.   Perform tube thoracostomy on the right side

VI-82. A 32-year-old man with a medical history of morbid obesity, active tobacco use, and hypertension is referred for a sleep study by his primary physician. The patient describes falling asleep at work almost every afternoon and is frequently drowsy when driving his car. His girlfriend notes that he snores heavily throughout the night, and seems to have intermittent episodes when he is not breathing at all. He undergoes the study, which reveals six to seven hypopneic events and two to three apneic events each hour. Which of the following is true regarding obstructive sleep apnea (OSA)?

    A.   85% of patients with OSA have a body mass index (BMI) >30 kg/m^2

    B.   Irregular breathing during sleep without daytime sleepiness qualifies as OSA

    C.   The male to female ratio is roughly equal in OSA

    D.   This patient does not meet criteria for OSA based on having too few apneic events per hour

    E.   This patient should be screened for diabetes mellitus

VI-83. In the intensive care unit, you are caring for a 36-year-old man with a cocaine overdose. He has pyrexia, tachycardia, and hypertensive urgency. He begins to have brief episodes of ventricular tachycardia but is awake but disoriented. Over the next hour, his ventricular tachycardia becomes more frequent and lasts longer each time. What is the appropriate management strategy for his arrhythmia?

    A.   Intravenous diazepam

    B.   Intravenous hydralazine

    C.   Intravenous norepinephrine

    D.   Intravenous propranolol

VI-84. Which of the following interstitial lung diseases is not associated with smoking?

    A.   Desquamative interstitial pneumonitis

    B.   Respiratory bronchiolitis–interstitial lung disease

    C.   Idiopathic pulmonary fibrosis

    D.   Bronchiolitis obliterans organizing pneumonia

    E.   Pulmonary Langerhans cell histiocytosis

VI-85. A 53-year-old male is seen in the emergency department with sudden-onset fever, chills, malaise, and shortness of breath but no wheezing. He has no significant past medical history and is a farmer. Of note, he worked earlier in the day stacking hay. PA and lateral chest radiography show bilateral upper lobe infiltrates. Which organism is most likely to be responsible for this presentation?

    A.   *Nocardia asteroides*

    B.   *Histoplasma capsulatum*

    C.   *Cryptococcus neoformans*

    D.   *Actinomyces*

    E.   *Aspergillus fumigatus*

VI-86. A 56-year-old woman presents for evaluation of dyspnea and cough for 2 months. During this time, she has also had intermittent fevers, malaise, and a 5.5 kg (12 lb) weight

VI-86. *(Continued)*

loss. She denies having any ill contacts and has not recently traveled. She works as a nurse, and a yearly PPD test performed 3 months ago was negative. She denies any exposure to organic dusts and does not have any birds as pets. She has a history of rheumatoid arthritis and is currently taking hydroxychloroquine, 200 mg twice daily. There has been no worsening in her joint symptoms. On physical examination, diffuse inspiratory crackles and squeaks are heard. A CT scan of the chest reveals patchy alveolar infiltrates and bronchial wall thickening. Pulmonary function testing reveals mild restriction. She undergoes a surgical lung biopsy. The pathology shows granulation tissue filling the small airways, alveolar ducts, and alveoli. The alveolar interstitium has chronic inflammation and organizing pneumonia. What is the most appropriate therapy for this patient?

A. Azathioprine, 100 mg daily
B. Discontinue hydroxychloroquine and observe
C. Infliximab IV once monthly
D. Methotrexate, 15 mg weekly
E. Prednisone, 1.5 mg/kg daily

VI-87. You are evaluating a patient with a chronic respiratory acidosis. Which of the following tests will be helpful in distinguishing a central nervous system cause of chronic hypoventilation from a pulmonary airway or pulmonary parenchymal cause?

A. Alveolar-arterial ($A - a$) oxygen gradient
B. Diaphragmatic EMG
C. Maximal expiratory pressure
D. Pa_{CO_2}
E. Pa_{O_2}

VI-88. A 72-year-old female with severe osteoporosis presents for evaluation of shortness of breath. She is a lifetime nonsmoker and has had no exposures. On physical examination you note marked kyphoscoliosis. All the following pulmonary abnormalities are expected *except*

A. restrictive lung disease
B. alveolar hypoventilation
C. obstructive lung disease
D. ventilation-perfusion abnormalities with hypoxemia
E. pulmonary hypertension

VI-89. A 39-year-old man comes to the emergency department for a persistent cough. He has had high fevers, chills, and a cough for 2 weeks. He was well until 2 weeks ago. He is visiting family locally and resides in Tennessee. Initially, the cough was nonproductive but has become productive as the rest of his symptoms have worsened. He complains of pleuritic chest pain and arthralgias. He works as a ranger in a wooded state park. On physical examination, he is thin but well nourished. He has no skin lesions. Chest auscultation reveals crackles throughout both lung fields. A chest radiograph shows alveolar infil-

VI-89. *(Continued)*

trates bilaterally with a cavity in the left middle lobe without adenopathy. His white blood cell count is 15,000/μL, hemoglobin is 12 g/dL, and platelets are 248,000/μL. Sodium is 136 meq/L, potassium 3.8 meq/L, bicarbonate 24 meq/L, and renal function is normal. Which diagnostic test is most likely to reveal the cause of this patient's pulmonary syndrome?

A. Acid-fast bacilli smear of the sputum
B. Bone marrow aspirate and culture
C. Sputum KOH stain
D. Sputum Quellung reaction
E. Urinary *Legionella* antigen

VI-90. A 45-year-old female with known rheumatoid arthritis complains of a 1-week history of dyspnea on exertion and dry cough. She had been taking hydroxychloroquine and prednisone 7.5 mg until 3 months ago, when low-dose weekly methotrexate was added because of active synovitis. The patient's temperature is 37.8°C (100°F), and her room air oxygen saturation falls from 95% to 87% with ambulation. Chest-x-ray shows new bilateral alveolar infiltrates.

Pulmonary function tests reveal the following:

FEV_1, 3.1 L (70% of predicted)
TLC, 5.3 L (60% of predicted)
FVC, 3.9 L (68% of predicted)
VC, 3.9 L (58% of predicted)
FEV_1/FVC, 79%
Diffusion capacity for carbon monoxide (DLCO), 62% of predicted

She had a normal pulmonary function test (PFT) 1 year ago. All but which of the following would be an appropriate next step?

A. Start broad-spectrum antibiotics.
B. Increase the methotrexate dose.
C. Perform bronchoalveolar lavage with transbronchial lavage.
D. Increase prednisone to 60 mg/d.
E. Discontinue methotrexate.

VI-91. All of the following are relative contraindications for the use of succinylcholine as a paralytic for endotracheal intubation *except*

A. acetaminophen overdose
B. acute renal failure
C. crush injuries
D. muscular dystrophy
E. tumor lysis syndrome

VI-92. A 32-year-old female presents with subjective complaints of paresthesias and weakness. She reports that she was well until 4 weeks ago, when she had a self-limited diarrheal illness that lasted 4 days. For the last week she has

VI-92. *(Continued)*

noted tingling in the fingers and toes. More recently she feels as if she is developing weakness to the extent where she has difficulty walking because she is unable to lift her toes. Additionally, she feels that she has lost significant grip strength. You suspect Guillain-Barré syndrome after a *Campylobacter* infection, and the patient is hospitalized and started on intravenous immunoglobulin. After the hospitalization, the patient's symptoms worsen so that she now is unable to lift her legs against gravity and is complaining of shortness of breath with a decreased voice. Which of the following is an indication for the initiation of mechanical ventilation in this patient with suspected diaphragmatic weakness?

A. Vital capacity below 20 mL/kg
B. Elevated Pa_{CO_2}
C. Maximum inspiratory pressure less than 30 cmH$_2$O
D. Maximum expiratory pressure less than 40 cmH$_2$O
E. All of the above

VI-93. A 38-year-old African-American woman is referred to the clinic for evaluation of an abnormal chest radiograph. She had been brought to the hospital after a motor vehicle accident and had a chest radiograph performed to evaluate for rib fracture. On radiography, she was found to have bilateral hilar lymphadenopathy. She has since recovered from her accident with no further chest pain. She otherwise states that she is in good health. She has had no shortness of breath, cough, or wheezing. She has never had prior lung disease. She denies recent acute illness, fevers, chills, night sweats, or weight loss. She has a history of hypertension and takes lisinopril. She lives in West Virginia. She does not smoke cigarettes. On physical examination, she appears well and in no distress. An oxygen saturation on room air is 97%. A thorough physical examination is normal. A CT of the chest is recommended and demonstrates bilateral enlargement of hilar lymph nodes and right paratracheal lymph node measuring up to 1.5 cm in size. The lung parenchyma is normal. Pulmonary function tests show a total lung capacity of 4.8 L (96% predicted) and a diffusion capacity of carbon monoxide of 13.4 (88% predicted). Spirometry is normal without obstruction. Bronchoscopy with transbronchial biopsies and transbronchial needle aspiration shows non-caseating granulomas. No fungal elements or acid-fast bacilli are seen, but cultures are pending. What is the best approach to therapy for this patient?

A. Isoniazid, pyrazinamide, rifampin, and ethambutol
B. Itraconazole
C. Prednisone 20 mg daily
D. Prednisone 1 mg/kg daily
E. Reassurance and close follow-up

VI-94. A 28-year-old man is brought to the emergency room by ambulance after being stung by several yellow

VI-94. *(Continued)*

jackets while cleaning out an old storage building at his home. He received four bites on his arms and neck. Immediately after being stung, he developed swelling at the sites and a diffuse pruritus. Within 15 min, diffuse urticaria and wheezing developed. His family called emergency services, and upon their arrival the patient was noted to be hypotensive (blood pressure 88/42 mmHg) and tachycardic (136 beats/min). There was swelling of the tongue with diffuse wheezing. Epinephrine, 0.3 mg, was given IM immediately. During transportation to the emergency room, the patient developed marked respiratory distress with use of accessory muscles and inspiratory stridor. Endotracheal intubation and mechanical ventilation were initiated for impending airway obstruction. A second dose of epinephrine, 0.3 mg, was administered IM. Upon arrival at the emergency department, the patient is sedated and remains paralyzed following his intubation. His current vital signs are: blood pressure 74/40 mmHg, heart rate 145 beats/min, respiratory rate 10 breaths/min, temperature 37.3°C, and Sa_{O_2} 100%. The ventilator settings are assist-control mode with a set rate of 10, Fi_{O_2} 1.0, tidal volume 500 mL, and positive end-expiratory pressure (PEEP) of 5 cmH$_2$O. There is diffuse urticaria and flushing of the skin. The lips and tongue are swollen. Diffuse expiratory wheezes are present and end prior to the start of the next inhalation. The cardiovascular examination demonstrates a regular tachycardia without murmurs. Bowel sounds are hyperactive. Neurologic examination is consistent with paralytic administration. Two 16-gauge IVs have been placed in the bilateral antecubital fossae. A liter of normal saline (0.9%) has been administered during transport to the hospital, and an infusion of normal saline is being continued at 1 L/h. The patient is receiving inhaled albuterol through the ventilator circuit. Which of the following is the best approach to ongoing management of this patient that is most likely to improve his hypotension?

A. Administer diphenhydramine, 50 mg, and ranitidine, 50 mg, IV.
B. Administer epinephrine, 0.1–0.3 mg IV.
C. Administer methylprednisolone, 125 mg IV.
D. Change the IV fluid solution from normal saline to lactated Ringer's solution and increase rate to 2 L/h.
E. Disconnect the patient from the ventilator to allow a full exhalation.

VI-95. Which of the following treatments has not been shown to improve mortality in septic shock?

A. Activated protein C (drotrecogin alpha)
B. Administration of antibiotics within 1 h of presentation
C. Bicarbonate therapy for severe acidosis
D. Early goal-directed therapy

VI-96. A 68-year-old male is seen in the clinic for evaluation of chronic cough that has lasted 4 months. He reports that the cough is dry and occurs at any time of the day. He denies hemoptysis or associated constitutional symptoms. Further, there is no wheezing, acid reflux symptoms, or postnasal drip. Past medical history is notable for a well-compensated ischemic cardiomyopathy that was diagnosed 6 months ago. His current medications include aspirin, carvedilol, furosemide, ramipril, amlodipine, and digoxin. He has no history of tobacco or alcohol abuse and denies occupational exposure. Physical examination shows a normal upper airway, clear lungs,

VI-96. (*Continued*)
and a normal cardiac examination with the exception of an enlarged point of maximal impulse. Plain radiography of the chest is normal with the exception of cardiomegaly. Which of the following is the most appropriate next step in his management?

A. Bronchoscopy
B. Changing furosemide to bumetanide
C. Discontinuing digoxin
D. Changing ramipril to valsartan
E. Giving azithromycin for 5 days

VI. DISORDERS OF THE RESPIRATORY SYSTEM

ANSWERS

VI-1. **The answer is C.** *(Chap. 35)* In the evaluation of cyanosis, the first step is to differentiate central from peripheral cyanosis. In central cyanosis, because the etiology is either reduced oxygen saturation or abnormal hemoglobin, the physical findings include bluish discoloration of both mucous membranes and skin. In contrast, peripheral cyanosis is associated with normal oxygen saturation but slowing of blood flow and an increased fraction of oxygen extraction from blood; subsequently, the physical findings are present only in the skin and extremities. Mucous membranes are spared. Peripheral cyanosis is commonly caused by cold exposure with vasoconstriction in the digits. Similar physiology is found in Raynaud's phenomenon. Peripheral vascular disease and deep venous thrombosis result in slowed blood flow and increased oxygen extraction with subsequent cyanosis. Methemoglobinemia causes abnormal hemoglobin that circulates systemically. Consequently, the cyanosis associated with this disorder is systemic. Other common causes of central cyanosis include severe lung disease with hypoxemia, right-to-left intracardiac shunting, and pulmonary arteriovenous malformations.

VI-2. **The answer is D.** *(Chap. 251)* Aspiration can lead to anaerobic infection and chemical pneumonitis. The etiologic differential diagnosis of community-acquired pneumonia (CAP) in a patient with a history of recent travel to the southwestern United States should include *Coccidioides*. *Aspergillus* has a worldwide distribution and is not a cause of CAP syndrome. Alcohol use predisposes patients to anaerobic infection, likely due to aspiration, as well as *S. pneumoniae*. *Klebsiella* is classically associated with CAP in alcoholic patients but in reality this is rarely seen. Patients with structural lung disease, such as cystic fibrosis or bronchiectasis, are at risk for a unique group of organisms including *P. aeruginosa* and *S. aureus*. Poor dental hygiene is associated with anaerobic infections.

VI-3. **The answer is A.** *(Chaps. 34, 255, and 312)* A variety of autoimmune diseases may cause pulmonary/renal disease, including Wegener's granulomatosis, microscopic polyangiitis, SLE, and cryoglobulinemia. Goodpasture's syndrome is characterized by the presence of anti–glomerular basement antibodies that cause glomerulonephritis with concurrent diffuse alveolar hemorrhage. The disease typically presents in patients over 40 years old with a history of cigarette smoking. These patients usually do not have fevers or joint symptoms. Among the listed options, antibodies to glutamic acid decarboxylase are seen in patients with type 1 diabetes or stiff-man syndrome, anti–smooth muscle antibodies in patients with autoimmune hepatitis, and anti–U1 RNP in those with mixed connective tissue disease. Antiphospholipid antibody syndrome may cause renal disease and alveolar hemorrhage, but this usually occurs in the context of a systemic illness with prominent thrombosis in other organ systems [extremities, central nervous system (CNS)].

VI-4. **The answer is E.** *(Chap. 249)* Multiple drugs have been associated with eosinophilic pulmonary reactions. They include nitrofurantoin, sulfonamides, NSAIDs, penicillins, thiazides, tricyclic antidepressants, hydralazine, and chlorpropramide, among others. Amiodarone can cause an acute respiratory distress syndrome with the initiation of the drug as well as a syndrome of pulmonary fibrosis. Eosinophilic pneumonia is not caused by amiodarone.

VI-5.   The answer is A. *(Chap. 31)* *Streptococcus pyogenes* is the most common cause of bacterial pharyngitis in adults, accounting for ~5–15% of cases of acute pharyngitis (the largest number being viral). Group A Streptococcus is an uncommon cause of pharyngitis after age 15. Cough and coryza are more suggestive of viral pharyngitis, as is a less severe sore throat. Pharyngeal exudates, tender cervical adenopathy, fever, and lack of cough are all more predictive of pharyngitis due to *S. pyogenes*. Some experts recommend empirical penicillin treatment without throat sampling for rapid antigen and culture if at least three or four of the above clinical criteria are met, while others recommend making a microbiologic diagnosis in all cases where streptococcal infection is being considered. The rapid streptococcal antigen test is indeed rapid but lacks complete sensitivity in a clinic setting. Sending streptococcal antigen–negative samples for culture that is more sensitive but takes 2–4 days to return is also controversial.

VI-6.   The answer is E. *(Chap. 31)* Nonspecific upper respiratory tract infections (URIs) are the leading cause of ambulatory care visits. By definition, they are characterized by no prominent localizing features, and symptoms include rhinorrhea (with or without purulence), nasal congestion, cough, and sore throat. Nearly all nonspecific URIs are caused by viral infections including rhinovirus (most common), influenza, parainfluenza, and adenovirus. Purulent secretions in the absence of other clinical features are a poor predictor of bacterial infection. Although decongestant medicines, antitussives, and nasal saline help temporarily ameliorate the symptoms of URI, no antibiotics, vitamin, or alternative medicine has consistently been shown in a randomized clinical trial to affect the duration of a cold.

VI-7.   The answer is A. *(Chap. 257)* Primary spontaneous pneumothorax is usually secondary to the rupture of small apical blebs that lie near the pleural surface. The typical patient is a thin young male who smokes. The presenting symptoms are chest pain and dyspnea. The recommended initial approach to treatment is needle aspiration of the pneumothorax. If this fails to fully expand the lung, placement of a small apical tube thoracostomy can be utilized to continue to drain the air. Large-bore chest tubes are not necessary to drain the air present in a pneumothorax. If ongoing air leak is present after ~5 days, then the patient should be referred for thoracoscopy to staple the blebs and perform pleural abrasion. This procedure is also recommended for those individuals who develop recurrent pneumothoraces, which occurs in ~50% of individuals with a primary spontaneous pneumothorax. If the pneumothorax is small (<15%), observation and administration of 100% oxygen is an option for treatment. Use of 100% oxygen speeds reabsorption of the pneumothorax by promoting diffusion of air that is composed of a nitrogen and oxygen mixture back into the lungs.

VI-8.   The answer is C. *(Chap. 273)* Primary pulmonary hypertension is an uncommon disease that usually affects young females. Early in the illness affected persons often are diagnosed as psychoneurotic because of the vague nature of the presenting complaints, for example, dyspnea, chest pain, and evidence of hyperventilation without hypoxemia on arterial blood gas testing. However, progression of the disease leads to syncope in approximately one-half of cases and signs of right heart failure on physical examination. Chest x-ray typically shows enlarged central pulmonary arteries with or without attenuation of peripheral markings. The diagnosis of primary pulmonary hypertension is made by documenting elevated pressures by right heart catheterization and excluding other pathologic processes. Lung disease of sufficient severity to cause pulmonary hypertension would be evident by history and on examination. Major differential diagnoses include thromboemboli and heart disease; outside the United States, schistosomiasis and filariasis are common causes of pulmonary hypertension, and a careful travel history should be taken.

Nomenclature and Classification of Pulmonary Hypertension

Diagnostic Classification

1. Pulmonary arterial hypertension

    Primary pulmonary hypertension: sporadic and familial

    Related to

        a. Collagen-vascular disease

        b. Congenital systemic to pulmonary shunts

        c. Portal hypertension

        d. HIV infection

        e. Drugs/toxins: anorexigens and other

        f. Persistent pulmonary hypertension of the newborn

        g. Other

2. Pulmonary venous hypertension

    Left-side atrial or ventricular heart disease

    Left-side valvular heart disease

    Extrinsic compression of central pulmonary veins: fibrosing mediastinitis and adenopathy/ tumors

    Pulmonary veno-occlusive disease

    Other

3. Pulmonary hypertension associated with disorders of the respiratory system and/or hypoxemia

Chronic obstructive pulmonary disease	Chronic exposure to high altitude
Interstitial lung disease	Neonatal lung disease
Sleep-disordered breathing	Alveolar-capillary dysplasia
Alveolar hypoventilatory disorders	Other

4. Pulmonary hypertension due to chronic thrombotic and/or embolic disease

    Thromboembolic obstruction of proximal pulmonary arteries

    Obstruction of distal pulmonary arteries

        a. Pulmonary embolism (thrombus, tumor, ova and/or parasites, foreign material)

        b. In-situ thrombosis

        c. Sickle cell disease

5. Pulmonary hypertension due to disorders directly affecting the pulmonary vasculature

    Inflammatory: Schistosomiasis; Sarcoidosis; other

    Pulmonary capillary hemangiomatosis

VI-9. **The answer is E.** *(Chap. 256)* This patient is presenting with massive pulmonary embolus with ongoing hypotension, right ventricular dysfunction, and profound hypoxemia requiring 100% oxygen. In this setting, continuing with anticoagulation alone is inadequate, and the patient should receive circulatory support with fibrinolysis, if there are no contraindications to therapy. The major contraindications to fibrinolysis include hypertension >180/110 mmHg, known intracranial disease or prior hemorrhagic stroke, recent surgery, or trauma. The recommended fibrinolytic regimen is recombinant tissue plasminogen activator (rTPA), 100 mg IV over 2 h. Heparin should be continued with the fibrinolytic to prevent a rebound hypercoagulable state with dissolution of the clot. There is a 10% risk of major bleeding with fibrinolytic therapy with a 1–3% risk of intracranial hemorrhage. The only indication approved by the U.S. Food and Drug Administration for fibrinolysis in pulmonary embolus (PE) is for massive PE presenting with life-threatening hypotension, right ventricular dysfunction, and refractory hypoxemia. In submassive PE presenting with preserved blood pressure and evidence of right ventricular dysfunction on echocardiogram, the decision to pursue fibrinolysis is made on a case-by-case situation. In addition to fibrinolysis, the patient should also receive circulatory support with vasopressors. Dopamine and dobutamine are the vasopressors of choice for the treatment of shock in PE. Caution should be taken with ongoing high-volume fluid administration as a poorly functioning right ventricle may be poorly tolerant of additional fluids. Ongoing fluids may worsen right ventricular ischemia and further dilate the right ventricle, displacing the interventricular septum to the left to worsen cardiac output and hypotension. If the patient had contraindications to fibrinolysis and was unable to be stabilized with vasopressor support, referral for surgical embolectomy should be considered. Referral for inferior vena cava filter placement is not indicated at this time. The patient should be stabilized hemodynamically as a first priority. The indications for inferior vena cava filter placement are active bleeding, precluding anticoagulation, and recurrent deep venous thrombosis on adequate anticoagulation.

VI-10, VI-11, VI-12, and VI-13. The answers are C, B, D, and A, respectively. *(Chap. 246)* Ventilatory function can be easily measured with lung volume measurement and the FEV_1/FVC ratio. A decreased FEV_1/FVC ratio diagnoses obstructive lung disease. Alternatively, low lung volumes, specifically decreased TLC, and occasionally decreased RV diagnose restrictive lung disease. With extensive air trapping in obstructive lung disease, TLC is often increased and RV may also be increased. VC is proportionally decreased. MIP measures respiratory muscle strength and is decreased in patients with neuromuscular disease. Thus, myasthenia gravis will produce low lung volumes and decreased MIP, whereas patients with idiopathic pulmonary fibrosis will have normal muscle strength and subsequently a normal MIP but decreased TLC and RV. In some cases of pulmonary parenchymal restrictive lung disease, the increase in elastic recoil results in an increased FEV_1/FVC ratio. The hallmark of obstructive lung disease is a decreased FEV_1/FVC ratio; thus, the correct answer for Q VI-13 is A.

VI-14. The answer is D. *(Chap. 257)* Thoracentesis is indicated for any patient presenting with pneumonia and a pleural effusion more than 10 mm thick on lateral decubitus imaging because a significant percentage of these patients will show evidence of bacterial invasion and require further intervention. Other indications for thoracentesis for pleural effusions that complicate pneumonias include loculation of the pleural fluid and evidence of thickened parietal pleura on chest CT. The pleural fluid should be sent for cell count, differential, pH, protein, LDH, glucose, and culture with Gram stain. This will allow one to differentiate a simple parapneumonic effusion from a complicated one or from empyema. All effusions complicating pneumonia should be exudative, meeting at least one of Light's criteria: (1) pleural fluid protein/serum protein over 0.5, (2) pleural fluid LDH/serum LDH over 0.6, and (3) pleural fluid LDH more than two-thirds of the normal upper limit for serum. Factors that increase the likelihood that tube thoracostomy will have to be performed include loculated pleural fluid, pH below 7.20, pleural fluid glucose below 60 mg/dL, positive Gram stain or culture of pleural fluid, and presence of gross pus on aspiration.

VI-15. The answer is C. *(Chap. 254)* The only therapy that has been proved to improve survival in patients with COPD is oxygen in the subset of patients with resting hypoxemia. This patient probably has resting hypoxemia resulting from the presence of an elevated jugular venous pulse, pedal edema, and an elevated hematocrit. Theophylline has been shown to increase exercise tolerance in patients with COPD through a mechanism other than bronchodilation. Glucocorticoids are not indicated in the absence of an acute exacerbation and may lead to complications if they are used indiscriminately. Atenolol and enalapril have no specific role in therapy for COPD but are often used when there is concomitant illness.

VI-16 and VI-17. The answers are E and E. *(Chap. 33)* The mountain climber is at risk for two well-described altitude-related conditions: high-altitude cerebral edema and high-altitude pulmonary edema. High-altitude pulmonary edema is a well-described subset of pulmonary edema. Other causes of pulmonary edema include cardiogenic, neurogenic, and noncardiogenic (as seen in acute respiratory distress syndrome). Although the exact mechanism of this disorder is unclear, one commonly accepted hypothesis suggests that increased cardiac output and hypoxic vasoconstriction with resultant pulmonary hypertension combine to cause high-pressure pulmonary edema. Persons less than 25 years old are more likely than are older persons to develop this condition, probably because hypoxic vasoconstriction of the pulmonary arteries is more pronounced in this population. Persons who regularly live at high altitudes are still at risk for high-altitude pulmonary edema when they descend to a lower altitude and then return to higher areas. Prevention can be achieved by means of prophylactic administration of acetazolamide and gradual ascent to higher altitudes. Once this condition develops, the most important therapy is to descend to a lower altitude. Other therapies include oxygen to decrease hypoxic pulmonary vasoconstriction and diuretic therapy as needed.

VI-18. **The answer is B.** *(Chap. 253)* Patients with cystic fibrosis are at risk for colonization and/or infection with a number of pathogens, and in general these infections have a temporal relationship. In childhood, the most frequently isolated organisms are *Haemophilus influenzae* and *Staphylococcus aureus*. As patients age, *Pseudomonas aeruginosa* becomes the predominant pathogen. Interestingly, *Aspergillus fumigatus* is found in the airways of up to 50% of cystic fibrosis patients. All these organisms merely colonize the airways but occasionally can also cause disease. *Burkholderia* (previously called *Pseudomonas*) *cepacia* can occasionally be found in the sputum of cystic fibrosis patients, where it is always pathogenic and is associated with a rapid decline in both clinical parameters and pulmonary function testing. Atypical mycobacteria can occasionally be found in the sputum but are often merely colonizers. *Acinetobacter baumannii* is not associated with cystic fibrosis; rather, it is generally found in nosocomial infections.

VI-19. **The answer is F.** *(Chap. 260)* The most common cause of mortality in patients who have undergone lung transplantation is chronic allograft rejection, also known as bronchiolitis obliterans syndrome (BOS). This disorder results from fibroproliferation of the small airways with resultant airflow obstruction. Histologically, there is an absence of acute inflammation. Clinically, the diagnosis is made by a sustained fall of 20% or more in FEV_1 in the setting of airflow limitation. Alternatively, the diagnosis can be made on lung biopsy. Risk factors for the development of BOS include acute rejection episodes and lymphocytic bronchiolitis. CMV pneumonitis has inconsistently been named as a risk factor as well. With a prevalence in lung transplant recipients of 50% at 3 years, this disorder is the main limitation on long-term survival after lung transplantation. These patients often have concurrent bacterial infection or colonization that may improve with therapy. When identified, chronic rejection or BOS generally is treated with increased immunosuppression. However, no controlled trials have shown consistent efficacy of this approach, and anecdotally the results appear to be poor.

VI-20. **The answer is B.** *(Chap. 250)* Asbestos was a commonly used insulating material from the 1940s to the mid-1970s, after which it was largely replaced by fiberglass and slag wool. Workers in many occupations had significant exposure and often did not use protective equipment. There are several pulmonary manifestations of asbestos exposure in the lungs, the most important of which are pleural plaques, benign asbestos pleural effusions, asbestosis, lung cancer, and mesothelioma. Pleural plaques, which appear as calcifications or thickening along the parietal pleura, simply suggest exposure and not pulmonary impairment. Benign pleural effusions can occur and are often bloody. They may regress or progress spontaneously. Asbestosis refers to interstitial lung disease, generally with fibrosis, seen in the lower lung fields of a chest radiogram or chest CT and an associated restrictive ventilatory defect. This patient does not have interstitial changes on chest radiography and has no restriction on pulmonary function tests; therefore, he does not have asbestosis. The risk of lung cancer, including squamous cell cancer and adenocarcinoma, is elevated in all patients with asbestos exposure but is amplified further by cigarette smoking. In contrast, mesothelioma risk, though elevated in patients with asbestos exposure, is not increased by cigarette smoking. Interestingly, despite the high risk of malignancies in this group of patients, no benefit has been ascribed to screening techniques, including biannual chest radiograms.

VI-21. **The answer is C.** *(Chap. 251)* The decision to hospitalize a patient with community-acquired pneumonia (CAP) must be individualized and considerate of the markedly increased cost of inpatient care. The CURB-65 criteria are a severity of illness score that can be helpful in identifying patients with low-risk disease who may not require hospitalization. The CURB-65 criteria include: *C*onfusion, *B*UN ≥20 mg/dL, *r*espiratory rate ≥30 breaths/min, *b*lood pressure ≤90 systolic or ≤60 diastolic, and age >*65*. Patients with a score of 0 or 1 have a <4% mortality. Patients with a score of 2 have a 30-day mortality of almost 10% and should likely be admitted to the hospital. Patients with a score of 3–5 have >20% 30-day mortality and may warrant ICU care. All of the patients except patient C have 0 or 1 scores and could be considered candidates for outpatient treatment. Patient

D may warrant further evaluation for her confusion. Another objective system, the Pneumonia Severity Index (PSI) requires 20 variables but is more widely studied. Its use has been associated with lower admission rates for less sick patients. Whatever objective scoring criteria are used, management and treatment decisions should be tempered by individual patient factors including underlying disease, adherence factors, social support, and other resources.

VI-22. **The answer is E.** *(Chap. 263)* Modes of ventilation differ in how breaths are triggered, cycled, and limited. The figure shows the ventilator pressure waveform in the top panel and volume delivered in the bottom panel. When considering the pressure waveforms, there are several breaths that are triggered by patient effort, which is indicated by a drop in the airway pressure below 0. In addition, the last breath in the figure shows no drop in airway pressure. This indicates a machine-triggered breath. Thus, the mode used allows both patient-triggered and machine-triggered ventilation. The volume waveform also provides additional information to determine the mode of mechanical ventilation that is depicted here. Two of the patient-triggered breaths are associated with small inspired tidal volumes, whereas the other two breaths (one patient-triggered and one machine-triggered) deliver the same tidal volume. The larger breaths are volume-cycled, and the smaller breaths reflect the spontaneous tidal volume of the patient. This type of ventilation is characteristic of synchronized intermittent mandatory ventilation (SIMV). SIMV allows spontaneous ventilation by the patient but delivers a mandatory prescribed minute ventilation. Often, SIMV is combined with pressure support ventilation so that the patient has ventilatory assistance during a spontaneous ventilatory effort. SIMV is sometimes used in ventilator weaning and in individuals with obstructive lung disease to prevent development of intrinsic positive end-expiratory pressure (PEEP) that may develop with assist control mode ventilation. With assist control mode ventilation, patient triggering of the ventilator results in delivery of the prescribed tidal volume with each breath. In patients with a high respiratory rate, this can result in hyperventilation and intrinsic PEEP due to inadequate time for exhalation of the full tidal volume.

Pressure-control and pressure-support ventilation are pressure-cycled, rather than volume-cycled, modes of ventilation. In pressure-control ventilation, the physician sets an inspiratory pressure level, and the tidal volume delivered may be variable on a breath-to-breath basis, as the machine will continue to deliver inspiratory volume until the preset pressure is reached. Breaths can be machine-triggered or patient-triggered in this mode of ventilation. With pressure-support ventilation, breaths are patient triggered. When the patient initiates a breath, the ventilator raises the inspiratory pressure to the level prescribed by the physician, assisting with ventilation. The pressure will remain at this level until the ventilator senses that the inspiratory flow has declined to a preset threshold determined by the ventilator.

Continuous positive airway pressure provides a set pressure that is usually between 5 and 10 cmH$_2$O throughout respiration. All respiratory efforts must be triggered by the patient, and the tidal volume relies on the inspiratory efforts of the patient. This is not a true support mode of ventilation and is frequently used to assess acceptability for extubation.

VI-23. **The answer is C.** *(Chap. 256)* In determining the appropriate regimen for venous thromboembolism prophylaxis, one must consider the risk associated with the patient and/or the procedure. High-risk patients include those who undergo orthopedic procedures involving the knee or pelvis, those with a hip or pelvis fracture, and those who have undergone gynecologic cancer surgery. Generally, these patients should receive an aggressive approach to thromboembolism prophylaxis, including warfarin with a goal INR of 2.0 to 2.5 for 4 to 6 weeks, twice-daily subcutaneous low-molecular-weight heparin, or intermittent pneumatic compression devices plus warfarin. Moderate-risk patients, including those undergoing gynecologic, urologic, thoracic, or abdominal surgery, and medically ill patients can be appropriately treated with subcutaneous unfractionated heparin plus graded compression stockings or intermittent pneumatic compression devices. Low-risk patients do not require medications or devices for prophylaxis but should be encouraged to ambulate frequently.

VI-24. The answer is D. *(Chap. 252)* The combination of infertility and recurrent sinopulmonary infections should prompt consideration of an underlying disorder of ciliary dysfunction that is termed primary ciliary dyskinesia. These disorders account for approximately 5 to 10% of cases of bronchiectasis. A number of deficiencies have been described, including malfunction of dynein arms, radial spokes, and microtubules. All organ systems that require ciliary function are affected. The lungs rely on cilia to beat respiratory secretions proximally and subsequently to remove inspired particles, especially bacteria. In the absence of this normal host defense, recurrent bacterial respiratory infections occur and can lead to bronchiectasis. Otitis media and sinusitis are common for the same reason. In the genitourinary tract, sperm require cilia to provide motility. Kartagener's syndrome is a combination of sinusitis, bronchiectasis, and situs inversus. It accounts for approximately 50% of patients with primary ciliary dyskinesia. Cystic fibrosis is associated with infertility and bilateral upper lobe infiltrates, it causes a decreased number of sperm or absent sperm on analysis because of the congenital absence of the vas deferens. Sarcoidosis, which is often associated with bihilar adenopathy, is not generally a cause of infertility. Water balloon–shaped heart is found in those with pericardial effusions, which one would not expect in this patient.

VI-25. The answer is C. *(Chap. 246)* In this patient presenting with multilobar pneumonia, hypoxemia is present that does not correct with increasing the concentration of inspired oxygen. The inability to overcome hypoxemia or the lack of a notable increase in Pa_{O_2} with increasing fraction of inspired oxygen (FI_{O_2}) physiologically defines a shunt. A shunt occurs when deoxygenated blood is transported to the left heart and systemic circulation without having the capability of becoming oxygenated. Causes of shunt include alveolar collapse (atelectasis), intraalveolar filling processes, intrapulmonary vascular malformations, or structural cardiac disease leading to right-to-left shunt. In this case, the patient has multilobar pneumonia leading to alveoli that are being perfused but unable to participate in gas exchange because they are filled with pus and inflammatory exudates. Acute respiratory distress syndrome is another common cause of shunt physiology. Ventilation-perfusion ($\dot{V}/\dot{Q}$) mismatch is the most common cause of hypoxemia and results when there are some alveolar units with low $\dot{V}/\dot{Q}$ ratios (low ventilation to perfusion) that fail to fully oxygenate perfused blood. When blood is returned to the left heart, the poorly oxygenated blood admixes with blood from normal $\dot{V}/\dot{Q}$ alveolar units. The resultant hypoxemia is less severe than with shunt and can be corrected with increasing the inspired oxygen concentration. Hypoventilation with or without other causes of hypoxemia is not present in this case as the Pa_{CO_2} <40 mmHg, indicating hyperventilation. The acidosis present in this case is of a metabolic rather than a pulmonary source. Because the patient is paralyzed, she is unable to increase her respiratory rate above the set rate to compensate for the metabolic acidosis.

VI-26. The answer is D. *(Chap. 164)* This patient presents with the classic findings of severe leptospirosis (Weil's syndrome). Leptospires are spirochetes that persist in the renal tubules of a variety of animal reservoirs. The most important reservoir is the rat, and humans are infected after exposure to rat urine. Exposure to rodent urine followed by a flulike illness approximately 1 week later is typical for anicteric leptospirosis. Many of these patients with mild disease have resolution of their symptoms within a week and then develop a recurrence after 1 to 3 days during the immune phase. It is during the immune phase that patients develop aseptic meningitis. A minority of patients with leptospirosis develop Weil's syndrome, which is characterized by severe jaundice without evidence of hepatocellular damage, acute renal failure, and respiratory failure. Conjunctival suffusion is a classic physical finding. Rhabdomyolysis, hemolysis, shock, and adult respiratory distress syndrome may develop. The diagnosis is usually established by serology; culture is performed in reference laboratories and takes weeks. In cases of presumptive severe leptospirosis, therapy with penicillin, amoxicillin, erythromycin, or doxycycline should be initiated. Newer-generation cephalosporins have in vitro activity, but no clinical studies have evaluated in vivo efficacy. Severe leptospirosis is epidemiologically and clinically similar to hantavirus infection.

VI-27.   **The answer is C.** *(Chap. 257)*   This patient is presenting with a large unilateral pleural effusion. By Light's criteria, the effusion is exudative in nature. Light's criteria are: (1) pleural fluid protein/serum protein >0.5; (2) pleural fluid LDH/serum LDH >0.6; (3) pleural fluid LDH >2/3 of the upper limits of normal. In addition, the pleural fluid has a lymphocytic predominance. In this patient who is a smoker with abnormal lymph nodes in the mediastinum, the most likely cause of an exudative effusion with excess lymphocytes is malignancy, likely due to a lung cancer. Of the choices listed, sending the pleural fluid for cytology is the best test to determine the cause of the pleural effusion. If this is unsuccessful, consideration of thoracoscopic biopsy of the pleura or bronchoscopic biopsy of the mediastinal lymph nodes should be considered. Mediastinoscopy could also be considered. The patient should receive screening mammography yearly as indicated by her age, but this is not the best choice for diagnosis of the pleural effusion. The patient has no symptoms to suggest an infection, and lymphocytic predominance in the pleural fluid is not consistent with a parapneumonic effusion. Thus, pleural fluid culture is unlikely to yield the diagnosis.

VI-28.   **The answer is B.** *(Chap. 31)*   Antibiotics are tremendously overprescribed for the presumptive diagnosis of acute sinusitis. Acute bacterial sinusitis is uncommon in patients with symptoms of less than 7 days' duration even in the presence of purulent discharge. Most cases are due to viral infections. Decongestants and nasal lavage should be prescribed initially. In a patient with a known history of allergic rhinitis, nasal corticosteroids may be added. Empirical antibiotic therapy may be prescribed for patients whose symptoms do not improve with conservative therapy after 1 week and patients with a known predisposition to sinus infection (e.g., cystic fibrosis). Imaging of the sinuses should not be performed in routine cases. For recurrent or persistent sinusitis, CT is preferred to standard sinus radiography. Aspiration should be performed when there is known opacification of a sinus and empirical therapy has not been effective or the patient is at risk of opportunistic infection. In the absence of nasal perforation, lung symptoms or signs, or renal disease that raises suspicion of vasculitis or Wegener's granulomatosis, measurement of serum ANCA is not warranted.

VI-29.   **The answer is C.** *(Chap. 246)*   The residual volume of the lung is the amount of gas that remains in the lung after a maximal expiratory effort. It is determined by airway closure. Residual volume is elevated in conditions that result in premature airway closure with expiration or due to inability to fully exhale due to muscle weakness or chest wall stiffness. Of the choices listed, only emphysema is associated with an increased residual volume. In emphysema, there is destruction of alveoli usually related to the effects of cigarette smoking. The destruction of alveoli leads to decreased traction on small airways and allows them to collapse at higher lung volumes, resulting in an increased residual volume. When emphysema occurs concomitantly with chronic bronchitis, the airway inflammation characteristic of chronic bronchitis also leads to increased residual volume due to decreased airway diameter. Other disorders that lead to increased residual volume include asthma, diaphragmatic weakness, and kyphoscoliosis. Idiopathic pulmonary fibrosis usually causes a decrease in residual volume due to airway stiffness. Obesity should not affect residual volume.

VI-30.   **The answer is A.** *(Chap. 192)*   This patient comes from an area where histoplasmosis is endemic (Ohio and Mississippi river valleys) and is complaining of classic, though nonspecific, symptoms. Usually acute histoplasmosis resolves without therapy in the immunocompetent patient. Acute pulmonary histoplasmosis is a moderate to severe illness that can be fatal if not diagnosed promptly. It usually occurs 2–4 weeks after heavy exposure and presents with a flulike illness. Parenchymal infiltrates with hilar and mediastinal adenopathy are typical. Fungal culture is the "gold standard," test but fungal staining will yield positive results in about half of cases. The figure shows the classic narrow budding yeast evident on silver stain. Symptomatic patients with respiratory histoplasmosis should be treated with lipid amphotericin for 1–2 weeks followed by 6–12 weeks of itraconazole. Glucocorticoids may be used as adjuvant therapy along with antifungals to decrease inflammation. Ciprofloxacin and piperacillin/tazobactam have no antifungal activity. Caspofungin is effective for treatment of candidiasis, not histoplasmosis.

VI-31.　The answers are 1-C; 2-B; 3-D; 4-A. *(Chaps. 264, 265, and 266)* A variety of vasopressor agents are available for hemodynamic support. The effects of these medications are dependent upon their effects on the sympathetic nervous system to produce changes in heart rate, cardiac contractility, and peripheral vascular tone. Stimulation of α-1 adrenergic receptors in the peripheral vasculature causes vasoconstriction and improves mean arterial pressure by increasing systemic vascular resistance. The β_1 receptors are located primarily in the heart and cause increased cardiac contractility and heart rate. The β_2 receptors are found in the peripheral circulation and cause vasodilatation and bronchodilation. Phenylephrine acts solely as an α-adrenergic agonist. It is considered a second-line agent in septic shock and is often used in anesthesia to correct hypotension following induction of anesthesia. Phenylephrine is also useful for spinal shock. The action of dopamine is dependent upon the dosage used. At high doses, dopamine has high affinity for the α receptor whereas at lower doses (<5 μg/kg per min) it does not. In addition, dopamine acts at β_1 receptors and dopaminergic receptors. The effect on these receptors is greatest at lower doses. Norepinephrine and epinephrine affect both α and β_1 receptors to increase peripheral vascular resistance, heart rate, and contractility. Norepinephrine has less β_1 activity than epinephrine or dopamine and, thus, has less associated tachycardia. Norepinephrine and dopamine are the recommended first-line therapies for septic shock. Epinephrine is the drug of choice for anaphylactic shock. Dobutamine is primarily a β_1 agonist with lesser effects at the β_2 receptor. Dobutamine increases cardiac output through improving cardiac contractility and heart rate. Dobutamine may be associated with development of hypotension because of its effects at the β_2 receptor causing vasodilatation and decreased systemic vascular resistance.

VI-32.　The answer is C. *(Chap. 28)* Obstructive sleep apnea (OSA) is a common sleep disorder affecting up to 20% of the population, and the incidence of OSA is expected to increase as the incidence of obesity has risen over the past 30 years. OSA is characterized by repetitive events during which the posterior oropharynx collapses with a marked decrease or absence of airflow despite ongoing respiratory effort. Obstructive events are often associated with marked disruptions in sleep continuity with frequent arousals. Recurrent oxygen desaturations, which may be very severe, also occur concurrently with obstructive sleep apnea events. The figure illustrates a typical obstructive sleep apnea event. In this figure, the nasal/oral airflow channel demonstrates a near absence of airflow despite ongoing respiratory effort. Each obstructive event depicted in this illustration is associated with a concomitant decrease in oxygen saturation from a baseline of 98% to 86–91% and lasts for about 20–30 s. Central sleep apnea is diagnosed when there is an absence of airflow in association with an absence of respiratory effort lasting for at least 10 s. Cheyne-Stokes respiration is a type of central sleep apnea characterized by a crescendo-decrescendo pattern of respiratory effort and airflow. A period of apnea is terminated by a period of hyperpnea. Unlike obstructive sleep apnea, arousals during Cheyne-Stokes respiration occur during the hyperpneic phase of respiration rather than at the termination of the apnea. Cheyne-Stokes respiration is frequently seen in congestive heart failure and following cerebrovascular events. Periodic limb movement disorder of sleep is characterized by recurrent leg movements during sleep. The typical periodic limb movement is dorsiflexion of the great toe and ankle. Periodic limb movements become increasingly frequent with age, and most are not associated with significant sleep disruption or arousals.

VI-33 and VI-34.　The answers are E and D. *(Chap. 255)* Pulmonary alveolar proteinosis (PAP) is a rare disorder with an incidence of approximately 1 in 1 million. The disease usually presents between ages 30 and 50 and is slightly more common in men. Three distinct subtypes have been described: congenital, acquired, and secondary (most frequently caused by acute silicosis or hematologic malignancies). Interestingly, the pathogenesis of the disease has been associated with antibodies to granulocyte-macrophage colony-stimulating factor (GM-CSF) in most cases of acquired disease in adults. The pathobiology of the disease is failure of clearance of pulmonary surfactant. These patients typically present with subacute dyspnea on exertion with fatigue and low-grade fevers. Associated laboratory abnormalities include polycythemia, hypergammaglobulinemia, and increased LDH levels. Classically, the CT appearance is described as "crazy pavement" with ground-glass alveolar infiltrates in a perihilar distribution and intervening areas of normal lung. Bronchoalveolar lavage is diagnostic, with large amounts of amorphous proteinaceous material seen. Macrophages filled with PAS-positive material are also frequently seen. The treatment of choice is whole-lung lavage through a double-lumen endotracheal tube. Survival at 5 years is higher than 95%, although some patients will need a repeat whole-lung lavage. Secondary infection, especially with *Nocardia,* is common, and these patients should be followed closely.

VI-35 and VI-36. The answers are B and C. *(Chap. 264)* Hypovolemic shock is the most common form of shock and occurs due to either hemorrhage or loss of plasma volume in the form of gastrointestinal, urinary, or insensible losses. Symptoms of hemorrhagic and nonhemorrhagic shock are indistinguishable. Mild hypovolemia is considered to be loss of <20% of the blood volume and usually presents with few clinical signs save for mild tachycardia. Loss of 20–40% of the blood volume typically induces orthostasis. Loss of >40% of the blood volume leads to the classic manifestations of shock: marked tachycardia, hypotension, oliguria, and finally obtundation. Central nervous system perfusion is maintained until shock becomes severe. Oliguria is a very important clinical parameter that should help guide volume resuscitation.

After assessing for an adequate airway and spontaneous breathing, initial resuscitation aims at reexpanding the intravascular volume and controlling ongoing losses. Volume resuscitation should be initiated with rapid IV infusion of isotonic saline or Ringer's lactate. In head-to-head trials, colloidal solutions have not added any benefit compared to crystalloid, and in fact appeared to increase mortality for trauma patients. Hemorrhagic shock with ongoing blood losses and a hemoglobin ≤10 g/dL should be treated with transfusion of packed red blood cells (pRBCs). Once hemorrhage is controlled, transfusion of packed RBCs should be performed only for hemoglobin ≤7 g/dL. Patients who remain hypotensive after volume resuscitation have a very poor prognosis. Inotropic support and intensive monitoring should be initiated in these patients.

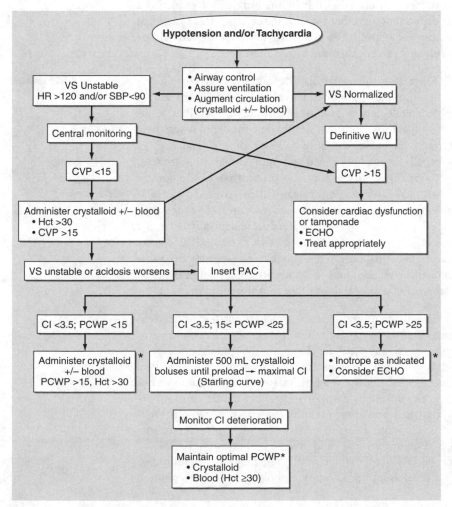

FIGURE VI-36 An algorithm for the resuscitation of the patient in shock. VS, vital signs; HR, heart rate; SBP, systolic blood pressure; W/U, work up; CVP, central venous pressure; Hct, hematocrit; ECHO, echocardiogram; PAC, pulmonary artery catheter; CI, cardiac index in (L/min) per m^2; PCWP, pulmonary capillary wedge pressure in mmHg. *Monitor SV_{O_2}, SVRI, and RVEDVI as additional markers of correction for perfusion and hypovolemia. Consider age-adjusted CI. SV_{O_2}, saturation of hemoglobin with O_2 in venous blood; SVRI, systemic vascular resistance index; RVEDVI, right-ventricular end-diastolic volume index.

VI-37. **The answer is B.** *(Chap. 246)* The patient in this presentation is presenting after a narcotic overdose, which leads to hypoxia because of hypoventilation. The major causes of hypoxemia are hypoventilation, shunt, and $\dot{V}/\dot{Q}$ mismatch. Diffusing defects can also cause hypoxemia but are a much less frequent cause. A final cause of hypoxemia to consider is decreased concentration of oxygen in inspired air, which is only present at altitude or in the setting of medical equipment malfunction. When evaluating a patient with hypoxia, it is important to consider whether the alveolar-arterial oxygen gradient is normal or elevated. Of the causes of hypoxia, only hypoventilation and decreased fraction of inspired oxygen will cause hypoxia with a normal A – a gradient. The formula for calculating the alveolar oxygen concentration is:

$$P_{A_{O_2}} = ((P_{atm} - P_{H_2O})^*(F_{I_{O_2}})) - (Pa_{CO_2}/R),$$
where P_{atm} = atmospheric pressure,
P_{H_2O} = water vapor pressure,
$F_{I_{O_2}}$ = fraction of inspired oxygen, and
R = respiratory quotient.

When values are substituted assuming usual conditions at sea level and with the patient breathing room air, the equation is simplified to:

$$P_{A_{O_2}} = (760 - 47)(0.21) - (Pa_{CO_2}/0.8) = 150 - Pa_{CO_2}/0.8$$

In this patient, the calculated $P_{A_{O_2}}$ is 50. Thus, the A – a gradient is 8 mmHg (normal value <15 mmHg) and is normal. Thus, the only correct answer is B.

VI-38. **The answer is D.** *(Chap. 246)* The functional residual capacity (FRC) is the volume of gas that remains within the lungs at the end of a normal tidal respiration. The FRC comprises the expiratory reserve volume (ERV) and the residual volume (RV). The ERV is the additional volume of gas that can be forcefully exhaled from the lung after completing a passive exhalation. The RV is the amount of gas that remains in the lung after a maximal expiratory effort. The lung volume at FRC reflects equilibrium between the lung elastic recoil pressure inward and the outward forces generated by the chest wall.

VI-39. **The answer is D.** *(Chap. 258)* Respiratory muscular disorders rarely cause chronic hypoventilation unless there is significant diaphragmatic weakness. Myasthenia gravis, muscular dystrophy, amyotrophic lateral sclerosis, and other chronic myopathies that involve peripheral musculature as well as the diaphragm should be considered when there are signs or symptoms of diaphragmatic weakness. Upright chest radiographs may show diaphragm elevation but are usually normal. When diaphragm weakness is present, forced vital capacity will be >10–15% lower in the supine position than in the upright position, and maximal inspiratory and expiratory pressures will be reduced. Transdiaphragmatic pressure gradients (esophageal minus gastric pressures) can also be measured as a confirmatory test. Diffusing capacity has little diagnostic value; it is mostly useful as a physiologic measure and a predictor of oxygen desaturation with exercise. It is usually normal in muscle weakness. A normal perfusion scan has a high negative predictive value for ruling out pulmonary embolism; an angiogram is not indicated. CT scan of the head would not be useful in diagnosing myasthenia gravis or other motor neuron diseases.

VI-40. **The answer is B.** *(Chap. 257)* The most common cause of pleural effusion is left ventricular failure. Pleural effusions occur in heart failure when there are increased hydrostatic forces increasing the pulmonary interstitial fluid and the lymphatic drainage is inadequate to remove the fluid. Right-sided effusions are more common than left-sided effusions in heart failure. Thoracentesis would show a transudative fluid. Pneumonia can be associated with a parapneumonic effusion or empyema. Parapneumonic effusions are the most common cause of exudative pleural effusions and are second only to heart failure as a cause of pleural effusions. Empyema refers to a grossly purulent pleural effusion. Malignancy is the second most common cause of exudative pleural effusion. Breast and lung cancers and lymphoma cause 75% of all malignant pleural effusions. On thoracentesis, the effusion is exudative. Cirrhosis and pulmonary embolus are far less common causes of pleural effusions.

VI-41. **The answer is D.** *(Chap. 264)* The patient above is in cardiogenic shock from an ST-elevation myocardial infarction. Shock is a clinical syndrome in which vital organs do not receive adequate perfusion. Understanding the physiology underlying shock is a crucial factor in determining appropriate management. Cardiac output is the major determinant of tissue perfusion and is the product of stroke volume and heart rate. In turn, stroke volume is determined by preload, or ventricular filling, afterload, or resistance to ventricular ejection, and contractility of the myocardium. In this patient, the hypoxic and damaged myocardium has suddenly lost much of its contractile function, and stroke volume will therefore decrease rapidly, dropping cardiac output. Systemic vascular resistance will increase in order to improve return of blood to the heart and increase stroke volume. Central venous pressure is elevated as a consequence of increased vascular resistance, decreased cardiac output and poor forward flow, and neuroendocrine-mediated vasoconstriction. The pathophysiology of other forms of shock is shown as a comparison.

TABLE VI-41   Physiologic Characteristics of the Various Forms of Shock

Type of Shock	CVP and PCWP	Cardiac Output	Systemic Vascular Resistance	Venous O_2 Saturation
Hypovolemic	↓	↓	↑	↓
Cardiogenic	↑	↓	↑	↓
Septic				
Hyperdynamic	↓↑	↑	↓	↑
Hypodynamic	↓↑	↓	↑	↑↓
Traumatic	↓	↓↑	↑↓	↓
Neurogenic	↓	↓	↓	↓
Hypoadrenal	↓↑	↓	=↓	↓

Note: CVP, central venous pressure; PCWP, pulmonary capillary wedge pressure.

VI-42. **The answer is A.** *(Chap. 256; Ridker et al, 1995.)* Many patients who develop pulmonary thromboembolism have an underlying inherited predisposition that remains clinically silent until they are subjected to an additional stress, such as the use of oral contraceptive pills, surgery, or pregnancy. The most frequently inherited predisposition to thrombosis is so-called activated protein C resistance. The inability of a normal protein C to carry out its anticoagulant function is due to a missense mutation in the gene coding for factor V in the coagulation cascade. This mutation, which results in the substitution of a glutamine for an arginine residue in position 506 of the factor V molecule, is termed the factor V Leiden gene. Based on the Physicians Health Study, about 3% of healthy male physicians carry this particular missense mutation. Carriers are clearly at an increased risk for deep venous thrombosis and also for recurrence after the discontinuation of warfarin. The allelic frequency of factor V Leiden is higher than that of all other identified inherited hypercoagulable states combined, including deficiencies of protein C, protein S, and antithrombin III and disorders of plasminogen.

VI-43. **The answer is B.** *(Chap. 260)* The optimal timing for lung transplantation is critical to improve survival and add quality-adjusted life years. Individuals with cystic fibrosis should be considered for lung transplantation when the FEV_1 is <30% predicted values or is rapidly falling. Other indications for referral in cystic fibrosis include Pa_{O_2} <50 mmHg on room air, Pa_{CO_2} >50 mmHg, pulmonary arterial hypertension, increasing hospitalization, and recurrent hemoptysis.

VI-44. **The answer is E.** *(Chap. 256)* Warfarin should not be used alone as initial therapy for the treatment of venous thromboembolic disease (VTE) for two reasons. First, warfarin does not achieve full anticoagulation for at least 5 days as its mechanism of action is to decrease the production of vitamin K–dependent coagulation factors in the liver. Secondly, a paradoxical reaction that promotes coagulation may also occur upon initiation of warfarin as it also decreases the production of the vitamin K–dependent anticoagulants protein C and protein S, which have shorter half-lives than the procoagulant factors. For many years, unfractionated heparin delivered IV was the treatment of choice for VTE. However, it requires frequent monitoring of aPTT levels and hospitalization until therapeutic INR is achieved with warfarin. There are now several safe and effective alternatives to unfractionated heparin that can be delivered SC. Low-molecular-weight heparins (enoxaparin, tinzaparin) are fragments of unfractionated heparin with a lower molecular weight. These compounds have a greater bioavailability, longer half-life, and more predictable onset of action. Their use in renal insufficiency should be considered with caution because low-molecular-weight heparins are renally cleared. Fondaparinux is a direct factor Xa inhibitor that, like low-molecular-weight heparins, requires no monitoring of anticoagulant effects and has been demonstrated to be safe and effective in treating both deep venous thrombosis and pulmonary embolism.

VI-45.   The answer is B. *(Chap. 158)* *M. tuberculosis* is spread by droplet nuclei that are aerosolized by coughing, sneezing, or speaking. The droplets dry quickly and may stay airborne and subject to inhalation for hours. The probability of acquiring tuberculosis is related to the degree of infectiousness and the intimacy and duration of contact. Smear-positive patients have the greatest infectivity. Patients with cavitary, laryngeal, or endobronchial disease produce the most infectious organisms. Patients with smear-negative/culture-positive or disseminated disease are less infectious. Patients with culture-negative (treated) or extrapulmonary tuberculosis are essentially noninfectious. Patients with tuberculosis who are HIV-infected also appear to be less infectious because of the lower frequency of cavitary disease. These factors emphasize the importance of public health measures to control the transmission of tuberculosis.

VI-46.   The answer is D. *(Chap. 255)* This patient's presentation is typical of pulmonary Langerhans cell histiocytosis (eosinophilic granulomas). Cigarette smoking is virtually universal among these patients. The disease may be found incidentally on radiograms or may present with respiratory and systemic complaints. Spontaneous pneumothorax is a common presentation and occurs in approximately 25% of these patients. The radiographic combination of small reticular/nodular opacities in the bases (with sparing of the costophrenic angle) and apical cysts is characteristic and virtually diagnostic. Pulmonary function testing will show a reduced DLCO. Lung volumes may be normal or reduced, depending on the severity. Approximately 33% of these patients improve with smoking cessation, but most develop progressive interstitial disease. Immunosuppressive agents do not appear to influence the course of disease. Intravenous α_1 antitrypsin may benefit patients with deficiency, who will present with lower lobe emphysema. Miliary tuberculosis radiographically appears with multiple small nodules, but cysts are not typical. *Pneumocystic carinii* pneumonia (PCP) may present with spontaneous pneumothorax in patients with HIV infection; however, this patient has no apparent risk factors, and the small nodules on CT are not typical.

VI-47.   The answer is E. *(Chap. 255)* This patient's clinical presentation and CT imaging are consistent with the diagnosis of idiopathic pulmonary fibrosis (IPF), which is manifested histologically as usual interstitial pneumonitis (UIP). On microscopic examination, UIP is characterized by a heterogeneous appearance on low magnification with normal-appearing alveoli adjacent to severely fibrotic alveoli. There is lymphocytic infiltrate and scattered foci of fibroblasts within the alveolar septae. End-stage fibrosis results in honeycombing with loss of all alveolar structure. The typical clinical presentation of IPF/UIP is slowly progressive exertional dyspnea with a nonproductive cough. Clinical examination reveals dry crackles and digital clubbing. Patients with IPF are usually >50 years, and more than two-thirds have a history of current or former tobacco use. A high-resolution CT scan of the chest can be diagnostic, in the typical clinical situation of an older individual, and shows subpleural pulmonary fibrosis that is greatest at the lung bases. As disease progresses, traction bronchiectasis and honeycombing are characteristic on CT scan. The cause of UIP is unknown, and no therapies have been shown to improve survival in this disease with the exception of lung transplantation. Mortality is 50% within 3 years of diagnosis. The presence of a dense periodic acid–Schiff positive amorphous material in alveolar spaces is characteristic of pulmonary alveolar proteinosis. Pulmonary alveolar proteinosis is an interstitial lung disease that presents with progressive dyspnea, and CT imaging shows characteristic "crazy paving" with ground-glass infiltrates and thickened alveolar septae. Fibrosis is not present. Alveolar destruction with emphysematous changes would be seen in chronic obstructive pulmonary disease (COPD). The presence of crackles without wheezing or hyperinflation on examination does not suggest COPD. Furthermore, clubbing is not seen in COPD. Diffuse alveolar damage is seen in acute interstitial pneumonitis and acute respiratory distress syndrome. These disorders present with a rapid acute course that is not present in this case. The formation of noncaseating granulomas is typical of sarcoidosis, a systemic disease that usually presents in younger individuals. It is more common in those of African-American race. A typical CT in sarcoidosis would show interstitial infiltrates and hilar lymphadenopathy. End-stage disease may result in pulmonary fibrosis, but it is greatest in the upper lobes.

VI-48. **The answer is D.** *(Chap. 263)* Determining when an individual is an appropriate candidate for a spontaneous breathing trial is important for the care of mechanically ventilated patients. An important initial step in determining if a patient is likely to be successfully extubated is to evaluate the mental status of the patient. This can be difficult if the patient is receiving sedation, and it is recommended that sedation be interrupted on a daily basis for a short period to allow assessment of mental status. Daily interruption of sedation has been shown to decrease the duration of mechanical ventilation. If the patient is unable to respond to any commands or is completely obtunded, this individual is at high risk for aspiration and unlikely to be successfully extubated. In addition, the patient's underlying medical condition should be stable, and the patient should be off vasopressor support. If these conditions are met, the patient should be on minimal ventilatory support. This includes the ability to maintain the pH between 7.35 and 7.40 and an Sa_{O_2} of >90% while receiving an FI_{O_2} ≤0.5 and a PEEP ≤5 cmH$_2$O.

VI-49. **The answer is B.** *(Chaps. 34 and 142)* *Bordetella pertussis* is becoming an increasingly common cause of cough in adolescents and adults. Some studies have shown that pertussis is associated with 12–30% of prolonged coughing illnesses lasting >2 weeks. The clinical manifestations of pertussis infection are classically described by a catarrhal phase followed by a paroxysmal phase. The catarrhal phase begins after a 7-to-10-day incubation period and lasts 1–2 weeks. This phase is marked by an upper respiratory illness that is similar in symptoms to the common cold, with low-grade fever, rhinitis, mild cough, and lacrimation. This is followed by a prolonged paroxysmal coughing phase during which coughing can become quite severe. The term *whooping cough* as a synonym for pertussis is derived from the spasms of coughing that occur during the paroxysmal phase that are often terminated by an audible whoop. Posttussive emesis is frequent. Between paroxysms of cough, the patient is otherwise well. Sleep is often disturbed as the cough tends to be worse at night. Usually this phase lasts from 2–4 weeks, with cough waning in severity after this point. The convalescent phase marks recovery from the illness and lasts from 1–3 months, during which time the cough gradually lessens in severity. Intercurrent viral illnesses that occur over the next year may cause a recurrence of paroxysmal cough. Diagnosis of pertussis in the paroxysmal phase of the illness relies on serologic testing of IgG and IgA antibodies to pertussis with evidence of a two- to fourfold increase in levels suggestive of recent infection. Increasingly, a single specimen for serology can be obtained and compared to established population values. Therapy is not indicated as it does not substantially alter the course of disease except in the catarrhal phase. Other common causes of chronic cough include asthma, allergic rhinitis with postnasal drip, and gastroesophageal reflux disease. Occasionally, asthma may present with cough alone. In these patients, a methacholine challenge test is used to confirm the diagnosis, especially in the setting of normal spirometry. Peak expiratory flow monitoring in the workplace is useful when an occupational cause of asthma or chronic cough is suggested. Typical clinical features include symptoms that increase over the work week and wane significantly during time off work. Individuals with allergic rhinitis often develop cough as a result of postnasal drip, which can become more severe after upper respiratory illnesses. However, the severity of the cough without prior history of chronic rhinitis in this case argues against allergic rhinitis. Thus skin testing for allergens is not indicated. Finally, gastroesophageal reflux disease may also be associated with chronic cough and would be diagnosed with a 24-h pH probe. The preceding illness and abrupt onset of severe symptoms, however, are inconsistent with this diagnosis.

VI-50.   **The answer is B.** *(Chap. 250)* The patient presents with typical asthma symptoms; however, the symptoms are escalating and now require nearly constant use of oral steroids. It is of note that the symptoms are worse during weekdays and better on weekends. This finding suggests that there is an exposure during the week that may be triggering the patient's asthma. Often textile workers have asthma resulting from the inhalation of particles. The first step in diagnosing a work-related asthma trigger is to check FEV_1 before and after the first shift of the workweek. A decrease in FEV_1 would suggest an occupational exposure. Skin testing for allergies would not be likely to pinpoint the work-related exposure. Although *A. fumigatus* can be associated with worsening asthma from allergic bronchopulmonary aspergillosis, this would not have a fluctuation in symptoms throughout the week. The patient does not require further testing to diagnose that he has asthma; therefore, a methacholine challenge is not indicated. Finally, the exercise physiology test is generally used to differentiate between cardiac and pulmonary causes or deconditioning as etiologies for shortness of breath.

VI-51.   **The answer is E.** *(Chap. 259)* While clinical history can suggest a diagnosis of obstructive sleep apnea and can be strengthened by the use of objective sleep questionnaires such as the Epworth Sleepiness Score, evidence of recurrent breathing disruptions during sleep is necessary to make the diagnosis. OSA is a condition requiring life-long therapy; diagnosis should be based on objective findings such as those obtained from polysomnography. Limited sleep studies that measure one or two parameters may be cost-effective when interpreted by experts; however, their predictive capacity does not compare favorably to a polysomnogram. Unfortunately there are at present no satisfactory pharmacologic options for patients with obstructive sleep apnea. Modafinil has shown marginal improvement in patients also using CPAP. It is expensive and not currently recommended as a first-line agent. CPAP ventilation has been shown in double-blind randomized clinical trials to improve virtually all aspects of disease in patients with OSA, including number of apneas and hypopneas, sleep quality, blood pressure, driving ability, mood, and quality of life. CPAP is often burdensome and uncomfortable at first. The benefits as well as the downsides of CPAP should be covered with patients. Another treatment option is the mandibular repositioning splint, which holds the tongue and lower jaw forward in order to widen the pharyngeal airway. These too can be difficult to use, and long-term compliance is poor. There are several surgical options for patients with narrowed airways that are effective in carefully selected patients.

VI-52 and VI-53.   The answers are C and D. *(Chap. 249)* The patient has a subacute presentation of hypersensitivity pneumonitis related to exposure to bird droppings and feathers at work. Hypersensitivity pneumonitis is a delayed-type hypersensitivity reaction that has a variety of presentations. Some people develop acute onset of shortness of breath, fevers, chills, and dyspnea within 6 to 8 h of antigen exposure. Others may present subacutely with worsening dyspnea on exertion and dry cough over weeks to months. Chronic hypersensitivity pneumonitis presents with more severe and persistent symptoms with clubbing. Progressive worsening is common with the development of chronic hypoxemia, pulmonary hypertension, and respiratory failure. The diagnosis relies on a variety of tests. Peripheral eosinophilia is not a feature of this disease, although neutrophilia and lymphopenia are frequently present. Other nonspecific markers of inflammation may be elevated, including the erythrocyte sedimentation rate, C-reactive protein, rheumatoid factor, and serum immunoglobulins. If a specific antigen is suspected, serum precipitins directed toward that antigen may be demonstrated. Chest radiography may be normal or show a diffuse reticulonodular infiltrate. High-resolution chest CT is the imaging modality of choice and shows ground-glass infiltrates in the lower lobes. Centrilobular infiltrates are often seen as well. In the chronic stages patchy emphysema is the most common finding. Histopathologically, interstitial alveolar infiltrates predominate, with a variety of lymphocytes, plasma cells, and occasional eosinophils and neutrophils seen. Loose, non-caseating granulomas are typical.

Treatment depends on removing the individual from exposure to the antigen. If this is not possible, the patient should wear a mask that prevents small-particle inhalation during exposure. In patients with mild disease, removal from antigen exposure alone may be sufficient to treat the disease. More severe symptoms require therapy with glucocorticoids at an equivalent prednisone dose of 1 mg/kg daily for 7 to 14 days. The steroids are then gradually tapered over 2 to 6 weeks.

VI-54. **The answer is D.** *(Chap. 252)* Bronchiectasis is defined as an abnormal and permanent dilatation of the bronchi. It can be focal or widespread in the lung. It typically affects older patients and is found more commonly in women than men. Bronchiectasis results from inflammation and destruction of the bronchial wall and is usually triggered by infection. Bacteria such as *Staphylococcus aureus* and *Klebsiella* are common causes. Adenovirus and influenza virus are the main viruses that can cause bronchiectasis. Mycobacteria, including tuberculosis, are major causes worldwide. Patients with impaired immunity to pulmonary infections, such as those with cystic fibrosis or ciliary dysfunction, are highly susceptible to bronchiectasis. Patients frequently complain of recurrent cough and purulent sputum. Frequent lung infections should raise suspicion of this diagnosis. Physical examination findings can be varied and are not sufficient alone for diagnosis. Rhonchi and wheezes can be heard over the affected area; severe cases may present with right-heart failure. Chest radiography often shows nonspecific findings. Honeycomb lung is characteristic of end-stage interstitial lung disease. High-resolution CT of the chest is considered the standard technique to confirm diagnosis of bronchiectasis. It will show the dilated airways beyond the central airways. If focal, it is most likely due to prior necrotizing infection; however, mycobacterial infection (*M. tuberculosis*, Mycobacteria other than tuberculosis) should be considered. Diffuse bronchiectasis may be due to cystic fibrosis, immunoglobulin deficiency, ciliary dysfunction syndromes, α_1 antitrypsin deficiency, allergic bronchopulmonary aspergillosis, collagen vascular disease, or HIV infection.

VI-55. **The answer is B.** *(Chap. 255)* Pulmonary complications are common in patients with systemic lupus erythematosus (SLE). The most common manifestation is pleuritis with or without effusion. Other possible manifestations include pulmonary hemorrhage, diaphragmatic dysfunction with loss of lung volumes (the so-called shrinking lung syndrome), pulmonary vascular disease, acute interstitial pneumonitis, and bronchiolitis obliterans organizing pneumonia. Other systemic complications of SLE also cause pulmonary complications, including uremic pulmonary edema and infectious complications. Chronic progressive pulmonary fibrosis is not a complication of SLE.

VI-56. **The answer is C.** *(Chaps. 157 and 251)* The radiograph describes a lung abscess that most likely is due to anaerobic infection. The anaerobes involved are most likely oral, but *Bacteroides fragilis* is isolated in up to 10% of cases. Vancomycin, ciprofloxacin, and cephalexin have no significant activity against anaerobes. Most oral anaerobic strains have the capacity to produce β-lactamase. For many years penicillin was considered the standard treatment for anaerobic lung infections. However, clinical studies have demonstrated the superiority of clindamycin over penicillin in the treatment of lung abscess. When there are contraindications to clindamycin, penicillin plus metronidazole is likely to be as effective as clindamycin.

VI-57. **The answer is E.** *(Chap. 257)* Pleural effusions are commonly associated with pneumonia and should be assessed via thoracentesis to determine whether the pleural fluid is also infected. A viscous, infected pleural fluid can become organized following pneumonia, resulting in development of empyema or chronic pleural effusion with trapped lung that is unable to reexpand. In order to prevent these complications, it is recommended that all pleural effusions separated from the chest wall by >10 mm undergo thoracentesis. Characteristics that predict increased likelihood of complications with a parapneumonic effusion include: loculated pleural fluid, pleural fluid pH <7.20, pleural fluid glucose <60 mg/dL, positive Gram stain or culture of the pleural fluid, and presence of frank pus (empyema) of the pleural space. Individuals whose pleural fluid has any of these characteristics should be considered for tube thoracostomy drainage of the pleural fluid.

VI-58.   The answer is C. *(Chap. 260)* Compared with other solid organ transplants, lung transplants have the highest mortality, with only a 50% survival after 5 years. The leading causes of death in the early posttransplant period are infectious complications. Primary graft failure occurs immediately after the transplant and is sometimes called ischemia-reperfusion injury. This can be fatal but can be treated with supportive care. Acute rejection occurs in ~50% of lung transplant patients within the first year but is rarely fatal. Posttransplant lymphoproliferative disorder is a B cell lymphoma associated with the Epstein-Barr virus and is related to the degree of immunosuppression. It is a rare complication of transplant. Bronchiolitis obliterans syndrome denotes chronic rejection and is the leading cause of late mortality in lung transplant.

VI-59.   The answer is D. *(Chap. 252)* This patient presents with a lung abscess in the setting of pneumonia. Lung abscess is defined as a pulmonary cavitation caused by infection. Aspiration is the predominant means of acquiring infection. The most common anatomic sites of aspiration (when people are lying on their back) and therefore lung abscess include the superior segment of the right lower lobe, posterior segment of the right upper lobe, and superior segment of the left lower lobe. Anaerobic bacteria are the most prevalent isolates from lung abscesses, as these are the most common bacteria aspirated from the mouth. Alcoholism is a known risk factor for aspiration. Necrotizing aerobic bacteria such as *Staphylococcus aureus*, *Klebsiella pneumoniae*, and *Nocardia* can cause lung abscesses but do so with much less frequency than do anaerobic bacteria. *Peptostreptococcus*, an anaerobic organism that is part of normal mouth flora, has been shown to be the most common organism isolated from lung abscesses. Polymicrobial culture results are not uncommon. Management includes antibiotics aimed at treating anaerobes, such as clindamycin.

VI-60.   The answer is C. *(Chap. 28)* This patient complains of symptoms that are consistent with restless legs syndrome (RLS). This disorder affects 1–5% of young to middle-aged individuals and as many as 20% of older individuals. The symptoms of restless legs syndrome are a nonspecific uncomfortable sensation in the legs that begin during periods of quiescence and are alleviated with movement. Patients frequently find it difficult to describe their symptoms, but usually describe the sensation as deep within the affected limb. Rarely is the sensation described as distinctly painful unless an underlying neuropathy is also present. The severity of the disorder tends to wax and wane over time and tends to worsen with sleep deprivation, caffeine intake, pregnancy, and alcohol. Renal disease, neuropathy, and iron deficiency are known secondary cause of RLS symptoms. In this patient, correcting the iron deficiency is the best choice for initial therapy as this may entirely relieve the symptoms of RLS. For individuals with primary RLS (not related to another medical condition), the dopaminergic agents are the treatment of choice. Pramipexole or ropinirole are recommended as first-line treatment. While carbidopa/levodopa is highly effective, individuals have a high risk of developing augmented symptoms over time, with increasingly higher doses needed to control the symptoms. Other options for treating RLS include narcotics, benzodiazepines, and gabapentin. Hormone replacement therapy has no role in the treatment of RLS.

VI-61.   The answer is C. *(Chap. 253)* This patient has a history suggestive of cystic fibrosis, with the exception of her age. The persistent asthma, airflow obstruction, and sputum cultures growing *P. aeruginosa* and *S. aureus* coupled with bilateral upper lobe infiltrates should prompt further investigation for this disease. The diagnosis of cystic fibrosis is based on clinical criteria plus laboratory evidence. The laboratory test of choice remains analysis of sweat chloride values. Patients with mutations in the cystic fibrosis transmembrane regulator (CFTR) will have increased amounts of chloride in their sweat, and a chloride value over 70 meq/L will generally be found. Approximately 1 to 2% of patients with cystic fibrosis will have normal results of sweat chloride testing, and in these cases the nasal transepithelial potential difference has been used for diagnosis. While the ΔF508 mutation accounts for the majority of patients with cystic fibrosis, more than 1000 other mutations that can cause this disorder have been described. Thus, the absence of this mutation does not rule out cystic fibrosis. Bronchoscopy with transbronchial biopsy probably will show bronchiectasis and chronic airway inflammation but will not be diagnostic. Similar findings probably will be found on a chest CT but are not diagnostic.

VI-62.   **The answer is A.** *(Chap. 158)* This patient has evidence of recent tuberculosis infection with the change from a negative to a positive PPD. A chest radiogram should be performed to rule out active disease and the presence of latent disease. If there is no abnormality, isoniazid should be prescribed to prevent subsequent development of active disease. The optimal duration of therapy is 6 to 12 months, with most recommending 9 months to achieve maximal protection from active disease. The major complication of this therapy is hepatitis. Isoniazid should not be given to patients with active liver disease. All these patients should be educated about the signs or symptoms of hepatitis and should be instructed to discontinue the medication if those symptoms develop. Patients should be questioned about symptoms monthly. Baseline liver function tests need be obtained only in patients with a history of liver disease or daily alcohol use. Serial measurement of liver function is not necessary in the absence of a history of liver disease or alcohol use.

VI-63.   **The answer is B.** *(Chap. 245)* This patient presents with subacute-onset dyspnea and an examination consistent with pleural effusion. Dullness to percussion can be seen with consolidation, atelectasis, and pleural effusion. With consolidation, voice transmission is increased during expiration so that one may hear whispered pectoriloquy or egophony. However, in both pleural effusion and atelectasis, breath sounds are diminished and there is no augmentation of voice transmission. Although this patient could have either atelectasis or pleural effusion, the lack of tracheal deviation points to pleural effusion. Atelectasis would have to be of many segments to account for these findings, and such significant airway collapse would generally cause ipsilateral tracheal deviation. The clinician would expect to find pleural effusion on chest film, and the most appropriate next management step would be thoracentesis to aid in the diagnosis of the etiology and for symptomatic relief. With a lack of symptoms to suggest infection, antibiotics are not indicated. Similarly, in the absence of wheezing or significant sputum production, bronchodilators and deep suctioning are unlikely to be helpful. Bronchoscopy may be indicated ultimately in the management of this patient, particularly if malignancy is suspected; however, the most appropriate first attempt at diagnosis is by means of thoracentesis.

VI-64.   **The answer is F.** *(Chap. 31)* Many experts suggest treatment for acute sinusitis if symptoms are severe and duration of illness is >7 days. However, even among patients who meet this criterion, only 40–50% are shown to have bacterial sinusitis. Yet, there is actually little way other than unduly invasive sinus aspiration to differentiate viral from bacterial sinusitis. CT has no value whatsoever in the workup of acute sinusitis but may be useful for chronic sinusitis where anatomic disease might be implicated in recurrent or persistent infection. Nasal culture is likely to pick up commensal bacterial flora and will not be representative of the flora seen in the anatomically sequestered sinus. Immunocompromised patients represent a distinct subset because of their predilection for fungal sinusitis. These patients should receive early otolaryngologic evaluation.

VI-65.   **The answer is A.** *(Chap. 260)* Lung transplantation has been successfully utilized in the treatment of end-stage lung disease since the early 1990s. Currently, ~1700 lung transplants are performed yearly worldwide. The most common reason for lung transplant is COPD, accounting for 38.5% of all lung transplants performed between 1995 and 2004. In addition, another 8.6% of lung transplants were performed because of emphysema due to α_1 antitrypsin deficiency. IPF and cystic fibrosis are the second and third most common reasons for lung transplantation, respectively. Pulmonary hypertension and sarcoidosis each account for <5% of all lung transplants. Single lung transplantation is an option for patients with COPD, IPF, and sarcoidosis. Patients with cystic fibrosis and pulmonary hypertension receive double lung transplants.

VI-66.   **The answer is D.** *[Chap. 251; LA Mandell et al: Clin Infect Dis 44(Suppl 2):S27, 2007]* The Infectious Diseases Society of America and the American Thoracic Society state that in the proper clinical context, a new infiltrate on chest imaging should be present to diagnose community acquired pneumonia (CAP). An accurate history is important because the differential diagnosis of CAP includes heart disease, chronic bronchitis, pulmonary embolism, and acute bronchitis. At least two clinical symptoms consistent with acute pulmonary infection (any combination of fever, cough, chest pain, or dyspnea) should be present for diagnosis. Cough is the most common symptom in patients presenting with CAP. Physical findings have a sensitivity and specificity of 60–70%, and therefore radiology is recommended to make the diagnosis. Similarly, laboratory studies including WBC count and measures of inflammation are neither sensitive nor specific enough to make a diagnosis. Antibiotics are not recommended for acute bronchitis. In some cases, follow-up radiograph or empirical therapy for CAP should be considered if clinical suspicion is high and the original chest x-ray is negative. The microbiologic basis of CAP can usually not be definitively determined on a clinical and radiographic basis. Except for the small minority of patients who are admitted to the intensive care unit, no data exist to show that specific pathogen-directed therapy is superior to empirical therapy. Microbiologic data are not components of the clinical diagnosis of CAP.

VI-67.   The answer is A. *(Chap. 246)* Spirometry does not measure total lung capacity because it cannot account for residual volume. The most frequently used and accurate measures of lung volumes are steady-state helium dilution lung volumes and body plethysmography. In helium dilution the patient inspires a known concentration of helium from a closed circuit of known volume. After the patient rebreathes in the closed circuit for a period of time, the concentration of helium equilibrates, and subsequently the lung volumes can be calculated by using Avogadro's law. This calculation assumes that gas in the circuit will rapidly equilibrate with the ventilated portions of the lung. However, if there are slowly emptying areas of the lung, as in cystic fibrosis patients, or parts of the lung that do not participate in gas exchange at all, as in bullous emphysema patients, helium dilution will underestimate true lung volumes. Subsequently, body plethysmography is the preferred method for lung volume measurement in these disease states. To perform body plethysmography, the patient sits in a sealed box and pants against a closed mouthpiece. Panting results in changes in the pressure of the box that, when compared with changes at the mouthpiece, can be used to calculate lung volumes. This method measures total thoracic gas volume and is more accurate than helium dilution. Helium lung volumes are easier to perform for patients and staff and give reliable results in most circumstances. Many centers measure a single-breath helium dilution lung volume when measuring the diffusing capacity of carbon monoxide, which has the same or greater limitations as the rebreathing method. Transdiaphragmatic pressure is used to measure respiratory muscle strength, not lung volumes.

VI-68.   The answer is E. *(Chap. 126)* Patients with lung transplants have the highest risk of pneumonia among all recipients of solid organ transplants. The pathogens causing pulmonary infections vary with the time after transplantation. The most common pathogens in the first 2 weeks (early period) after surgery are the gram-negative bacteria, particularly Enterobacteriaceae and *Pseudomonas, Staphylococcus, Aspergillus,* and *Candida.* Between 1 and 6 months (middle period), most infections are due to either primary activation or reactivation of CMV. CMV pneumonia is often difficult to distinguish from acute transplant rejection. More than 6 months after a transplant (late period), the chronic suppression of cell-mediated immunity places patients at risk of infection from *Pneumocystis, Nocardia, Listeria,* other fungi, and intracellular pathogens. Pretransplant lung donor cultures often guide posttransplant empirical antibiotic choices. Prophylaxis against CMV in seropositive donors or recipients and *Pneumocystis* is routine after lung transplantation.

VI-69.   The answer is A. *(Chap. 28)* Narcolepsy is a sleep disorder characterized by excessive sleepiness with intrusion of rapid-eye-movement (REM) sleep into wakefulness. Narcolepsy affects ~1 in 4000 individuals in the United States with a genetic predisposition. Recent research has demonstrated that narcolepsy is associated with low or undetectable levels of the neurotransmitter hypocretin (orexin) in the cerebrospinal fluid. This neurotransmitter is released from a small number of neurons in the hypothalamus. Given the association of narcolepsy with the MHC antigen HLA DQB1*0602, it is thought that narcolepsy is an autoimmune process that leads to destruction of the hypocretin-secreting neurons in the hypothalamus. The classic symptom tetrad of narcolepsy is: (1) cataplexy;

(2) hypnagogic or hypnopompic hallucinations; (3) sleep paralysis; and (4) excessive daytime somnolence. Of these symptoms, cataplexy is the most specific for the diagnosis of narcolepsy. Cataplexy refers to the sudden loss of muscle tone in response to strong emotions. It most commonly occurs with laughter or surprise but may be associated with anger as well. Cataplexy can have a wide range of symptoms, from mild sagging of the jaw lasting for a few seconds to a complete loss of muscle tone lasting several minutes. During this time, individuals are aware of their surroundings and are not unconscious. This symptom is present in 76% of individuals diagnosed with narcolepsy and is the most specific finding for the diagnosis. Hypnagogic and hypnopompic hallucinations and sleep paralysis can occur from anything that causes chronic sleep deprivation, including sleep apnea and chronic insufficient sleep. Excessive daytime somnolence is present in 100% of individuals with narcolepsy but is not specific for the diagnosis as this symptom may be present with any sleep disorder as well as with chronic insufficient sleep. The presence of two or more REM periods occurring during a daytime multiple sleep latency test is suggestive but not diagnostic of narcolepsy. Other disorders that may lead to presence of REM during short daytime nap periods include sleep apnea, sleep phase delay syndrome, and insufficient sleep.

VI-70. **The answer is B.** *(Chap. 28; http://www.sleepfoundation.org/site/c.huIXKjM0IxF/b.2417355/ k.143E/2002_Sleep_in_America_Poll.htm, accessed December 27, 2007)* Insomnia is the most common sleep disorder in the population. In the 2002 Sleep in America Poll, 58% of respondents reported at least one symptom of insomnia on a weekly basis, and a third of individuals experience these symptoms on a nightly basis. Insomnia is defined clinically as the inability to fall asleep or stay asleep, which leads to daytime sleepiness or poor daytime function. These symptoms occur despite adequate time and opportunity for sleep. Obstructive sleep apnea is thought to affect as many as 10–15% of the population and is currently underdiagnosed in the United States. In addition, because of the rising incidence of obesity, obstructive sleep apnea is also expected to increase in incidence over the coming years. Obstructive sleep apnea occurs when there is ongoing effort to inspire against an occluded oropharynx during sleep. It is directly related to obesity and also has an increased incidence in men and in older populations. Narcolepsy affects 1 in 4000 people and is due to a deficit of hypocretin (orexin) in the brain. Symptoms of narcolepsy include sudden loss of tone in response to emotional stimuli (cataplexy), hypersomnia, sleep paralysis, and hallucinations with sleep onset and waking. Physiologically, there is intrusion or persistence of rapid-eye-movement sleep during wakefulness that accounts for the classic symptoms of narcolepsy. Restless legs syndrome is estimated to affect 1–5% of young to middle-aged adults and as many as 10–20% of the elderly. Restless legs syndrome is marked by uncomfortable sensations in the legs that are difficult to describe. The symptoms have an onset with quiescence, especially at night, and are relieved with movement. Delayed sleep phase syndrome is a circadian rhythm disorder that commonly presents with a complaint of insomnia and accounts for as much as 10% of individuals referred to the sleep clinic for evaluation of insomnia. In delayed sleep phase syndrome, the intrinsic circadian rhythm is delayed such that sleep onset occurs much later than normal. When allowed to sleep according to the intrinsic circadian rhythm, individuals with delayed sleep phase syndrome sleep normally and do not experience excessive somnolence. This disorder is most common in adolescence and young adulthood.

VI-71. **The answer is B.** *(Chap. 258)* The physiologic effects of hypoventilation are typically magnified during sleep because of a further reduction in central respiratory drive. Hypercapnia causes cerebral vasodilation, which manifests as headache upon wakening. The headache typically resolves soon after awakening as the Pa_{CO_2} decreases with increased ventilation and cerebral vascular tone returns to normal. Patients with frequent arousals from sleep and hypoventilation commonly complain of daytime somnolence and may also exhibit confusion and fatigue. Hypoventilation causes an increase in Pa_{CO_2} and an obligatory fall in PA_{O_2}. The hypoxemia can stimulate erythropoiesis and result in polycythemia. With central hypoventilation disorders, patients may also have impaired cranial nerve reflexes or muscular function, causing aspiration.

VI-72. The answer is C. *(Chap. 28)* Parasomnias are abnormal behaviors or experiences that arise from stages 3 and 4 sleep. Also known as confusional arousals, the electroencephalogram during a parasomnia event frequently shows persistence of slow-wave (delta) sleep into arousal. Non-REM (NREM) parasomnias may also include more complex behavior, including eating and sexual activity. Treatment of NREM parasomnias is usually not indicated, and a safe environment should be assured for the patient. In cases where injury is likely to occur, treatment with a drug that decreases slow-wave sleep will treat the parasomnia. Typical treatment is a benzodiazepine. There are no typical parasomnias that arise from stage I or stage II sleep. REM parasomnias include nightmare disorder and REM-behavior disorder. REM-behavior disorder is increasingly recognized as associated with Parkinson's disease and other Parkinsonian syndrome. This disorder is characterized by lack of decreased muscle tone in REM sleep, which leads to the acting out of dreams, sometimes resulting in violence and injury.

VI-73. The answer is E. *(Chap. 250)* Passive cigarette smoking, or secondhand smoking, has been associated in the last 15 years with many adverse outcomes. A correlation has been demonstrated between the number of smokers in a house and the concentration of respirable particulate load. Furthermore, meta-analyses of the best data have shown that persons who receive passive cigarette smoke have a 25% increase in mortality associated with lung cancer, respiratory illness, and cardiac disease compared with persons without such an exposure. Children with smoking parents have been shown to have an increased prevalence of respiratory illness and decreased lung function compared with nonexposed children.

VI-74. The answer is C. *(Chap. 265)* The annual incidence of sepsis has increased to >700,000 individuals yearly in the United States, and sepsis accounts for >200,000 deaths yearly. Approximately two-thirds of the cases of sepsis occur in individuals with other significant comorbidities, and the incidence of sepsis increases with age and preexisting comorbidities. In addition, the incidence of sepsis is thought to be increasing as a result of several other factors. These include increased longevity of individuals with chronic disease, including AIDS, and increased risk for sepsis in individuals with AIDS. The practice of medicine has also influenced the risk of sepsis, with an increased risk of sepsis related to the increased use of antimicrobial drugs, immunosuppressive agents, mechanical ventilation, and indwelling catheters and other hardware.

VI-75 and VI-76. The answers are A and B. *(Chap. 251)* The first patient is a candidate for outpatient therapy because of his CURB-65 score of 0. As shown below, an oral macrolide (azithromycin, clarithromycin) is the best choice. Respiratory fluoroquinolones may be used in the presence of comorbidities or recent antibiotics. The second patient has a CURB-65 score of 3 (age, respiratory rate, BUN) and merits consideration for inpatient therapy. Of the listed choices, a β-lactam (ceftriaxone) plus a macrolide (clarithromycin) is best. A respiratory fluoroquinolone may also be used as a single agent unless the patient goes to the intensive care unit, when a β-lactam should also be used. Fluconazole does not have a role for community-acquired pneumonia (CAP); it is used to treat candidal infections. Piperacillin/tazobactam is a consideration when *Pseudomonas* infection is considered likely, such as in patients with cystic fibrosis or bronchiectasis. Vancomycin is only a consideration for CAP when epidemiologic considerations make methicillin-resistant *Staphylococcus aureus* a likely pathogen.

VI-77. The answer is A. *(Chap. 263)* Patients initiated on mechanical ventilation require a variety of supportive measures. Sedation and analgesia with a combination of benzodiazepines and narcotics are commonly used to maintain patient comfort and safety while mechanically ventilated. In addition, patients are immobilized and are thus at high risk for development of deep venous thrombosis and pulmonary embolus. Prophylaxis with unfractionated heparin or low-molecular-weight heparin SC should be administered. Prophylaxis against diffuse gastrointestinal mucosal injury is also indicated, particularly in individuals with neurologic insult or those with severe respiratory failure and adult respiratory distress syndrome. Gastric acid suppression can be managed with H_2-receptor antagonists, proton pump inhibitors, and carafate. It is also recommended that individuals who are expected to be intubated for >72 hours receive nutritional support. Prokinetic agents are often required. A final supportive measure that should be instituted in all intensive care units is to maintain a protocol that includes frequent positional changes and surveillance for prevention of decubitus ulcers. In the past, frequent ventilator circuit changes had been studied as a measure for prevention of ventilator-associated pneumonia, but they were ineffective and may even have increased the risk of ventilator-associated pneumonia.

VI-78. **The answer is B.** *(Chap. 265; RP Dellinger et al: Crit Care Med 32: 858, 2004)* Sepsis is a systemic inflammatory response that develops in response to a microbial source. To diagnose the systemic inflammatory response syndrome (SIRS), a patient should have two or more of the following conditions: (1) fever or hypothermia; (2) tachypnea; (3) tachycardia; or (4) leukocytosis, leukopenia, or >10% band forms. This patient fulfills the criteria for sepsis with septic shock as she meets the above criteria for SIRS with the presence of organ dysfunction and ongoing hypotension despite fluid resuscitation. The patient has received 2 L of IV colloid and now has a central venous pressure of 18 cmH$_2$O. Ongoing large-volume fluid administration may result in pulmonary edema as the central venous pressure is quite high. At this point, fluid administration should continue, but at a lower infusion rate. In this patient, who is receiving chronic glucocorticoids for an underlying inflammatory condition, stress-dose steroids should be administered because adrenal suppression will prevent the patient from developing the normal stress response in the face of SIRS. Glucocorticoids may be given while waiting for results of the cosyntropin stimulation test. If the patient fails to respond to glucocorticoids, she should be started on vasopressor therapy. A single small study has suggested that norepinephrine may be preferred over dopamine for septic shock, but these data have not been confirmed in other trials. The "Surviving Sepsis" guidelines state that either norepinephrine or dopamine should be considered as first-line agent for the treatment of septic shock. Transfusion of red blood cells in the critically ill has been associated with a higher risk for development of acute lung injury, sepsis, and death. A threshold hemoglobin value of 7 g/dL has been shown to be as safe as a value of 10 g/dL and is associated with fewer complications. In this patient, a blood transfusion is not currently indicated, but may be considered if the central venous oxygen saturation is <70% in order to improve oxygen delivery to tissues. An alternative to blood transfusion in this setting is the use of dobutamine to improve cardiac output.

VI-79. **The answer is D.** *(Chap. 265)* Sepsis is responsible for >200,000 deaths yearly in the United States, and the incidence of sepsis has been increasing over the past 20 years. Approximately two-thirds of patients have underlying comorbidities, and the incidence of sepsis increases markedly with age. Pathophysiologically, sepsis occurs as a result of the inflammatory reaction that develops in response to an infection. Microbial invasion of the bloodstream is not necessary for the development of severe sepsis. In fact, blood cultures are positive in only 20–40% of cases of severe sepsis and in only 40–70% of septic shock. The systemic response to infection classically has been demonstrated by the response to lipopolysaccharide (LPS), which is also called endotoxin. LPS binds to receptors on the surfaces of monocytes, macrophages, and neutrophils, causing activation of these cells to produce a variety of inflammatory mediators including tumor necrosis factor α (TNF-α). This process amplifies the LPS signal, stimulating a process of inflammation that leads to complement activation, increase in procoagulant factors, and cellular injury. The end result of this systemic inflammatory process is widespread intravascular thrombosis. This process is meant to wall off invading microorganisms to prevent infection from spreading to other tissues, but in cases of severe sepsis, this leads to tissue hypoxia and ongoing cellular injury. In addition, systemic hypotension develops as a reaction to inflammatory mediators and occurs despite increased levels of plasma catecholamines. Physiologically, this is manifested as a marked decrease in systemic vascular resistance despite evidence of increased sympathetic activation. Survival in sepsis has improved in the past decades largely due to advances in supportive care in the intensive care unit. Activated protein C is the only medication currently approved for treatment of sepsis and has been demonstrated to cause a 33% relative risk mortality reduction.

VI-80. **The answer is D.** *(Chap. 263)* Mechanical ventilation is frequently used to support ventilation in individuals with both hypoxemic and hypercarbic respiratory failure. Mechanical ventilators provide warm, humidified gas to the airways in accordance with preset ventilator settings. The ventilator serves as the energy source for inspiration, whereas expiration is a passive process, driven by the elastic recoil of the lungs and chest wall. Positive end-expiratory pressure (PEEP) may be used to prevent alveolar collapse on expiration. The physiologic consequences of PEEP include decreased preload and decreased afterload. Decreased preload occurs because PEEP decreases venous return to the right atrium and may manifest as hypotension, especially in an individual who is volume-depleted. In addition, PEEP is transmitted to the heart and great vessels. This complicated interaction leads to a decrease in afterload and may be beneficial to individuals with depressed cardiac function. When utilizing mechanical ventilation, the physician should also be cognizant of other potential physiologic consequences of the ventilator settings. Initial settings chosen by the physician include mode of ventilation, respiratory rate, fraction of inspired oxygen, and tidal volume, if volume-cycled ventilation is used, or maximum pressure, if pressure-cycled ventilation is chosen. The respiratory therapist also has the ability to alter the inspiratory flow rate and waveform for delivery of the chosen mode of ventilation. These choices can have important physiologic consequences for the patient. In individuals with obstructive lung disease, it is important to maximize the time for exhalation. This can be done by decreasing the respiratory rate or decreasing the inspiratory time (increase the I:E ratio, prolong expiration), which is accomplished by increasing the inspiratory flow rate. Care must also be taken in choosing the inspired tidal volume in volume-cycled ventilatory modes as high inspired tidal volumes can contribute to development of acute lung injury due to overdistention of alveoli.

VI-81. **The answer is B.** *(Chap. 263)* Patients intubated for respiratory failure due to obstructive lung disease (asthma or chronic obstructive pulmonary disease) are at risk for the development of intrinsic positive end-expiratory pressure (auto-PEEP). Because these conditions are characterized by expiratory flow limitation, a long expiratory time is required to allow a full exhalation. If the patient is unable to exhale fully, auto-PEEP develops. With repeated breaths, the pressure generated from auto-PEEP continues to rise and impedes venous return to the right ventricle. This results in hypotension and also increases the risk for pneumothorax. Both of these conditions should be considered when evaluating this patient. However, because breath sounds are heard bilaterally, pneumothorax is less likely, and tube thoracostomy is not indicated at this time. Development of auto-PEEP has most likely occurred in this patient because the patient is currently agitated and hyperventilating as the effects of the paralytic agent wear off. In AC mode ventilation, each respiratory effort will deliver the full tidal volume of 550 mL and there is a decreased time for exhalation allowing auto-PEEP to occur. Immediate management of this patient should include disconnecting the patient from the ventilator to allow the patient to fully exhale and decrease the auto-PEEP. A fluid bolus may temporarily increase the blood pressure but would not eliminate the underlying cause of the hypotension. After treatment of the auto-PEEP by disconnecting the patient from the ventilator, sedation is important to prevent further occurrence of auto-PEEP by decreasing the respiratory rate to the set rate of the ventilator. Sedation can be accomplished with a combination of benzodiazepines and narcotics or propofol. Initiation of vasopressor support is not indicated, unless other measures fail to treat the hypotension and it is suspected that sepsis is the cause of hypotension.

VI-82. **The answer is E.** *(Chap. 259)* Obstructive sleep apnea is defined by excessive daytime sleepiness and at least five obstructed breathing events (hypopnea or apnea) per hour of sleep. Apneic events are pauses in breathing that last ≥10 s. Hypopneic events occur when ventilation is reduced by 50% for ≥10 s. It should be stressed that there are two components to diagnosis: symptoms of daytime sleepiness combined with obstructive breathing while asleep. Patients with disordered breathing at night who are asymptomatic while awake *do not have* OSA. The central pathogenesis of sleep apnea is pharyngeal narrowing that leads to airway obstruction when somnolent. Risk factors include male gender, obesity, and a shortened mandible or maxilla. It remains unclear whether smoking is an independent risk factor. The disorder is twice as common in men as in women. About 50% of patients with OSA have a BMI of >30 kg/m². There appears to be an association between diabetes mellitus and OSA that is independent of obesity. Insulin resistance has been shown to be related to increasing frequency of apneas and hypopneas. Based on his other cardiac risk factors, including smoking, obesity, and hypertension, as well as his new diagnosis of OSA, this patient should be screened for diabetes mellitus.

VI-83. **The answer is D.** *(Chap. 389; RL Lange: N Engl J Med 345:351, 2001.)* Cocaine overdose is a potentially lethal condition that should be managed in the intensive care unit setting. These patients are in a hyperadrenergic state characterized by hypertension, tachycardia, tonic-clonic seizures, dyspnea and ventricular arrhythmias. Ventricular arrhythmias have been managed with IV nonselective beta-receptor blockers such as propranolol. There is concern with giving beta-blockers in patients with cocaine-induced chest pain or myocardial ischemia because of the potential for unopposed alpha activity provoking coronary vasospasm. Calcium channel blockers are often used in patients with cocaine intoxication and potential coronary ischemia to avoid this effect. Tonic-clonic seizures have been managed with IV diazepam infusions, but it would not benefit the ventricular ectopy. Hydralazine may manage the hypertension but would have no effect on the ventricular arrhythmia and might cause a reflex tachycardia. Cardioversion is not indicated for this patient who is in nonsustained ventricular tachycardia. Also, without addressing the underlying disorder prompting the arrhythmia (i.e., increased norepinephrine in the presynaptic space), the tachycardia is likely to recur. Norepinephrine would be contraindicated as it would exacerbate the hyperadrenergic state.

VI-84. **The answer is D.** *(Chap. 255)* Desquamative interstitial pneumonitis, respiratory bronchiolitis–interstitial lung disease, pulmonary Langerhans cell histiocytosis, Goodpasture's disease, and pulmonary alveolar proteinosis are almost always associated with cigarette smoking. In addition, 67 to 75% of patients with idiopathic pulmonary fibrosis also have a history of cigarette use. Bronchiolitis obliterans organizing pneumonia (BOOP), or cryptogenic organizing pneumonia, is often an idiopathic syndrome that presents in the fifth to sixth decade of life with dyspnea on exertion, cough, fevers, malaise, and weight loss. The cause in most instances is unknown, although BOOP may occur concomitantly with primary pulmonary disorders as a nonspecific reaction to lung injury. BOOP usually responds to steroid therapy, which induces clinical recovery in two-thirds of patients. It is not associated with previous tobacco use.

VI-85. **The answer is D.** *(Chap. 250)* The patient presents with acute-onset pulmonary symptoms, including wheezing, with no other medical problems. He is a farmer and was recently handling hay. The clinical presentation and radiogram are consistent with farmer's lung, a hypersensitivity pneumonitis caused by *Actinomyces*. In this disorder moldy hay with spores of actinomycetes are inhaled and produce a hypersensitivity pneumonitis. The disorder is seen most commonly in rainy periods, when the spores multiply. Patients present generally 4 to 8 h after exposure with fever, cough, and shortness of breath without wheezing. Chest radiograms often show patchy bilateral, often upper lobe infiltrates. The exposure history will differentiate this disorder from other types of pneumonia.

VI-86. **The answer is E.** *(Chap. 255)* This patient with rheumatoid arthritis (RA) is presenting with pulmonary symptoms, and the biopsy shows a pattern of cryptogenic organizing pneumonia (COP), a known pulmonary manifestation of rheumatoid arthritis. COP (formerly bronchiolitis obliterans organizing pneumonia, BOOP) usually presents in the fifth or sixth decades with a flulike illness. Symptoms include fevers, malaise, weight loss, cough, and dyspnea. Inspiratory crackles are common, and late inspiratory squeaks may also be heard. Pulmonary function testing reveals restrictive lung disease. The typical pattern on high-resolution chest CT is patchy areas of airspace consolidation, nodular opacities, and ground-glass opacities that occur more frequently in the lower lung zones. Pathology shows the presence of granulation tissue plugging airways, alveolar ducts, and alveoli. There is frequently chronic inflammation in the alveolar interstitium. Treatment with high-dose steroids is effective in two-thirds of individuals, with most individuals being able to be tapered to lower doses over the first year. Azathioprine is an immunosuppressive therapy that is commonly used in interstitial lung disease due to usual interstitial pneumonitis. While it may be considered in COP unresponsive to glucocorticoids, it would not be a first-line agent used without concomitant steroid therapy. RA has multiple pulmonary complications. However, therapy with infliximab or methotrexate, which are useful for severe RA, are not used in the treatment of COP. Methotrexate also has pulmonary side effects and may cause pulmonary fibrosis. Hydroxychloroquine is frequently useful for joint symptoms in autoimmune disorders. Its major side effect is retinal toxicity, and it is not known to cause COP.

VI-87. **The answer is A.** *(Chap. 258)* Disorders of the respiratory drive, respiratory muscular system, some chest wall disorders and upper airways obstruction may produce an elevated Pa_{CO_2} despite having normal pulmonary function. In this setting, the alveolar-arterial (A – a) oxygen gradient will be normal but the minute ventilation is low, producing a respiratory acidosis. In pulmonary parenchymal or airways diseases associated with respiratory acidosis (pulmonary fibrosis, chronic obstructive pulmonary disease), the Pa_{CO_2} is elevated, the A – a gradient is commonly increased, and minute ventilation is either elevated or normal. Any cause of respiratory acidosis may produce an obligatory fall in Pa_{O_2}. Diaphragmatic dysfunction and maximal inspiratory or expiratory pressures are commonly impaired with respiratory neuromuscular dysfunction but may be normal in other disorders of central hypoventilation such as stroke.

VI-88. **The answer is C.** *(Chap. 257)* Severe kyphoscoliosis causes pulmonary symptoms in up to 3% of patients with this condition. The physical abnormalities caused by the forward and lateral curvature of the spine result in abnormal pulmonary mechanics. This is manifested primarily as restrictive lung disease with chronic alveolar hypoventilation. This in turn leads to ventilation-perfusion imbalances that result in hypoxic vasoconstriction and may cause the eventual development of pulmonary hypertension.

VI-89. **The answer is C.** *(Chap. 194)* This patient lives in a part of the country where *Blastomyces* infection is found. Other endemic regions in North America are the Mississippi and Ohio River basins, the Great Lake states, and areas along the St. Lawrence River. The subacute course after an abrupt onset, arthralgias, and alveolar infiltrates with a cavity are all suggestive of *Blastomyces* infection, given the region from which the patient originates. Pleural effusions and mediastinal adenopathy are uncommon. Respiratory failure and disseminated infection are more common in immunocompromised patients who may have a mortality of >50%. *Legionella* pneumonia may present in a similar fashion, but those patients usually have a predisposing condition such as diabetes, advanced age, end-stage renal disease, immunosuppression, or advanced lung disease. Hyponatremia may be seen in *Legionella* pneumonia but is more common in Legionnaire's disease. Although a bone marrow aspirate may grow *Blastomyces*, isolation from more accessible material (i.e., sputum, pus) usually makes bone marrow aspiration unnecessary. The KOH stain of expectorated sputum is positive in >80% of cases of *Blastomyces* pneumonia. The Quellung reaction is used to diagnose infection with *Streptococcus pneumoniae*. However, the time course of this infection is prolonged for pneumococcal pneumonia, and necrotizing infection causing cavitation is rare. The time course of the infection is too rapid for pulmonary tuberculosis, although tuberculosis should be considered in the evaluation of cavitary lesions of the lung.

VI-90. **The answer is B.** *(Chap. 255)* This patient's clinical-radiologic presentation, in addition to the lung function information, which revealed a moderate restrictive defect and a moderate gas transfer defect, suggests an acute pneumonitis. The differential diagnosis includes various causes of diffuse alveolar hemorrhage, idiopathic bronchiolitis obliterans organizing pneumonia, acute eosinophilic pneumonia, interstitial lung disease secondary to connective tissue disorders [systemic lupus erythematosus (SLE), rheumatoid arthritis, polymyositis], and diffuse alveolar damage secondary to other causes (sepsis, drugs, toxins, infections, etc.). Methotrexate has been associated with an idiosyncratic drug reaction, with particular risk in the elderly and in patients with decreased creatinine clearance. Discontinuing the medicine and in some cases adding high-dose steroids constitute the initial management. Initiating empirical broad-spectrum antibiotics until a more definite result could be obtained via a bronchoscopy would be a reasonable approach.

VI-91.　**The answer is A.** *(Chap. 263)* To obtain a stable airway for invasive mechanical ventilation, patients must safely undergo endotracheal intubation. In most patients, paralytic agents are used in combination with sedatives to accomplish endotracheal intubation. Succinylcholine is a depolarizing neuromuscular blocking agent with a short half-life and is one of the most commonly used paralytic agents. However, because it depolarizes the neuromuscular junction, succinylcholine cannot be used in individuals with hyperkalemia because the drug may cause further increases in the potassium level and potentially fatal cardiac arrhythmias. Some conditions in which it is relatively contraindicated to use succinylcholine because of the risk of hyperkalemia include acute renal failure, crush injuries, muscular dystrophy, rhabdomyolysis, and tumor lysis syndrome. Acetaminophen overdose is not a contraindication to the use of succinylcholine unless concomitant renal failure is present.

VI-92.　**The answer is E.** *[Chap. 257; Arch Neurol 58(6):893–898, 2001.]* Patients with Guillain-Barré syndrome (acute inflammatory demyelinating polyneuropathy) are at high risk of developing respiratory failure, with up to 30% requiring mechanical ventilation during the course of their illness. Patients with this syndrome should be hospitalized and followed for evidence of respiratory failure. The most common means of doing this is serial measurements of vital capacity and maximum inspiratory pressure. Once the vital capacity has fallen to less than 20 mL/kg body weight, mechanical ventilation is indicated. Other measures of impending ventilatory failure include a maximum inspiratory pressure less than 30 cmH$_2$O and a maximum expiratory pressure less than 40 cmH$_2$O. Although rising Pa$_{CO_2}$ provides clear evidence of ventilatory failure and is an indication for the initiation of mechanical ventilation, ideally these other measures will identify these individuals before their progression to overt ventilatory failure.

VI-93.　**The answer is E.** *(Chap. 322)* Sarcoidosis is an inflammatory disorder of unknown cause that is characterized by the presence of noncaseating granulomas. The worldwide prevalence of sarcoidosis is estimated to be 20–60 per 100,000 population. The highest incidence occurs in the Nordic population, but in the United States, the incidence of sarcoidosis is highest in African Americans. Sarcoidosis typically occurs in young, otherwise-healthy adults. Up to 20% of cases can be found incidentally on chest radiograph in asymptomatic individuals, as in this case presentation. When present, typical symptoms are most commonly cough and dyspnea. However, sarcoidosis can affect any organ system. After the respiratory symptoms, skin disease and ocular findings are the most commonly seen manifestations of sarcoidosis. Lung involvement is seen in >90% of individuals with sarcoidosis, and staging of pulmonary sarcoidosis is based upon findings on chest radiograph. Stage I disease refers to patients with hilar adenopathy only. In stage II disease, hilar adenopathy is present with pulmonary infiltrates. Stage III disease has no evidence of hilar adenopathy, but interstitial pulmonary disease is present; stage IV disease consists of pulmonary fibrosis. Occasionally, the term *stage 0 disease* is used to refer to individuals with extrapulmonary sarcoidosis and no lung involvement. Definitive diagnosis of sarcoidosis relies upon demonstration of noncaseating granulomas on biopsy of affected tissue without other cause for granulomatous disease. In this case, transbronchial needle aspiration of a hilar lymph node demonstrated noncaseating granulomas, as did transbronchial tissue biopsies. Even without overt involvement of lung parenchyma, granulomas are frequently found on transbronchial tissue biopsies. Treatment of sarcoidosis is largely based upon symptoms. In this patient without symptomatic disease and normal lung function, no treatment is necessary. She should receive reassurance and close follow-up for development of symptomatic disease. In stage I disease, between 50 and 90% will resolve spontaneously without treatment. When treatment is necessary, prednisone is the treatment of choice initially. Usually doses of 20–40 mg are effective, but with cardiac or neurologic involvement, higher doses of prednisone, up to 1 mg/kg, are often necessary. For severe manifestations of sarcoidosis, addition of azathioprine, methotrexate, or cyclophosphamide may be required. Joint and dermatologic manifestations often respond well to hydroxychloroquine. This patient has no evidence of infection by clinical history, with a biopsy that is negative for fungal and mycobacterial organisms. Treatment with antifungal or mycobacterial therapy is not indicated.

VI-94. The answer is B. *(Chap. 311; P Lieberman et al: J Allergy Clin Immunol 115:S483, 2005)*
This patient is presenting with severe anaphylaxis manifested by respiratory failure and sustained hypotension not responsive to initial treatment with IM epinephrine and IV fluids. At this point, management should focus upon establishing and maintaining blood pressure for adequate organ perfusion. Life-threatening anaphylaxis is an immediate IgE-mediated hypersensitivity reaction that usually appears within minutes of exposure to a sensitized antigen. However, most individuals who die of anaphylaxis related to insect stings are unaware of their sensitization. Symptoms of anaphylaxis include urticaria, angioedema, laryngospasm, bronchospasm, and vascular collapse. Nausea, vomiting, and diarrhea may also occur. With the onset of anaphylactic shock, massive vasodilatation and capillary leak occur. In one study, it was estimated that there was a 50% decrease in intravascular volume within the first few minutes of anaphylactic shock *(MM Fisher: Anaesth Intens Care 14(1):17, 1986)*. The first step in treating anaphylaxis is to administer epinephrine 0.3 to 0.5 mg (0.3–0.5 mL of a 1:1000 solution) IM or SC. In severe anaphylaxis, the IM route is preferred. Additional doses can be given as needed every 5 min, and there is no absolute contraindication to ongoing treatment with epinephrine in anaphylaxis. If anaphylaxis fails to improve quickly with administration of epinephrine, establishment of a secure airway and delivery of oxygen should be paramount. In addition, rapid bolus of 1–2 L of intravenous fluids through large-bore IVs is indicated to replace intravascular volume. Previous studies have demonstrated no difference between colloid and crystalloid solutions for initial volume resuscitation in anaphylaxis. However, lactated Ringer's solution should not be used because of an increased risk of metabolic acidosis. Ongoing shock that is refractory to the above therapies is best treated with ongoing administration of large volumes of IV fluids, as described in the scenario, as well as continued administration of epinephrine via the IV route. Initial doses of IV epinephrine range from 0.1–0.3 mg administered over several minutes, and institution of a continuous infusion of epinephrine at a rate of 0.2–2 mg/min can be considered. Other vasopressor therapy such as dopamine or vasopressin can be added to maintain blood pressure if the shock is refractory to epinephrine infusion. Antihistamine therapy with H_1 and H_2 blockers are considered second-line therapy after epinephrine, as these agents have a slower onset of action. Antihistamine therapy alone should not be given for treatment of anaphylactic shock. Glucocorticoids have no role in the acute therapy of anaphylaxis, but should be administered once the patient is stabilized to prevent late-phase reactions with recurrent anaphylaxis. Disconnecting the patient from the ventilator would be appropriate for the treatment of hypotension due to the development of intrinsic positive end-expiratory pressure. However, in this case, the patient is set at a low respiratory rate. In addition, it is noted that the wheezing stops prior to the next inhalation, suggesting that the patient is fully exhaling the inspired tidal volume. Thus, it is unlikely that intrinsic-PEEP is occurring.

VI-95. The answer is C. *(Chap. 265)* As the mortality from sepsis has increased over the past 20 years, more research has been performed to attempt to limit mortality. Specific therapies have been developed to target the inflammatory response to sepsis, particularly the effect of the inflammatory response on the coagulation system. Activated protein C was the first drug approved by the U.S. Food and Drug Administration for the treatment of septic shock. This drug is an anticoagulant that may also have antiapoptotic and anti-inflammatory properties. In a randomized controlled trial, activated protein C was associated with an absolute reduction in mortality of 6.1%, and the effect of the drug on mortality was greatest in those who were most critically ill. However, in those individuals who are less severely ill, activated protein C may increase mortality. While it is unethical to randomize individuals to a trial assessing the appropriate timing of antibiotic delivery, retrospective analyses have demonstrated an increased risk of death if antibiotics are not given within 1 h of presentation. A single-center trial of early goal-directed therapy in septic shock showed a survival advantage when this approach was taken. Early goal-directed therapy developed a protocol for fluid administration, institution of vasopressors, and blood transfusion based on physiologic parameters, including mean arterial pressure, central venous oxygen saturation, and presence of acidosis among others. Bicarbonate therapy is commonly used when severe metabolic acidosis (pH <7.2) is present in septic shock. However, there is no evidence that bicarbonate improves hemodynamics, response to vasopressors, or outcomes in septic shock.

VI-96.   **The answer is D.** *(Chap. 34)* The patient presents with chronic cough as it has lasted for more than 3 weeks. He denies symptoms of the most common causes of chronic cough, such as asthma, gastroesophageal reflux disease, and postnasal drip. However, he does take an angiotensin-converting enzyme (ACE) inhibitor, which is known to cause chronic cough in 5 to 20% of the patients who take this class of medications. Cough that is due to ACE inhibitors generally begins between 1 week and 6 months after medication initiation. The most appropriate diagnostic and therapeutic step at this point is to discontinue the ramipril. Angiotensin receptor blockers can be used instead of the ACE inhibitor to improve cardiac outcomes but are generally not recommended as first-line therapy. In light of this patient's lack of risk factors for malignancy and lack of sputum production, bronchoscopy would not be helpful in this case. Furosemide and digoxin are not associated with cough. As the patient denies having infectious or constitutional symptoms, empirical courses of antibiotics are not warranted.

VII. DISORDERS OF THE URINARY AND KIDNEY TRACT

QUESTIONS

DIRECTIONS: Choose the **one best** response to each question.

VII-1. A clinic patient who has a diagnosis of polycystic kidney disease has been doing research on the Internet. She is asymptomatic and has no significant family history. She asks you for screening for intracranial aneurysms. You recommend which of the following?

A. Head CT scan without contrast
B. CT angiogram
C. Cerebral angiogram
D. Magnetic resonance angiogram
E. No further testing

VII-2. Which of the following is the most potent stimulus for hypothalamic production of arginine vasopressin?

A. Hypertonicity
B. Hyperkalemia
C. Hypokalemia
D. Hypotonicity
E. Intravascular volume depletion

VII-3. A 28-year-old woman with HIV on antiretroviral therapy complains of abdominal pain in the emergency department. Laboratory data show a creatinine of 3.2 mg/dL; her baseline creatinine is 1.0 mg/dL. Urinalysis shows large numbers of white blood cells and red blood cells without epithelial cells, leukocyte esterase, or nitrites. Which test is indicated to diagnose the cause of her acute renal failure?

A. Acid-fast stain of the urine
B. Anti-GBM (glomerular base membrane) antibodies
C. Renal angiogram
D. Renal ultrasound
E. Urine electrolytes

VII-4. You are evaluating a 40-year-old patient admitted to the hospital with cirrhosis and an upper gastrointestinal bleed. The bleeding was treated with endoscopy and photocoagulation, and the patient is now stable. He required two units of packed red blood cells. He was briefly hypotensive upon admission but has remained stable for the past 5 days. He is becoming oliguric. Laboratory data show a creatinine of 4.0 mg/dL, whereas his baseline is 0.8–1.1 mg/dL. So-

VII-4. *(Continued)*
dium is 140 meq/L, BUN is 49 mg/dL. Urine sediment shows rare granular casts. His urine sodium is 50 meq/L, urine osmolality 287 mosmol and urine creatinine is 35 mg/dL. What is the cause of this patient's acute renal failure?

A. Acute interstitial nephritis
B. Acute tubular necrosis
C. Glomerulonephritis
D. Hepatorenal syndrome
E. Prerenal azotemia

VII-5. The pain associated with acute urinary tract obstruction is a result of which of the following?

A. Compensatory natriuresis
B. Decreased medullary blood flow
C. Increased renal blood flow
D. Vasodilatory prostaglandins

VII-6. Preoperative assessment of a 55-year-old male patient going for coronary angiography shows an estimated glomerular filtration rate of 33 mL/min per 1.73 m^2 and poorly controlled diabetes. He is currently on no nephrotoxic medications, and the nephrologist assures you that he does not currently have acute renal failure. The case is due to begin in 4 h, and you would like to prevent contrast nephropathy. Which agent will definitely reduce the risk of contrast nephropathy?

A. Dopamine
B. Fenoldopam
C. Indomethacin
D. *N*-acetylcysteine
E. Sodium bicarbonate

VII-7. All the following forms of glomerulonephritis (GN) have associated normal serum complement C4 levels *except*

A. lupus nephritis stage IV
B. poststreptococcal GN
C. hemolytic-uremic syndrome
D. membranoproliferative GN type II
E. endocarditis-associated GN

VII-8. An 84-year-old female nursing home resident is brought to the emergency department due to lethargy. At the nursing home, she was found to have a blood pressure of 85/60 mmHg, heart rate 101 beats/min, temperature 37.8°C. Laboratory data are obtained: sodium 137 meq/L, potassium 2.8 meq/L, HCO_3^- 8 meq/L, chloride 117 meq/L, BUN 17 mg/dL, creatinine 0.9 mg/dL. An arterial blood gas shows Pa_{O_2} 80 mmHg, P_{CO_2} 24 mmHg, pH 7.29. Her urine analysis is clear and has a pH of 4.5. What is the acid-base disorder?

A. Anion-gap metabolic acidosis
B. Non-anion gap metabolic acidosis
C. Non-anion-gap metabolic acidosis and respiratory alkalosis
D. Respiratory acidosis

VII-9. What is the most likely cause of the acid-base disorder of the patient in the preceding scenario?

A. Diarrhea
B. Diuretic use
C. Hyperacute renal failure
D. Hypoaldosteronism
E. Proximal renal tubular acidosis

VII-10. A 79-year-old male with a history of dementia is brought to the emergency department because of an 8-h history of lethargy. For the last 2 days he has been complaining of lower abdominal pain. His oral intake was normal until the last 8 h. The patient takes no medications. Temperature is normal, blood pressure is 150/90 mmHg, heart rate is 105/min, and respirations are 20/min. Physical examination is notable for elevated neck veins and diffuse lower abdominal pain with normal bowel sounds. The bladder is percussed to the umbilicus, and there is an enlarged prostate. He is lethargic but responsive. Serum chemistries are notable for sodium of 128 meq/L, potassium of 5.7 meq/L, BUN of 100 mg/dL, and creatinine of 2.2 mg/dL. Two months ago his laboratory studies were normal. A Foley catheter is placed, yielding 1100 mL of urine. Which of the following statements regarding his clinical condition is true?

A. His renal function probably will return to normal within the next week.
B. He will need aggressive volume resuscitation over the next 24 h.
C. He will have oliguria over the next 24 h.
D. Immediate dialysis is indicated.
E. Urinalysis will reveal hypertonic urine.

VII-11. A 71-year-old woman is transferred to your hospital with new-onset renal failure requiring hemodialysis. On hospital day 1 at the outside hospital, she was admitted with a Killip class III inferior myocardial infarction. She underwent percutaneous coronary intervention on day 1 with successful angioplasty. On day 2, she spiked a

VII-11. *(Continued)*
fever and was started on gentamicin and a fluoroquinolone for pneumonia. A chest x-ray showed pulmonary vascular congestion on day 3, which was treated with IV loop diuretic. She complained of leg pain on day 4 which responded well to potassium repletion and ibuprofen. She is transferred to you with a urinalysis that shows 17 white blood cells, 1 red blood cell, 0 epithelial cells, no leukocyte esterase. Hansel's stain is positive for eosinophils. Serum laboratory studies show a creatinine of 4.2 mg/dL and undetectable complement levels. It is now hospital day 7. On which hospital day was her renal failure caused?

A. 1
B. 2
C. 3
D. 4

VII-12. A 57-year-old man is admitted to the hospital for dehydration and confusion. In the emergency department he complained of excessive thirst and he was found to have a serum sodium of 162 meq/L and a newly elevated creatinine of 2.2 mg/dL. After receiving IV fluid, his sensorium clears and the patient relays to you that he drinks large amounts of fluid each day and makes about 2 L of urine each day. He has noticed that his urine output has no relation to the amount of fluid he drinks. His sodium remains elevated at 150 meq/L, and his urine osmolality returns at 80 mosmol/kg. After careful water restriction, you administer 10 µg of desmopressin intranasally and remeasure his urine osmolality. The osmolality is now 94 mosmol/kg. What is the most likely cause of his hypernatremia?

A. Chronic hyperventilation
B. Diabetes insipidus
C. Excessive solute intake
D. Gastrointestinal losses
E. Surreptitious use of diuretics

VII-13. What is the correct long-term treatment for the patient in the preceding scenario?

A. Arginine vasopressin (AVP) analogues
B. Brain imaging and, if indicated, resection
C. Lithium carbonate
D. Narcotics
E. Salt restriction and diuretics

VII-14. A 53-year-old female with long-standing depression and a history of rheumatoid arthritis is brought in by her daughter, who states that she found an empty bottle of acetylsalicylic acid by her mother's bedside. The patient is found to be confused and lethargic and is unable to provide a definitive history. What is the most likely set of laboratory values?

VII-14. *(Continued)*

	Na$^+$	K$^+$	Cl$^-$	HCO$_3^-$	Serum Creatinine	Room Air ABG		
						P$_{O_2}$	P$_{CO_2}$	pH
	(Serum, meq/L)				μmol/L (mg/dL)			
A	140	3.9	85	26	141 (1.6)	100	40	7.40
B	140	3.9	85	16	141 (1.6)	100	20	7.40
C	140	5.8	100	20	141 (1.6)	100	34	7.38
D	150	2.9	100	36	141 (1.6)	80	46	7.50
E	116	3.7	85	22	141 (1.6)	80	46	7.50

VII-15. You are evaluating a 28-year-old man from Peru with abdominal pain. As part of the diagnostic workup, an abdominal ultrasound shows bilateral hydronephrosis and hydroureters. Which of the following conditions is least likely in this patient?

A. Lymphoma
B. Meatal stenosis
C. Phimosis
D. Retroperitoneal fibrosis

VII-16. A 45-year-old male with a diagnosis of ESRD secondary to diabetes mellitus is being treated with peritoneal dialysis. This is being carried out as a continuous ambulatory peritoneal dialysis (CAPD). He undergoes four 2-L exchanges per day and has been doing so for approximately 4 years. Complications of peritoneal dialysis include which of the following?

A. Hypotension after drainage of dialysate
B. Hypoalbuminemia
C. Hypercholesterolemia
D. Hypoglycemia
E. Left pleural effusion

VII-17. While on rotation in a rural clinic, you are asked to evaluate a 70-year-old man with fever, shortness of breath and a productive cough. You appreciate increased fremitus with egophony over the right lower lung field and make a presumptive diagnosis of community-acquired pneumonia. Blood pressure is 138/74 mmHg, heart rate 99 beats/min, temperature 38.6°C and weight 72 kg. He has a history of a nephrectomy, and he tells you that his "kidneys don't work at 100%." Before prescribing antibiotics, you would like to know his renal function. What additional data do you need in order to calculate his creatinine clearance using the Cockcroft-Gault formula?

A. Plasma creatinine
B. Plasma and urine creatinine
C. Race and plasma creatinine
D. Race, plasma creatinine, and urine creatinine

VII-18. You are able to send the patient to the local hospital to get laboratory values drawn. His serum creatinine is

1.5 mg/dL, sodium 138 meq/L, potassium 3.8 meq/L, urine creatinine is 12 mmol. Using the Cockcroft-Gault equation, what is this patient's creatinine clearance?

A. 27 mL/min
B. 47 mL/min
C. 70 mL/min
D. 105 mL/min

VII-19. All of these findings are consistent with a chronic unilateral urinary tract obstruction *except*

A. anemia
B. dysuria
C. hypertension
D. pain with micturition
E. pyuria

VII-20. A 72-year-old male develops acute renal failure after cardiac catheterization. Physical examination is notable for diminished peripheral pulses, livedo reticularis, epigastric tenderness, and confusion. Laboratory studies include (mg/dL) BUN 131, creatinine 5.2, and phosphate 9.5. Urinalysis shows 10 to 15 white blood cells (WBC), 5 to 10 red blood cells (RBC), and one hyaline cast per high-power field (HPF). The most likely diagnosis is

A. acute interstitial nephritis caused by drugs
B. rhabdomyolysis with acute tubular necrosis
C. acute tubular necrosis secondary to radiocontrast exposure
D. cholesterol embolization
E. renal arterial dissection with prerenal azotemia

VII-21. A 34-year-old male is brought to the hospital with altered mental status. He has a history of alcoholism. He is somnolent and does not answer questions. Physical examination reveals blood pressure 130/80, heart rate 105/min, respiratory rate 24/min, and temperature 37°C (98.6°F). The remainder of the physical examination is unremarkable. Microscopic analysis of urine is shown below. Which of the following most likely will be found on further diagnostic evaluation?

VII-21. *(Continued)*

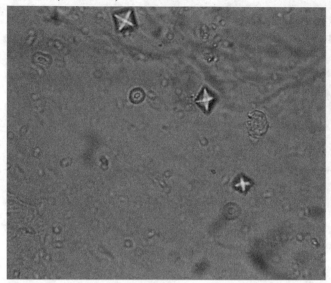

FIGURE VII-21

A. More than 10,000 bacterial colonies on urine culture
B. Anion gap metabolic acidosis
C. Hydronephrosis on ultrasound
D. Nephrolithiasis on CT scan
E. Positive antinuclear antibodies (ANA)

VII-22. A 52-year-old man is found at home hypotensive and confused. In the emergency department, his blood pressure is 82/60 mmHg and his heart rate is 115 beats/min. He is confused and lethargic. Laboratory data show: Sodium 133 meq/L, potassium 2.4 meq/L, chloride 70 meq/L, HCO_3^- 50 meq/L, BUN 44 mg/dL, creatinine 1.7 mg/dL. An arterial blood gas shows P_{O_2} of 62 mmHg, P_{CO_2} 49 mmHg, pH 7.66. What acid-base disorder is present?

A. Anion gap metabolic acidosis
B. Metabolic alkalosis
C. Metabolic alkalosis plus respiratory acidosis
D. Respiratory acidosis
E. Respiratory alkalosis

VII-23. What is the most likely cause of the acid-base disorder for the patient in the preceding scenario?

A. Acute myocardial infarction
B. Bartter syndrome
C. Cushing's disease
D. Mineralocorticoid excess
E. Vomiting

VII-24. A 52-year-old diabetic patient is referred to the emergency department from the endoscopy suite. The patient has diabetes and a history of colon cancer that was removed 3 years ago. He also has hyperlipidemia, which is well controlled on atorvastatin. He presented to the Endoscopy suite for a scheduled surveillance colonoscopy. Blood drawn upon arrival to shows a sodium of 121 meq/L and the patient seemed disoriented. On physical examination, mu-

VII-24. *(Continued)*
cous membranes are dry and there is no axillary moisture. Serum osmolality is checked and is 270 mosmol/kg. What is the most likely cause of this patient's hyponatremia?

A. Diabetes insipidus
B. Hyperglycemia
C. Hyperlipidemia
D. Hypovolemia
E. Syndrome of inappropriate secretion of antidiuretic hormone (SIADH)

VII-25. You are evaluating a patient with stage 5 chronic kidney disease (CKD) who has an estimated glomerular filtration rate of 12 mL/min per 1.73 m². She has no complaints and takes all of her medications on schedule. Physical examination reveals a woman in no acute distress. There is no pericardial rub, and reflexes and mental status are intact. She has trace peripheral edema. Laboratory data show a creatinine of 6.3 mg/dL, potassium 4.8 meq/L, HCO_3^- 20 meq/L. She has known proteinuria. What is best next step in the management of this patient's CKD?

A. Check serum blood urea nitrogen (BUN)
B. Continue current management
C. Referral to the emergency department for initiation of dialysis
D. Renal biopsy
E. Urine analysis

VII-26. Your clinic patient presents to your office complaining of numbness and tingling in her hands and around her mouth. On physical examination, you illicit Chovstek's sign (twitching of the circumoral muscles in response to gently tapping on the facial nerve) and Trousseau's sign (carpal spasm induced by inflation of a blood pressure cuff to 20 mmHg above the patient's systolic blood pressure for 3 min. You make a presumptive diagnosis of hypocalcemia. What laboratory test is the next step in diagnosing the cause of her hypocalcemia?

A. 1,25(OH₂)D
B. Ionized calcium
C. Parathyroid hormone (PTH)
D. Serum magnesium
E. Thyroid-stimulating hormone

VII-27. A 25-year-old man comes to your clinic because of a change in the color of his urine. He states that his urine has become red-tinged and has the foaminess of beer in the bowl. He has no abdominal pain or respiratory complaints. He has no cough, although he does report unintentional weight loss of 2–7 kg over the past month. He has no past medical history. In your office, you perform a urinalysis and dipstick which shows red blood cell (RBC) casts and RBCs (including dysmorphic cells). He has no white blood cells and no bacteria. The urine dipsick is 2+, with a spot protein-to-creatinine ratio of 850. What is the next step in this patient's evaluation?

VII-27. *(Continued)*

A. Measure antineutrophilic cytoplasmic antibody levels
B. Cystoscopy
C. Initiate therapy with an angiotensin-converting enzyme (ACE) inhibitor with close follow-up
D. Measure urine microalbumin
E. Renal CT scan

VII-28. A 10-year-old girl complaining of profound weakness, occasional difficulty walking, and polyuria is brought to the pediatrician. Her mother is sure the girl has not been vomiting frequently. The girl takes no medicines. She is normotensive, and no focal neurologic abnormalities are found. Serum chemistries include Na^+ 142 mmol/L, K^+ 2.5 mmol/L, HCO_3^- 32 mmol/L, and Cl^- 100 mmol/L. A 24-h urine collection on a normal diet reveals Na^+ 200 mmol/d, K^+ 50 mmol/d, and Cl^- 30 mmol/d. Renal ultrasound demonstrates symmetrically enlarged kidneys without hydronephrosis. A stool phenolphthalein test and a urine screen for diuretics are negative. Plasma renin levels are found to be elevated. Which of the following conditions is most consistent with these data?

A. Conn's syndrome
B. Chronic ingestion of licorice
C. Bartter's syndrome
D. Wilms' tumor
E. Proximal renal tubular acidosis

VII-29. A 56-year-old male is evaluated in the clinic after complaining of inability to maintain an erection. He reports good sexual function until 4 months ago. Since that time he has noted that he cannot maintain erections. The patient awakens three times weekly with an erection that is unchanged compared with his previous status. He states that his libido is unchanged but that he loses his erection within minutes. He has been married for 25 years and denies any extramarital affairs. He does not smoke. Recently the patient has had increased stressors in his life when he was laid off his job as a worker in an oil refinery. Past medical history is significant for hypertension, which is being treated with atenolol. On physical examination, blood pressure is 136/76 mmHg and heart rate is 64/min. The patient has normal secondary sexual characteristics without gynecomastia. There is no liver enlargement. The testes are firm and rubbery without masses and have an estimated volume of 35 mL by orchiometry. The penis is circumcised and without fibrotic plaques. Rectal examination reveals a normal prostate and normal anal sphincter tone. The bulbocavernosus reflex is intact. Prostate specific antigen (PSA) is 4.12 ng/mL. The testosterone level is 537 ng/dL. What is the best way to treat this patient's erectile dysfunction?

A. Discontinue atenolol.
B. Start sildenafil.
C. Initiate therapy with transdermal testosterone.

VII-29. *(Continued)*

D. Initiate therapy with intraurethral injection of alprostadil.
E. Further explore the patient's psychosocial history for evidence of anxiety and depression and consider referral for psychotherapy.

VII-30. A 32-year-old patient presents to your clinic complaining of right-sided flank pain and dark urine. He states that these symptoms began about a month ago. He denies any burning on urination and has had no fevers. He has not suffered any trauma and has not been sexually active recently. On review of systems he reports early satiety and describes a burning sensation in his chest when he lies down. An ultrasound of his right flank is performed and reveals >20 cysts of varying sizes in his right kidney. Which of the following statements is true?

A. Adult-onset polycystic kidney disease (PCKD) will lead to end-stage renal disease in 100% of patients by age 70.
B. Aortic stenosis is present in 25% of patient with PCKD.
C. 40% of patients with PCKD will have hepatic cysts by age 60.
D. PCKD is inherited as an autosomal recessive trait in adults.
E. There is a significantly increased risk of embolic stroke in patients with PCKD.

VII-31. In patients with chronic renal failure, which of the following is the most important contributor to renal osteodystrophy?

A. Impaired renal production of 1,25-dihydroxyvitamin D_3 [$1,25(OH)_2D_3$]
B. Hypocalcemia
C. Hypophosphatemia
D. Loss of vitamin D and calcium via dialysis
E. The use of calcitriol

VII-32. A 74-year-old female sees her physician for a follow-up visit for hypertension. One week ago she was started on an oral medication for hypertension. She takes no other medications. Blood pressure is 125/80 mmHg, and heart rate is 72/min. Serum chemistries reveal a sodium of 132 meq/L. Two weeks ago serum chemistries were normal. Which of the following medications most likely was initiated 1 week ago?

A. Enalapril
B. Furosemide
C. Hydrochlorothiazide
D. Metoprolol
E. Spironolactone

VII-33. Laboratory evaluation of a 19-year-old male who is being worked up for polyuria and polydipsia yields the following results:

VII-33. *(Continued)*

Serum electrolytes (meq/L): Na$^+$ 144, K$^+$ 4.0, Cl$^-$ 107, HCO$_3^-$ 25

BUN: 6.4 mmol/L (18 mg/dL)

Blood glucose: 5.7 mmol/L (102 mg/dL)

Urine electrolytes (mmol/L): Na$^+$ 28, K$^+$ 32

Urine osmolality: 195 mosmol/kg water

After 12 h of fluid deprivation, body weight has fallen by 5%. Laboratory testing now reveals the following:

Serum electrolytes (meq/L): Na$^+$ 150, K$^+$ 4.1, Cl$^-$ 109, HCO$_3^-$ 25

BUN: 7.1 mmol/L (20 mg/dL)

Blood glucose: 5.4 mmol/L (98 mg/dL)

Urine electrolytes (mmol/L): Na$^+$ 24, K$^+$ 35

Urine osmolality: 200 mosmol/kg water

One hour after the subcutaneous administration of 5 units of arginine vasopressin urine values are as follows:

Urine electrolytes (meq/L): Na$^+$ 30, K$^+$ 30

Urine osmolality: 199 mosmol/kg water

The likely diagnosis is

A. nephrogenic diabetes insipidus
B. osmotic diuresis
C. salt-losing nephropathy
D. psychogenic polydipsia
E. none of the above

VII-34. A 28-year-old man is diagnosed with acute myelogenous leukemia and has a white blood cell count of 168,000/µL. He initiates chemotherapy with cytarabine, etoposide, and daunorubicin. Within 24 h, his creatinine has increased from 1.0 mg/dL to 2.5 mg/dL, and he is oliguric. Pretreatment with which of the following medications may have prevented this complication?

A. Allopurinol
B. Colchicine
C. Furosemide
D. Prednisone
E. Sodium bicarbonate

VII-35. A 37-year-old man is brought to the emergency department by his wife from home. He was painting their garage and became unconscious. He has no past medical history. CT scan of the head is normal. Urine and serum toxicology screen, including ethanol and acetaminophen, are negative. Laboratory data show: Sodium 138 meq/L, potassium 4.4 meq/L, HCO$_3^-$ 5 meq/L, chloride 102 meq/L, BUN 15 mg/dL, calcium 9.7 mg/dL, glucose 94 mg/dL. An arterial blood gas on room air shows Pa$_{O_2}$ 95 mmHg, P$_{CO_2}$ 20 mmHg, pH 7.02. A urine analysis is unremarkable. On physical examination his blood pressure is 110/72 mmHg. He is barely arousable but responds to painful

VII-35. *(Continued)*

stimuli. Otherwise, he has no focal abnormalities. What is the acid-base disorder?

A. Anion-gap metabolic acidosis
B. Anion-gap metabolic acidosis with respiratory alkalosis
C. Non-anion-gap metabolic acidosis
D. Respiratory acidosis

VII-36. The "dose" of dialysis is currently defined as

A. the counter-current flow rate of the dialysate
B. the fractional urea clearance
C. the hours per week of dialysis
D. the number of sessions actually completed in a month

VII-37. A patient with a diagnosis of scleroderma who has diffuse cutaneous involvement presents with malignant hypertension, oliguria, edema, hemolytic anemia, and renal failure. You make a diagnosis of scleroderma renal crisis (SRC). What is the recommended treatment?

A. Captopril
B. Carvedilol
C. Clonidine
D. Diltiazem
E. Nitroprusside

VII-38. Your patient with end-stage renal disease on hemodialysis has persistent hyperkalemia. He has a history of total bilateral renal artery stenosis, which is why he is on hemodialysis. He only has electrocardiogram changes when his potassium rises above 6.0 meq/L, which occurs a few times per week. You admit him to the hospital for further evaluation. Your laboratory evaluation, nutrition counseling, and medication adjustments have not impacted his serum potassium. What is the next reasonable step to undertake for this patient?

A. Adjust the dialysate.
B. Administer a daily dose of furosemide.
C. Perform "sodium modeling."
D. Implant an automatic defibrillator.
E. Perform bilateral nephrectomy.

VII-39. A 63-year-old male is brought to the emergency department after having a seizure. He has a history of an unresectable lung mass treated with palliative radiation therapy. He is known to have a serum sodium of 128 meq/L chronically. The patient's wife reports that on the night before admission he was somnolent. This morning, while she was trying to awaken him, he developed a generalized tonic-clonic seizure lasting approximately 1 min. In the emergency room he is unresponsive. Vital signs and physical examination are otherwise normal. Serum sodium is 111 meq/L. He is treated with 3% saline and transferred to the intensive care unit. One day later serum sodium is 137 meq/L. He has had no further seizures since admission and is awake but is barely able to move

VII-39. *(Continued)*

his extremities and is dysarthric. Which of the following studies is most likely to explain his current condition?

A. Arteriogram showing a vertebral artery thrombus
B. CT of the head showing metastases
C. EEG showing focal seizures
D. MRI of the brainstem showing demyelination
E. Transesophageal echocardiogram showing left atrial thrombus

VII-40. A 25-year-old female with nephrotic syndrome from minimal-change disease is seen in the emergency department with increased right leg swelling. Ultrasound of the leg shows thrombosis of the superficial femoral vein. Which of the following is not a mechanism of hypercoagulability in this disorder?

A. Increased platelet aggregation
B. Low serum levels of protein C and protein S
C. Chronic disseminated intravascular coagulation
D. Hyperfibrinogenemia
E. Low serum levels of antithrombin III

VII-41. It is hospital day 5 for a 65-year-old patient with prerenal azotemia secondary to dehydration. His creatinine was initially 3.6 mg/dL on admission, but it has improved today to 2.1 mg/dL. He complains of mild lower back pain, and you prescribe naproxen to be taken intermittently. By what mechanism might this drug further impair his renal function?

A. Afferent arteriolar vasoconstriction
B. Afferent arteriolar vasodilatation
C. Efferent arteriolar vasoconstriction
D. Proximal tubular toxicity
E. Ureteral obstruction

VII-42. A 63-year-old male with a history of diabetes mellitus is found to have a lung nodule on chest radiography. To stage the disease further he undergoes a contrast-enhanced CT scan of the chest. One week before the CT scan, his BUN is 26 mg/dL and his creatinine is 1.8 mg/dL. Three days after the study he complains of dyspnea, pedal edema, and decreased urinary output. Repeat BUN is 86 mg/dL and creatinine is 4.4 mg/dL. The most likely mechanism of the acute renal failure is

A. acute tubular necrosis
B. allergic hypersensitivity
C. cholesterol emboli
D. immune-complex glomerulonephritis
E. ureteral outflow obstruction

VII-43. In the patient in Question VII-42 the urinalysis is most likely to show

A. granular casts
B. red blood cell casts
C. urinary eosinophils

VII-43. *(Continued)*

D. urinary neutrophils
E. white blood cell casts

VII-44. A 35-year-old female presents with complaints of bilateral lower extremity edema, polyuria, and moderate left-sided flank pain that began approximately 2 weeks ago. There is no past medical history. She is taking no medications and denies tobacco, alcohol, or illicit drug use. Examination shows normal vital signs, including normal blood pressure. There is 2+ edema in bilateral lower extremities. The 24-h urine collection is significant for 3.5 g of protein. Urinalysis is bland except for the proteinuria. Serum creatinine is 0.7 mg/dL, and ultrasound examination shows the left kidney measuring 13 cm and the right kidney measuring 11.5 cm. You are concerned about renal vein thrombosis. What test do you choose for the evaluation?

A. Computed tomography of the renal veins
B. Contrast venography
C. Magnetic resonance venography
D. ^{99}Tc-labeled pentetic acid (DPTA) imaging
E. Ultrasound with Doppler evaluation of the renal veins

VII-45. The posterior pituitary secretes arginine vasopressin (antidiuretic hormone) under which of the following stressors?

A. Hyperosmolarity
B. Hypernatremia
C. Volume depletion
D. A and B
E. A and C

VII-46. A 29-year-old man is admitted to the hospital with a severe asthma exacerbation. He is taken to the intensive care unit (ICU) and treated with continuous aerosolized β-adrenergic agonists and glucocorticoids. He requires bilevel positive airway pressure mechanical respiration. After 18 h of this therapy, his respiratory status begins to improve. He begins to complain of fatigue and myalgias in his legs. He has difficulty ambulating and on neurologic examination he has three out of five symmetric weakness in the lower extremities. On the cardiac monitor, you notice flattened T waves, ST depression, and a prolonged QT interval. What is the cause of this patient's neurologic and cardiac findings?

A. Adrenal insufficiency
B. ICU psychosis
C. Medication effect
D. Myocardial infarction with congestive heart failure
E. Todd's paralysis

VII-47. A 33-year-old male is brought for medical attention after completing an ultramarathon. Upon finishing he was disoriented and light-headed. His normal weight

VII-47. *(Continued)*

is 60 kg. Physical examination reveals a body temperature of 38.3°C (100.9°F), blood pressure of 85/60 mmHg, and heart rate of 125/min. The patient's neck veins are flat, and skin turgor is poor. Laboratory studies are notable for a serum sodium of 175 meq/L. The patient's estimated free water deficit is

A. 0.75 L
B. 1.5 L
C. 7.5 L
D. 15 L
E. 22.5 L

VII-48. A 66-year-old woman is being treated with penicillin for mitral valve endocarditis due to *Streptococcus viridans*. She initially improved with resolution of her fever after 7 days, but now comes to the emergency room complaining of fever and rash during week 4 of her treatment. She continues to receive penicillin IV via a central line equipped with an infusion system. She has had no drainage from the site of her central line and has otherwise been feeling well until she developed a diffuse pruritic rash over her entire body, beginning on her trunk. She also has had a fever to as high as 38.3°C at home. On examination, she has an erythematous maculopapular rash over her trunk and legs. In many areas, it has coalesced to form raised plaques. She currently has a temperature of 39°C. Her laboratory values shows a white blood cell count of 12,330/μL with 72% polymorphonuclear cells, 12% lymphocytes, 5% monocytes, and 11% eosinophils. Her BUN is 65 mg/dL, and creatinine is 2.5 mg/dL. At the time of her hospital discharge, the patient's BUN was 24

VII-48. *(Continued)*

mg/dL and creatinine was 1.2 mg/dL. Which test is most likely to yield the diagnosis of her acute renal failure?

A. 24-h urine protein level
B. Antistreptolysin O titers
C. Blood culture for aerobic and anaerobic bacteria
D. Echocardiogram
E. Hansel's stain for eosinophils in the urine

VII-49. All the following are complications during hemodialysis *except*

A. anaphylactoid reaction
B. fever
C. hyperglycemia
D. hypotension
E. muscle cramps

VII-50. A 42-year-old man with a history of pulmonary sarcoidosis is admitted to the intensive care unit with confusion and nausea. His family reports that he has had polyuria and polydipsia for some time but it has increased dramatically in the past week. On physical examination, his mucous membranes are dry and he is orthostatic by pulse. In the Emergency room, his blood glucose is 90 mg/dL. An electrocardiogram (ECG) taken at that time is shown below.

What is the cause of this patient's symptoms?

A. Hypercalcemia
B. Hyperkalemia
C. Hypocalcemia
D. Hypokalemia

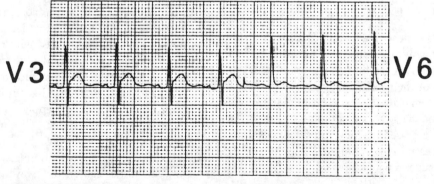

FIGURE VII-50

VII-51. The patient in the preceding scenario is found to have a serum calcium of 12.1 mg/dL. Of the following interventions, what therapy is most appropriate in this patient?

A. Glucocorticoids
B. Intravenous loop diuretic
C. Intravenous phosphate
D. Oral calcitriol
E. Zoledronic acid

VII-52. You are consulting to advise on another antihypertensive agent for a patient with difficult-to-control hypertension. Despite high doses of a beta blocker, the patient remains hypertensive. The estimated glomerular filtration rate (GFR) is 75 mL/min per 1.73 m². On physical examination, there is no exophthalmos and no thyroid bruit. The great vessels are without bruit as well. Abdominal examination reveals bruits loudest in bilateral flanks

VII-52. *(Continued)*

as well as a left femoral bruit. Peripheral pulses are intact. An ultrasound confirms the presence of bilateral renal artery stenosis. Which medication class would *not* be a good choice to add to this patient's regimen?

A. Thiazide diuretic
B. Calcium-channel blocker
C. Angiotensin II receptor blocker
D. Central acting alpha blocker

VII-53. Which of the following patients in need of dialysis would receive the greatest benefit from placing a peritoneal dialysis catheter rather than a hemodialysis catheter?

A. High-peritoneal transporters
B. Patients in developing countries
C. Patients older than 65
D. Patients with no residual kidney function
E. Patients with prior abdominal surgery

VII-54. A patient with a history of Sjögren's syndrome has the following laboratory findings: plasma sodium 139 meq/L, chloride 112 meq/L, bicarbonate 15 meq/L, and potassium 3.0 meq/L; urine studies show a pH of 6.0, sodium of 15 meq/L, potassium of 10 meq/L, and chloride of 12 meq/L. The most likely diagnosis is

A. type I renal tubular acidosis (RTA)
B. type II RTA
C. type III RTA
D. type IV RTA
E. chronic diarrhea

VII-55. The condition of a 50-year-old obese female with a 5-year history of mild hypertension controlled by a thiazide diuretic is being evaluated because proteinuria was noted during her routine yearly medical visit. Physical examination disclosed a height of 167.6 cm (66 in.), weight of 91 kg (202 lb), blood pressure of 130/80 mmHg, and trace pedal edema. Laboratory values are as follows:

Serum creatinine: 106 μmol/L (1.2 mg/dL)
BUN: 6.4 mmol/L (18 mg/dL)
Creatinine clearance: 87 mL/min
Urinalysis: pH 5.0; specific gravity 1.018; protein 3+; no glucose; occasional coarse granular cast
Urine protein excretion: 5.9 g/d

A renal biopsy demonstrates that 60% of the glomeruli have segmental scarring by light microscopy, with the remainder of the glomeruli appearing unremarkable (see following figure).

VII-55. *(Continued)*

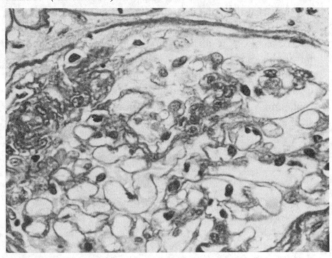

FIGURE VII-55

The most likely diagnosis is

A. hypertensive nephrosclerosis
B. focal and segmental sclerosis
C. minimal-change (nil) disease
D. membranous glomerulopathy
E. crescentic glomerulonephritis

VII-56. A 20-year-old college student seeks medical attention for light-headedness. He just completed a rigorous tennis match and did not drink any water or fluids. Supine blood pressure is 110/70 mmHg, and heart rate is 105/min. Upright, the blood pressure is 95/60 mmHg with a heart rate of 125/min. Temperature and mental status are normal. Which of the following laboratory results is most likely in this patient?

A. Serum BUN/creatinine ratio <20
B. Serum sodium <140 meq/L
C. Urine potassium <20 meq/L
D. Urine sodium <20 meq/L
E. Urine red blood cell casts

VII-57. A 50-year-old male is admitted to the hospital with pneumonia. He does well after the administration of antibiotics, but his sodium is noted to rise from 140 to 154 meq/L over 2 days. He reports thirst and has had a urine output of approximately 5 L per day. Which of the following is the most appropriate next step to evaluate the patient's disorder?

A. Measurement of serum osmolality
B. Measurement of serum vasopressin level
C. 24-h measurement of urinary sodium
D. Trial of arginine vasopressin
E. Trial of free water restriction

VII-58. A 16-year-old female star gymnast presents to your office complaining of fatigue, diffuse weakness, and muscle cramps. She has no previous medical history and denies tobacco, alcohol, or illicit drug use. There is no significant family history. Examination shows a thin female with normal blood pressure. Body mass index (BMI) is 18 kg/m². Oral examination shows poor dentition. Muscle tone is normal, and neurologic examination is normal. Laboratory studies show hematocrit of 38.5%, creatinine of 0.6 mg/dL,

VII-58. *(Continued)*
serum bicarbonate of 30 meq/L, and potassium of 2.7 meq/L. Further evaluation should include which of the following?

A. Urinalysis and urine culture
B. Plasma renin and aldosterone levels
C. Urine toxicology screen for opiates
D. Urine toxicology screen for diuretics
E. Serum magnesium level

VII. DISORDERS OF THE URINARY AND KIDNEY TRACT

ANSWERS

VII-1. **The answer is E.** *(Chap. 278)* Intracranial aneurysms are present in 5 to 10% of asymptomatic patients with ADPKD. Screening of all ADPKD patients is not recommended. Any presenting symptoms or a family history of subarachnoid hemorrhage or sudden death should prompt further screening with magnetic resonance angiography (MRA) or CT angiography or consideration of cerebral angiography.

VII-2. **The answer is A.** *(Chap. 46)* Excretion of water is tightly regulated at the collecting duct by arginine vasopressin (AVP, formerly antidiuretic hormone). An increase in plasma tonicity is sensed by hypothalamic osmoreceptors, causing AVP secretion from the posterior pituitary. AVP binding to the collecting duct leads to insertion of water channels (aquaporin-2) into the luminal membrane, promoting water reabsorption. Serum sodium is the principal extracellular solute, and so effective osmolality is determined predominantly by the plasma sodium concentration. Plasma osmolality normally is regulated within 1 to 2% of normal (280 to 290 mosmol/kg). The sensitivity of the baroreceptors for AVP release is far less than that of the osmoreceptors. Depletion of intravascular volume sufficient to decrease mean arterial pressure is necessary to stimulate AVP secretion.

VII-3. **The answer is D.** *(Chaps. 45 and 273)* In the evaluation of azotemia, the initial diagnostic modalities are a urine analysis and renal ultrasound. Renal ultrasound is important so that obstructive causes can be corrected urgently with urologic evaluation. This patient may have an obstructive nephropathy due to nephrolithiasis, as certain HIV medications can cause nephrolithiasis. Patients with nephrolithiasis can often have pyuria and hematuria. Urine electrolytes are useful to establish prerenal azotemia but should be performed only after urine analysis is unremarkable and renal ultrasound shows normal-sized kidneys. Anti-GBM antibodies are an important component of the evaluation of glomerulonephritis. Angiogram is useful when renal vascular disease is suspected.

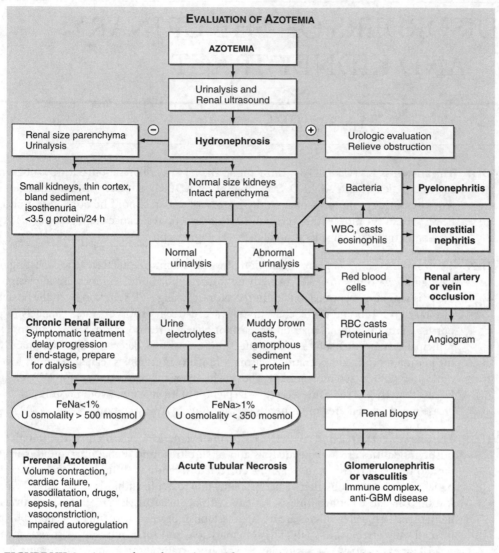

FIGURE VII-3   Approach to the patient with azotemia. WBC, white blood cell; RBC, red blood cell; GBM, glomerular basement membrane.

VII-4.   **The answer is B.** *(Chaps. 45 and 273)*   Acute renal failure with urine sediment showing muddy brown (granular) casts or an amorphous sediment in the absence of white blood cells, red blood cells, eosinophils or severe proteinuria has a high likelihood of being acute tubular necrosis. This is particularly true when an episode of renal hypoperfusion (hypotension) is present. It is possible to differentiate between prerenal azotemia and acute tubular necrosis by calculating the fractional excretion of sodium (FeNa) and by measuring the BUN/creatinine ratio, urine sodium, urine osmolality, and the urine/plasma creatinine ratio (see Figure VII-3, above). In this case, the BUN/creatinine ratio is <20, the urine sodium is >40 meq/L, urine osmolality <350 mosmol, FeNa 4%, and urine/plasma creatinine <20, indicating that this is acute renal failure with tubular injury. Pyuria is present in 75% of cases of acute interstitial nephritis (AIN) and there is no proximate drug exposure to suggest AIN. Hepatorenal syndrome is excluded by the elevated urine sodium. Glomerulonephritis is unlikely given the absence of red cell casts on urine analysis and the clinical situation.

VII-5.   **The answer is C.** *(Chap. 283)*   In acute urinary tract obstruction, pain is due to distention of the collecting system or renal capsule. Acutely, there is a compensatory increase in renal blood flow when kidney function is impaired by obstruction, which further exacerbates capsular stretch. Eventually, vasodilatory prostaglandins act to preserve renal function when glomerular filtration rate has decreased. Medullary blood flow decreases as the pressure of the obstruction further inhibits the renal parenchyma from perfusing; however, the ensuing chronic renal destruction may occur without substantial pain. When an obstruction has been relieved, there is a postobstructive diuresis that is mediated by relief of tubular pressure, increased solute load (per nephron), and natriuretic factors. There can be an extreme amount of diuresis, but this is not painful.

VII-6. **The answer is E.** *(Chap. 273)* Radiocontrast agents cause renal injury through intrarenal vasoconstriction and through generation of oxygen radicals causing acute tubular necrosis. These medications cause an acute decrease in renal blood flow and glomerular filtration rate. Patients with chronic kidney disease, diabetes mellitus, heart failure, multiple myeloma, and volume depletion are at highest risk of contrast nephropathy. It is clear that hydration with normal saline is an effective measure to prevent contrast nephropathy. Of the other measures mentioned here, only sodium bicarbonate or N-acteylcysteine could be recommended for clinical use to reduce the risk of contrast nephropathy. Dopamine has been proven an ineffective agent to prevent contrast nephropathy. Fenoldopam, a D_1-receptor agonist, has been tested in several clinical trials and does not appear to reduce the incidence of contrast nephropathy. Although several small clinical studies have suggested a clinical benefit to the use of N-acetylcysteine, a meta-analysis has been inconclusive, and the medication should be administered well in advance of the procedure. Sodium bicarbonate begun within 1 h of the procedure has shown a significant benefit in a single-center, randomized controlled trial. Due to the time limitations, and based on the evidence, only sodium bicarbonate would be helpful in this patient.

VII-7. **The answer is A.** *(Chap. 277)* In different disease processes the complement pathway is activated either by classical pathway activation or by alternative pathway activation. If the classical pathway is activated, as in lupus nephritis, the serum complement measures of C3, C4, and CH50 are low. If the alternative pathway is activated, C3 and CH50 may be low but C4 is at normal levels. When acute GN is suspected, measurement of serum complement levels will often limit the differential diagnosis. Other conditions with normal C4 include ANCA-associated diseases. Low C4 may be seen with membranoproliferative GN types I and III. Type I disease also may be associated with cryoglobulinemia.

VII-8. **The answer is B.** *(Chap. 48)* The pH is <7.35, therefore the primary process is an acidosis. The HCO_3^- is low and the P_{CO_2} is low, excluding a primary respiratory acidosis. The anion gap is normal at 12. The expected P_{CO_2} is between 24 and 16 mmHg for appropriate respiratory compensation. The P_{CO_2} in this example represents normal respiratory compensation for a metabolic acidosis.

VII-9. **The answer is A.** *(Chap. 48)* Metabolic acidosis occurs because of endogenous acid production or loss of bicarbonate. The anion gap is elevated in the presence of unmeasured anions (or, less commonly, a loss of unmeasured cations) and is normal with bicarbonate loss. A fall in the serum albumin of 1 g/dL from normal lowers the expected anion gap by 2.5 meq/L. The differential diagnosis for a non-anion gap metabolic acidosis includes gastrointestinal losses, renal acidosis, and drug-induced and other less common causes. Nursing home residents are at risk for institutionally acquired diarrheas, often infectious. The urine pH is usually high in proximal renal tubular acidosis, and the patients usually younger. Defects in the renin-angiotensin system, such as hypoaldosteronism, cause hyperkalemia, not hypokalemia. This patient has no evidence of renal failure. Diuretic use will usually cause a metabolic alkalosis.

VII-10. **The answer is A.** *(Chap. 283)* The prognosis for the return of normal renal function is excellent in patients with acute bilateral renal obstruction, such as an obstruction that is due to prostate enlargement. With relief of the obstruction, the prognosis depends on whether irreversible renal damage has occurred. Return of GFR usually follows relief of obstruction lasting 1 to 2 weeks provided that there has been no intercurrent infection. After 8 weeks of obstruction recovery is unlikely. Acute relief of bilateral obstruction commonly results in polyuria. An osmotic diuresis caused by excretion of retained urea and resolution of volume expansion contributes to the diuresis. The urine is hypotonic. The diuresis usually abates with resolution of normal extracellular volume, and so aggressive volume resuscitation is generally not necessary unless hypotension or overt volume depletion develops. Indications for acute hemodialysis are those for the usual complications of acute renal failure, including electrolyte disturbances, uremia, and inability to control volume.

VII-11. The answer is A. *(Chap. 273)* Atheroembolic disease can cause acute renal failure (ARF) after manipulation of the aorta or renal arteries during angiography. Cholesterol crystals embolize to the renal vasculature and lodge in small- to medium-sized vessels inciting a fibrotic reaction in the vessel wall, narrowing the lumen. Diagnostic clues to atheroembolic ARF are recent manipulation of the aorta or renal vessels, eosinophiluria, and low complement levels. The ARF usually occurs days to weeks after the inciting event. Aminoglycosides, diuretics, or nonsteroidal anti-inflammatory drugs can cause renal failure but it does not classically present with eosinophiluria or hypocomplementemia. Atheroembolic ARF is usually irreversible.

VII-12. The answer is B. *(Chap. 46)* The differential diagnosis for hypernatremia is fairly narrow as it results in a relative loss of water. Water is lost via renal or nonrenal mechanisms. The urine osmolality is a key historic piece of data. If the patient is excreting the minimum amount of maximally concentrated urine, gastrointestinal (osmotic diarrhea), insensible (skin or respiratory loss), or remote renal losses (diabetes mellitus) are the cause. This patient is excreting a large amount of dilute urine. He is not excreting >750 mosms in his urine daily, which would suggest diuretic use. Either central or nephrogenic diabetes insipidus (DI) must be the cause. In this patient, the lack of response to desmopressin indicates nephrogenic DI.

VII-13. The answer is E. *(Chap. 46)* The patient in the preceding scenario has nephrogenic diabetes insipidus (NDI). Causes of NDI include drugs (particularly lithium carbonate), hypercalcemia, hypokalemia, papillary necrosis, or congenital disorders. Symptomatic polyuria due to NDI can be treated with a low-sodium diet and thiazide diuretics, which induce mild volume depletion and enhanced proximal reabsorption of salt and water. Narcotics may be useful in patients with gastrointestinal hypermotility and water loss as a result thereof. AVP analogues are used to treat central diabetes insipidus and would have no impact on NDI. If a patient is found to have central diabetes insipidus, brain imaging should be obtained to rule out destruction of the neurohypophysis. Lithium carbonate is a cause of NDI and should be discontinued if causing symptomatic NDI.

VII-14. The answer is B. *(Chap. 48; N Engl J Med 338:26–34, 1998.)* A respiratory alkalosis with a combined metabolic acidosis is typical of salicylate toxicity. Salicylate intoxication can result in respiratory alkalosis, mixed respiratory alkalosis and metabolic acidosis, or, less commonly, a simple metabolic acidosis. Respiratory alkalosis is caused by direct stimulation of the respiratory center by salicylate. The accumulation of lactic acid and ketoacids leads to the concomitant metabolic acidosis. The severity of the neurologic manifestations largely depends on the concentration of salicylate in the central nervous system. Therapy is directed at limiting further drug absorption by administering activated charcoal and promoting the exit of salicylate from the CNS. This can be accomplished by alkalinizing the serum, typically by means of the addition of intravenous fluids with sodium bicarbonate, with the goal of raising the serum pH to between 7.45 and 7.50. Increasing the GFR will also enhance salicylate excretion. Hemodialysis is reserved for severe cases, especially those involving fulminant renal failure.

VII-15. The answer is D. *(Chap. 283)* The level of obstruction is important when considering urinary tract obstruction. Bilateral hydronephrosis and hydroureter suggest either a systemic process or mechanical obstruction at or below the level of the uretero-vesical junctions. While retroperitoneal fibrosis can cause such a picture, it is most common among middle-aged men. In patients of reproductive age, genital tract infections can cause meatal stenosis if left untreated or if infections are recurrent. Retroperitoneal lymphomas can cause bilateral hydroureter, as can more distal obstructions like phimosis. In the developing world, one may also consider schistosomiasis and genitourinary tuberculosis.

VII-16.   The answer is B. *(Chap. 275; Rubin et al: JAMA 291:697–703, 2004.)* Peritonitis is the most common serious complication of peritoneal dialysis. These patients typically present with abdominal pain, fever, and a cloudy peritoneal dialysate. Persistent or recurrent peritonitis may require the removal of the catheter. Further complications include losses of amino acids as well as albumin, which may be as much as 5 to 15 g/d. In addition, patients can absorb glucose through the peritoneal dialysate, resulting in hyperglycemia, not hypoglycemia. The resulting hyperglycemia can cause a hypertriglyceridemia, especially in patients with diabetes mellitus. Leakage of the dialysate fluid into the pleural space can also occur, more frequently on the right than on the left. It can be diagnosed by analysis of the pleural fluid, which typically has an elevated glucose concentration. Rapid fluid shifts are uncommon with peritoneal dialysis, and this approach may be favored for patients with congestive heart failure or unstable angina. A recent report suggested improved patient satisfaction with peritoneal dialysis compared with hemodialysis.

VII-17.   The answer is A. *(Chap. 45)* The serum creatinine is widely used as a reflection of renal function because metabolism of creatinine from muscle varies little in the steady state and it is a freely filtered small solute. Therefore, creatinine clearance is used as a reflection of glomerular filtration rate. However, many factors such as loss of muscle from aging, chronic disease, or malnutrition can mask significant changes in creatinine clearance with small changes in serum creatinine. Two formulas, the Cockcroft-Gault formula and the MDRD (modification of diet in renal disease), are often used to calculate creatinine clearance. The Cockcroft-Gault formula requires age, lean body weight, plasma creatinine, and sex to calculate the creatinine clearance. The more cumbersome and more accurate MDRD uses plasma creatinine, sex, race, and age. Urine creatinine is not a variable in either the Cockcroft-Gault or the MDRD formulas. Race is a variable only in the MDRD equation.

VII-18.   The answer is B. *(Chap. 45)*

$$\text{Creatinine clearance} = [(140 - \text{age}) \times \text{lean weight (kg)}]/\text{creatinine (mg/dL)} \times 72$$

Using the Cockcroft-Gault formula, this patient's creatinine clearance is 47 mL/min. This patient would have moderate (stage 3) renal insufficiency. This information may be important for drug dosing.

VII-19.   The answer is D. *(Chap. 283)* Erythrocytosis can develop in an obstructive uropathy as a result of increased erythropoietin production. Anemia in kidney disease occurs as a result of progressive renal parenchymal destruction. As the kidney attempts to preserve renal function and expand blood volume, renin levels increase and can cause a secondary hypertension. Dysuria can be seen in cases of chronic urinary tract obstruction due to urinary stasis and the propensity to develop urolithiasis. Pain with micturition is a hallmark of vesicoureteral reflux, which causes a chronic functional obstructive uropathy. Pyuria is common, as is urinary tract infection. Stasis promotes the growth of bacteria and urinary tract infection.

VII-20.   The answer is D. *(Chap. 273)* Cholesterol embolization (also known as atheroembolic renal disease) is characterized by pyuria, progressive renal failure (usually nonoliguric), and associated organ dysfunction (including bowel, pancreas, and CNS). Hypocomplementemia and eosinophiluria also may be seen. The urinalysis is not compatible with acute tubular necrosis because of the absence of granular casts.

VII-21.   The answer is B. *(Chaps. 45 and 48)* The octahedral, or envelope-shaped, crystals are due to the presence of calcium oxalate in the urine. Calcium oxalate crystals are classically seen in ethylene glycol ingestion, which also causes a high anion gap metabolic acidosis. White blood cell casts indicate an upper urinary tract infection associated with a positive urine culture. Uric acid (rhomboid shapes) or struvite ("coffin lids") crystals may be seen in cases of nephrolithiasis that causes hydronephrosis. Red blood cell casts are indicative of glomerular disease, often associated with a positive ANA.

VII-22. **The answer is B.** *(Chap. 48)* The pH is high and the plasma bicarbonate is high. This is indicative of a metabolic alkalosis, not a primary acidosis. A respiratory alkalosis is not consistent with an elevated P_{CO_2}. Similarly, the P_{CO_2} is elevated appropriately to compensate for the metabolic alkalosis, excluding a primary respiratory acidosis. The respiratory compensation for a metabolic alkalosis is limited by the hypoxic drive. When the P_{CO_2} rises into the 40s and 50s, the hypoxic drive maintains a Pa_{O_2} of >55–60 mmHg, preventing further hypoventilation to additionally increase P_{CO_2}.

VII-23. **The answer is E.** *(Chap. 48)* The differential diagnosis for a metabolic alkalosis can be divided into those disorders with extracellular fluid contraction and normotension (or hypotension) and those with extracellular fluid expansion and hypertension (see Table VII-23). Cushing's disease and mineralocorticoid excess cause a metabolic alkalosis with hypertension. Patients with Bartter syndrome are normotensive. This patient has evidence of hypovolemia with altered mental status, hypotension, and tachycardia. Myocardial infarction causing cardiogenic shock would result in an anion gap metabolic acidosis due to lactate accumulation.

TABLE VII-23   Causes of Metabolic Acidois

I. Exogenous HCO_3^- loads
   A. Acute alkali administration
   B. Milk-alkali syndrome
II. Effective ECFV contraction, normotension, K^+ deficiency, and secondary hyperreninemic hyperaldosteronism
   A. Gastrointestinal origin
      1. Vomiting
      2. Gastric aspiration
      3. Congenital chloridorrhea
      4. Villous adenoma
   B. Renal origin
      1. Diuretics
      2. Posthypercapnic state
      3. Hypercalcemia/hypoparathyroidism
      4. Recovery from lactic acidosis or ketoacidosis
      5. Nonreabsorbable anions including penicillin, carbenicillin
      6. Mg^{2+} deficiency
      7. K^+ depletion
      8. Bartter's syndrome (loss of function mutations in TALH)
      9. Gitelman's syndrome (loss of function mutation in Na^+-Cl^- cotransporter in DCT)
III. ECFV expansion, hypertension, K^+ deficiency, and mineralocorticoid excess
   A. High renin
      1. Renal artery stenosis
      2. Accelerated hypertension
      3. Renin-secreting tumor
      4. Estrogen therapy
   B. Low renin
      1. Primary aldosteronism
         a. Adenoma
         b. Hyperplasia
         c. Carcinoma
      2. Adrenal enzyme defects
         a. 11 β-Hydroxylase deficiency
         b. 17 α-Hydroxylase deficiency
      3. Cushing's syndrome or disease
      4. Other
         a. Licorice
         b. Carbenoxolone
         c. Chewer's tobacco
IV. Gain-of-function mutation of renal sodium channel with ECFV expansion, hypertension, K^+ deficiency, and hyporeninemic-hypoaldosteronism
   A. Liddle's syndrome

Note: ECFV, extracellular fluid volume; TALH, thick ascending limb of Henle's loop; DCT, distal convoluted tubule.

VII-24. **The answer is D.** *(Chap. 46)* This patient is most likely hypovolemic from the osmotic preparation for his colonoscopy. Physical examination supports hypovolemic hyponatremia. Hyperglycemia and hyperlipidemia can cause hyponatremia, but these conditions would be associated with a high and normal plasma osmolality, respectively. SIADH is unlikely to be causing the hyponatremia if the extracellular volume status is decreased. Diabetes insipidus is a hypernatremic disorder caused by excess water loss.

VII-25. **The answer is B.** *(Chap. 275)* Commonly accepted criteria for initiating patients on maintenance dialysis include uremic symptoms, hyperkalemia unresponsive to conservative measures, persistent extracellular fluid expansion despite diuretic therapy, acidosis refractory to medical therapy, a bleeding diathesis, and a creatinine clearance <10 mL/min per 1.73 m². This patient has none of those indications. Without symptoms of uremia, an elevated BUN is not sufficient to initiate maintenance dialysis. A urine analysis is unlikely to be helpful in deciding when to initiate dialysis for this patient. Renal biopsy does not usually have a role in stage 5 disease.

VII-26. **The answer is C.** *(Chap. 47)* Determining the PTH level is central to the evaluation of hypocalcemia (see Table VII-26). A suppressed or "inappropriately low" PTH level in the setting of hypocalcemia establishes absent or reduced PTH secretion as the cause. Hypomagnesemia may suppress PTH secretion and contribute to hypocalcemia. In contrast, an elevated PTH should direct attention to the vitamin D axis as the cause of hypocalcemia. Thyroid-stimulating hormone levels will not elucidate the proximate cause of hypocalcemia in the absence of PTH levels. In patients with suspected nutritional deficiency, the 25(OH)D should be checked. In patients with renal insufficiency or suspected vitamin D resistance, serum 1,25(OH)₂D levels are informative. An ionized calcium is a better marker of the true serum calcium levels but will not assist with diagnosis. Hypomagnesemia should be repleted along with hypocalcemia when both are present.

TABLE VII-26   Causes of Hypocalcemia

Low Parathyroid Hormone Levels (Hypoparathyroidism)
Parathyroid agenesis
Isolated
DiGeorge syndrome
Parathyroid destruction
Surgical
Radiation
Infiltration by metastases or systemic diseases
Autoimmune
Reduced parathyroid function
Hypomagnesemia
Activating CaSR mutations

High Parathyroid Hormone Levels (Secondary Hyperparathyroidism)
Vitamin D deficiency or impaired 1,25(OH)₂D production/action
Nutritional vitamin D deficiency (poor intake or absorption)
Renal insufficiency with impaired 1,25(OH)₂D production
Vitamin D resistance, including receptor defects
Parathyroid hormone resistance syndromes
PTH receptor mutations
Pseudohypoparathyroidism (G protein mutations)
Drugs
Calcium chelators
Inhibitors of bone resorption (bisphosphonates, plicamycin)
Altered vitamin D metabolism (phenytoin, ketoconazole)
Miscellaneous causes
Acute pancreatitis
Acute rhabdomyolysis
Hungry bone syndrome after parathyroidectomy
Osteoblastic metastases with marked stimulation of bone formation (prostate cancer)

Note: CaSR, calcium sensor receptor; PTH, parathyroid hormone.

VII-27. **The answer is A.** *(Chap. 45)* A key point in the diagnostic evaluation of hematuria is the presence of dysmorphic RBCs or RBC casts in the urine. This finding is strongly suspicious for glomerulonephritis. This diagnosis requires prompt evaluation and therapy to avoid irreversible renal failure. Concerning aspects of this patient's presentation for glomerulonephritis are the presence of RBC casts and >500 mg/24 h of protein in the urine. In the evaluation of proteinuria with hematuria, these features should prompt a serologic and hematologic evaluation and strong consideration of renal biopsy. A CT scan is unlikely to reveal the cause of this patient's hematuria because he has a glomerular problem. An ACE inhibitor may treat his proteinuria but will not address the underlying cause. Since it is already apparent that this patient has proteinuria, ultrasensitive testing for microalbumin is not necessary. Cystoscopy is performed when the source of bleeding is thought to be from the bladder, after renal sources have been eliminated as causes.

VII-28. **The answer is C.** *(Chaps. 46 and 278)* The evaluation of patients with hypokalemia should first include a consideration of redistribution of body potassium into cells such as that which occurs in alkalosis, β_2-agonist excess with refeeding syndrome and/or insulin therapy, vitamin B_{12} therapy, pernicious anemia, and periodic paralysis. In periodic paralysis serum bicarbonate is normal. If the patient is hypertensive and plasma renin is elevated, renovascular hypertension or a renin-secreting tumor (including Wilms) must be considered and appropriate imaging studies must be carried out. If plasma renin levels are low, mineralocorticoid effect may be high as a result of either endogenous hormone (glucocorticoid overproduction or aldosterone overproduction as in Conn's syndrome) or exogenous agents (licorice or steroids). In a normotensive patient a high serum bicarbonate excludes renal tubular acidosis. High urine chloride excretion makes gastrointestinal losses less likely and implies primary renal potassium loss, as may be seen in diuretic abuse (ruled out by the urine screen) or Bartter's syndrome. In Bartter's syndrome, hyperplasia of the granular cells of the juxtaglomerular apparatus leads to high renin levels and secondary aldosterone elevations. Such hyperplasia appears to be secondary to chronic volume depletion caused by a hereditary (autosomal recessive) defect that interferes with salt reabsorption in the thick ascending loop of Henle. Chronic potassium depletion, which frequently presents initially in childhood, leads to polyuria and weakness.

VII-29. **The answer is E.** *(Chap. 49)* The presence of unchanged nocturnal tumescence suggests psychogenic factors as the cause of the patient's erectile dysfunction (ED). Nocturnal tumescence occurs during REM sleep, and intact neurologic and circulatory systems are necessary for this to occur. Erectile dysfunction is reported in 52% of men between ages 40 and 70. The incidence of ED is higher in men with diabetes mellitus, heart disease, and hypertension and in tobacco users. Additionally, medications are frequently involved, especially many antihypertensive agents, including beta blockers, thiazide diuretics, calcium channel blockers, and angiotensin converting-enzyme (ACE) inhibitors. A thorough history and physical examination with limited laboratory testing usually yields the appropriate diagnosis.

VII-30. **The answer is C.** *(Chap. 278)* Polycystic kidney diseases are the most common life-threatening inherited diseases. Adult-onset disease is typically inherited in autosomal dominant fashion. It is a systemic disease caused by mutations in either the *PKD-1* or *PKD-2* gene. Phenotypic presentation is varied. Most patients are not symptomatic until middle age. Typical presentations include abdominal discomfort, hematuria, urinary tract infections, or hypertension. Most patients experience a steady decline in renal function over one to two decades following diagnosis. About 60% of patients will develop end-stage renal disease by age 70. Hypertension precedes renal failure. Risk factors for disease progression include male gender, African-American race, hypertension, and the presence of the polycystin-1 mutation. Patients are at an increased risk of subarachnoid and cerebral hemorrhage due to aneurysm formation. Cardiac abnormalities are present in 25% of patients, and most commonly include mitral valve prolapse and aortic regurgitation. Hepatic cysts are common and are found in 40% of patients by the age of 60. Renal ultrasound is the diagnostic test of choice and is 100% sensitive in patients older than

30 who have a positive family history. Treatment of PCKD is supportive; control of hypertension and close evaluation of kidney function are paramount.

VII-31.   The answer is A. *(Chap. 283; Ifudu: N Engl J Med 339:1054–1062, 1998.)* Renal osteodystrophy is a common complication of chronic renal disease and the most common complication secondary to impaired renal production of $1,25(OH)_2D_3$. This leads to a decreased calcium absorption in the gut as well as impaired renal phosphate excretion. The resulting hyperphosphatemia causes a secondary hyperparathyroidism. The hyperparathyroidism is subsequently worsened by hypocalcemia, which is present because of the hyperphosphatemia and the decreased enzymatic conversion of 25-hydroxyvitamin D to $1,25(OH)_2D_3$. Finally, $1,25(OH)_2D_3$ deficiency worsens hyperparathyroidism as the former is a direct inhibitor of parathyroid hormone secretion into the bone. The resultant decreased serum calcium concentration leads to secondary hyperparathyroidism. In addition, other causes of renal osteodystrophy include chronic metabolic acidosis resulting from dissolution of bone buffers and decalcification and the long-term administration of aluminum-containing antacids. No significant loss of vitamin D or calcium is associated with currently employed dialysis techniques, and the treatment of renal osteodystrophy often includes calcitriol.

VII-32.   The answer is C. *(Chap. 46)* Diuretic-induced hyponatremia almost always is due to thiazide diuretics. It occurs mostly in the elderly. The reduction in serum sodium may be severe and cause symptoms. Loop diuretics such as furosemide cause hyponatremia far less often than do thiazide diuretics. Thiazide diuretics inhibit sodium and potassium reabsorption in the distal tubule, leading to Na^+ and K^+ depletion and AVP-mediated water retention. In contrast, loop diuretics impair maximal urinary concentrating capacity, limiting AVP-mediated water retention. Many drugs may cause hyponatremia by promoting AVP secretion or action at the collecting duct; however, metoprolol and enalapril are not significant causes of SIADH. Spironolactone is a competitive antagonist of aldosterone at the mineralocorticoid receptor. It has weak natriuretic activity and is most likely to cause hyperkalemia.

VII-33.   The answer is A. *(Chaps. 46 and 334)* Failure to concentrate urine despite substantial hypertonic dehydration suggests a diagnosis of diabetes insipidus. A nephrogenic origin will be postulated if there is no increase in urine concentration after exogenous vasopressin. The only useful mode of therapy is a low-salt diet and the use of a thiazide or amiloride, a potassium-sparing distal diuretic agent. The resultant volume contraction presumably enhances proximal reabsorption and thereby reduces urine flow.

VII-34.   The answer is A. *(Chap. 279)* Individuals with acute leukemia and other myeloproliferative disorders are at risk for the development of tumor lysis syndrome following institution of chemotherapy. Tumor lysis syndrome results from rapid cell death with resultant increases in serum potassium, phosphate, and uric acid levels. Renal failure develops due to acute uric acid nephropathy, and pathology demonstrates deposition of uric acid crystals in the kidneys and the collecting system. The clinical picture is one of rapidly progressive renal failure, with oliguria and rapidly rising creatinine. Markedly elevated levels of serum uric acid would be expected in acute uric acid nephropathy, but hyperuricemia occurs in any cause of renal failure. A urine uric acid/creatinine ratio of >1 mg/mg confirms hyperuricemia and uric acid nephropathy as the cause of renal failure. This complication can largely be prevented by institution of allopurinol, 200–800 mg daily, prior to chemotherapy. Once hyperuricemia develops, however, efforts should be focused on preventing deposition of uric acid in the kidney. These measures include forced diuresis with furosemide or mannitol and alkalination of the urine with sodium bicarbonate. Dialysis may be required. Colchicine is used to treat the inflammation in acute gouty arthritis but has no effects on serum uric acid levels. It has no role in the treatment of uric acid nephropathy. Prednisone may be used in the chemotherapeutic regimens of some individuals with hematologic malignancies, but does not prevent development of hyperuricemia.

VII-35. **The answer is A.** *(Chap. 48)* Since the pH is low, the primary process is an acidosis. A low serum bicarbonate tells us that it is a metabolic acidosis. The anion gap [Na − (Cl + HCO$_3^-$)] is between 8 and 12 meq/L. In this example, the anion gap is elevated to 31 meq/L. The P$_{CO_2}$ decreases from a normal of 40 mmHg by 1 to 1.5 for each 1-meq decrease in serum bicarbonate. In this example, the serum bicarbonate has decreased by 19 meq/L (normal is 24 meq/L) and the expected P$_{CO_2}$ is between 11.5 and 21 mmHg. This is an example of an anion-gap metabolic acidosis with appropriate respiratory compensation. Respiratory acidosis is ruled out by the low P$_{CO_2}$. If this patient had a concomitant respiratory alkalosis, the P$_{CO_2}$ would be lower.

VII-36. **The answer is B.** *(Chap. 275)* Although the dose is currently defined as a derivation of the fractional urea clearance, factors that are also important include patient size, residual kidney function, dietary protein intake, comorbid conditions, and the degree of anabolism/catabolism. The efficiency of dialysis depends on the counter-current flow rate of the dialysate. The number of hours/sessions prescribed for a patient are derived from the dialysis dose and is individualized.

VII-37. **The answer is A.** *(Chap. 280)* The prognosis for patients with scleroderma renal disease is poor. In SRC patients prompt treatment with an ACE inhibitor may reverse acute renal failure. In recent studies the initiation of ACE inhibitor therapy resulted in 61% of patients having some degree of renal recovery and not needing chronic dialysis support. The survival rate is estimated to be 80 to 85% at 8 years. Among patients who needed dialysis, when treated with ACE inhibitors, over 50% were able to discontinue dialysis after 3 to 18 months. Therefore, ACE inhibitors should be used even if the patient requires dialysis support.

VII-38. **The answer is A.** *(Chap. 275)* The potassium concentration of dialysate is usually 2.5 meq/L but may be varied depending on the predialysis serum potassium. This patient may need a lower dialysate potassium concentration. Sodium modeling is an adjustment of the dialysate sodium that may lessen the incidence of hypotension at the end of a dialysis session. Aldosterone defects, if present, are not likely to play a role in this patient since his kidneys are not being perfused. Therefore, nephrectomy is not likely to control his potassium. Similarly, since the patient is likely anuric, there is no efficacy in utilizing loop diuretics to effect kaluresis. This patient has no approved indications for implantation of a defibrillator.

VII-39. **The answer is D.** *(Chaps. 46 and 334)* Rapid correction (or overcorrection) of hyponatremia may lead to the development of the osmotic demyelination syndrome. The relative hypertonicity of the extracellular fluid without time for intracellular compensation or osmotic compensation causes osmotic shrinkage of brain cells and demyelination. This syndrome usually occurs in patients with chronic hyponatremia who have osmotically equilibrated the intracellular space. These patients have flaccid paralysis, dysarthria, and dysphagia. Brain MRI will show demyelination, particularly in the brainstem (central pontine myelinolysis). Head CT scans will not demonstrate these lesions. The presence of bilateral extremity with minimal cranial nerve abnormalities would make a posterior circulation stroke less likely

VII-40. **The answer is C.** *(Chap. 45)* It is important to note that nephrotic syndrome with any cause can be associated with hypercoagulability. Antithrombin III and proteins C and S are lost in the urine, with concomitantly decreased serum levels. Increased platelet aggregation has been described, and hyperfibrinogenemia is thought to result from an inflammatory response and increased liver synthetic activity caused by urinary protein losses. Additionally, IgG is lost in the urine, and occasionally these patients develop low serum levels with associated immunocompromise. Chronic disseminated intravascular coagulation is not a mechanism of hypercoagulability in patients with the nephrotic syndrome.

VII-41. **The answer is A.** *(Chap. 273)* Nonsteroidal anti-inflammatory drugs (NSAIDs) do not alter glomerular filtration rate in normal individuals. However, in states of mild to moderate hypoperfusion (as in prerenal azotemia) or in the presence of chronic kidney disease, glomerular perfusion and filtration fraction are preserved through several compensatory mechanisms. In response to a reduction in perfusion pressures, stretch receptors in afferent arterioles trigger a cascade of events that lead to afferent arteriolar dilatation and efferent arteriolar vasoconstriction, thereby preserving glomerular filtration fraction. These mechanisms are partly mediated by the vasodilators prostaglandin E_2 and prostacyclin. NSAIDs can impair the kidney's ability to compensate for a low perfusion pressure by interfering with local prostaglandin synthesis and inhibiting these protective responses. Ureteral obstruction is not the mechanism by which NSAID impairs renal function in this scenario. NSAIDs are not known to be proximal tubule toxins.

VII-42 and VII-43. The answers are A and A. *(Chap. 273; R Solomon: Kidney Int 53:230, 1998.)* Radiocontrast agents are a common cause of acute renal failure and may result in acute tubular necrosis (contrast nephropathy). It is common for patients receiving intravenous contrast to develop a transient increase in serum creatinine. These agents cause renal failure by inducing intrarenal vasoconstriction and reducing renal blood flow, mimicking prerenal azotemia, and by directly causing tubular injury. The risk of contrast nephropathy may be reduced by initiating newer isoosmolar agents and minimizing the dose of contrast. When the reduction in renal blood flow is severe or prolonged, tubular injury develops, causing acute renal failure. Patients with intravascular volume depletion, diabetes, congestive heart failure, multiple myeloma, or chronic renal failure have an increased risk of contrast nephropathy. The urine sediment is bland in mild cases, but with acute tubular necrosis, muddy brown granular casts may be seen. Saline hydration plus *N*-acetylcysteine may decrease the risk and severity of contrast nephropathy. Red cell casts indicate glomerular disease, and white cell casts suggest upper urinary tract infection. Urinary eosinophils are seen in allergic interstitial disease caused by many drugs.

TABLE VII-42, -43   Guidelines for Use of Intravenous Contrast in Patients with Impaired Renal Function

Serum Creatinine, μmol/L (mg/dL)[a]	Recommendation
<133 (<1.5)	Use either ionic or nonionic at 2 mL/kg to 150 mL total
133–177 (1.5–2.0)	Nonionic; hydrate diabetics 1 mL/kg per hour × 10 h
>177 (>2.0)	Consider noncontrast CT or MRI; nonionic contrast if required
177–221 (2.0–2.5)	Nonionic only if required (as above); contraindicated in diabetics
>265 (>3.0)	Nonionic IV contrast given only to patients undergoing dialysis within 24 h

[a]Risk is greatest in patients with rising creatinine levels.
Note: CT, computed tomography; MRI, magnetic resonance imaging.

VII-44.   The answer is C. *(Chap. 280)* Renal vein thrombosis occurs in 10 to 15% of patients with nephrotic syndrome accompanying membranous glomerulopathy and oncologic disease. The clinical manifestations can be variable but may be characterized by fever, lumbar tenderness, leukocytosis, and hematuria. Magnetic resonance venography is the most sensitive and specific noninvasive form of imaging to make the diagnosis of renal vein thrombosis. Ultrasound with Doppler is operator-dependent and therefore may be less sensitive. Contrast venography is the gold standard for diagnosis, but it exposes the patient to a more invasive procedure and contrast load. Nuclear medicine screening is not performed to make this diagnosis.

VII-45.   The answer is D. *(Chaps. 46 and 334)* Arginine vasopressin is a neurohormone released from the posterior pituitary gland to help maintain water balance in the body. Also known as antidiuretic hormone, vasopressin is primarily released under conditions of hyperosmolarity and volume depletion. Although sodium is the main determinant of hyperosmolarity, sodium is not the only stimulus that affects the secretion of vasopressin. Other, less potent stimuli of vasopressin release include pregnancy, nausea, pain, stress, and hypoglycemia. In addition, many drugs can cause stimulation of the inappropriate secretion of vasopressin. This hormone acts on the principal cell in the distal convoluted tubule of the kidney to cause resorption of water. This occurs through nuclear mechanisms encoded by the aquaporin-2 gene that cause water channels to be inserted into the luminal membrane. The net effect is to cause the passive resorption of water along the osmotic gradient in the distal convoluted tubule.

VII-46.   The answer is C. *(Chap. 46)* β-Adrenergic agonists such as those used to treat bronchospasm are a common cause of hypokalemia. Activation of $β_2$-adrenergic receptors induces cellular uptake of potassium and promotes insulin secretion by pancreatic islet β cells. Clinical manifestations include fatigue, myalgias and muscular weakness. Severe hypokalemia leads to progressive weakness, hypoventilation and eventually complete paralysis. The electrocardiogram findings are common but do not correlate with the degree of hypokalemia in the serum. Todd's paralysis occurs after seizures. Neither myocardial infarction with failure nor ICU psychosis would present with objective lower extremity weakness without other more common indicators of these conditions. Adrenal insufficiency will generally cause hyperkalemia, not hypokalemia.

VII-47.   The answer is C. *(Chap. 46)* In addition to correction of hypernatremia, patients such as this who are volume-depleted require restoration of extracellular fluid volume. The quantity of water required to correct a free water deficit in hypernatremic patients can be estimated from the following equation:

$$\text{Water deficit} = [(\text{plasma Na} - 140)/140] \times \text{total body water}$$

Total body water is approximately 50% of lean body mass in men and 40% of lean body mass in women. In calculating the rate of water replacement, ongoing losses should be accounted for and plasma Na^+ should be lowered by no more than 0.5 meq/L an hour over the first 24 h. More rapid administration of water and normalization of serum sodium concentration may result in a rapid influx of water into cells that have already undergone osmotic normalization. The resulting cellular edema in the central nervous system (CNS) may cause seizures or neurologic damage.

VII-48.   The answer is E. *(Chap. 279)* The most likely cause of acute renal failure in this patient is allergic interstitial nephritis (AIN) due to penicillin. Many drugs can cause AIN including β-lactams, sulfonamides, fluoroquinolones, thiazide and loop diuretics, nonsteroidal anti-inflammatory drugs (NSAIDs), and cyclooxygenase-2 (COX-2) inhibitors. Most individuals have been taking the culprit drug for several weeks before the development of AIN and present with fevers, rash, and eosinophilia. This triad is present in only 10% of patients, however. Examination of the urine sediment shows hematuria and eosinophilia. Urine eosinophils can be seen with the use of a Hansel's stain. Proteinuria is usually mild except in cases where AIN is due to NSAIDs or COX-2 inhibitors, and 24-h urine collection for protein would be nonspecific. Renal imaging may suggest enlarged kidneys, and histology would show interstitial edema with infiltration of large numbers of inflammatory cells including eosinophils, lymphocytes, and PMNs. The main differential diagnosis is acute glomerulonephritis, but if an individual is on a culprit drug, the drug should be discontinued as an initial step. Discontinuation of the drug usually leads to complete reversal of the renal injury, although in severe cases, prednisone may be used to improve recovery. The clinical picture does not suggest relapse of endocarditis, worsening valvular dysfunction, or new infectious process such as a infection of the central venous catheter. Thus, blood cultures and echocardiogram are not useful in this situation. Antistreptolysin O titers are elevated in cases of poststreptococcal glomerulonephritis due to group A streptococcus, but would not be elevated in *S. viridans* endocarditis.

VII-49.   The answer is C. *(Chap. 275)* Hypotension is the most common complication during hemodialysis. The risk factors for developing hypotension during hemodialysis include excessive ultrafiltration, reduced intravascular volume before dialysis, impaired autonomic responses, osmolar shifts, food intake before dialysis, impaired cardiac function, and use of antihypertensive agents. The hypotension is usually managed with fluid administration and by decreasing the ultrafiltration rate. Muscle cramps are a decreasingly common complication of hemodialysis as a result of improvements in dialysis technique. Anaphylactoid reactions to the dialyzer once were common but are also decreasing in frequency with the use of newer-generation dialysis membranes. Fever is not a usual complication of hemodialysis but suggests the presence of an infection of the dialysis access site. Blood cultures should be obtained. Hyperglycemia is a complication of peritoneal dialysis, not of hemodialysis.

VII-50. **The answer is A.** *(Chap. 47)* Hypercalcemia causes characteristic changes on the ECG including bradycardia, atrioventricular block, and a shortened QT interval. Symptoms of hypercalcemia depend on the severity and time course of its development. Mild hypercalcemia is usually asymptomatic. Patients may progress to complain of vague neuropsychiatric symptoms including trouble concentrating, personality changes, and depression. Severe hypercalcemia, particularly if it develops acutely, may result in lethargy, stupor, or coma. Changes on the ECG of hypokalemia would include prominent U waves and a prolonged QU interval. Hyperkalemia acutely shows prominent T waves and PR depression. Hypocalcemia causes a prolongation of the QT interval.

VII-51. **The answer is A.** *(Chap. 47)* In sarcoidosis, similar to other granulomatous diseases such as tuberculosis and silicosis, there is increased conversion of 25(OH)D to the potent 1, 25(OH)$_2$D. 1,25(OH)$_2$D enhances intestinal calcium absorption, resulting in hypercalcemia and suppressed parathyroid hormone. Glucocorticoids decrease 1,25(OH)$_2$D production. Initial treatment for this patient should include IV fluids to restore extracellular fluid volume. Only after volume has been restored should loop diuretics be used to decrease serum calcium. Zoledronic acid is indicated if there is increased calcium mobilization from bone, as in malignancy or severe hyperparathyroidism. Intravenous phosphate is not indicated as it chelates calcium and may deposit in tissue and cause extensive organ damage if the calcium-phosphate product is >65. The mechanism of the hypercalcemia of sarcoidosis is related to excess vitamin D, therefore calcitriol would be contraindicated.

VII-52. **The answer is C.** *(Chap. 273)* In bilateral renal artery stenosis (or unilateral stenosis in a patient with a single kidney), GFR is preserved by the actions of angiotensin II: afferent arteriolar vasodilatation and efferent arteriolar vasoconstriction. Angiotensin-converting enzyme inhibitors and angiotensin II receptor blockers blunt these responses and can precipitate acute renal failure in this setting. Thiazide diuretics, calcium channel blockers, or centrally acting alphablockers are better choices for an antihypertensive agent in a patient with bilateral renal artery stenosis.

VII-53. **The answer is B.** *(Chap. 275)* In peritoneal dialysis, 1.5–3.0 L of dextrose-containing fluid is allowed to dwell in the peritoneum to remove toxic materials and volume. Factors such as infection, drugs, position, and exercise impact solute and water clearance. In the developed world, hemodialysis is often the preferred method for renal replacement for patients. However, in poorer countries where access to hemodialysis centers is limited, peritoneal dialysis is used more commonly. Residual renal function alters the dose of dialysis but does not impact the mode of dialysis. Moreover, patients with no residual renal function who receive peritoneal dialysis are at higher risk of uremia than patients on hemodialysis. High-transporters through the peritoneum require more frequent doses of peritoneal dialysis, potentially negating the benefit of this modality. In the developed world, the patient's age does not impact the mode of dialysis. Patients with prior abdominal surgeries often have difficulty with peritoneal dialysis catheter placement and dialysate delivery.

VII-54. **The answer is A.** *(Chap. 278)* This patient has a normal anion gap metabolic acidosis (anion gap = 12). The calculated urine anion gap (Na$^+$ + K$^+$– Cl$^-$) is +3; thus, the acidosis is unlikely to be due to gastrointestinal bicarbonate loss. In this patient the diagnosis is type I renal tubular acidosis, or distal RTA. This is a disorder in which the distal nephron does not lower pH normally. It is associated with a urine pH >5.5, hypokalemia, and lack of bicarbonaturia. This condition may be associated with calcium phosphate stones and nephrocalcinosis. Type II RTA, or proximal RTA, includes a pH <5.5, hypokalemia, a positive urine anion gap, bicarbinaturia, hypophosphatemia, and hypercalciuria. This condition results from defective resorption of bicarbonate. Type III RTA is rare and most commonly is seen in children. Type IV

RTA is also referred to as hyperkalemic distal RTA. Hyporeninemic hypoaldosteronism is the most common cause of type IV RTA and is usually associated with diabetic nephropathy.

VII-55. **The answer is B.** *(Chap. 277)* The characteristic pattern of focal (not all glomeruli) and segmental (not the entire glomerulus) glomerular scarring is shown. The history and laboratory features are also consistent with this lesion: some associated hypertension, diminution in creatinine clearance, and a relatively inactive urine sediment. The "nephropathy of obesity" may be associated with this lesion secondary to hyperfiltration; this condition may be more likely to occur in obese patients with hypoxemia, obstructive sleep apnea, and right-sided heart failure. Hypertensive nephrosclerosis exhibits more prominent vascular changes and patchy, ischemic, totally sclerosed glomeruli. In addition, nephrosclerosis seldom is associated with nephrotic-range proteinuria. Minimal-change disease usually is associated with symptomatic edema and normal-appearing glomeruli as demonstrated on light microscopy. This patient's presentation is consistent with that of membranous nephropathy, but the biopsy is not. With membranous glomerular nephritis all glomeruli are uniformly involved with subepithelial dense deposits. There are no features of crescentic glomerulonephritis present.

VII-56. **The answer is D.** *(Chap. 46)* This patient has a reduction in extracellular fluid (ECF) volume as evidenced by the resting tachycardia and orthostatic fall in blood pressure. In response (to maintain ECF volume), there is renal arteriolar vasoconstriction that causes a decrease in the glomerular filtration rate and filtered sodium. Tubular reabsorption of sodium increases as a result of the decreased filtered load and the effects of angiotensin II. These changes result in low (<20 meq/L) urine sodium excretion. There will also be an *increase* in the ratio of BUN to creatinine because of increased BUN reabsorption. As a result of the effects of aldosterone and the avid sodium reabsorption, urine potassium will be higher than urine sodium. Sweat is hypotonic relative to serum, and so patients with excessive sweating are more likely to be hypernatremic than hyponatremic. Red blood cell casts indicate glomerular disease. Prolonged hypotension caused by ECF contraction may cause tubular injury, leading to granular or epithelial cell casts.

VII-57. **The answer is B.** *(Chap. 45)* The patient's polyuria and thirst with rising sodium suggest diabetes insipidus. Although primary polydipsia can present similarly with thirst and polyuria, it does not cause hypernatremia; instead, hyponatremia results from increased extracellular water. Often patients with diabetes insipidus are able to compensate as outpatients when they have ready access to free water, but once hospitalized and unable to receive water freely, they develop hypernatremia. The first step in the evaluation of diabetes insipidus is to determine if it is central or nephrogenic. This is easily accomplished through measurement of the vasopressin level. In central diabetes insipidus it is low because of a failure of secretion from the posterior pituitary gland, whereas it is elevated in nephrogenic disease, in which the kidneys are insensitive to vasopressin. After measurement of the vasopressin level, a trial of nasal arginine vasopressin may be attempted. Generally nephrogenic diabetes insipidus will not improve significantly with this drug. Free water restriction, which will help with primary polydipsia, will cause worsening hypernatremia in patients with diabetes insipidus. Serum osmolality and 24-h urinary sodium excretion will not help in the diagnosis or management of this patient at this time.

VII-58. **The answer is D.** *(Chap. 278)* In any patient with hypokalemia the use of diuretics must be excluded. This patient has multiple warning signs for the use of agents to alter her weight, including her age, gender, and participation in competitive sports. Her BMI is low, and the oral examination may suggest chronic vomiting. Chronic vomiting may be associated with a low urine chloride level. Once diuretic use and vomiting are excluded, the differential diagnosis of hypokalemia and metabolic alkalosis includes magnesium deficiency, Liddle's syndrome, Bartter's syndrome, and Gittleman's syndrome. Liddle's syndrome is associated with hypertension and undetectable aldosterone and renin levels. It is a rare autosomal dominant disorder. Classic Bartter's syndrome has a presentation similar to that of this patient. It may also include polyuria and nocturia because of hypokalemia-induced diabetes insipidus. Gittleman's syndrome can be distinguished from Bartter's syndrome by hypomagnesemia and hypocalciuria.

VIII. DISORDERS OF THE GASTROINTESTINAL SYSTEM

QUESTIONS

DIRECTIONS: Choose the **one best** response to each question.

VIII-1. A 46-year-old man is admitted to the hospital for upper gastrointestinal (GI) bleeding. He has a known history of peptic ulcer disease, for which he takes a proton-pump inhibitor. His last admission for upper GI bleeding was 4 years ago. After fluid resuscitation, he is hemodynamically stable and his hematocrit has not changed in the past 8 h. Upper endoscopy is performed. Which of the following findings at endoscopy is most reassuring that the patient will not have a significant rebleeding episode within the next 3 days?

A. Adherent clot on ulcer
B. Clean-based ulcer
C. Gastric ulcer with arteriovenous malformations
D. Visible bleeding vessel
E. Visible nonbleeding vessel

VIII-2. Which of the following statements about alcoholic liver disease is *not* true?

A. Pathologically, alcoholic cirrhosis is often characterized by diffuse fine scarring with small regenerative nodules.
B. The ratio of AST to ALT is often higher than 2.
C. Serum aspartate aminotransferase levels are often greater than 1000 U/L.
D. Concomitant hepatitis C significantly accelerates the development of alcoholic cirrhosis.
E. Serum prothrombin times may be prolonged, but activated partial thromboplastin times are usually not affected.

VIII-3. A 47-year-old woman presents to the emergency room with severe mid-abdominal pain radiating to her back. The pain began acutely and is sharp. She denies cramping or flatulence. She has had two episodes of emesis of bilious material since the pain began, but this has not lessened the pain. She currently rates the pain as a 10 out of 10 and feels the pain is worse in the supine position. For the past few months, she has had intermittent episodes of right upper and mid-epigastric pain that occur after eating but subside over a few

VIII-3. *(Continued)*

hours. These are associated with a feeling of excess gas. She denies any history of alcohol abuse. She has no medical history of hypertension or hyperlipidemia. On physical examination, she is writhing in distress and slightly diaphoretic. Vital signs are: heart rate 127 beats/min, blood pressure 92/50 mmHg, respiratory rate 20 breaths/min, temperature 37.9°C, Sa_{O_2} 88% on room air. Her body mass index is 29 kg/m^2. The cardiovascular examination reveals a regular tachycardia. The chest examination shows dullness to percussion at bilateral bases with a few scattered crackles. On abdominal examination, bowel sounds are hypoactive. There is no rash or bruising evident on inspection of the abdomen. There is voluntary guarding on palpation. The pain with palpation is greatest in the periumbilical and epigastric area without rebound tenderness. There is no evidence of jaundice, and the liver span is about 10 cm to percussion. Amylase level is 750 IU/L, and lipase level is 1129 IU/L. Other laboratory values include: aspartate amino transferase (AST) 168 U/L, alanine aminotransferase (ALT) 196 U/L, total bilirubin 2.3 mg/dL, alkaline phosphatase level 268 U/L, lactate dehydrogenase LDH 300 U/L, and creatinine 1.9 mg/dL. The hematocrit is 43%, and white blood cell (WBC) count is 11,500/µL with 89% neutrophils. An arterial blood gas shows a pH of 7.32, Pa_{CO_2} 32 mmHg, and a Pa_{O_2} of 56 mmHg. An ultrasound confirms a dilated common bile duct with evidence of pancreatitis manifested as an edematous and enlarged pancreatitis. A CT scan shows no evidence of necrosis. After 3 L of normal saline, her blood pressure comes up to 110/60 mmHg with a heart rate of 105 beats/min. Which of the following statements best describes the pathophysiology of this disease?

A. Intrapancreatic activation of digestive enzymes with autodigestion and acinar cell injury
B. Chemoattraction of neutrophils with subsequent infiltration and inflammation

VIII-3. *(Continued)*

    C.   Distant organ involvement and systemic inflammatory response syndrome related to release of activated pancreatic enzymes and cytokines

    D.   All of the above

VIII-4. In the case vignette presented above, which of the following factors at presentation predicts a poor outcome and increased risk of death in acute pancreatitis?

    A.   Body mass index (BMI) >25 kg/m^2

    B.   Hematocrit ≥40%

    C.   Lipase >1000 IU/L

    D.   Pa$_{O_2}$ <60 mmHg

    E.   WBC count >10,000/μL

VIII-5. A 22-year old woman presents to the emergency department with abdominal pain and malaise. Her symptoms began about 8 h prior to presentation, and she has no diarrhea. The pain is mostly in the right flank currently but began in the periumbilical area. She has nausea and vomiting. Temperature is 100.3°C, blood pressure 129/90 mmHg, heart rate 101 beats/min. Physical examination shows only mild diffuse abdominal tenderness. The abdomen is soft and bowel sounds are diminished. She is tender in the right flank without costovertebral angle tenderness. The genitourinary and pelvic examinations are normal. White blood cell count is 10,000/μL. Urine analysis shows 2 white blood cells per high powered field, no epithelial cells, and 1 red blood cell per high powered field. A serum pregnancy test is negative. She has no past medical history and has never had similar symptoms. She is not sexually active. Which of the following is the most likely diagnosis?

    A.   Abdominal aortic aneurysm rupture

    B.   Acute appendicitis

    C.   Pyelonephritis

    D.   Mesenteric lymphadenitis

    E.   Pelvic inflammatory disease

VIII-6. A 28-year-old male with HIV and a CD4 count of 4/μL is admitted to the hospital with several days of epigastric boring abdominal pain radiating to the back with associated nausea and bilious vomiting. He has a history of disseminated mycobacterial disease, cryptococcal pneumonia, and injection drug use. His current medications include fluconazole, trimethoprim-sulfamethoxazole, clarithromycin, ethambutol, and rifabutin. On physical examination he has normal vital signs, decreased bowel sounds, and tender epigastrium without rebound or guarding. Rectal exam is guaiac-negative. The remainder of the examination is normal. Amylase and lipase are elevated. The patient is treated conservatively with intravenous fluids and bowel rest, with resolution of symptoms. Right upper quadrant ultrasound is normal, and calcium and triglycerides are normal. Which of the following changes to his medical regimen should be recommended on discharge?

VIII-6. *(Continued)*

    A.   Discontinue rifabutin.

    B.   Substitute azithromycin for clarithromycin.

    C.   Substitute dapsone for trimethoprim-sulfamethoxazole.

    D.   Substitute amphotericin for fluconazole.

    E.   Discontinue trimethoprim-sulfamethoxazole.

VIII-7. All of the following necessitate sending bacterial stool cultures in patients with diarrhea for 2 days severe enough to keep them home from work *except*

    A.   age >75

    B.   bloody stools

    C.   dehydration

    D.   recent lung transplantation

    E.   temperature >38.5°C

VIII-8. While doing rounds in the intensive care unit, you see a 70-year-old male patient with multisystem organ failure who is postoperative day 3. Review of his history reveals that he had a perforated appendix due to a delay in the diagnosis of acute appendicitis. Prior to his surgical intervention, he was noted to be delirious. His preoperative laboratory results showed: sodium, 133 meq/dL, potassium, 5.2 meq/dL, chloride, 98 meq/dL, bicarbonate, 14 meq/dL, blood urea nitrogen 85 mg/dL, creatinine, 3.2 mg/dL. Urine analysis had no red cells, white cells, and trace protein. An electrocardiogram showed ST-segment depression in an area of an old myocardial infarct. Preoperative troponin I level was 0.09 mg/dL. He had no history of chronic renal insufficiency. What is the most likely etiology of this patient's renal failure?

    A.   Acute interstitial nephritis

    B.   Congestive heart failure

    C.   Glomerulonephritis

    D.   Ureteral injury

    E.   Volume depletion

VIII-9. All the following are causes of diarrhea *except*

    A.   diabetes

    B.   hypercalcemia

    C.   hyperthyroidism

    D.   irritable bowel syndrome

    E.   metoclopramide

VIII-10. A 55-year-old white male with a history of diabetes presents to your office with complaints of generalized weakness, weight loss, nonspecific diffuse abdominal pain, and erectile dysfunction. The examination is significant for hepatomegaly without tenderness, testicular atrophy, and gynecomastia. Skin examination shows a diffuse slate-gray hue slightly more pronounced on the face and neck. Joint examination shows mild swelling of the second and third metacarpophalangeal

VIII-10. *(Continued)*

joints on the right hand. What is the recommended test for diagnosis?

- A.   Serum ferritin
- B.   Serum iron studies, including transferrin saturation
- C.   Urinary iron quantification in 24-h collection
- D.   Genetic screen for *HFE* gene mutation (C282Y and H63D)
- E.   Liver biopsy

VIII-11.   All the following are associated with an increased risk for cholelithiasis *except*

- A.   chronic hemolytic anemia
- B.   obesity
- C.   high-protein diet
- D.   pregnancy
- E.   female sex

VIII-12.   A 28-year-old man is admitted to the hospital with a large perianal abscess. He is taken to the operating room for incision and drainage, which he tolerates well, and he is discharged home with a 2-week course of antibiotics. He returns to the hospital 2 months later for a rash on his shins. On examination, he has discrete red swollen nodules on both of his shins without fluctuance. They measure ~2 cm in diameter. He has no respiratory complaints, and the rest of his skin examination is normal. Laboratory data show a white blood cell count of 12,000 with a normal differential. Erythrocyte sedimentation rate is 64 mm/h. A chest radiograph is normal. Thyroid-stimulating hormone is 3.27 mU/L, and a glycosylated hemoglobin is 5.3%. Which of the following conditions is he also likely to have?

- A.   Giant cell arteritis
- B.   *Pneumocystis jirovecii* pneumonia
- C.   Sarcoidosis
- D.   Type 1 diabetes
- E.   Uveitis

VIII-13.   A 55-year-old male with cirrhosis is seen in the clinic to follow up a recent hospitalization for spontaneous bacterial peritonitis. He is doing well and finishing his course of antibiotics. He is taking propranolol and lactulose; besides complications of end-stage liver disease, he has well-controlled diabetes mellitus and had a basal cell carcinoma resected 5 years ago. The cirrhosis is thought to be due to alcohol abuse, and his last drink of alcohol was 2 weeks ago. He and his wife ask if he is a liver transplant candidate. He can be counseled in which of the following ways?

- A.   He is not a transplant candidate as he has a history of alcohol dependence.
- B.   He is not a transplant candidate now, but may be after a sustained period of proven abstinence from alcohol.
- C.   Because he has diabetes mellitus he is not a transplant candidate.

VIII-13. *(Continued)*

- D.   Because he had a skin cancer he is not a transplant candidate.
- E.   He is appropriate for liver transplantation and should be referred immediately.

VIII-14.   A 16-year-old woman had visited your clinic 1 month ago with jaundice, vomiting, malaise, and anorexia. Two other family members were ill with similar symptoms. Based on viral serologies, including a positive anti-hepatitis A virus (HAV) IgM, a diagnosis of hepatitis A was made. The patient was treated conservatively, and 1 week after first presenting, she appeared to have made a full recovery. She returns to your clinic today complaining of the same symptoms she had 1 month ago. She is jaundiced, and an initial panel of laboratory tests returns elevated transaminases. Which of the following offers the best explanation of what has occurred in this patient?

- A.   Co-infection with hepatitis C
- B.   Hepatitis A recurrence
- C.   Inappropriate treatment of initial infection
- D.   Incorrect initial diagnosis; this patient likely has hepatitis B
- E.   Relapsing hepatitis

VIII-15.   A male patient with inflammatory bowel disease (IBD) comes to your office as a new patient. Reviewing the medical records, you note that he has had primarily rectal disease. Macroscopic photographs from his most recent colonoscopy show a lumpy, bumpy, hemorrhagic mucosa with ulcerations. Histology shows a process that is limited to the mucosa, with the deep layers unaffected. There are crypt abscesses. Which historic feature would be surprising in a patient with this form of IBD?

- A.   Age 15–30
- B.   Current smoker
- C.   Fraternal twin sister does not have IBD
- D.   Identical twin brother does not have IBD
- E.   Intact appendix

VIII-16.   A 26-year-old male presents with persistent perianal pain for 2 months that is worse with defecation. The patient notes that he occasionally sees small amounts of red blood on the toilet tissue. He never has had blood staining the toilet bowl. He reports persistent constipation but has not had any incontinence. He denies anal trauma. On physical examination there is a linear ulceration with raised edges with a skin tag at the distal end. Circular fibers of the hypertrophied internal sphincter are visible. What is the most appropriate treatment of this disease?

- A.   Sitz baths
- B.   Placement of a mechanical loop followed by surgical resection
- C.   Steroid enemas
- D.   Nitroglycerin ointment
- E.   Mesalamine enemas

VIII-17. A 76-year-old man complains of frequent small stools that are not abnormally liquid or hard. There is some pain with passing the stool. He has no abdominal pain, nausea, melena, vomiting, or fever. He has approximately eight to ten bowel movements per day, which interferes with his quality of life, though there is no fecal incontinence. What is a possible diagnosis to explain his complaints?

A. Hypothyroidism
B. Neuromuscular disorder
C. Proctitis
D. Ulcerative colitis
E. Viral gastroenteritis

VIII-18. Which of the following proteins does not cause secretion of gastric acid?

A. Acetylcholine
B. Caffeine
C. Gastrin
D. Histamine
E. Somatostatin

VIII-19. A 62-year-old female has a 3-month history of diffuse crampy abdominal pain and watery diarrhea and has lost 14 lb over this period. There is no prior history of abdominal or gynecologic disease. She is on no regular medications, is a nonsmoker, and does not consume alcohol. Colonoscopy reveals normal colonic mucosa. Biopsies of the colon reveal inflammation with extensive subepithelial collagen deposition and lymphocytic infiltration of the epithelium. Which of the following is the most likely diagnosis?

A. Collagenous colitis
B. Crohn's disease
C. Ischemic colitis
D. Lymphocytic colitis
E. Ulcerative colitis

VIII-20. A 29-year-old woman who recently immigrated to the United States from South America presents to a local emergency room with severe abdominal pain, jaundice, and fever. No one else at home is ill. She is unsure how long her symptoms have been going on, but describes a sudden worsening over the past 3 days. She has been unable to get out of bed and has not been eating well over that period of time. She has had nausea and vomiting. She denies alcohol or illicit drug use. She is rapidly triaged and on initial laboratory studies is found to have an ALT and AST in the thousands. She is to be admitted for inpatient management, and viral hepatitis serologies are sent. In a patient with acute hepatitis B, which of the following would be the first indication of infection?

A. Anti-HBc (antibody to hepatitis B core antigen)
B. Clinical symptoms such as fever, jaundice, and abdominal pain
C. HBeAg (hepatitis B e antigen)

VIII-20. *(Continued)*
D. HBsAg (hepatitis B surface antigen)
E. Increased transaminases

VIII-21. The patient described above has the following laboratory results: HBsAg is positive, Anti-HBc IgM is positive, and HBeAg is positive. All other serologies are negative. She is diagnosed with acute hepatitis B. When interpreting hepatitis B serology results, the term "window period" refers to the time between which of the following?

A. Anti-HBs and anti-HBc positivity
B. Clinical symptoms and anti-HBs
C. HBsAg and anti-HBs positivity
D. HBsAg and HBeAg positivity
E. Increased transaminases and HBsAg

VIII-22. A 57-year-old man with peptic ulcer disease experiences transient improvement with *Helicobacter pylori* eradication. However, 3 months later, symptoms recur despite acid-suppressing therapy. He does not take nonsteroidal anti-inflammatory agents. Stool analysis for *H. pylori* antigen is negative. Upper GI endoscopy reveals prominent gastric folds together with the persistent ulceration in the duodenal bulb previously detected and the beginning of a new ulceration 4 cm proximal to the initial ulcer. Fasting gastrin levels are elevated and basal acid secretion is 15 meq/h. What is the best test to perform to make the diagnosis?

A. No additional testing is necessary.
B. Blood sampling for gastrin levels following a meal.
C. Blood sampling for gastrin levels following secretin administration.
D. Endoscopic ultrasonography of the pancreas.
E. Genetic testing for mutations in the MEN1 gene.

VIII-23. A 29-year-old woman comes to see you in clinic because of abdominal discomfort. She feels abdominal discomfort on most days of the week, and the pain varies in location and intensity. She notes constipation as well as diarrhea, but diarrhea predominates. In comparison to 6 months ago, she has more bloating and flatulence than she has had before. She identifies eating and stress as aggravating factors, and her pain is relieved by defecation. You suspect irritable bowel syndrome (IBS). Laboratory data include: white blood cell (WBC) count 8000/μL, hematocrit, 32%, platelets, 210,000/μL, and erythrocyte sedimentation rate (ESR) of 44 mm/h. Stool studies show the presence of lactoferrin but no blood. Which intervention is appropriate at this time?

A. Antidepressants
B. Ciprofloxacin
C. Colonoscopy
D. Reassurance and patient counseling
E. Stool bulking agents

VIII-24. After a careful history and physical and a cost-effective workup, you have diagnosed your patient with IBS. What other condition would you expect to find in this patient?

VIII-24. *(Continued)*

A. Abnormal brain anatomy
B. Autoimmune disease
C. History of sexually transmitted diseases
D. Hypersensitivity to peripheral stimuli
E. Psychiatric diagnosis

VIII-25. Which of the following statements about cardiac cirrhosis is true?

A. Prolonged passive congestion from right-sided heart failure results first in congestion and necrosis of portal triads, resulting in subsequent fibrosis.
B. AST and ALT levels may mimic the very high levels seen in acute hepatitis infection or acetaminophen toxicity.
C. Budd-Chiari syndrome cannot be distinguished clinically from cardiac cirrhosis.
D. Venoocclusive disease is a major cause of morbidity and mortality in patients undergoing liver transplantation.
E. Echocardiography is the gold standard for diagnosing constrictive pericarditis as a cause of cirrhosis.

VIII-26. A patient with known peptic ulcer disease presents with sudden abdominal pain to the emergency department. She is thought to have peritonitis but refuses an abdominal examination due to the discomfort caused by previous examinations. Which of the following maneuvers will provide reasonably specific evidence of peritonitis without manual palpation of the abdomen?

A. Bowel sounds are absent on auscultation.
B. Forced cough elicits abdominal pain.
C. Hyperactive bowel sounds are heard on auscultation.
D. Pain is elicited with gentle pressure at the costovertebral angle.
E. Rectal examination reveals heme-positive stools.

VIII-27. In chronic hepatitis B virus (HBV) infection, presence of hepatitis B e antigen (HBeAg) signifies which of the following?

A. Development of liver fibrosis leading to cirrhosis
B. Dominant viral population is less virulent and less transmissible
C. Increased likelihood of an acute flare in the next 1–2 weeks
D. Ongoing viral replication
E. Resolving infection

VIII-28. A 42-year-old male presents for evaluation of recurrent sharp substernal chest pain that occurs primarily at rest and radiates to both arms and the sides of the chest. He notes that the pain is worse with eating and emotional stress. The pain lasts approximately 10 min before resolving entirely. He has undergone a full cardiac evaluation, including negative exercise echocardiography for inducible ischemia. You suspect diffuse esophageal

VIII-28. *(Continued)*

spasm and order a barium swallow for further evaluation. Which of the following findings would best correlate with your suspected diagnosis?

A. Proximal esophageal dilatation with tapered beak-like appearance distally near the gastroesophageal junction
B. Uncoordinated distal esophageal contractions resulting in a corkscrew appearance of the esophagus
C. Dilation of the esophagus with loss of peristaltic contractions in the middle and distal portions of the esophagus
D. Reflux of barium back into the distal portion of the esophagus
E. A tapered narrowing in the distal esophagus with an apple core–like lesion

VIII-29. A 26-year-old woman presents to your clinic and is interested in getting pregnant. She seeks your advice regarding vaccines she should obtain, and in particular asks about the hepatitis B vaccine. She works as a receptionist for a local business, denies alcohol or illicit drug use, and is in a monogamous relationship. Which of the following is true regarding hepatitis B vaccination?

A. Hepatitis B vaccine consists of two intramuscular doses 1 month apart.
B. Only patients with defined risk factors need be vaccinated.
C. Pregnancy is not a contraindication to the hepatitis B vaccine.
D. This patient's hepatitis serologies should be checked prior to vaccination.
E. Vaccination should not be administered to children under 2 years old.

VIII-30. A 41-year-old female presents to your clinic with a week of jaundice. She notes pruritus, icterus, and dark urine. She denies fever, abdominal pain, or weight loss. The examination is unremarkable except for yellow discoloration of the skin. Total bilirubin is 6.0 mg/dL, and direct bilirubin is 5.1 mg/dL. AST is 84 U/L, and ALT is 92 U/L. Alkaline phosphatase is 662 U/L. CT scan of the abdomen is unremarkable. Right upper quadrant ultrasound shows a normal gallbladder but does not visualize the common bile duct. What is the most appropriate next management step?

A. Antibiotics and observation
B. Endoscopic retrograde cholangiopancreatography (ERCP)
C. Hepatitis serologies
D. HIDA scan
E. Serologies for antimitochondrial antibodies

VIII-31. A 46-year-old woman with a past medical history of osteoporosis presents to the hospital because of hematemesis. She reports having bright-red bloody emesis

VIII-31. *(Continued)*

for 2 h as well as seeing "coffee-grounds" in her emesis. However, you do not witness any vomiting in the emergency department. She takes calcium, vitamin D, and alendronate. Blood pressure is 108/60 mmHg, heart rate 93 beats/min, and temperature 37.6°C. Her hematocrit is 30% (baseline 37%). You request an emergent upper endoscopy and resuscitate the patient with fluids. What is the role for immediate IV proton-pump inhibitor (PPI) therapy in this patient?

A. It is contraindicated given her history of osteoporosis.
B. It should be initiated as this will decrease further bleeding.
C. It should be initiated only if high-risk ulcers are identified at the time of endoscopy.
D. It will decrease her bleeding risk, length of hospitalization, likelihood to need surgery, and overall mortality.
E. There is no indication for immediate IV PPI therapy.

VIII-32. While waiting for endoscopy, you recheck her hematocrit 2 h later and it remains 30%. Vital signs are unchanged. You perform a gastric lavage, which returns clear fluid. Test of occult blood in the lavage is negative. What is the most appropriate intervention at this time?

A. Perform a CT scan of the abdomen.
B. Continue current management and plan.
C. Perform another gastric lavage.
D. Recheck another hematocrit in 2 h.
E. Request psychiatric consultation for factitious bleeding.

VIII-33. A 34-year-old male reports "yellow eyes" for the last 2 days during a routine employment examination. He states that since his early twenties he has had similar episodes of yellow eyes lasting 2 to 4 days. He denies nausea, abdominal pain, dark urine, light-colored stools, pruritus, or weight loss. He has not sought prior medical attention because of finances, lack of symptoms, and the predictable resolution of the yellow eyes. He takes a multivitamin and some herbal medications. On examination he is mildly obese. He is icteric. There are no stigmata of chronic liver disease. The patient's abdomen is soft and nontender, and there is no organomegaly. Laboratory examinations are normal except for a total bilirubin of 3 mg/dL. Direct bilirubin is 0.2 mg/dL. AST, ALT, and alkaline phosphatase are normal. Hematocrit, lactate dehydrogenase (LDH), and haptoglobin are normal. Which of the following is the most likely diagnosis?

A. Crigler-Najjar syndrome type 1
B. Cholelithiasis
C. Dubin-Johnson syndrome
D. Gilbert's syndrome
E. Medication-induced hemolysis

VIII-34. What is the appropriate next management step for this patient?

VIII-34. *(Continued)*

A. Genotype studies
B. Peripheral blood smear
C. Prednisone
D. Reassurance
E. Right upper quadrant ultrasound

VIII-35. A 45-year-old male says that for the last year he occasionally has regurgitated particles from food eaten several days earlier. His wife complains that his breath has been foul-smelling. He has had occasional dysphagia for solid foods. The most likely diagnosis is

A. gastric outlet obstruction
B. scleroderma
C. achalasia
D. Zenker's diverticulum
E. diabetic gastroparesis

VIII-36. All the following cancers commonly metastasize to the liver *except*

A. breast
B. colon
C. lung
D. melanoma
E. prostate

VIII-37. A 38-year-old male presents to his physician with 4 to 6 months of weight loss and joint complaints. He reports that his appetite is good, but he has had diarrhea with six to eight loose, foul-smelling stools each day. He has also had migratory pain in the knees and shoulders. Stool studies demonstrate steatorrhea. Which of the following diagnostic tests is most likely to be positive in this patient?

A. Serum IgA antiendomysial antibodies
B. Serum IgA antigliadin antibodies
C. Serum PCR for *Tropheryma whippelii*
D. Small bowel biopsy showing reduced villous height and crypt hyperplasia
E. Stool *Clostridium difficile* toxin

VIII-38. Inflammatory bowel disease (IBD) may be caused by exogenous factors. Gastrointestinal flora may promote an inflammatory response or may inhibit inflammation. Probiotics have been used to treat IBD. Which of the following organisms has been used in the treatment of IBD?

A. *Campylobacter* spp.
B. *Clostridium difficile*
C. *Escherichia* spp.
D. *Lactobacillus* spp.
E. *Shigella* spp.

VIII-39. A 61-year-old male is admitted to your service for swelling of the abdomen. You detect ascites on clinical examination and perform a paracentesis. The results show a white blood cell count of 300 leukocytes/μL with

VIII-39. *(Continued)*

35% polymorphonuclear cells. The peritoneal albumin level is 1.2 g/dL, protein is 2.0 g/dL, and triglycerides are 320 mg/dL. Peritoneal cultures are pending. Serum albumin is 2.6 g/dL. Which of the following is the most likely diagnosis?

A. Congestive heart failure
B. Peritoneal tuberculosis
C. Peritoneal carcinomatosis
D. Chylous ascites
E. Bacterial peritonitis

VIII-40. A 78-year-old female nursing home resident complains of rectal pain and profuse watery diarrhea for 2 days. Her nurse reports 2 weeks of constipation prior to this. A physician sent a *Clostridium difficile* stool antigen test that returned negative. What is the next step in establishing a diagnosis?

A. Colonoscopy
B. Digital rectal examination
C. Repeat *C. difficile* stool antigen test
D. Rotavirus stool antigen
E. Stool culture

VIII-41. Which of the following is the most common cause of acute pancreatitis in the United States?

A. Alcohol
B. Drugs
C. Gallstones
D. Hypercalcemia
E. Hyperlipidemia

VIII-42. A 24-year-old woman with a history of irritable bowel syndrome (IBS) has been treated with loperamide, psyllium, and imipramine. Because of continued abdominal pain, bloating, and alternating constipation/diarrhea, she is started on alosetron, 0.5 mg bid. Five days later she is brought to the emergency department with severe abdominal pain. On examination she is in severe discomfort. Her temperature is 39°C, blood pressure 90/55 mmHg, heart rate 115 beats/min, respiratory rate 22 breaths/min, and oxygen saturation normal. Abdominal examination is notable for hypoactive bowel sounds, diffuse tenderness, and guarding without rebound tenderness. Her stool is heme positive. Laboratory studies are notable for a white blood cell count of 15,800 with a left shift and a slight anion gap metabolic acidosis. Which of the following is the most likely diagnosis?

A. Appendicitis
B. *Clostridium difficile* colitis
C. Crohn's disease
D. Ischemic colitis
E. Perforated duodenal ulcer

VIII-43. An 88-year-old woman is brought to your clinic by her family because she has become increasingly so-

VIII-43. *(Continued)*

cially withdrawn. The patient lives alone and has been reluctant to visit or be visited by her family. Family members, including seven children, also note a foul odor in her apartment and on her person. She has not had any weight loss. Alone in the examining room, she only complains of hemorrhoids. On mental status examination, she does have signs of depression. Which of the following interventions is most appropriate at this time?

A. Head CT scan
B. Initiate treatment with an antidepressant medication
C. Physical examination including genitourinary and rectal examination
D. Screening for occult malignancy
E. Serum thyroid-stimulating hormone

VIII-44. You are asked to consult on a 62-year-old white female with pruritus for 4 months. She has noted progressive fatigue and a 5-lb weight loss. She has intermittent nausea but no vomiting and denies changes in her bowel habits. There is no history of prior alcohol use, blood transfusions, or illicit drug use. The patient is widowed and had two heterosexual partners in her lifetime. Her past medical history is significant only for hypothyroidism, for which she takes levothyroxine. Her family history is unremarkable. On examination she is mildly icteric. She has spider angiomata on her torso. You palpate a nodular liver edge 2 cm below the right costal margin. The remainder of the examination is unremarkable. A right upper quadrant ultrasound confirms your suspicion of cirrhosis. You order a complete blood count and a comprehensive metabolic panel. What is the most appropriate next test?

A. 24-h urine copper
B. Antimitochondrial antibodies (AMA)
C. Endoscopic retrograde cholangiopancreatography (ERCP)
D. Hepatitis B serologies
E. Serum ferritin

VIII-45. Your 33-year-old patient with Crohn's disease (CD) has had a disappointing disease response to glucocorticoids and 5-ASA agents. He is interested in steroid-sparing agents. He has no liver or renal disease. You prescribe once-weekly methotrexate injections. In addition to monitoring hepatic function and complete blood count, what other complication of methotrexate therapy do you advise the patient of?

A. Disseminated histoplasmosis
B. Lymphoma
C. Pancreatitis
D. Pneumonitis
E. Primary sclerosing cholangitis

VIII-46. Which of the following is potentially associated with constipation?

- A. Colon cancer
- B. Depression
- C. Eating disorder
- D. Hypothyroidism
- E. Irritable bowel syndrome
- F. Pharmaceutical agents
- G. All of the above

VIII-47. A 23-year-old Turkish female presents to the emergency department for evaluation of acute abdominal pain. She reports that she has had multiple episodes of severe abdominal pain since age 15. These episodes have been very severe, once prompting exploratory laparotomy at age 18 with removal of the appendix, which was histologically benign. She reports that the pain lasts approximately 2 or 3 days and then resolves entirely without intervention. There are no clear triggers for the pain. Past evaluation has included normal upper and lower endoscopy, normal small bowel series, and multiple CT scans that have shown only small amounts of free fluid in the abdominal cavity. In addition, the patient recently developed a migratory arthritis affecting her knees and ankles. The patient is currently on no medications. Multiple other family members have similar complaints. On physical examination the patient appears in moderate distress, lying very still. Temperature is 39.8°C (103.6°F). Heart rate is 130, and blood pressure is 112/66. She has evidence of a pleural effusion on the right with decreased breath sounds and dullness to percussion of half the lung field. She has a regular tachycardia without murmurs. Bowel sounds are hypoactive, and there is moderate diffuse abdominal tenderness. There is mild rebound tenderness diffusely throughout the abdomen without guarding. Her left knee is swollen and erythematous with an effusion. Laboratory studies show a white blood cell count of 15,300/mm³ (90% neutrophils). Erythrocyte sedimentation rate is 110 s. Arthrocentesis reveals a white blood cell count of 68,000 with 98% neutrophils. Culture is negative at 1 week. The patient's symptoms resolve over the course of 72 h. What is the best therapy for prevention of the patient's symptoms?

- A. Azathioprine
- B. Colchicine
- C. Hemin
- D. Indomethacin
- E. Prednisone

VIII-48. An 18-year-old man presents to a rural clinic with nausea, vomiting, anorexia, abdominal discomfort, myalgias, and jaundice. He describes occasional alcohol use and is sexually active. He describes using heroin and cocaine "a few times in the past." He works as a short-order cook in a local restaurant. He has lost 15.5 kg (34 lb) since his last visit to clinic and appears emaciated and ill-

VIII-48. (Continued)
appearing. On examination he is noted to have icteric sclerae and a palpable, tender liver below the right costal margin. In regard to acute hepatitis, which of the following is true?

- A. A distinction between viral etiologies cannot be made using clinical criteria alone.
- B. Based on age and risk factors, he is likely to have hepatitis B infection.
- C. He does not have hepatitis E virus, as this infects only pregnant women.
- D. This patient cannot have hepatitis C because his presentation is too acute.
- E. This patient does not have hepatitis A because his presentation is too fulminant.

VIII-49. A 22-year-old pregnant woman presents to the emergency department with abdominal pain and malaise. Her symptoms began about 8 h prior to presentation and she has no diarrhea. Her pain is mostly in the right flank currently but began in the periumbilical area. She has nausea and vomiting. She has had an uncomplicated pregnancy and she is at 24 weeks' gestation. She receives regular obstetric care, and her last examination, including an echo, was normal 1 week ago. Temperature is 100.3°C, blood pressure 129/90 mmHg, and heart rate 105 beats/min. Physical examination shows only mild abdominal tenderness. The abdomen is soft and bowel sounds are diminished. She is tender in the right lower quadrant without costovertebral angle tenderness. The genitourinary examination is normal, and she has a closed os. Fetal monitoring shows a normal fetal heart rate. White blood cell count is 10,000/μL. Urine analysis shows 2 white blood cells per high powered field, no epithelial cells, and 1 red blood cell per high powered field. What is the most likely diagnosis?

- A. Acute appendicitis
- B. Fitz-Hugh–Curtis syndrome
- C. Mittelschmerz
- D. Nephrolithiasis
- E. Pyelonephritis

VIII-50. A 54-year-old male presents with 1 month of diarrhea. He states that he has 8 to 10 loose bowel movements a day. He has lost 8 lb during this time. Vital signs and physical examination are normal. Serum laboratory studies are normal. A 24-h stool collection reveals 500 g of stool with a measured stool osmolality of 200 mosmol/L and a calculated stool osmolality of 210 mosmol/L. Based on these findings, what is the most likely cause of this patient's diarrhea?

- A. Celiac sprue
- B. Chronic pancreatitis
- C. Lactase deficiency
- D. Vasoactive intestinal peptide tumor
- E. Whipple's disease

VIII-51. All the following are risk factors for developing cholangiocarcinoma *except*

A. choledochal cyst
B. cholelithiasis
C. liver flukes
D. sclerosing cholangitis
E. working in the rubber industry

VIII-52. A 34-year-old female presents to your clinic with 5 weeks of right upper quadrant pain. She denies nausea, changes in bowel habits, or weight loss. Her past medical history is unremarkable. Her only medications are a multivitamin and oral contraceptives. The examination is notable for a palpable liver mass 2 cm below the right costal margin. Serum α fetoprotein is normal. An abdominal CT scan shows two 3-cm hypervascular lesions in the right hepatic lobe that are suggestive of hepatocellular adenoma. What is the most appropriate next management step?

A. Observation
B. Discontinuation of oral contraceptives
C. Referral for surgical excision
D. Radiofrequency ablation (RFA)
E. CT-guided biopsy

VIII-53. A 50-year-old male without a significant past medical history or recent exposure to alcohol presents with midepigastric abdominal pain, nausea, and vomiting. The physical examination is remarkable for the absence of jaundice and any other specific physical findings. Which of the following is the best strategy for screening for acute pancreatitis?

A. Measurement of serum amylase
B. Measurement of serum lipase
C. Measurement of both serum amylase and serum lipase
D. Isoamylase level analysis
E. Magnetic resonance imaging

VIII-54. A 43-year-old man with alcohol dependence presents with a sharp epigastric pain radiating to the back. He also has had nausea with bilious emesis on three occasions in the past 24 h. He has had no bright red blood or coffee-ground material in his vomitus, nor has he had melena. His last alcohol intake was yesterday, and he normally drinks a gallon of whiskey on a daily basis. He has a history of acute pancreatitis due to alcohol. On physical examination, he appears uncomfortable, writhing in bed. His vital signs are: heart rate 112 beats/min, blood pressure 156/92 mmHg, temperature 37.8°C, respiratory rate 24 breaths/min, and Sa$_{O_2}$ 96% on room air. The abdominal examination reveals decreased bowel sounds and is tympanitic to percussion. There is diffuse tenderness to palpation in the midepigastrium without rebound. Voluntary guarding is present. The liver span is 15 cm to percussion, and a smooth liver edge is palpated 5 cm below the right costal margin. No spleen tip is palpable. The

VIII-54. *(Continued)*
amylase is 580 U/L, and lipase is 690 U/L. Liver function testing reveals an AST of 280 U/L, ALT 184 U/L, alkaline phosphatase 89 U/L, and albumin 2.6 g/dL. Fecal occult blood testing is negative. Which of the following best reflects the current recommendations on treatment of acute pancreatitis in this patient?

A. A nasogastric tube with intermittent suctioning is necessary to prevent ongoing stimulation of pancreatic enzyme release by gastric secretions.
B. Early oral alimentation decreases the risk of infection and speeds recovery
C. Placement of a nasojejunal feeding tube will allow early institution of oral feeding and reduce hospital length of stay.
D. Total parenteral nutrition is indicated because the patient has evidence of chronic malnutrition and is expected to be unable to tolerate oral alimentation for >1 week.
E. Treatment with analgesia, IV fluid resuscitation, and avoidance of oral feeding will result in improvement in 3–7 days.

VIII-55. A 38-year-old male is seen in the urgent care center with several hours of severe abdominal pain. His symptoms began suddenly, but he reports several months of pain in the epigastrium after eating, with a resultant 10-lb weight loss. He takes no medications besides over-the-counter antacids and has no other medical problems or habits. On physical examination temperature is 38.0°C (100.4°F), pulse 130/min, respiratory rate 24/min, and blood pressure 110/50 mmHg. His abdomen has absent bowel sounds and is rigid with involuntary guarding diffusely. A plain film of the abdomen is obtained and shows free air under the diaphragm. Which of the following is most likely to be found in the operating room?

A. Necrotic bowel
B. Necrotic pancreas
C. Perforated duodenal ulcer
D. Perforated gallbladder
E. Perforated gastric ulcer

VIII-56. Which of the following is the source of this patient's peritonitis?

A. Blood
B. Bile
C. Foreign body
D. Gastric contents
E. Pancreatic enzymes

VIII-57. A 37-year-old female presents with a chief complaint of difficulty swallowing. She reports that she feels as if food gets stuck in her midchest. She notices no difference between liquids or solids but does note that the symptoms worsen when she eats hurriedly. She has had a 15-lb weight loss and reports regurgitation of undigested

VIII-57. *(Continued)*

food after eating. The patient undergoes barium swallow. What is the most likely diagnosis?

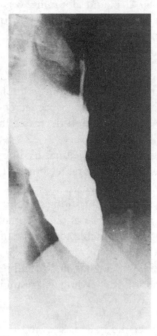

FIGURE VIII-57

A.   Esophageal stricture
B.   Esophageal spasm
C.   Achalasia
D.   Esophageal cancer
E.   CREST syndrome

VIII-58. Which of the following extraintestinal manifestations of inflammatory bowel disease typically worsens with exacerbations of disease activity?

A.   Ankylosing spondylitis
B.   Arthritis
C.   Nephrolithiasis
D.   Primary sclerosing cholangitis
E.   Uveitis

VIII-59. A 62-year-old male is evaluated in the emergency department for a complaint of vomiting and inability to tolerate oral intake. These symptoms have gradually progressed from occasional episodes of emesis after meals to an extent where the patient has not been able to tolerate solid foods for the last week. He notes no significant sensation of nausea before the emesis. Instead, the patient describes vomiting partially digested foods within a half hour of eating. The patient notes no abdominal pain. He has experienced an unintentional 30-lb weight loss over 6 months. The patient has a history of diabetes mellitus that is poorly controlled, with a glycosylated hemoglobin level of 8.9%. The patient underwent partial gastrectomy for peptic ulcer disease at age 52. His only medication is insulin therapy. On physical examination the patient is cachectic with a body mass index (BMI) of 17. He has

VIII-59. *(Continued)*

temporal wasting. The abdominal examination reveals no masses and is nontender. The bowel sounds are normoactive, and the patient's stool is hemoccult-negative. An abdominal film shows an enlarged gastric bubble with decompressed small intestinal loops. What is the most likely diagnosis?

A.   Small bowel obstruction
B.   Gastroparesis
C.   Esophageal stricture
D.   Gastric outlet obstruction
E.   Cholelithiasis

VIII-60. The patient in Question VIII-59 undergoes upper endoscopy for further evaluation, and a large mass is seen in the fundus of the stomach. Biopsy shows gastric adenocarcinoma. All the following are risk factors for the development of this disease *except*

A.   atrophic gastritis
B.   alcoholism
C.   *Helicobacter pylori* infection
D.   high consumption of salted and smoked food
E.   juvenile hamartomatous polyps

VIII-61. A 25-year-old female with cystic fibrosis is diagnosed with chronic pancreatitis. She is at risk for all of the following complications *except*

A.   vitamin B_{12} deficiency
B.   vitamin A deficiency
C.   pancreatic carcinoma
D.   niacin deficiency
E.   steatorrhea

VIII-62. All of the following statements regarding fat malabsorption are true *except*

A.   90% of pancreatic exocrine function must be lost before malabsorption ensues.
B.   Celiac disease is a commonly overlooked cause of nonspecific, gastrointestinal symptoms and fat malabsorption.
C.   Nutritional deficiencies are uncommon.
D.   Steatorrhea is formally established with >7 g of fat in stool over 24 h.
E.   Symptoms include greasy, foul-smelling stools that are difficult to flush.

VIII-63. A 64-year-old man seeks evaluation from his primary care physician because of chronic diarrhea. He reports that he has two or three large loose bowel movements daily. He describes them as markedly foul-smelling, and they often leave an oily ring in the toilet. He also notes that the bowel movements often follow heavy meals, but if he fasts or eats low-fat foods, the stools are more formed. Over the past 6 months, he has lost about 18 kg (40 lb). In this setting, he reports intermittent episodes of abdominal pain that can be quite se-

VIII-63. *(Continued)*

vere. He describes the pain as sharp and in a mid-epigastric location. He has not sought evaluation of the pain previously, but when it occurs, he will limit his oral intake and treat the pain with nonsteroidal antiinflammatory drugs. He notes the pain has not lasted for >48 h and is not associated with meals. His past medical history is remarkable for peripheral vascular disease and tobacco use. He currently smokes one pack of cigarettes daily. In addition, he drinks two to six beers daily. He has stopped all alcohol intake for up to a week at a time in the past without withdrawal symptoms. His current medications are aspirin, 81 mg daily, and albuterol metered dose inhaler (MDI) on an as-needed basis. On physical examination, the patient is thin but appears well. His body mass index is 18.2 kg/m^2. Vital signs are normal. Cardiac and pulmonary examinations are normal. The abdominal examination shows mild epigastric tenderness without rebound or guarding. The liver span is 12 cm to percussion and palpable 2 cm below the right costal margin. There is no splenomegaly or ascites present. There are decreased pulses in the lower extremities bilaterally. An abdominal radiograph demonstrates calcifications in the epigastric area, and CT scan confirms that these calcifications are located within the body of the pancreas. No pancreatic ductal dilatation is noted. An amylase level is 32 U/L, and lipase level is 22 U/L. What is the next most appropriate step in diagnosing and managing this patient's primary complaint?

A. Advise the patient to stop all alcohol use and prescribe pancreatic enzymes.
B. Advise the patient to stop all alcohol use and prescribe narcotic analgesia and pancreatic enzymes.
C. Perform angiography to assess for ischemic bowel disease.
D. Prescribe prokinetic agents to improve gastric emptying.
E. Refer the patient for endoscopic retrograde cholangiopancreatography (ERCP) for sphincterotomy

VIII-64. A 52-year-old male with chronic hepatitis C presents to your clinic with worsening right upper quadrant pain. Examination shows a palpable right upper quadrant mass. CT scan shows a large 5 × 5 cm mass in the right lobe of the liver. Serum α fetoprotein is elevated. A CT-guided liver biopsy confirms the suspected diagnosis of hepatocellular carcinoma. All the following are appropriate management steps *except*

A. referral for surgical resection
B. referral for radiofrequency ablation
C. referral for liver transplantation
D. systemic chemotherapy
E. chemoembolization

VIII-65. What is the most common cause of chronic secretory diarrhea in the United States?

VIII-65. *(Continued)*

A. Carcinoid tumor
B. Crohn's disease with ileitis
C. Lactose intolerance
D. Lymphocytic colitis
E. Medications

VIII-66. A 26-year-old female presents to the emergency room after ingesting "lots of pills." Her boyfriend discovered her crying on the floor of their bedroom, found numerous open bottles of acetaminophen scattered throughout the apartment, and called 911. He does not know when she first took the pills but had last seen her 4 h before finding her on the floor. She is nauseated and vomits once in the emergency room. Vital signs are stable. On examination she is alert and oriented. She has some epigastric tenderness to deep palpation. Otherwise the examination is unremarkable. Her acetaminophen level is 400 µg/mL. Liver function tests are normal. Which of the following statements regarding her clinical condition is *not* true?

A. *N*-acetylcysteine is the treatment of choice for acetaminophen toxicity.
B. Alkalinization of the urine is not effective as a treatment for acetaminophen toxicity.
C. The patient should be admitted and observed for 48 to 72 h as her hepatic injury may manifest days after the initial ingestion.
D. Liver transplantation is the only option for patients who develop fulminant hepatic failure from acetaminophen.
E. Normal liver function tests at presentation make significant liver injury unlikely.

VIII-67. A 37-year-old woman presents with abdominal pain, anorexia, and fever of 4 days' duration. The abdominal pain is mostly in the left lower quadrant. Her past medical history is significant for irritable bowel syndrome, diverticulitis treated 6 months ago, and status post-appendectomy. Since her last bout of diverticulitis she has increased her fiber intake and avoids nuts and popcorn. Review of systems is positive for weight loss, daily chills and sweats, and "bubbles" in her urinary stream. Her temperature is 39.6°C. A limited CT scan shows thickened colonic wall (5 mm) and inflammation with pericolic fat stranding. She is admitted with a presumptive diagnosis of diverticulitis. What is the most appropriate management for this patient?

A. A trial of rifaximin and a high-fiber diet
B. Bowel rest, ciprofloxacin, metronidazole, and ampicillin
C. Examination of the urine sediment
D. Measurement of 24-h urine protein
E. Surgical removal of the affected colon and exploration

VIII-68. A 69-year-old patient presents to the emergency department with hematochezia of 4 h duration. The patient is pale but alert and oriented. Blood pressure is 107/82 mmHg, respiratory rate is 24 breaths/min and heart rate is 96 beats/min. The hematocrit is 24%, with a baseline of 32%. Which of the following represents the best approach for localization of this patient's intestinal bleeding?

A. Angiography is most appropriate for this massive gastrointestinal (GI) bleed.
B. Angiography is of little utility since the patient is not stable.
C. Colonoscopy is better suited to localize bleeding, if it is massive.
D. Colonoscopy can be diagnostic and therapeutic in this mild GI bleed.
E. Immediate surgery with intraoperative localization is appropriate.

VIII-69. Chronic active hepatitis is most reliably distinguished from chronic persistent hepatitis by the presence of

A. extrahepatic manifestations
B. hepatitis B surface antigen in the serum
C. antibody to hepatitis B core antigen in the serum
D. a significant titer of anti-smooth-muscle antibody
E. characteristic liver histology

VIII-70. All the following are causes of bloody diarrhea *except*

A. *Campylobacter*
B. *Cryptosporidia*
C. *Escherichia coli*
D. *Entamoeba*
E. *Shigella*

VIII-71. A 36-year-old female with AIDS and a CD4 count of 35/mm^3 presents with odynophagia and progressive dysphagia. The patient reports daily fevers and a 20-lb weight loss. The patient has been treated with clotrimazole troches without relief. On physical examination the patient is cachectic with a body mass index (BMI) of 16 and a weight of 86 lb. The patient has a temperature of 38.2°C (100.8°F). She is noted to be orthostatic by blood pressure and pulse. Examination of the oropharynx reveals no evidence of thrush. The patient undergoes EGD, which reveals serpiginous ulcers in the distal esophagus without vesicles. No yellow plaques are noted. Multiple biopsies are taken that show intranuclear and intracytoplasmic inclusions in large endothelial cells and fibroblasts. What is the best treatment for this patient's esophagitis?

A. Ganciclovir
B. Thalidomide
C. Glucocorticoids
D. Fluconazole
E. Foscarnet

VIII-72. A 32-year-old man who recently returned from a vacation in Thailand presents with the acute onset of jaundice, abdominal pain, and vomiting. He is able to tolerate small amounts of food. His vital signs are normal, and an abdominal examination reveals a nontender liver edge palpable 2 cm below the right costal margin. His transaminases are elevated in the thousands, hepatitis B surface (anti-HBs) antigen is positive, and antibody to hepatitis B surface antigen is negative. He has no previous medical history and abstains from alcohol use. He has never received a hepatitis B vaccine series. Which of the following do you recommend as first-line management?

A. Conservative management and close follow-up
B. Hepatitis B vaccine series
C. Hospital admission and initiation of a liver transplant workup
D. Immediate entecavir treatment until anti-HBs is positive
E. Immediate lamivudine treatment for a planned 6-month course

VIII-73. A 48-year-old male seeks evaluation for diarrhea and malabsorptive symptoms. Approximately 5 years ago the patient underwent partial gastrectomy with gastrojejunostomy for a perforated duodenal ulcer. He had done well since that time until 5 months ago, when he developed abdominal pain and bloating after eating. In addition, the patient has had profound diarrhea that occurs after eating and is worse after he eats fatty foods. He notes that the diarrhea is foul-smelling and often leaves a greasy film in the toilet. On physical examination the patient is thin with a body mass index of 19. The examination is unremarkable. His stool is hemoccult-negative. Laboratory studies are remarkable except for an albumin of 3.1 g/dL. He is noted to have a hemoglobin of 9.6 mg/dL and a mean corpuscular volume (MCV) of 106. What is the most likely diagnosis?

A. Dumping syndrome
B. Bile reflux gastropathy
C. Afferent loop syndrome
D. Postvagotomy diarrhea
E. Zollinger-Ellison syndrome

VIII-74. A 17-year-old Asian student complains of abdominal bloating and diarrhea, particularly after eating ice cream and other milk products. Her parents have similar symptoms. The patient denies any weight loss or systemic symptoms. The physical examination is normal. Treatment with which of the following medications is most likely to reduce her symptoms?

A. Cholestyramine
B. Metoclopramide
C. Omeprazole
D. Viokase®
E. None of the above

VIII-75. A 36-year-old male presents with fatigue and tea-colored urine for 5 days. Physical examination reveals jaundice and tender hepatomegaly but is otherwise unremarkable. Laboratories are remarkable for an aspartate aminotransferase (AST) of 2400 U/L and an alanine aminotransferase (ALT) of 2640 U/L. Alkaline phosphatase is 210 U/L. Total bilirubin is 8.6 mg/dL. Which of the following is *least* likely to cause this clinical picture and these laboratory abnormalities?

A. Acute hepatitis A infection
B. Acute hepatitis B infection
C. Acute hepatitis C infection
D. Acetaminophen ingestion
E. Budd-Chiari syndrome

VIII-76. A 69-year-old man with Parkinson's disease is admitted to the intensive care unit from a long-term care facility for diarrhea, fever, and hypotension. He initially developed diarrhea 2 days ago, and this morning was found to have a blood pressure of 72/44 mmHg, heart rate of 130 beats/min, and temperature of 38.9°C. He began to receive IV fluids and was transferred to the emergency department. Upon arrival, he is lethargic and minimally responsive. He remains febrile and hypotensive with blood pressure 78/44 mmHg and heart rate 122 beats/min after 1 L of normal saline. His abdomen is tense and distended, with hypoactive bowel sounds. A plain radiograph of the abdomen shows "thumbprinting" or free air, but the colon is dilated to 8 cm. Stool is positive for occult blood. The patient undergoes colonoscopy, and the results are shown in Figure VIII-76 (Color Atlas). What is the most likely diagnosis?

A. Diverticulitis
B. Ischemic colitis
C. Pseudomembranous colitis
D. Salmonella infection
E. Ulcerative colitis

VIII-77. One week after removal of a biliary mass, a patient still has an elevated total bilirubin. The patient is recovering well and imaging of the hepatobiliary system shows no remaining pathology. The conjugated bilirubin is decreasing but remains elevated out of proportion to the patient's recovery. What is the best explanation for this finding?

A. Bilirubin bound to albumin
B. Gilbert's syndrome
C. Hibernating hepatocytes
D. Incomplete resection
E. Occult hemolysis

VIII-78. Which of the following statements regarding bilirubin metabolism is true?

A. Bacterial β-glucuronidases unconjugate the conjugated bilirubin that reaches the distal ileum.
B. Bilirubin solubilizes in the serum after conversion from biliverdin in the reticuloendothelial system.

VIII-78. *(Continued)*
C. Conjugated bilirubin is passively transported into the bile canalicular system.
D. Glutathione S-transferase B facilitates conjugated bilirubin's transport into the bile canalicular system.
E. Most bilirubin that reaches the terminal ileum is reabsorbed as urobilinogen.

VIII-79. A patient with alcoholic cirrhosis has increasing ascites despite dietary sodium control and diuretics. A paracentesis shows clear, turbid fluid. There are 2300 white blood cells (WBCs) and 150 red blood cells per microliter. The WBC differential shows 75% lymphocytes. Fluid protein is 3.2 g/dL and the serum-ascites albumin gradient (SAAG) is 1.0 g/dL. What is the most appropriate next study in this patient's management?

A. Adenosine deaminase activity of the ascitic fluid
B. CT scan of the liver
C. Peritoneal biopsy
D. None; consider transplant evaluation

VIII-80. A 24-year-old patient is admitted to the intensive care unit with obtundation and jaundice over 1–2 days. No further history is available. The following laboratory findings are obtained:

Total bilirubin 7.2 mg/dL
Direct bilirubin 4.0 mg/dL
AST: 1478 U/L
ALT: 1056 U/L
Alkaline phosphatase: 132 U/L
INR: 3.1
Albumin: 3.6 g/dL

All of the following tests are indicated *except*

A. antinuclear antibody (ANA)
B. ceruloplasmin
C. endoscopic retrograde cholangiopancreatography (ERCP)
D. hepatitis B surface antigen
E. toxicology screen

VIII-81. A defect in which of the following bilirubin metabolic processes will give rise to bilirubinuria?

A. Conjugation of bilirubin to glucuronic acid
B. Conversion of biliverdin to bilirubin
C. Transport of conjugated bilirubin into bile canaliculi
D. Transport of unconjugated bilirubin into hepatocytes

VIII-82. An 85-year-old woman is brought to a local emergency room by her family. She has been complaining of abdominal pain off and on for several days, but this morning states that this is the worst pain of her life. She is able to describe a sharp, stabbing pain in her abdomen. Her family reports that she has not been eating and seems to have no appetite. She has a past medical history of atrial fibrillation and hypercholesterolemia.

VIII-82. *(Continued)*

She has had two episodes of vomiting and in the ER experiences diarrhea that is hemoccult positive. On examination she is afebrile, with a heart rate of 105 beats/min and blood pressure of 111/69 mmHg. Her abdomen is mildly distended and she has hypoactive bowel sounds. She does not exhibit rebound tenderness or guarding. She is admitted for further management. Several hours after admission she becomes unresponsive. Blood pressure is difficult to obtain and at best approximation is 60/40 mmHg. She has a rigid abdomen. Surgery is called and the patient is taken for emergent laparotomy. She is found to have acute mesenteric ischemia. Which of the following is true regarding this diagnosis?

A. Mortality for this condition is >50%.
B. Risk factors include low-fiber diet and obesity.
C. The "gold standard" for diagnosis is CT scan of the abdomen.
D. The lack of acute abdominal signs in this case is unusual for mesenteric ischemia.
E. The splanchnic circulation is poorly collateralized.

VIII-83. The differential diagnosis of an isolated unconjugated (indirect) hyperbilirubinemia is limited. In a patient with isolated unconjugated hyperbilirubinemia, which of these historic findings would be unlikely?

A. Calcium bilirubinate gallstones
B. Cryoglobulinemia
C. History of gout
D. Spherocytosis
E. Recurrent long-bone pain crises

VIII-84. Which of the following statements regarding pancreatic cancer is true?

A. Five-year survival is ~5%.
B. Most cases present with locally confined disease amenable to a surgical cure.
C. Pancreatic adenocarcinomas occur most frequently in the pancreatic tail.
D. The median age of diagnosis is 49 years.
E. The most common tumor type is an islet cell tumor.

VIII-85. In a patient with ascites, which of the following physical examination findings suggests a superior vena cava obstruction instead of intrinsic hepatic cirrhosis?

A. Bulging flanks
B. Collateral venous flow downward toward the umbilicus
C. Everted umbilicus
D. Pulsatile liver
E. Venous hum at the umbilicus

VIII-86. You are managing a patient with stage IV pancreatic adenocarcinoma. The patient has been treated with gemcitabine for 16 weeks, and a recent CT scan confirms growth of the mass in the head of the pancreas over that time period. The patient has had biliary stents placed without complication for obstructive jaundice. The patient's weight is stable and he is able to perform activities of daily living independently. The patient wants to know what "the next step" is now that gemcitabine has seemed to fail. What is the most appropriate recommendation at this time?

A. Initiate treatment with 5-fluorouracil.
B. Make a referral to home hospice care.
C. Refer for debulking surgery.
D. Refer for external beam radiation as an adjunct to chemotherapy.
E. Suggest enrolling in a clinical trial.

VIII-87. All of the following physical examination clues are helpful for differentiating jaundice caused by hyperbilirubinemia from other causes *except*

A. greenish discoloration of the skin
B. involvement of the nasolabial folds
C. predominant involvement of palms, soles, and forehead
D. sparing of non-sun-exposed areas of the body
E. sparing of the sclera

VIII-88. When evaluating a patient with chronic ascites, a high (>1.1 g/dL) serum-ascites albumin gradient (SAAG) is consistent with all of the following diagnoses *except*

A. cirrhosis
B. congestive heart failure
C. constrictive pericarditis
D. hepatic vein thrombosis
E. nephrosis

VIII-89. You are managing a patient who complains of abdominal pain. The pain is located in the epigastric area and radiates to the back. Leaning forward improves the pain. The rest of the physical examination is unremarkable and there is no jaundice. The total bilirubin is 0.7 mg/dL and CA 19-9 level is within the normal range. An ultrasound of the abdomen shows a 2.5-cm well-circumscribed mass in the tail of the pancreas. There is no ductal dilation. A CT scan confirms the presence of a 2.5-cm spiculated mass in the tail of the pancreas with no surrounding lymphadenopathy or local extension. What is the next most appropriate step in this patient's management?

A. Magnetic resonance cholangiopancreatography
B. Refer for surgical resection
C. Serial CA 19-9 measurement
D. Ultrasound-guided biopsy

VIII. DISORDERS OF THE GASTROINTESTINAL SYSTEM

ANSWERS

VIII-1. **The answer is B.** *(Chap. 42)* Upper GI bleeding has an in-hospital mortality rate of 5–10%, with most people dying from their underlying disease rather than exsanguination. Peptic ulcers are the most common cause of upper GI bleeding requiring hospitalization, accounting for ~50% of cases. Other causes include variceal bleeding, Mallory-Weiss tears, erosive disease of the upper GI tract, malignancy, and unidentified. Characteristics of the ulcer at endoscopy provide important prognostic information. One-third of patients with an active bleeding vessel or a nonbleeding visible vessel will have rebleeding that requires surgery. Any finding other than a clean-based ulcer should prompt admission and monitoring for 3 days, as most rebleeding occurs within 3 days. Finding a clean-based ulcer is reassuring, and if the patient is stable and has no other indication for hospitalization, he may be safely discharged.

VIII-2. **The answer is C.** *(Chap. 302)* Alcoholic cirrhosis is the most common type of cirrhosis encountered in North America. Unlike some other causes of cirrhosis, pathologically it is characterized by small, fine scarring and small regenerative nodules. Therefore, it sometimes is referred to as micronodular cirrhosis. There is clear evidence that excessive alcohol use in the setting of chronic hepatitis C strongly increases the risk of development of cirrhosis; therefore, screening and appropriate counseling are essential. Ethanol results in proportionally greater inhibition of ALT synthesis than AST synthesis. Therefore, serum AST is usually disproportionately elevated relative to ALT, resulting in a ratio greater than 2. The liver is the site of vitamin K–dependent carboxylation of coagulation factors II, VII, IX, and X. Therefore, with progressive deterioration in liver function, elevations in serum prothrombin time result, as the extrinsic pathway of coagulation is primarily dependent on tissue factor and factor II. The intrinsic pathway contains many other unaffected factors, and the activated partial thromboplastin time is often normal. Unlike the case in acute viral hepatitis, acetaminophen toxicity, and vascular congestion, alcoholic injury to the liver rarely elevates the transaminases above levels in the hundreds. Elevations in the AST above 500 to 600 U/L should prompt a search for alternative or coincident diagnoses.

VIII-3. **The answer is D.** *(Chap. 307)* The pathophysiology of acute pancreatitis evolves in three phases. During the initial phase, pancreatic injury leads to intrapancreatic activation of digestive enzymes with subsequent autodigestion and acinar cell injury. Acinar injury is primarily attributed to activation of zymogens (proenzymes), particularly trypsinogen, by lysosomal hydrolases. Once trypsinogen is converted to trypsin, the activated trypsin further perpetuates the process by activating other zymogens to further autodigestion. The inflammation initiated by intrapancreatic activation of zymogens leads to the second phase of acute pancreatitis, with local production of chemokines that causes activation and sequestration of neutrophils in the pancreas. Experimental evidence suggests that neutrophilic inflammation can also cause further activation of trypsinogen, leading to a cascade of increasing acinar injury. The third phase of acute pancreatitis reflects the systemic processes that are caused by release of inflammatory cytokines and activated proenzymes into the systemic circulation. This process can lead to the systemic inflammatory response syndrome with acute respiratory distress syndrome, extensive third-spacing of fluids, and multiorgan failure.

VIII-4. The answer is D. *(Chap. 307)* Several risk factors have been identified that predict an increased risk of death in acute pancreatitis. Pancreatic necrosis and evidence of multiorgan failure have been the strongest predictors of death in multiple case series. This includes the presence of shock, hypoxemia (Pa_{O_2} <60 mmHg), renal failure (creatinine >2.0 mg/dL), hemoconcentration with a hematocrit >44%, and gastrointestinal bleeding. In addition, other clinical factors including obesity (BMI >30 kg/m^2) and age >70 predict poorer outcomes. Values of amylase and lipase have not been shown to predict the course of acute pancreatitis, and amylase can be spuriously elevated in the presence of a pH <7.32. The Ranson criteria include a variety of biochemical markers at admission and at 48 h that predict outcome in acute pancreatitis. This patient does not meet any of the Ranson criteria at admission (age >55, WBC count >16,000/μL, glucose >200 mg/dL, AST >250 U/L, LDH >350 U/L). A reevaluation at 48 h would be necessary to use Ranson criteria to assess the patient's risk of death to see if any of the six additional criteria had been fulfilled.

VIII-5. The answer is B. *(Chap. 294)* In acute appendicitis, tenderness is invariably present at some point in the development of the disorder. Tenderness to palpation will often occur at McBurney's point, anatomically located on a line one-third of the way between the anterior iliac spine and the umbilicus. Abdominal tenderness may be completely absent if there is a retrocecal or pelvic appendix, in which case the sole physical finding may be tenderness in the flank. This is the case with the patient in this scenario. The pain which began in the periumbilical region is pathognomonic for appendicitis. The differential diagnosis of acute appendicitis includes pelvic inflammatory disease, mesenteric lymphadenitis, ruptured ovarian follicle, nephrolithiasis, and pyelonephritis. Pelvic inflammatory disease is less likely because of the history and negative pelvic examination. The urinalysis does not suggest pyelonephritis. There is no history of chronic gastrointestinal disorder (e.g., Crohn's disease) associated with mesenteric lymphadenitis. Ruptured aortic aneurysm is not likely in a young person with no history of congenital atherosclerosis and would most likely present with shock, not inflammatory symptoms.

VIII-6. The answer is C. *(Chap. 307)* A diagnosis of pancreatitis is made in an appropriate clinical setting with abdominal pain radiating to the back and elevated amylase and lipase. Although there are many causes of acute pancreatitis, among the most common are medications, alcohol, and gallstones. This patient does not drink alcohol and right upper quadrant ultrasound does not show cholelithiasis, leaving medications as the likely etiology. Commonly associated drugs are sulfonamides, estrogens, 6-mercaptopurine, azathioprine, anti-HIV medications, and valproic acid. The patient was taking sulfamethoxazole, which is a sulfonamide. He should be advised to discontinue this medication, and different *Pneumocystis carinii* pneumonia prophylaxis should be prescribed. Alternative regimens include dapsone, aerosolized pentamidine, and atovaquone. Discontinuation of all *Pneumocystis* pneumonia prophylaxis with his degree of immune suppression is unadvisable.

VIII-7. The answer is C. *(Chap. 40)* Most causes of acute diarrhea are infectious. Dehydration is a feature of all infectious diarrheas and does not suggest bacterial etiology. Fever and bloody diarrhea are more suggestive. Immunocompromised hosts and the elderly are at greater risk for developing bacteremia and sepsis with certain pathogens, and they also may be less likely to have symptoms suggesting a bacterial pathogen. Stool cultures are typically sent in these populations unless symptoms are mild. See Figure VIII-7.

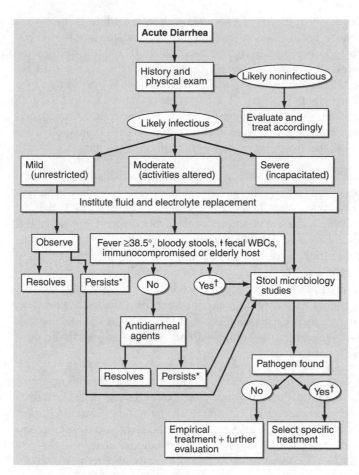

FIGURE VIII-7 Algorithm for the management of acute diarrhea. Consider empirical Rx before evaluation with (*) metronidazole and with (†) quinolone. WBCs, white blood cells.

VIII-8. **The answer is E.** *(Chap. 294)* This patient had acute peritonitis secondary to a ruptured appendix. Acute peritonitis is associated with decreased intestinal motor activity, resulting in distention of the intestinal lumen with gas and fluid. The accumulation of fluid in the bowel together with the lack of oral intake leads to rapid intravascular volume depletion. In the presence of systemic inflammation, there is also widespread third space loss. In the current case, this manifested as acute renal failure as well as in the cardiac and central nervous systems. Ureteral injury is a complication of abdominal surgery, but this patient's renal failure predated the procedure. Glomerulonephritis and acute interstitial nephritis are causes of acute renal failure; however, there is no evidence of red cell casts or pyuria. While not mentioned, it is likely that the urine specific gravity was elevated.

VIII-9. **The answer is B.** *(Chap. 40)* Rapid transit may accompany many diarrheas as a secondary or contributing process, but primary dysmotility is an unusual cause of diarrhea. Hormonal and metabolic processes may result in increased motility. Hyperthyroidism is often clinically accompanied by complaints of diarrhea. Medications are a common cause of diarrhea either as a primary cause of motility as in the case of "prokinetic" agents such as metoclopramide and erythromycin or as a side effect of bacterial overgrowth as in the case of prolonged antibiotic administration. Diabetes results in microvascular complications of peripheral and autonomic neuropathies and may result in gastroparesis and intestinal dysmotility. Irritable bowel syndrome is extremely common. It is characterized by disturbed intestinal and colonic motor and sensory responses to various stimuli. Clinically, it is characterized by episodes of constipation and diarrhea. Although disturbances in electrolytes may cause changes in intestinal motility, hypercalcemia is typically associated with constipation, not diarrhea.

VIII-10. **The answer is D.** *(Chap. 351)* Hemochromatosis is a common disorder of iron storage in which inappropriate increases in intestinal iron absorption result in excessive deposition in multiple organs but predominantly in the liver. There are two forms: hereditary hemochromatosis, in which the majority of cases are associated with mutations of the *HFE* gene, and secondary iron overload, which usually is associated with iron-loading anemias such as thalassemia and sideroblastic anemia. Serum ferritin testing and plasma iron studies can be very suggestive of the diagnosis, with the ferritin often >500 μg/L and transferrin saturation of 50 to 100%. However, these tests are not conclusive, and further testing is still required for the diagnosis. Although liver biopsy and evaluation for iron deposition or a hepatic iron index (μg/g dry weight)/56 × age > 2 is the definitive diagnosis, genetic testing is widely available today, and because of the high prevalence of *HFE* gene mutations associated with hereditary hemochromatosis, it is recommended for diagnostic evaluation. If the genetic testing is inconclusive, the invasive liver biopsy evaluation may be indicated.

VIII-11. **The answer is C.** *(Chap. 305)* Gallstones are very common, particularly in Western countries. Cholesterol stones are responsible for 80% of cases of cholelithiasis; pigment stones account for the remaining 20%. Cholesterol is essentially water-insoluble. Stone formation occurs in the setting of factors that upset cholesterol balance. Obesity, cholesterol-rich diets, high-calorie diets, and certain medications affect biliary secretion of cholesterol. Intrinsic genetic mutations in certain populations may affect the processing and secretion of cholesterol in the liver. Pregnancy results in both an increase in cholesterol saturation during the third trimester and changes in gallbladder contractility. Pigment stones are increased in patients with chronic hemolysis, cirrhosis, Gilbert's syndrome, and disruptions in the enterohepatic circulation. Although rapid weight loss and low-calorie diets are associated with gallstones, there is no evidence that a high-protein diet confers an added risk of cholelithiasis.

VIII-12. **The answer is E.** *(Chap. 291)* Anorectal abscess is more prevalent in immunocompromised patients such as those with diabetes, inflammatory bowel disease (IBD), or hematologic disorders and in persons who are HIV-positive. They are more common in men than women and typically occur in young patients. The greatly elevated erythrocyte sedimentation rate (ESR) (corrected for age) suggests an inflammatory state, and the skin nodules would suggest erythema nodosum. IBD often presents with perianal abscesses and is associated with an elevated ESR, erythema nodosum, and uveitis, among other extraintestinal manifestations. Giant cell arteritis would be uncommon in a patient this young. A normal glycosylated hemoglobin makes type 1 diabetes less likely. Acute sarcoidosis may present with erythema nodosum (Lofgrens syndrome), but there is typically mediastinal adenopathy. There is no association between sarcoidosis and perianal abscess. While patients with HIV infection commonly develop anorectal abscess, *Pneumocystis* pneumonia would typically present with respiratory complaints and an abnormal radiograph, not erythema nodosum.

VIII-13. **The answer is B.** *(Chap. 304)* The patient has advanced cirrhosis with a high risk of mortality as evidenced by his episode of spontaneous bacterial peritonitis. His diabetes and remote skin cancers are not absolute contraindications for liver transplantation, but active alcohol abuse is. The other absolute contraindications to transplantation are life-threatening systemic disease, uncontrolled infections, preexisting advanced cardiac or pulmonary disease, metastatic malignancy, and life-threatening congenital malignancies. Ongoing drug or alcohol abuse is an absolute contraindication, and patients who would otherwise be suitable candidates should immediately be referred to appropriate counseling centers to achieve abstinence. Once that is achieved for an acceptable period of time, transplantation can be considered. Indeed, alcoholic cirrhosis accounts for a substantial portion of the patients who undergo liver transplantation.

VIII-14. **The answer is E.** *(Chap. 298)* Hepatitis A is an acute, self-limited virus that is acquired almost exclusively via the fecal-oral route. It is classically a disease of poor hygiene and overcrowding. Outbreaks have been traced to contaminated water, milk, frozen raspberries and strawberries, green onions, and shellfish. Infection occurs mostly in children and young adults. It almost invariably resolves spontaneously and results in lifelong immunity. Fulminant disease occurs in ≤0.1% of cases, and there is no chronic form (in contrast to hepatitis B and C). Diagnosis is made by demonstrating a positive IgM antibody to HAV, as described in the case above. An IgG antibody to HAV indicates immunity, obtained by previous infection or vaccination. A small proportion of patients will experience relapsing hepatitis weeks to months after a full recovery to HAV infection. This too is self-limited. There is no approved antiviral therapy for hepatitis A disease. An inactivated vaccine has decreased the incidence of the disease, and it is recommended for all U.S. children, for high-risk adults, and for travelers to endemic areas. Passive immunization with immune globulin is also available, and it is effective in preventing clinical disease before exposure or during the early incubation period.

VIII-15.   **The answer is B.** *(Chap. 289)* The location and description of this form of IBD, without mention of other parts of the gastrointestinal tract involved and superficial involvement of the mucosa, is highly suggestive of ulcerative colitis (UC). The effects of cigarette smoking are different on UC and Crohn's disease (CD). The risk of UC in smokers is less than half that of nonsmokers. In contrast, smoking is associated with a twofold risk of CD. UC is equally common in males and females, whereas CD is more common in women. The age distribution is similar for UC and CD. Appendectomy is protective in UC. There is 0% concordance for dizygotic twins in UC and only 6% concordance for monozygotic disease. CD has a substantially higher concordance in monozygotic twins, but a 5% concordance in dizygotic twins.

VIII-16.   **The answer is D.** *(Chap. 291)* The patient has a chronic anal fissure. Anal fissures are often diagnosed by history alone, with severe anal pain made worse with defecation. There is often mild associated bleeding, but less than that seen with hemorrhoidal bleeding. The blood is usually described as staining the toilet paper or coating the stool. Associated conditions include constipation, trauma, Crohn's disease, and infections, including tuberculosis and syphilis. Acute anal fissures appear like a linear laceration, whereas chronic fissures show evidence of hypertrophied anal papillae at the proximal end with a skin tag at the distal end. Often the circular fibers of the internal anal sphincter can be seen at the base of the fissure. Acute anal fissures are treated conservatively with increased dietary fiber intake, topical anesthetics or glucocorticoids, and sitz baths. Treatment for chronic anal fissures is aimed at finding methods to decrease anal sphincter tone. Topical nitroglycerin or botulinum toxin injections may be used. In some cases surgical therapy becomes necessary with lateral internal sphincterotomy and dilatation.

VIII-17.   **The answer is C.** *(Chap. 40)* Diarrhea is loosely defined as passage of abnormally liquid or unformed stools and an increased frequency. This patient has pseudodiarrhea, based on frequent stools, but not diarrhea as they are not loose. Rectal urgency is a common complaint in pseudodiarrhea. The differential diagnosis for pseudodiarrhea includes proctitis and irritable bowel syndrome. Neuromuscular syndromes are linked most closely with fecal incontinence, and hypothyroid most commonly leads to constipation. Ulcerative colitis presents with a broad spectrum of symptoms and cannot be entirely ruled out, but bloody diarrhea, fevers, and pain are more typical. Viral gastroenteritis is acute, self-resolving, and causes diarrhea and often nausea.

VIII-18.   **The answer is E.** *(Chap. 287)* Gastric parietal cells create hydrochloric acid through a process of oxidative phosphorylation involving the H^+-K^+-ATPase pump. For each molecule of hydrochloric acid produced, a bicarbonate ion is released into the gastric venous circulation, creating the "bicarbonate tide." Control of gastric acid secretion is primarily under the control of the parasympathetic system. Postganglionic vagal fibers stimulate muscarinic receptors on parietal cells to increase acid secretion. In addition, cholinergic stimulation increases gastrin release from antral G cells as well as increasing the sensitivity of parietal cells to circulating gastrin. Gastrin is the most potent stimulus of gastric acid secretion and is released from antral G cells in response to cholinergic stimuli. Histamine is also a potent stimulus for gastric acid secretion. It is stored in enterochromaffin-like cells in the oxyntic glands of the stomach. Stimuli for histamine release include gastrin and acetylcholine. Finally, caffeine stimulates gastrin release and thus increases acid secretion.

The most important protein produced in the stomach for inhibition of acid secretion is somatostatin. It is produced in the D cells of the antrum, and its release is stimulated by a fall in the gastric pH to less than 3.0. Further inhibition of gastric acid secretion is mediated by intestinal peptides secreted from the duodenum in response to acid pH. These peptides include gastric inhibitory peptide and vasoactive intestinal peptide. Finally, hyperglycemia and hypertonic fluids in the duodenum also inhibit gastric acid secretion through mechanisms that are unknown.

VIII-19.   The answer is A.   *[Chap. 289; Am J Gastroenterol 98(12 Suppl):S31– S36, 2003.]*   Collagenous colitis is one of the two atypical (microscopic) colitides that should be included in the differential diagnosis of inflammatory bowel disease. The other atypical colitis is lymphocytic colitis. These diseases present typically with watery diarrhea in 50-to 60-year-old patients. Collagenous colitis is markedly more common in women, whereas lymphocytic colitis has an equal sex distribution. Both have normal endoscopic appearances and require biopsy for diagnosis. Collagenous colitis features increased subepithelial collagen deposition and inflammation with increased intraepithelial lymphocytes. In lymphocytic colitis, there is no collagen deposition and there are greater numbers of intraepithelial lymphocytes than is the case in collagenous colitis. Treatment for collagenous colitis ranges from sulfasalazine or mesalamine to glucocorticoids, depending on severity. Lymphocytic colitis is usually treated with 5-ASA or prednisone.

VIII-20 and VIII-21.   The answers are D and C.   *(Chap. 298)*   The clinical hallmarks of acute hepatitis are rarely subtle and consist of general malaise, abdominal discomfort, nausea, vomiting, anorexia, weight loss, headache, fever, and jaundice. After viral infection due to hepatitis B occurs, HBsAg begins to circulate in the blood and is the first viral marker present. HBsAg precedes elevated transaminases and clinical symptoms by several weeks. It becomes undetectable within several months of the onset of jaundice. The replicative stage of hepatitis B virus (HBV) infection is the time of maximal infectivity and liver-injury. HBeAg is a qualitative marker of this phase. HBV DNA is a quantitative marker of the infectivity and liver injury phase. Anti-HBc is typically the next detectable viral marker and precedes anti-HBs by weeks to months. As the appearance of anti-HBs is variable, some patients will experience a period of time in which the only detectable serum marker of hepatitis B infection will be anti-HBc. In other words, there is a gap, or "window period," between the disappearance of HBsAg and the appearance of anti-HBs. As more sensitive immunoassays have been developed, this window period has become less prevalent. The figure below demonstrates the time course of serum markers and clinical symptoms in acute hepatitis B.

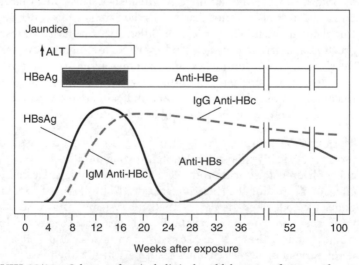

FIGURE VIII-20/21   Scheme of typical clinical and laboratory features of acute hepatitis B.

VIII-22.   The answer is C.   *(Chap. 287)*   Fasting gastrin levels can be elevated in a variety of conditions including atrophic gastritis with or without pernicious anemia, G-cell hyperplasia, and acid suppressive therapy (gastrin levels increase as a consequence of loss of negative feedback). The diagnostic concern in a patient with persistent ulcers following optimal therapy is Zollinger-Ellison syndrome (ZES). The result is not sufficient to make a diagnosis because gastrin levels may be elevated in a variety of conditions. Elevated basal acid secretion also is consistent with ZES, but up to 12% of patients with peptic ulcer disease may have basal acid secretion as high as 15 meq/h. Thus, additional testing is necessary. Gastrin levels may go up with a meal (>200%) but this test does not distinguish G-cell hyperfunction from ZES. The best test in this setting is the secretin stimulation test. An increase in gastrin levels >200 pg within 15 min of administering 2 µg/kg of secretin by intravenous bolus has a sensitivity and specificity of >90% for ZES. Endoscopic ultrasonography is useful in locating the gastrin-secreting tumor once the positive secretin test is obtained. Genetic testing for mutations in the gene that encodes the menin protein can detect the fraction of patients with gastrinomas that are a manifestation of Multiple Endocrine Neoplasia type I (Wermer's syndrome). Gastrinoma is the second most common tumor in this syndrome behind parathyroid adenoma, but its peak incidence is generally in the third decade.

VIII-23. **The answer is C.** *(Chap. 290)* Although this patient has signs and symptoms consistent with IBS, the differential diagnosis is large. Few tests are required for patients who have typical IBS symptoms and no alarm features. In this patient, alarm features include anemia, an elevated ESR, and evidence of WBCs in the stool. Alarm features warrant further investigation to rule out other gastrointestinal disorders such as diverticular disease or inflammatory bowel disease. Reassurance, stool bulking agents, and antidepressants are all therapies to consider if a patient does indeed have IBS

VIII-24. **The answer is E.** *(Chap. 290)* Up to 80% of patients with IBS also have abnormal psychiatric features; however, no single psychiatric diagnosis predominates. The mechanism is not well understood but may involve altered pain thresholds. Although these patients are hypersensitive to colonic stimuli, this does not carry over to the peripheral nervous system. Functional brain imaging shows disparate activation in, for example, the mid-cingulate cortex, but brain anatomy does not discriminate IBS patients from those without IBS. An association between a history of sexual abuse and IBS has been reported but not with sexually transmitted diseases. Patients with IBS do not have an increased risk of autoimmunity.

VIII-25. **The answer is B.** *(Chap. 302)* Severe right-sided heart failure may lead to chronic liver injury and cardiac cirrhosis. Elevated venous pressure leads to congestion of the hepatic sinusoids and of the central vein and centrilobular hepatocytes. Centrilobular fibrosis develops, and fibrosis extends outward from the central vein, not the portal triads. Gross examination of the liver shows a pattern of "nutmeg liver." Although transaminases are typically mildly elevated, severe congestion, particularly associated with hypotension, may result in dramatic elevation of AST and ALT 50- to 100-fold above normal. Budd-Chiari syndrome, or occlusion of the hepatic veins or inferior vena cava, may be confused with congestive hepatopathy. However, the signs and symptoms of congestive heart failure are absent in patients with Budd-Chiari syndrome, and these patients can be easily distinguished clinically from those with heart failure. Venoocclusive disease may result from hepatic irradiation and high-dose chemotherapy in preparation for hematopoietic stem cell transplantation. It is not a typical complication of liver transplantation. Although echocardiography is a useful tool for assessing left and right ventricular function, findings may be unimpressive in patients with constrictive pericarditis. A high index of suspicion for constrictive pericarditis (e.g., prior episodes of pericarditis, mediastinal irradiation) should lead to a right-sided heart catheterization with demonstration of "square root sign," limitation of right heart filling pressure in diastole that is suggestive of restrictive cardiomyopathy. Cardiac magnetic resonance imaging may also be helpful in determining which patients should proceed to cardiac surgery.

VIII-26. **The answer is B.** *(Chap. 14)* The pain of peritoneal inflammation is steady, aching, and localized predominantly over the affected area(s). Somatic nerves supplying the parietal peritoneum transmit the pain stimulus, allowing localization. The pain of peritoneal inflammation is invariably accentuated by pressure or changes in tension of the peritoneum. Asking a patient to cough will increase the intraabdominal pressure and lead to rebound tenderness without palpating the abdomen. Another characteristic of peritoneal inflammation is the tonic reflex spasm of the abdominal musculature. Costovertebral angle tenderness, a sign suggestive of pyelonephritis, and heme-positive stools are neither sensitive nor specific for peritonitis. The presence or quality of bowel sounds are not reliable physical examination findings to distinguish an acute abdomen from a more benign diagnosis.

VIII-27. **The answer is D.** *(Chap. 300)* In the course of acute hepatitis B, HBeAg positivity is common and usually transient. Persistence of HBeAg in the serum for >3 months indicates an increased likelihood of development of chronic hepatitis B. In chronic hepatitis B, presence of HBeAg in the serum indicates ongoing viral replication and increased infectivity. It is also a surrogate for inflammatory liver injury but not fibrosis. The development of antibody to HBeAg (anti-HBe) is indicative of the nonreplicative phase of HBV infection. During this phase, intact virions do not circulate and infectivity is less. Currently, quantification of HBV DNA with polymerase chain reaction allows risk stratification as $<10^3$ virions/μL is the approximate threshold for liver injury and infectivity.

VIII-28. **The answer is B.** *(Chap. 286)* Diffuse esophageal spasm is a disorder of esophageal motility marked by disorganized nonperistaltic contractions. The contractions are due to dysfunction of the inhibitory nerves, with pain correlating with contractions of long duration and large amplitude. Clinically, patients present with sharp substernal chest pain that may mimic cardiac disease with radiation to the arms, chest, and jaw. Symptoms last for a few seconds to minutes and may be related to swallowing or emotional stress. Dysphagia with or without pain often coexists. The presence of cardiac disease needs to be evaluated before consideration of a noncardiac cause of chest pain. The diagnostic procedure of choice is barium swallow, which shows loss of normal peristaltic contractions below the level of the aortic arch. Instead, there are numerous uncoordinated simultaneous contractions that produce multiple ripples in the esophageal wall with sacculation and pseudodiverticula. This creates the characteristic appearance of a "corkscrew" esophagus. Treatment is aimed primarily at preventing these contractions with medications that cause smooth muscle relaxation, such as nitrates and calcium channel blockers. The other options listed describe other diseases of the esophagus. A beaklike appearance of the distal esophagus is characteristic of achalasia. Scleroderma causes atrophy of the smooth muscle within the lower two-thirds of the esophagus and is represented on barium swallow as dilation of the distal esophagus with loss of peristaltic contractions. Gastroesophageal reflux disease is a common disorder that affects 15% of persons at least once per week and is marked by loss of lower esophageal sphincter tone with reflux of barium back into the distal esophagus. Esophageal narrowing with apple-core lesions is typical of esophageal cancer.

VIII-29. **The answer is C.** *(Chap. 298)* The current hepatitis B vaccine is a recombinant vaccine consisting of yeast-derived hepatitis B surface antigen particles. A strategy of vaccinating only high-risk individuals in the United States has been shown to be ineffective, and universal vaccination against hepatitis B is now recommended. Pregnancy is *not* a contraindication to vaccination. Vaccination should ideally be performed in infancy. Routine evaluation of hepatitis serologies is not cost-effective and is not recommended. The vaccine is given in three divided intramuscular doses at 0, 1, and 6 months.

VIII-30. **The answer is B.** *(Chap. 305)* The clinical presentation is consistent with a cholestatic picture. Painless jaundice always requires an extensive workup, as many of the underlying pathologies are ominous and early detection and intervention often offers the only hope for a good outcome. The gallbladder showed no evidence of stones and the patient shows no evidence of clinical cholecystitis, and so a HIDA scan is not indicated. Similarly, antibiotics are not necessary at this point. The cholestatic picture without significant elevation of the transaminases on the liver function tests makes acute hepatitis unlikely. Antimitochondrial antibodies are elevated in cases of primary biliary cirrhosis (PBC), which may present in a similar fashion. However, PBC is far more common in women than in men, and the average age of onset is the fifth or sixth decade. The lack of an obvious lesion on CT scan does not rule out a source of the cholestasis in the biliary tree. Malignant causes such as cholangiocarcinoma and tumor of the ampulla of Vater and nonmalignant causes such as sclerosing cholangitis and Caroli's disease may be detected only by direct visualization with ERCP. ERCP is useful both diagnostically and therapeutically as stenting procedures may be done to alleviate the obstruction.

VIII-31. **The answer is C.** *(Chap. 42)* Randomized controlled trials of IV PPI therapy for upper gastrointestinal (GI) bleeding have shown that this therapy decreased further bleeding, but not mortality, for patients with high-risk ulcers (active bleeding, visible vessel, adherent clot) at the time of endoscopy. Instituting IV PPI for all patients with upper GI bleeding does not significantly improve outcomes. Studies have shown a link between long-term usage of PPIs and osteoporosis, but this does not preclude the acute use of PPI in an osteoporotic patient if there is a compelling indication.

VIII-32. **The answer is B.** *(Chap. 42)* Hemoglobin/hematocrit levels often do not change acutely in acute GI bleeding. It may take up to 72 hours to see the hemoglobin fall. Moreover, gastric lavage can be non-bloody in 18% of cases of upper GI bleeding. This is seen when there is a duodenal source of bleeding or when the nasogastric tube does not enter the stomach. Testing non-bloody gastric aspirates for occult blood is not useful. Therefore, when there is a clinical suspicion for an upper GI bleed, endoscopy should be performed. CT scanning the abdomen will not be helpful in evaluating an upper GI bleed in the absence of other findings. Rechecking another hematocrit will not alter the indication for upper endoscopy.

VIII-33 and VIII-34. **The answers are D and D.** *(Chap. 297)* Gilbert's syndrome is characterized by a mild unconjugated hyperbilirubinemia. UGT1A1 activity is typically reduced to 10 to 35% of normal, resulting in impaired conjugation. Diagnosis occurs during young adulthood. Exacerbations occur during times of stress, fatigue, alcohol use, or decreased caloric intake. Episodes are self-limited and benign. No treatment is required, and patient reassurance is recommended. Crigler-Najjar syndrome type 1 is a congenital disease characterized by more dramatic elevations in bilirubin that occur first in the neonatal period. Dubin-Johnson syndrome is another congenital hyperbilirubinemia. However, it is a predominantly conjugated hyperbilirubinemia. Medications and toxins may produce jaundice in the setting of cholestasis or hepatocellular injury. Similarly, medications may induce hemolysis; however, the normal hematocrit, LDH, and haptoglobin eliminate hemolysis as a possibility. Obstructive cholelithiasis is characterized by right upper quadrant pain that is often exacerbated by fatty meals. The absence of symptoms or elevation in other liver function tests also makes this diagnosis unlikely.

VIII-35. **The answer is D.** *(Chaps. 39 and 286)* A Zenker's diverticulum typically causes halitosis and regurgitation of saliva and particles of food consumed several days earlier. When a Zenker's diverticulum fills with food, it may produce dysphagia by compressing the esophagus. Gastric outlet obstruction can cause bloating and regurgitation of newly ingested food. Gastrointestinal disorders associated with scleroderma include esophageal reflux, the development of wide-mouthed colonic diverticula, and stasis with bacterial overgrowth. Achalasia typically presents with dysphagia for both solids and liquids. Gastric retention caused by the autonomic neuropathy of diabetes mellitus usually results in postprandial epigastric discomfort and bloating.

VIII-36. **The answer is E.** *(Chaps. 88 and 295)* The liver is particularly vulnerable to invasion by tumor cells because of its dual blood supply by the portal vein and the hepatic arteries. Most patients with liver metastases present with symptoms from the primary tumor. Sometimes hepatic involvement is suggested by features of active hepatic disease, including abdominal pain, hepatomegaly, and ascites. Liver biochemical tests are often the first clue to metastatic disease, but the elevations are often mild and nonspecific. Typically, alkaline phosphatase is the most sensitive indicator of metastatic disease. Lung, breast, and colon cancer are the most common tumors that metastasize to the liver. Melanoma, particularly ocular melanoma, also commonly seeds the hepatic circulation. Prostate cancer is a much less common cause of hepatic metastases.

VIII-37.   The answer is C. *(Chap. 288)*   The combination of steatorrhea, weight loss, and migratory large joint arthralgias is consistent with the diagnosis of Whipple's disease. Whipple's disease may also cause cardiac and central nervous system (CNS) disease, including dementia. It is caused by chronic infection with *T. whippelii*. The disease occurs predominantly in middle-aged white men. Whipple's disease may also be diagnosed by a small bowel (or other involved organ) showing macrophages staining positive for PAS and containing the small Whipple's bacillus. Treatment for Whipple's disease requires prolonged (1 year) therapy with trimethoprim-sulfamethoxazole or chloramphenicol. Antiendomysial antibodies, antigliadin IgA antibodies, and the small bowel biopsy findings described above are characteristic of celiac sprue. Antibiotic-associated colitis caused by *C. difficile* does not cause steatorrhea.

VIII-38.   The answer is D. *[Chap. 289, Cochrane Database Syst Rev 2007 Oct 17;(4)]*   Despite being described as a clinical entity for over a century, the etiology of IBD remains cryptic. Current theory is related to an interplay between inflammatory stimuli in genetically predisposed individuals. Recent studies have identified a group of genes or polymorphisms that confer risk of IBD. Multiple microbiologic agents, including some that reside as "normal" flora, may initiate IBD by triggering an inflammatory response. Anaerobic organisms (e.g., *Bacteroides* and *Clostridia* spp.) may be responsible for the induction of inflammation. Other organisms, for unclear reasons, may have the opposite effect. These "probiotic" organisms include *Lactobacillus* spp., *Bifidobacterium* spp., *Taenia suis* and *Saccharomyces boulardii*. *Shigella*, *Escherichia*, and *Campylobacter* spp. are known to promote inflammation. Studies of probiotic therapy in adults and children with IBD have shown potential benefit for reducing disease activity.

VIII-39.   The answer is A. *(Chaps. 44 and 296)*   Diagnostic paracentesis is part of the routine evaluation in a patient with ascites. Fluid should be examined for its gross appearance, protein content, cell count and differential, and albumin. Cytologic and culture studies should be performed when one suspects infection or malignancy. The serum-ascites albumin gradient (SAG) offers the best correlation with portal pressure. A high gradient (>1.1 g/dL) is characteristic of uncomplicated cirrhotic ascites and differentiates ascites caused by portal hypertension from ascites not caused by portal hypertension in more than 95% of cases. Conditions that cause a low gradient include more "exudative" processes such as infection, malignancy, and inflammatory processes. Similarly, congestive heart failure and nephrotic syndrome cause high gradients. In this patient the SAG is 1.5 g/dL, indicating a high gradient. The low number of leukocytes and polymorphonuclear cells makes bacterial or tubercular infection unlikely. Chylous ascites often is characterized by an opaque milky fluid with a triglyceride level greater than 1000 mg/dL in addition to a low SAG.

VIII-40.   The answer is B. *(Chap. 40)*   This patient is most likely to have fecal impaction with overflow diarrhea around the impacted area. Colonoscopy is not necessary for diagnosis and may not be needed therapeutically depending on the success of manual disimpaction. *C. difficile* infection should always be considered in institutionalized persons, particularly the elderly, even in the absence of antecedent diarrhea. However, a negative stool antigen carries very good negative predictive value. Stool culture is indicated in the elderly with moderate to severe diarrhea, but in this case the more likely diagnosis should be ruled out before this is done. Viral gastroenteritis is also possible, but a pathogen is typically not sought as these syndromes self-resolve and there is no available antiviral agent.

VIII-41.   The answer is C. *(Chap. 307)*   All of the listed choices are causes of acute pancreatitis. Gallstone disease remains the most common cause, responsible for 30–60% of all acute pancreatitis. The second most common cause of acute pancreatitis is alcohol (15–30%). The risk of pancreatitis in alcoholics is quite low, with only 5 cases of pancreatitis per 100,000 individuals. All of the other possible answers each account for <10% of all acute pancreatitis.

VIII-42. **The answer is D.** *(Chap. 290)* Serotonin receptor antagonists enhance the sensitivity of the afferent neurons projecting from the gut. Alosetron, a 5-HT$_3$ receptor antagonist, reduces perception of painful visceral stimulation, induces rectal relaxation, and delays colonic transport in patients with IBS. Clinical studies have shown the long-term efficacy of alosetron for IBS. However, in postrelease surveillance, 84 cases of ischemic colitis were reported soon after patients were placed on alosetron. Of these, 44 cases required surgery and 4 patients died. Most cases developed within 30 days of starting the medication, and many were within 1 week. Alosetron was withdrawn voluntarily in 2000 but has been reintroduced with a strict monitoring program. Given the temporal relation and compatible clinical presentation, that is the most likely diagnosis in this case. A CT scan would likely show diffuse colitis. Therapy involves discontinuation of the drug, supportive therapy, and possible surgical resection. The other diagnoses may present with a similar clinical picture and should be on the differential diagnosis.

VIII-43. **The answer is C.** *(Chap. 291)* This patient has symptoms (social isolation), signs (foul odor), and risk factors (multiparity) for procidentia (rectal prolapse) and fecal incontinence. Procidentia is far more common in women than men and is often associated with pelvic floor disorders. It is not uncommon for these patients to become socially withdrawn and suffer from depression because of the associated fecal incontinence. The foul odor is a result of poor perianal hygiene due to the prolapsed rectum. Although depression in the elderly is an important medical problem, it is too premature in the evaluation to initiate medical therapy for depression. Occult malignancy and thyroid abnormalities may cause fecal incontinence and depression, but a physical examination would be diagnostic and avoid costly tests. Often patients are concerned they have a rectal mass or carcinoma. Examination after an enema often makes the prolapse apparent. Medical therapy is limited to stool bulking agents or fiber. Surgical correction is the mainstay of therapy.

VIII-44. **The answer is B.** *(Chap. 302)* The presence of cirrhosis in an elderly woman with no prior risk factors for viral or alcoholic cirrhosis should raise the possibility of primary biliary cirrhosis (PBC). It is characterized by chronic inflammation and fibrous obliteration of intrahepatic ductules. The cause is unknown, but autoimmunity is assumed as there is an association with other autoimmune disorders, such as autoimmune thyroiditis, CREST syndrome, and the sicca syndrome. The vast majority of patients with symptomatic disease are women. AMA is positive in over 90% of patients with PBC and only rarely is positive in other conditions. This makes it the most useful initial test in the diagnosis of PBC. Since there are false-positives, if AMA is positive, a liver biopsy is performed to confirm the diagnosis. The 24-h urine copper collection is useful in the diagnosis of Wilson's disease. Hepatic failure from Wilson's disease typically occurs before age 50 years. Hemochromatosis may result in cirrhosis. It is associated with lethargy, fatigue, loss of libido, discoloration of the skin, arthralgias, diabetes, and cardiomyopathy. Ferritin levels are usually increased, and the most suggestive laboratory abnormality is an elevated transferrin saturation percentage. Although hemochromatosis is a possible diagnosis in this case, PBC is more likely in light of the clinical scenario. Although chronic hepatitis B and hepatitis C are certainly in the differential diagnosis and must be ruled out, they are unlikely because of the patient's history and lack of risk factors.

VIII-45. **The answer is D.** *(Chap. 289)* Methotrexate, azathioprine, cyclosporine, tacrolimus, or anti-tumor necrosis factor (TNF) antibody are reasonable options for patients with CD, depending on the extent of macroscopic disease. Pneumonitis is a rare but serious complication of methotrexate therapy. Primary sclerosing cholangitis is an extraintestinal manifestation of inflammatory bowel disease (IBD). Pancreatitis is an uncommon complication of azathioprine, and IBD patients treated with azathioprine are at fourfold increased risk of developing a lymphoma. Anti-TNF antibody therapy is associated with an increased risk of tuberculosis, disseminated histoplasmosis, and a number of other infections.

VIII-46. **The answer is G.** *(Chap. 40)* Chronic constipation occurs from inadequate fiber or fluid consumption, disordered colonic transit, disordered anorectal function due to a neurogastroenterologic disorder, drugs, or systemic disorders that impact the gastrointestinal tract. Constipation is more often addressed from a therapeutic position by clinicians. Yet it is important not to overlook the fact that constipation can be a presenting feature of a large number of medical, surgical, and psychiatric conditions. Therefore, new or severe constipation should prompt a complete history and physical examination to ensure a key diagnosis is not being overlooked.

TABLE VIII-46   Causes of Constipation in Adults

Types of Constipation and Causes	Examples
Recent onset	
Colonic obstruction	Neoplasm; stricture: ischemic, diverticular, inflammatory
Anal sphincter spasm	Anal fissure, painful hemorrhoids
Medications	
Chronic	
Irritable bowel syndrome	Constipation-predominant, alternating
Medications	Ca^{2+} blockers, antidepressants
Colonic pseudo-obstruction	Slow-transit constipation, megacolon (rare Hirschsprung's, Chagas)
Disorders of rectal evacuation	Pelvic floor dysfunction; anismus; descending perineum syndrome; rectal mucosal prolapse; rectocele
Endocrinopathies	Hypothyroidism, hypercalcemia, pregnancy
Psychiatric disorders	Depression, eating disorders, drugs
Neurologic disease	Parkinsonism, multiple sclerosis, spinal cord injury
Generalized muscle disease	Progressive systemic sclerosis

VIII-47. **The answer is B.** *(Chap. 291)* This is a classic presentation of familial Mediterranean fever, an inherited disease most common in Armenians, Arabs, Turks, and non-Ashkenazi Jews. Febrile episodes begin in early childhood, with more than 90% of patients experiencing the first attack by age 20. Fever is invariably a feature of an acute attack. Other common features include severe serositis presenting most frequently as peritonitis or pleuritis. The pain is often so severe that exploratory laparotomy may be performed to search for a source of peritonitis. CT imaging shows only small amounts of free fluid in the abdomen or pleural space. On laboratory testing this fluid represents sterile neutrophilia in response to the intense serosal inflammation. Other manifestations of the disease include acute monoarthritis with large sterile, neutrophilic effusions and a rash that resembles erysipelas on the lower extremity. The attacks are self-limited and resolve within 72 h, although the joint symptoms may persist. Amyloidosis as a result of chronic inflammation is a common manifestation late in the disease. Laboratory studies are nonspecific, showing changes expected with acute inflammation. Diagnosis usually can be made with clinical criteria alone, although there is gene testing available for the most common mutations that cause the disease. Treatment is targeted at preventing attacks with colchicine, a drug that inhibits microtubule formation and has been demonstrated to decrease the frequency and intensity of the attacks. In addition, it can prevent the development of amyloidosis. There are no alternative therapies available, although investigations into the use of interferon and tumor necrosis factor inhibitors are ongoing.

VIII-48. **The answer is A.** *(Chap. 298)* A clear distinction between viral etiologies of acute hepatitis cannot be made on clinical or epidemiologic features alone. This patient is at risk of many forms of hepatitis due to his lifestyle. Given his occupation in food services, from a public health perspective it is important to make an accurate diagnosis. Serologies must be obtained to make a diagnosis. While hepatitis C virus typically does not present as an acute hepatitis, this is not absolute. Hepatitis E virus infects men and women equally and resembles hepatitis A virus in clinical presentation. This patient should be questioned regarding IV drug use, and in addition to hepatitis serologies, an HIV test should be performed.

VIII-49. **The answer is A.** *(Chap. 294)* Appendicitis occurs in every 500–2000 pregnancies and tends to be most common during the second trimester. It is important to consider acute appendicitis in this population due to the frequent occurrence of mild abdominal discomfort, nausea, and vomiting during pregnancy. The unremarkable urine analysis makes pyelonephritis or nephrolithiasis less likely. Rupture of a Graafian follicle (mittelschmerz) occurs during menses, not pregnancy. Fitz-Hugh–Curtis (perihepatitis) syndrome could present with these symptoms during pregnancy; however, there is no cervicitis on examination, and the initial periumbilical pain makes appendicitis more likely.

VIII-50. **The answer is D.** *(Chap. 288)* This patient has a stool osmolality gap (measured stool osmolality – calculated stool osmolality) of <50 mosmol/L, suggesting a secretory rather than an osmotic cause for diarrhea. Secretory causes of diarrhea include toxin-mediated diarrhea (cholera, enterotoxigenic *Escherichia coli*) and intestinal peptide–mediated diarrhea in which the major pathophysiology is a luminal or circulating secretagogue. The distinction between secretory diarrhea and osmotic diarrhea aids in forming a differential diagnosis. Secretory diarrhea will not decrease substantially during a fast and has a low osmolality gap. Osmotic diarrhea will generally decrease during a fast and has a high (>50 mosmol/L) osmolality gap. Celiac sprue, chronic pancreatitis, lactase deficiency, and Whipple's disease all cause an osmotic diarrhea.

VIII-51. **The answer is B.** *(Chaps. 88 and 305)* Cholangiocarcinoma occurs most commonly in the sixth and seventh decades of life. Patients often present with symptoms and signs of biliary obstruction, including right upper quadrant pain, jaundice, and cholangitis. Unfortunately, most patients present with unresectable disease, and 5-year survival is dismal. Diagnosis is often made by cholangiography. Chronic infection with the liver flukes *Opisthorchis* and *Clonorchis* confers an added risk of cholangiocarcinoma. Similarly, exposure to toxic dyes in the automobile and rubber industries, primary sclerosing cholangitis, and congenital malformations of the biliary tree such as choledochal cysts and Caroli disease predispose to the development of cholangiocarcinoma. Cholelithiasis is not clearly a predisposing factor.

VIII-52. **The answer is B.** *(Chaps. 88 and 295)* Hepatic adenomas are benign tumors of the liver found in women in the third and fourth decades. Hormones are thought to play an essential pathophysiologic role. The risk of adenomas is increased among those taking oral contraceptives, anabolic steroids, and exogenous androgens. These adenomas typically occur in the right lobe and are often asymptomatic and are discovered incidentally. Clinical features may include pain or a palpable mass. Diagnosis is usually made by a combination of modalities, including ultrasound, CT, MRI, and nuclear medicine. The risk of malignant transformation is low. Surveillance is recommended for asymptomatic small lesions. However, since this patient has significant pain, an intervention is necessary. In light of the relationship with hormones and the low risk of malignant transformation, the first option would be discontinuation of oral contraceptive therapy and follow-up in 4 to 6 weeks. Tumors that do not shrink after discontinuation of oral contraceptives may require surgical excision. RFA has no established role, and biopsy is not indicated as the clinical picture is highly suggestive of a benign lesion. Advice should be given to patients with large adenomas that pregnancy may exacerbate symptoms and promote hemorrhage.

VIII-53. **The answer is C.** *(Chap. 307)* Though it is widely used as a screening test to rule out acute pancreatitis in a patient with acute abdominal or back pain, only about 85% of patients with acute pancreatitis have an elevated serum amylase level. Confounding issues include delay between symptoms and the obtaining of blood samples, the presence of chronic pancreatitis, and hypertriglyceridemia, which can falsely lower levels of both amylase and lipase. Because the serum amylase level may be elevated in other conditions, such as renal insufficiency, salivary gland lesions, tumors, burns, and diabetic ketoacidosis, as well as in other abdominal diseases, such as intestinal obstruction and peritonitis, amylase isoenzyme levels have been used to distinguish among these possibilities. Therefore, the pancreatic isoenzyme level can be used to diagnose acute pancreatitis more specifically in the setting of a confounding condition. The serum lipase assay is less subject to confounding variables. However, the sensitivity of the serum lipase level for acute pancreatitis may be as low as 70%. Therefore, recommended screening for acute pancreatitis includes both serum amylase and serum lipase.

VIII-54. **The answer is E.** *(Chap. 307)* This patient present with acute pancreatitis related to alcohol use and has a past history of similar episodes. His presentation does not suggest severe pancreatitis. In this setting, 85–90% of patients will recover spontaneously in 3–7 days with conservative management. Analgesics should be given to control pain and will likely also aid in decreasing this patient's blood pressure. In addition, patients with pancreatitis are frequently volume-depleted due to a variety of factors, including decreased oral intake, vomiting, and third-spacing of fluid with increased vascular permeability. Intravenous volume repletion should be initially given at a high rate to replace volume loss on presentation. After initial volume resuscitation, IV fluids containing glucose should be continued until the patient is able to tolerate oral feeding. In mild pancreatitis, no oral alimentation is recommended until pain has adequately resolved, because the time period that NPO status is maintained is expected to be ≤1 week. In severe cases of pancreatitis, individuals are hypermetabolic and are frequently expected to remain NPO for extended periods. In this setting, alimentation with nasojejunal feeding is preferred over total parenteral nutrition as there appears to be less infection with use of the enteral feedings. This is thought to be due to better maintenance of the gut mucosal barrier function with enteral feeding. Use of nasogastric suctioning offers no clinical benefit in mild pancreatitis, and its use is considered elective.

VIII-55 and VIII-56. **The answers are C and D.** *(Chap. 294)* The patient presents with several months of epigastric abdominal pain that is worse after eating. His symptoms are highly suggestive of peptic ulcer disease, with the worsening pain after eating suggesting a duodenal ulcer. The current presentation with acute abdomen and free air under the diaphragm diagnoses perforated viscus. Perforated gallbladder is less likely in light of the duration of symptoms and the absence of the significant systemic symptoms that often accompany this condition. As the patient is relatively young with no risk factors for mesenteric ischemia, necrotic bowel from an infarction is highly unlikely. Pancreatitis can have a similar presentation, but a pancreas cannot perforate and liberate free air. Peritonitis is most commonly associated with bacterial infection, but it can be caused by the abnormal presence of physiologic fluids, for example, gastric contents, bile, pancreatic enzymes, blood, or urine, or by foreign bodies. In this case peritonitis most likely is due to the presence of gastric juice in the peritoneal cavity after perforation of a duodenal ulcer has allowed these juices to leave the gut lumen.

VIII-57. **The answer is C.** *(Chap. 286)* The patient has typical symptoms of and barium findings for achalasia, an esophageal disease marked by abnormal motility and failure of the lower esophageal sphincter to relax normally with swallowing. The underlying abnormality is loss of the intramural neurons that control the inhibitory neurotransmitters. Other diseases that can cause secondary achalasia through destruction of these neurons include Chagas' disease, malignancy, and viral infections. Typical clinical symptoms of achalasia include dysphagia with both solids and liquids equally and worsening of symptoms with emotional stressors and rapid eating. Aspiration and regurgitation of undigested food are also common. The presence of esophageal reflux symptoms is inconsistent with the diagnosis of achalasia. The course is usually progressive, with weight loss occurring over several months. Diagnosis can be made from the classic appearance on barium swallow of esophageal dilatation with a beaklike appearance of the lower esophagus representing the failure of the lower esophageal sphincter (LES) to relax. Other diagnostic maneuvers include manometry demonstrating increased LES tone, and endoscopy should be performed to exclude coincident carcinoma. Treatment is often difficult. Nitrates and calcium channel blockers offer short-term benefits for relief of symptoms but lose efficacy over time. Endoscopic injections of botulinum toxin are also effective for short periods but may lead to fibrosis with repeated injections. Balloon dilatation is effective in approximately 85% of patients with the side effect of perforation or bleeding. Finally, some patients ultimately require surgical intervention with myotomy, which has equal success compared to balloon dilatation.

VIII-58. **The answer is B.** *(Chap. 289)* Arthritis, typically involving the large joints of the upper and lower extremities, develops in 15 to 20% of patients with inflammatory bowel disease (IBD). It is more common in Crohn's disease (CD) than in ulcerative colitis (UC) and flares with disease activity. Treatment is focused on controlling bowel inflammation. Erythema nodosum and venous thromboembolism also generally correlate with intestinal disease activity. In contrast, the other extraintestinal manifestations of IBD listed above typically do not correlate with disease activity. Ankylosing spondylitis is more common in CD than in UC and may occur in up to 10% of these patients. The course is often progressive and debilitating. Nephrolithiasis occurs more frequently in CD with ileal disease resulting from calcium oxalate stones. Primary sclerosing cholangitis (PSC) occurs in 1 to 5% of patients with IBD. Most patients with PSC have IBD. PSC may be detected before active bowel disease and may even occur years after proctocolectomy in patients with UC. Ten percent of patients with PSC will develop cholangiocarcinoma. Uveitis is associated with UC and CD and may occur during remission or after bowel resection. Without timely treatment with corticosteroids, vision loss may ensue.

VIII-59. **The answer is D.** *(Chap. 39)* The patient's symptoms are most consistent with an obstructive process. The progressive and gradual nature of the process is evident in worsening tolerance for solid foods over the course of months. The patient's prior partial gastrectomy predisposes him to gastric outlet obstruction as a result of stricture at the previous anastomosis. In addition, gastric ulcers often undergo malignant transformation. Although the patient has no current symptoms of peptic ulcer disease, underlying malignancy with gastric outlet obstruction must be considered as gastric ulcers may develop into cancerous lesions if left untreated. Other factors that support the diagnosis of gastric outlet obstruction are the abdominal x-ray findings of dilated gastric bubble and the lack of air in the small bowel. Small bowel obstruction presents acutely with abdominal distention, pain, and vomiting. One would expect to find dilated small bowel loops with air-fluid levels. Gastroparesis is common in poorly controlled diabetic patients, symptomatically affecting approximately 10% of those patients. Frequent vomiting of poorly digested food is reported, as in this patient. However, no abnormal findings are associated on standard radiography. Finally, cholelithiasis is most often asymptomatic but can present as biliary colic. There should be associated pain in the right upper quadrant and epigastrium with eating. Again, the abdominal radiogram is normal in this condition with the possible exception of stones seen within the gallbladder.

VIII-60. **The answer is E.** *(Chap. 39)* Juvenile hamartomatous polyps are lesions that consist of lamina propria and dilated cystic glands. They are at increased risk of bleeding, but not malignant transformation. Other polyposis syndromes including familial adenomatous polyposis, Peutz-Jeghers syndrome, and Gardner's syndrome confer increased malignant potential throughout the GI tract. Gastric adenocarcinoma remains a prevalent malignancy worldwide despite significant decline in incidence over the last 50 years. The highest incidence of gastric cancer occurs in Japan. A major pathophysiologic risk appears to be related to bacterial conversion of ingested nitrites into carcinogens in the stomach. Risk factors for the development of gastric cancer include long-term ingestion of foods with high concentrations of nitrite (dried, smoked, salted foods) and conditions that promote bacterial colonization/infection in the stomach, such as *Helicobacter* infection, chronic gastritis, and achlorhydria. Duodenal ulcers are not a risk factor for gastric carcinoma.

VIII-61. **The answer is D.** *(Chap. 307)* Chronic pancreatitis is a common disorder in any patient population with relapsing acute pancreatitis, especially patients with alcohol dependence, pancreas divisum, and cystic fibrosis. The disorder is notable for both endocrine and exocrine dysfunction of the pancreas. Often diabetes ensues as a result of loss of islet cell function; though insulin-dependent, it is generally not as prone to diabetic ketoacidosis or coma as are other forms of diabetes mellitus. As pancreatic enzymes are essential to fat digestion, their absence leads to fat malabsorption and steatorrhea. In addition, the fat-soluble vitamins, A, D, E, and K, are not absorbed. Vitamin A deficiency can lead to neuropathy. Vitamin B_{12}, or cobalamin, is often deficient. This deficiency is hypothesized to be due to excessive binding of cobalamin by cobalamin-binding proteins other than intrinsic factor that are normally digested by pancreatic enzymes. Replacement of pancreatic enzymes orally with meals will correct the vitamin deficiencies and steatorrhea. The incidence of pancreatic adenocarcinoma is increased in patients with chronic pancreatitis, with a 20-year cumulative incidence of 4%. Chronic abdominal pain is nearly ubiquitous in this disorder, and narcotic dependence is common. Niacin is a water-soluble vitamin, and absorption is not affected by pancreatic exocrine dysfunction.

VIII-62. The answer is C. *(Chap. 40)* Greasy, foul-smelling stools that are difficult to flush are classic for fat malabsorption. The diarrhea is caused by the osmotic effects of fatty acids and neutral fats. Fat malabsorption syndromes classically lead to weight loss and many vitamin deficiencies, including iron, vitamin B_{12}, vitamin D, and vitamin K. Pancreatic insufficiency must be considered in cases of malabsorption, but destruction of the organ must be near total for this to occur, usually in the setting of long-standing alcohol abuse. Celiac disease affects 1% of Americans, often presents with symptoms similar to those of irritable bowel syndrome, and requires an endoscopy with biopsy to confirm the diagnosis. Other causes of steatorrhea include bacterial overgrowth, bariatric surgery, liver disease, and Whipple's disease. A 24-h stool collection is a formal way to confirm steatorrhea, though a consistent patient history may be adequate to begin evaluation. Small-intestinal disease typically will result in fecal fat of ~15–25 g/day, and pancreatic exocrine insufficiency may result in >30 g/day.

VIII-63. The answer is A. *(Chap. 307)* This patient likely has chronic pancreatitis related to long-standing alcohol use, which is the most common cause of chronic pancreatitis in adults in the United States. Chronic pancreatitis can develop in individuals who consume as little as 50 g of alcohol daily (equivalent to ~30–40 ounces of beer). The patient's description of his loose stools is consistent with steatorrhea, and the recurrent bouts of abdominal pain are likely related to his pancreatitis. In most patients, abdominal pain is the most prominent symptom. However, up to 20% of individuals with chronic pancreatitis present with symptoms of maldigestion alone. The evaluation for chronic pancreatitis should allow one to characterize the pancreatitis as large- vs. small-duct disease. Large-duct disease is more common in men and is more likely to be associated with steatorrhea. In addition, large-duct disease is associated with the appearance of pancreatic calcifications and abnormal tests of pancreatic exocrine function. Women are more likely to have small-duct disease, with normal tests of pancreatic exocrine function and normal abdominal radiography. In small-duct disease, the progression to steatorrhea is rare, and the pain is responsive to treatment with pancreatic enzymes. The characteristic findings on CT and abdominal radiograph of this patient are characteristic of chronic pancreatitis, and no further workup should delay treatment with pancreatic enzymes. Treatment with pancreatic enzymes orally will improve maldigestion and lead to weight gain, but they are unlikely to fully resolve maldigestive symptoms. Narcotic dependence can frequently develop in individuals with chronic pancreatitis due to recurrent and severe bouts of pain. However, as this individual's pain is mild, it is not necessary to prescribe narcotics at this point in time. An ERCP or magnetic resonance cholangiopancreatography (MRCP) may be considered to evaluate for a possible stricture that is amenable to therapy. However, sphincterotomy is a procedure performed via ERCP that may be useful in treating pain related to chronic pancreatitis and is not indicated in the patient. Angiography to assess for ischemic bowel disease is not indicated as the patient's symptoms are not consistent with intestinal angina. Certainly, weight loss can occur in this setting, but the patient usually presents with complaints of abdominal pain after eating and pain that is out of proportion with the clinical examination. Prokinetic agents would likely only worsen the patient's malabsorptive symptoms and are not indicated.

VIII-64. The answer is D. *(Chaps. 88 and 300)* Hepatocelluar carcinoma (HCC) is one of the most common tumors in the world. Its high prevalence in Asia and sub-Saharan Africa is related to the prevalence of chronic hepatitis B infection in those areas. The rising incidence in the United States is related to the presence of chronic hepatitis C. It is more common in men than in women and usually arises from a cirrhotic liver. The incidence peaks in the fifth and sixth decades of life in Western countries but one to two decades earlier in regions of Asia and Africa. Chronic liver disease with other etiologies, such as hemochromatosis, primary biliary cirrhosis, and alcoholic cirrhosis, also carries an increased risk of HCC. Patients often present with an enlarging abdomen in the setting of chronic liver failure. α Fetoprotein levels may be elevated. The primary treatment modality is surgery. Surgical resection offers the best hope for a cure. In cases in which there are multiple lesions or resection is technically not feasible, other options, such as radiofrequency ablation, may be tried. Liver transplantation in selected patients offers a survival that is the same as the survival after transplantation for nonmalignant liver disease. Chemoembolization may confer a survival benefit in patients with nonresectable disease. Systemic chemotherapy is generally not effective and is reserved for palliation when other, more local strategies have been tried.

VIII-65.   **The answer is E.**   *(Chap. 40)*   Diarrhea lasting >4 weeks is considered chronic. Most causes of chronic diarrhea are noninfectious. They can be grouped into secretory, osmotic, steatorrheal, inflammatory, dysmotility, factitious, and iatrogenic causes. Secretory diarrheas are due to altered fluid or electrolyte transport across the enterocolonic mucosa. They typically are large-volume stools that persist with fasting and occur during the night. Stimulant laxatives such as bisacodyl, cascara, castor oil, and senna are very common offending agents for secretory diarrhea. Therefore, the patient's complete (not just prescribed) medication list should always be reviewed before engaging on an expensive search for causes of chronic diarrhea. Countless medications may cause diarrhea; common offenders include antibiotics and antihypertensives. Lactose intolerance is a common cause of osmotic diarrhea. Carcinoid, vasoactive intestinal polypeptide-secreting tumors, medullary thyroid carcinoma, gastrinoma, and villous adenoma are uncommon tumors that are on the differential diagnosis of secretory diarrhea. Crohn's disease can lead to bile salt–induced secretory diarrhea as a presenting feature, but this is less common than its usual presentation as an inflammatory diarrhea. Lymphocytic colitis is an inflammatory disease that causes diarrhea in the elderly.

VIII-66.   **The answer is E.**   *(Chaps. 299 and e35)*   Drug-induced liver injury is common. Acetaminophen is one of the most common causes of drug-induced injury. It is often ingested in suicide attempts or accidentally by children. Acetaminophen is metabolized by a phase II reaction to innocuous sulfate and glucuronide metabolites. However, a small proportion of acetaminophen is metabolized by a phase I reaction to a hepatoxic metabolite, *N*-acetylbenzoquinone-imide (NAPQI). When excessive amounts of NAPQI are formed, glutathione levels are depleted and covalent binding of NAPQI is thought to occur, with hepatocyte macromolecules leading to hepatic injury. Patients often present with confusion, abdominal pain, and sometimes shock. Treatment includes gastric lavage, activated charcoal, and supportive measures. The risk of toxicity is derived from a nomogram plot where acetaminophen plasma levels are plotted against time after ingestion. In this patient the level was above 200 μg/mL at 4 h, indicating a risk of toxicity. Therefore, *N*-acetylcysteine, a sulfhydryl compound, is administered as a reservoir of sulfhydryl groups to support the reserves of glutathione. Normal liver function tests at the time of presentation do not indicate a benign course. Rather, patients must be observed for a period of days as the hepatic toxicity and transaminitis may manifest 4 to 6 days after the initial ingestion. Alkalinization plays no role. However, in patients who develop signs of hepatic failure (e.g., progressive jaundice, coagulopathy, confusion), liver transplantation is the only established option.

VIII-67.   **The answer is E.**   *(Chap. 291)*   Surgical therapy is indicated in all low-risk surgical patients with complicated diverticular disease. Patients with at least two episodes of diverticulitis requiring hospitalization, with disease that does not respond to medical therapy, or who develop intra-abdominal complications are considered to have complicated disease. Complicating this patient's relapse of diverticulitis is probably an enterovesicular fistula causing pneumaturia. Studies indicate that younger patients (<50 years) may experience a more aggressive form of the disease than older patients, and therefore waiting for more than two attacks before considering surgery is not recommended. Rifaximin is a poorly absorbed broad-spectrum antibiotic that, when combined with a fiber-rich diet, is associated with less frequent symptoms in patients with uncomplicated diverticular disease. Pneumaturia represents a potential surgical urgency and should not be confused with proteinuria.

VIII-68.   The answer is A. *(Chap. 291)* Hemorrhage from a colonic diverticulum is the most common cause of hematochezia in patients >60 years of age. Patients with atherosclerosis, hypertension, and increased bleeding risk are most commonly affected. Most bleeds are intense, but are self-limited and stop spontaneously. They usually arise from the right colon. The lifetime risk of rebleeding is 25%. While colonoscopy can be both diagnostic and therapeutic in lower GI bleeding, the ability to visualize the mucosa is limited when the bleeding is brisk. Angiography can localize the bleeding and, if the patient is stable, bleeding is best managed by mesenteric angiography. If identified, the bleeding vessel may be successfully occluded with a coil in 80% of cases with <10% risk of colonic ischemia. This patient is normotensive and has a normal heart rate, suggesting that he is stable for angiography. Surgery is reserved for patients with unstable bleeding or a >6 unit/24 h bleeding episode.

VIII-69.   The answer is E. *(Chap. 300)* Although chronic active hepatitis may be associated with extraintestinal manifestations (e.g., arthritis) and the presence in the serum of autoantibodies (e.g., anti-smooth-muscle antibody), these factors are not invariably present. The distinction between chronic active hepatitis and chronic persistent hepatitis can be established only by doing a liver biopsy. In chronic active hepatitis there is piecemeal necrosis (erosion of the limiting plate of hepatocytes surrounding the portal triads), hepatocellular regeneration, and extension of inflammation into the liver lobule; these features are not seen in chronic persistent hepatitis. Both diseases may be associated with serologic evidence of hepatitis B infection.

VIII-70.   The answer is B. *(Chap. 40)* *Campylobacter* and *Shigella* are associated with bloody diarrhea. Fecal-oral transmission and exposure to undercooked poultry products are routes of transmission. Although bloody diarrhea is a common occurrence in amebic dysentery, patients may develop extraintestinal manifestations in the liver, lungs, heart, and brain. Enterotoxigenic *E. coli* causes a watery diarrhea, but enterohemorrhagic *E. coli* O157:H7 (often from undercooked hamburger) may cause a severe dysentery and the development of hemolytic-uremic syndrome. Cryptosporidiosis is a common cause of diarrhea in immunodeficient individuals. It causes a profuse watery diarrhea with mucus, but blood and fecal leukocytes are extremely rare.

VIII-71.   The answer is A. *(Chap. 286)* This patient has symptoms of esophagitis. In patients with HIV various infections can cause this disease, including herpes simplex virus (HSV), cytomegalovirus (CMV), varicella zoster virus (VZV), *Candida*, and HIV itself. The lack of thrush does not rule out *Candida* as a cause of esophagitis, and EGD is necessary for diagnosis. CMV classically causes serpiginous ulcers in the distal esophagus that may coalesce to form large giant ulcers. Brushings alone are insufficient for diagnosis, and biopsies must be performed. Biopsies reveal intranuclear and intracytoplasmic inclusions with enlarged nuclei in large fibroblasts and endothelial cells. Intravenous ganciclovir is the treatment of choice, and valganciclovir is an oral preparation that has been introduced recently. Foscarnet is useful in treating ganciclovir-resistant CMV.

Herpes simplex virus manifests as vesicles and punched-out lesions in the esophagus with the characteristic finding on biopsy of ballooning degeneration with ground-glass changes in the nuclei. It can be treated with acyclovir or foscarnet in resistant cases. *Candida* esophagitis has the appearance of yellow nodular plaques with surrounding erythema. Treatment usually requires fluconazole therapy. Finally, HIV alone can cause esophagitis that can be quite resistant to therapy. On EGD these ulcers appear deep and linear. Treatment with thalidomide or oral glucocorticoids is employed, and highly active antiretroviral therapy should be considered.

VIII-72.   The answer is A. *(Chap. 298)* In healthy adults without a previous history of liver disease, complete recovery from acute hepatitis B infection occurs in about 99% of cases. In this population, including the patient described above, antiviral treatment is unlikely to improve this excellent prognosis and should be avoided. A resolved infection will induce lifelong immunity, and a vaccine series is not necessary. Based on experience with antiviral therapy for chronic hepatitis B infection, some practitioners will treat severe cases of acute hepatitis B with antivirals such as lamivudine or entecavir, though there are no clinical trials in this patient population.

VIII-73. **The answer is C.** *(Chap. 288)* The patient's symptoms are consistent with bacterial overgrowth in the afferent loop. These patients complain of abdominal bloating and pain 20 min to 1 h after eating. There may be associated vomiting. In addition, malabsorptive diarrhea is common and ceases with fasting. The report of foul-smelling diarrhea that floats should prompt an evaluation for fat malabsorption. This patient also has a macrocytic anemia, which can result from vitamin B_{12} deficiency.

Many other complications have been noted after surgery for peptic ulcer disease. Dumping syndrome refers to a spectrum of vasomotor symptoms that occur after peptic ulcer surgery, including tachycardia, light-headedness, and diaphoresis. It can occur within 30 min of eating and is related to rapid delivery of hyperosmolar contents to the proximal small intestine, resulting in large fluid shifts. A late dumping syndrome can also occur, with similar symptoms developing 90 min to 3 h after eating. It is related to meals containing large amounts of simple carbohydrates and thus causes insulin surges and hypoglycemia. Bile reflux gastropathy presents after partial gastrectomy with abdominal pain, early satiety, and vomiting. Histologic examination reveals minimal inflammation but extensive epithelial injury. Treatment consists of prokinetic agents and bile acid sequestrants. Finally, postvagotomy diarrhea occurs in 10% of patients after peptic ulcer surgery. These patients usually complain of severe diarrhea that occurs 1 to 2 h after meals. Abdominal bloating and malabsorption are not usually part of this syndrome.

VIII-74. **The answer is E.** *(Chap. 288)* This patient most likely has primary lactase deficiency. Carbohydrates in the diet are composed of starches, disaccharides (lactose, sucrose), and glucose. Only monosaccharides (glucose, galactose) are absorbed in the small intestine so that starches and disaccharides must be digested before absorption. Starches are digested by amylase (pancreatic > salivary). Lactose, the disaccharide present in milk, requires digestion by brush border lactase into glucose and galactose. Lactase is present in the intestinal brush border in all species during the postnatal period but disappears except in humans. There are marked racial differences in the persistence of lactase, with Asians having among the highest prevalence of lactase deficiency and Northern Europeans having the lowest prevalence. In primary lactase deficiency other aspects of intestinal nutrient absorption and brush border function are normal. Symptoms usually arise in adolescence or adulthood and consist of diarrhea, abdominal pain, cramps, bloating, and flatus after the consumption of milk products. The differential diagnosis includes irritable bowel syndrome. Treatment involves avoidance of foods with a high lactose content (milk, ice cream) and use of oral galactosidase ("lactase") enzyme replacement. The efficacy of the enzyme replacement treatments varies with the product, the food, and the individual. Cholestyramine is useful in cases of bile acid diarrhea. Viokase is used in patients with chronic pancreatic insufficiency (chronic pancreatitis, resection, cystic fibrosis) and contains amylase, protease, and lipase. Metoclopramide is a promotility agent and will not help symptoms of lactase deficiency. Omeprazole is a proton pump inhibitor and will decrease gastric acid secretion.

Primary Lactase Deficiency in Different Adult Ethnic Groups	
Ethnic Group	Prevalence of Lactase Deficiency, %
Northern European	5–15
Mediterranean	60–85
African black	85–100
American black	45–80
American Caucasian	10–25
Native American	50–95
Mexican American	40–75
Asian	90–100

Source: From FJ Simons: The geographic hypothesis and lactose malabsorption. A weighing of the evidence. Am J Dig Dis 23:963, 1978.

VIII-75. **The answer is C.** *(Chaps. 298 and 300)* Causes of extreme elevations in serum transaminases generally fall into a few major categories, including viral infections, toxic ingestions, and vascular/hemodynamic causes. Both acute hepatitis A and hepatitis B infections may be characterized by high transaminases. Fulminant hepatic failure may occur, particularly in situations in which acute hepatitis A occurs on top of chronic hepatitis C infection or if hepatitis B and hepatitis D are cotransmitted. Most cases of acute hepatitis A or B infection in adults are self-limited. Hepatitis C is an RNA virus that does not typically cause acute hepatitis. However, it is associated with a high probability of chronic infection. Therefore, progression to cirrhosis and hepatoma is increased in patients with chronic hepatitis C infection. Extreme transaminitis is highly unlikely with acute hepatitis C infection. Acetaminophen remains one of the major causes of fulminant hepatic failure and is managed by prompt administration of N-acetylcysteine. Budd-Chiari syndrome is characterized by posthepatic thrombus formation. It often presents with jaundice, painful hepatomegaly, ascites, and elevated transaminases.

VIII-76.   The answer is C. *(Chap. e25)*   The endoscopic picture demonstrates typical pseudomembranous colitis with yellow adherent pseudomembranes that appear raised and measure up to 1 cm. Pseudomembranous colitis is the pathologic manifestation of extensive infection with *Clostridium difficile*, as not all patients who develop diarrheal illness due to *C. difficile* will show evidence of colitis, with or without pseudomembranes present. Pathologically pseudomembranes consist of fibropurulent debris that adheres to the damaged colonic mucosa. Pseudomembranes may develop in other causes of colitis, including ischemic colitis. The pseudomembranes of *C. difficile* colitis are unique, however, because of features seen by microscopic examination. The surface epithelium is denuded, and the underlying colonic mucosa is diffusely infiltrated with neutrophils. The colonic crypts are distended by mucopurulent material that becomes the pseudomembranes when the crypts rupture. Ischemic colitis may rarely form pseudomembranes that appear similar on colonoscopy, and it may be difficult to differentiate pseudomembranous colitis from ischemic colitis from that caused by *C. difficile*. However, in this case, the patient's clinical presentation is more consistent with *C. difficile* colitis than ischemic colitis. In addition, the recent administration of fluoroquinolone antibiotics should raise the suspicion of *C. difficile* infection. A more typical appearance of ischemic colitis on colonoscopy is patchy mucosal edema with bluish discoloration and subepithelial hemorrhage. Salmonella causes ileitis and colitis with marked mucosal edema and enlargement of Peyer's patches. Pseudomembrane formation is not common. Ulcerative colitis and Crohn's disease would not typically produce pseudomembranes, but would be associated with deep ulcerations of the mucosa, which are not apparent here. Diverticular disease is not demonstrated on the endoscopic picture.

VIII-77.   The answer is A. *(Chap. 43)*   The van den Bergh reaction is commonly used to identify the concentration of conjugated (direct) and total bilirubin. One shortcoming of this method is the inability to differentiate the fraction of conjugated bilirubin that is bound to albumin. Albumin-linked bilirubin (biliprotein) has a longer half-life (12–14 days) in the serum than the free form (4 h), which accounts for one of the enigmas of jaundiced patients with liver disease: the elevated serum bilirubin level declines more slowly than expected in some patients who are otherwise recovering well. Hepatobiliary function is not impaired in these patients.

VIII-78.   The answer is A. *(Chap. 43)*   Biliverdin is converted to bilirubin in the reticuloendothelial system. Bilirubin is insoluble in serum and must be bound to albumin before it can be transported to the liver. At the hepatocyte, bilirubin is able to passively be absorbed and reach the endoplasmic reticulum. The enzyme glutathione S-transferase B appears to reduce efflux of bilirubin out of the hepatocyte. In the endoplasmic reticulum, bilirubin is conjugated to glucuronic acid yielding bilirubin mono- and diglucuronide. Conjugated bilirubin is transported into the bile canalicular system via an active process by multiple drug resistance protein 2. In the terminal ileum, bacterial glucuronidases unconjugate the conjugated bilirubin. Unconjugated bilirubin is further reduced into urobilinogen in the terminal ileum. Most (80–90%) of the urobilinogen is excreted in the feces. The remaining 10–20% are passively absorbed into the portal venous blood and either reexcreted by the liver or the kidney.

VIII-79.   The answer is A. *(Chap. 44)*   In patients with chronic cirrhosis who develop new or worsening ascites without dietary or medication nonadherence, another occult disorder may be the reason. Common disorders that cause this phenomenon include portal vein thrombosis, hepatocellular carcinoma, portal vein thrombosis, bacterial peritonitis, alcoholic hepatitis, viral infection, and peritoneal tuberculosis. An elevated WBC count is more common when there is a neoplasm, bacterial peritonitis, or tuberculosis. The predominance of lymphocytes raises the suspicion for tuberculosis. The SAAG is classically low in cases of tuberculous peritonitis but may be high when there is concomitant cirrhosis and transudative ascites. The sensitivity of the adenosine deaminase activity is characteristically poor in patients with cirrhosis due to poor T cell–mediated response, therefore, peritoneal biopsy or visual diagnosis during laparoscopy are likely to be required for diagnosis.

VIII-80. **The answer is C.** *(Chap. 43)* When evaluating a patient with jaundice, initial steps include determining whether the hyperbilirubinemia is predominantly unconjugated or conjugated and whether there is any other laboratory evidence of hepatobiliary dysfunction. When there are associated biochemical liver abnormalities, further discrimination into a predominantly cholestatic or hepatocellular pattern is possible. A hepatocellular pattern, as in this example characterized by ALT/AST elevated out of proportion to the alkaline phosphatase, should prompt a search for viral, autoimmune, toxicologic, and abnormal deposition disease. Acetaminophen is a common cause of mental status change, jaundice, and hepatocellular injury in the intensive care unit. Liver biopsy may ultimately become necessary. Anatomic abnormalities are more common when there is a cholestatic pattern of injury characterized by an elevated alkaline phosphatase out of proportion to the AST/ALT. In those cases, ultrasound and possible ERCP may be indicated.

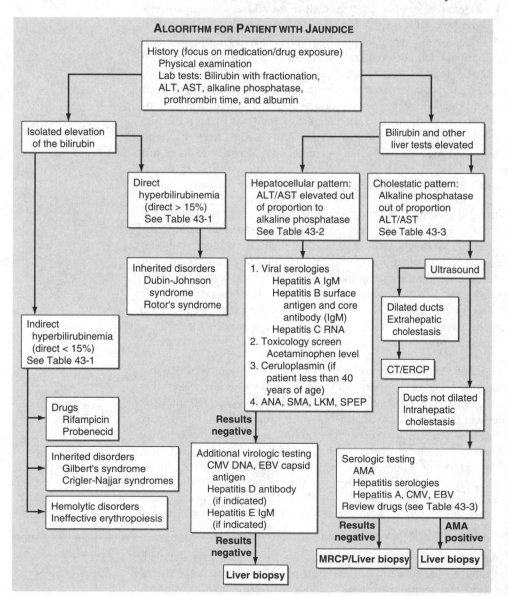

FIGURE VIII-80 Evaluation of the patient with jaundice. MRCP, magnetic resonance cholangiopancreatography; ALT, alanine aminotransferase; AST, aspartate aminotransferase; SMA, smooth-muscle antibody; AMA, antimitochondrial antibody; LKM, liver-kidney microsomal antibody; SPEP, serum protein electrophoresis; CMV, cytomegalovirus; EBV, Epstein-Barr virus. Tables cited are from Harrison's, 17e, Chap. 43.

VIII-81. **The answer is C.** *(Chap. 43)* Unconjugated bilirubin is always bound to albumin in the serum, is not filtered by the kidney, and is not found in the urine. Therefore, any bilirubin found in the urine must be conjugated to glucuronic acid. The presence of bilirubinuria implies the presence of liver disease. Defects that cause elevated levels of unconjugated bilirubin will not cause bilirubinuria. A defect in bilirubin production will not cause bilirubinuria.

VIII-82. **The answer is A.** *(Chap. 292)* Mesenteric ischemia is a relatively uncommon and highly morbid illness. Acute mesenteric ischemia is usually due to arterial embolus (usually from the heart) or from thrombosis in a diseased vascular bed. Major risk factors include age, atrial fibrillation, valvular disease, recent arterial catheterization, and recent myocardial infarction. Ischemia occurs when the intestines are inadequately perfused by the splanchnic circulation. This blood supply has extensive collateralization and can receive up to 30% of the cardiac output, making poor perfusion an uncommon event. Patients with acute mesenteric ischemia will frequently present with pain out of proportion to their initial physical examination. As ischemia persists, peritoneal signs and cardiovascular collapse will follow. Mortality is >50%. While radiographic imaging can suggest ischemia, the gold standard for diagnosis is laparotomy.

VIII-83. **The answer is B.** *(Chap. 43)* Causes of isolated unconjugated (indirect) hyperbilirubinemia include inherited (sickle cell disease, spherocytosis, glucose-6-phosphate dehydrogenase deficiency) and acquired (microangiopathic hemolytic anemia, paroxysmal nocturnal hemoglobinuria, immune hemolysis) hemolytic disorders, ineffective erythropoiesis (nutritional deficiencies), inherited conditions (Gilbert's syndrome, Crigler-Najjar types I and II), and drugs (probenecid, ribavirin, rifampicin). Inherited hemolytic disorders with chronic hemolysis carry a high risk of developing calcium bilirubinate gallstones. Patients with hemolytic disorders that cause excessive heme production seldom have a serum bilirubin >5 mg/dL. Higher levels may occur during acute hemolytic conditions (sickle cell crisis) or with concomitant renal or hepatocellular disease. Probenecid (used to treat gout) and rifampicin cause unconjugated hyperbilirubinemia by diminishing hepatic uptake of bilirubin. Cryoglobulinemia is associated with hepatitis C infection which, if present, is associated with a mild hepatocellular pattern of injury and an elevated direct bilirubin.

VIII-84. **The answer is A.** *(Chap. 89)* Ductal adenocarcinomas of the exocrine pancreas are the most common type (>90%) of pancreatic neoplasm. The pancreatic head is the most common site. The median age of diagnosis is 72 years, with the peak incidence between 65 and 85 years. The incidence is slightly higher in men than women and in African Americans than Caucasians. Pancreatic carcinoma is uncommon below the age of 50. These tumors are aggressive and usually present with locally inoperable disease with local and distal metastases. The 5-year survival is only about 5%. It is the fourth leading cause of cancer death. Other less common types of pancreatic neoplasms include islet cell tumors and neuroendocrine tumors.

VIII-85. **The answer is B.** *(Chap. 44)* A carefully performed physical examination can reveal important clues concerning the etiology of abdominal swelling. Ascites and increased intraperitoneal pressure will produce stretched skin, bulging flanks, and an everted umbilicus regardless of the etiology of the ascites. Auscultating a venous hum at the umbilicus may signify portal hypertension with increased collateral blood flow around the liver but may not distinguish distal hepatic venous or superior vena cava obstruction. Prominent abdominal venous pattern with the direction of flow away from the umbilicus often reflects portal hypertension. Collateral venous flow from the lower abdomen to the umbilicus suggests inferior vena cava obstruction. Flow from the upper abdomen downward toward the umbilicus suggests superior vena cava obstruction. A pulsatile liver is classically described in severe tricuspid regurgitation.

VIII-86. **The answer is E.** *(Chap. 89)* When first-line therapy for pancreatic cancer has failed, fit patients should be referred for enrollment in clinical trials to identify novel therapeutic agents. Gemcitabine has been shown to be superior to treatment with 5-fluorouracil. Patients with little life expectancy or who have a poor functional status may benefit by incorporating palliative or hospice care into their treatment plan. External beam chemoradiotherapy may be helpful when the disease is locally advanced and causing significant morbidity. Debulking surgery has no role in the treatment of advanced pancreatic cancer since the risk of the procedure is similar to that of a curative resection and offers no survival benefit. Biliary stenting is useful for relieving obstructive jaundice.

VIII-87. The answer is D. *(Chap. 43)* Jaundice that is not due to hyperbilirubinemia may be caused by excessive carotene ingestion, the use of quinacrine, and excessive exposure to phenols. In carotenoderma, the ingested pigment is predominantly deposited in the palms, soles, forehead, and nasolabial folds. The jaundice of carotenoderma, but not quinacrine usage, spares the sclera. The nasolabial folds can be involved in any cause of jaundice. When there is jaundice, skin pigment deposition does not depend on sun exposure. Over time, with bilirubin deposition, sun exposure oxidizes bilirubin to biliverdin causing a green discoloration of the skin in light-skinned patients.

VIII-88. The answer is E. *(Chap. 44)* The serum-ascites albumin gradient correlates directly with portal pressure. A SAAG >1.1 g/dL is characteristic of portal hypertension with >97% accuracy. A low SAAG (<1.1 g/dL) indicates the patient does not have portal hypertension with >97% accuracy. Occult cirrhosis, intrahepatic sinusoidal destruction, massive hepatic metastases, Budd-Chiari syndrome, right-sided cardiac valve disease, right-sided heart failure, and constrictive pericarditis should be considered when evaluating new-onset ascites with a high SAAG without clear etiology.

TABLE VIII-88   Characteristics of Ascitic Fluid in Various Disease States

Condition	Gross Appearance	Protein, g/L	Serum-Ascites Albumin Gradient, g/dL	Cell Count Red Blood Cells, >10,000/μL	Cell Count White Blood Cells, per μL	Other Tests
Cirrhosis	Straw-colored or bile-stained	<25 (95%)	>1.1	1%	<250 (90%)[a]; predominantly mesothelial	
Neoplasm	Straw-colored, hemorrhagic, mucinous, or chylous	>25 (75%)	<1.1	20%	>1000 (50%); variable cell types	Cytology, cell block, peritoneal biopsy
Tuberculous peritonitis	Clear, turbid, hemorrhagic, chylous	>25 (50%)	<1.1	7%	>1000 (70%); usually >70% lymphocytes	Peritoneal biopsy, stain and culture for acid-fast bacilli
Pyogenic peritonitis	Turbid or purulent	If purulent, >25	<1.1	Unusual	Predominantly polymorphonuclear leukocytes	Positive Gram's stain, culture
Congestive heart failure	Straw-colored	Variable, 15–53	>1.1	10%	<1000 (90%); usually mesothelial, mononuclear	
Nephrosis	Straw-colored or chylous	<25 (100%)	<1.1	Unusual	<250; mesothelial, mononuclear	If chylous, ether extraction, Sudan staining
Pancreatic ascites (pancreatitis, pseudocyst)	Turbid, hemorrhagic, or chylous	Variable, often >25	<1.1	Variable, may be blood-stained	Variable	Increased amylase in ascitic fluid and serum

[a]Because the conditions of examining fluid and selecting patients were not identical in each series, the percentage figures (in parentheses) should be taken as an indication of the order of magnitude rather than as the precise incidence of any abnormal finding.

VIII-89.   The answer is B.   *(Chap. 89)*   Patients with a suspicious pancreatic lesion seen on imaging that may be curable with local resection are often taken to surgery without further tissue characterization. Transcutaneous biopsy carries with it the theoretical risk of seeding the surrounding tissues as the needle is passed. Endoscopic ultrasound-guided fine-needle aspiration is increasing being utilized for biopsies as there is less risk of intraperitoneal spread of tumor. A negative biopsy or fine-needle aspiration may not be sufficient to rule out a neoplasm when the lesion is small. The dismal prognosis for advanced disease calls for prompt surgical referral for potentially curable lesions. An elevated CA 19-9 level is suggestive of pancreatic cancer but may also be elevated in cases of jaundice without pancreatic cancer. The reported sensitivity and specificity of the CA 19-9 assay for pancreatic cancer is reported between 80 and 90%, but it should not be used to confirm or exclude pancreatic cancer when the clinical scenario suggests the diagnosis.

IX. RHEUMATOLOGY AND IMMUNOLOGY

QUESTIONS

DIRECTIONS: Choose the **one best** response to each question.

IX-1. A 73-year-old woman with a medical history of obesity and diabetes mellitus presents to your clinic complaining of right knee pain that has been progressive and is worse with walking or standing. She has taken over-the-counter nonsteroidal anti-inflammatory drugs without relief. She wants to know what is wrong with her knee and what may have caused it. X-rays are performed and reveal cartilage loss and osteophyte formation. Which of the following represents the most potent risk factor for the development of osteoarthritis?

A. Age
B. Gender
C. Genetic susceptibility
D. Obesity
E. Previous joint injury

IX-2. A 42-year-old obese male presents to your office with complaints of paresthesias in the right hand that are worst in the fourth and fifth fingers. Symptoms have been present intermittently for the last 4 months. He has no other past medical history and takes no medications. The examination is significant for an intact neurologic examination of the right upper extremity but mild wasting of the intrinsic muscles on inspection of the right hand. Laboratories show a normal white blood cell count, hemoglobin, and sedimentation rate. Electrolytes and creatinine and liver function tests are normal except for a serum glucose of 148 mg/dL. What is the most likely etiology of this patient's symptoms?

A. Diabetes mellitus
B. Cholesterol emboli
C. Churg-Strauss disease
D. Cervical spondylosis
E. Neurogenic thoracic outlet syndrome

IX-3. A 54-year-old man is admitted for persistent lower abdominal and groin pain that began 7 months previously. Two months before his present admission, he required exploratory laparoscopy for acute abdominal pain and presumed cholecystitis. This revealed necrotic omental tissue

IX-3. *(Continued)*
and pericholecystitis necessitating omentectomy and cholecystectomy. However, the pain continued unchanged. He currently describes it as periumbilical and radiating into his groin and legs. It becomes worse with eating. The patient has also had episodic severe testicular pain, bowel urgency, nausea, vomiting, and diuresis. He has lost ~22.7 kg over the preceding 6 months. His past medical history is significant of hypertension that has recently become difficult to control.

Medications on admission include aspirin, hydrochlorothiazide, hydromorphone, lansoprazole, metoprolol, and quinapril. On physical examination, the patient appears comfortable. His blood pressure is 170/100 mmHg, his heart rate is 88 beats/min, and he is afebrile. He has normal first and second heart sounds without murmurs, and an S_4 is present. There are no carotid, renal, abdominal, or femoral bruits.

His lungs are clear to auscultation. Bowel sounds are normal. Abdominal palpation demonstrates minimal diffuse tenderness without rebound or guarding. No masses are present, and the stool is negative for occult blood. During the examination, the patient develops Raynaud's phenomenon in his right hand that persists for several minutes. His neurologic examination is intact. Admission laboratory studies reveal an erythrocyte sedimentation rate of 72 mm/h, a BUN of 17 mg/dL, and a creatinine of 0.8 mg/dL. The patient has no proteinuria or hematuria. Tests for antinuclear antibodies, anti-double-stranded-DNA antibodies, and antineutrophil cytoplasmic antibodies are negative. Liver function tests are abnormal with an AST of 89 IU/L and an ALT of 112 IU/L. Hepatitis B surface antigen and e antigen are positive. Mesenteric angiography demonstrates small beaded aneurysms of the superior and inferior mesenteric veins. What is the most likely diagnosis?

A. Hepatocellular carcinoma
B. Ischemic colitis
C. Microscopic polyangiitis
D. Mixed cryoglobulinemia
E. Polyarteritis nodosa

IX-4. A 64-year-old African-American male is evaluated in the hospital for congestive heart failure, renal failure, and polyneuropathy. Physical examination on admission was notable for these findings and raised waxy papules in the axilla and inguinal region. Admission laboratories showed a BUN of 90 mg/dL and a creatinine of 6.3 mg/dL. Total protein was 9.0 g/dL, with an albumin of 3.2 g/dL. Hematocrit was 24%, and white blood cell and platelet counts were normal. Urinalysis was remarkable for 3+ proteinuria but no cellular casts. Further evaluation included an echocardiogram with a thickened left ventricle and preserved systolic function. Which of the following tests is most likely to diagnose the underlying condition?

A.   Bone marrow biopsy
B.   Electromyogram (EMG) with nerve conduction studies
C.   Fat pad biopsy
D.   Right heart catheterization
E.   Renal ultrasound

IX-5. A 31-year-old woman presents to your clinic complaining of painful arthritis that is worse in the mornings when she wakes up. She was recently evaluated by an ophthalmologist for uveitis in her right eye. A recent laboratory report shows an erythrocyte sedimentation rate of 48 mm/h. Which of the following will be helpful in distinguishing relapsing polychondritis from rheumatoid arthritis (RA)?

A.   Arthritis associated with RA is nonerosive.
B.   Eye inflammation is absent in relapsing polychondritis.
C.   Relapsing polychondritis will not present with vasculitis.
D.   Relapsing polychondritis will present with high-titer rheumatoid factor.
E.   The arthritis of relapsing polychondritis is asymmetric.

IX-6. A 66-year-old woman with a history of rheumatoid arthritis and frequent pseudogout attacks in her left knee presents with night sweats and a 2-day history of left knee pain. On physical examination, her temperature is 38.6°C, heart rate is 110 beats/min, blood pressure is 104/78 mmHg, and oxygen saturation is 97% on room air. Her left knee is swollen, red, painful, and warm. With 5° of flexion or extension, she develops extreme pain. She has evidence of chronic joint deformity in her hands, knees, and spine. Peripheral white blood cell (WBC) count is 16,700 cells/μL with 95% neutrophils. A diagnostic tap of her left knee reveals 168,300 WBCs per microliter, 99% neutrophils, and diffuse needle-shaped birefringent crystals present. Gram stain shows rare gram-positive cocci in clusters. Management includes all of the following *except*

A.   blood cultures
B.   glucocorticoids
C.   needle aspiration of joint fluid
D.   orthopedic surgery consult
E.   vancomycin

IX-7. A 58-year-old female presents complaining of right shoulder pain. She does not recall any prior injury but notes that she feels that the shoulder has been getting progressively more stiff over the last several months. She previously had several episodes of bursitis of the right shoulder that were treated successfully with NSAIDs and steroid injections. The patient's past medical history is also significant for diabetes mellitus, for which she takes metformin and glyburide. On physical examination, the right shoulder is not warm or red but is tender to touch. Passive and active range of motion is limited in flexion, extension, and abduction. A right shoulder radiogram shows osteopenia without evidence of joint erosion or osteophytes. What is the most likely diagnosis?

A.   Adhesive capsulitis
B.   Avascular necrosis
C.   Bicipital tendinitis
D.   Osteoarthritis
E.   Rotator cuff tear

IX-8. A 44-year-old woman presents for evaluation of dry eyes and mouth. She first noticed these symptoms >5 years ago and the symptoms have worsened over time. She describes her eyes as gritty-feeling, as if there were sand in her eyes. Sometimes her eyes burn, and she states that it is difficult to be outside in bright sunlight. In addition, her mouth is quite dry. In her job, she is frequently asked to give business presentations and finds it increasingly difficult to complete a 30- to 60-minute presentation. She usually has water with her at all times. Although she reports good dental hygiene without any recent changes, her dentist has had to place fillings twice in the past 3 years for dental caries. Her only other past medical history is treated tuberculosis that she contracted while in the Peace Corp in Southeast Asia when in her twenties. She takes no medication regularly and does not smoke. Ocular examination reveals punctuate corneal ulcerations on Rose Bengal stain, and the Schirmer test shows <5 mm of wetness after 5 min. Her oral mucosa is dry with thick mucous secretions, and the parotid glands are enlarged bilaterally. Laboratory examination reveals positive antibodies to Ro and La (SS-A and SS-B). In addition, her chemistries reveal a sodium of 142 mEq/L, potassium 2.6 mEq/L, chloride 115 mEq/L, and bicarbonate of 15 mEq/L. What is the most likely cause of the hypokalemia and acidemia in this patient?

A.   Diarrhea
B.   Distal (type I) renal tubular acidosis
C.   Hypoaldosteronism
D.   Purging with underlying anorexia nervosa
E.   Renal compensation for chronic respiratory alkalosis

IX-9. A patient with end-stage renal disease on hemodialysis presents to your office with hand pain and you diagnose carpal tunnel syndrome. A serum thyroid-stimulating hormone level is normal. You also note bilateral knee effusions,

IX-9. *(Continued)*

which the patient states have been there for many months. Suspecting an amyloid deposition disease, you perform a fat pad biopsy. Which protein do you expect to find on immunohistochemical staining?

A. β_2-Microglobulin
B. Fibrinogen α-chain
C. Immunoglobulin light chain
D. Serum amyloid A
E. Transthyretin

IX-10. A 41-year-old female presents to your clinic with 3 weeks of weakness, lethargy. and depressed mood. She notes increasing difficulty with climbing steps, rising from a chair, and combing her hair. She has no difficulty buttoning her blouse or writing. The patient also notes some dyspnea on exertion and orthopnea. She denies rash, joint aches, or constitutional symptoms. She is on no medications, and the past medical history is otherwise uninformative. The family history is notable only for coronary artery disease. The physical examination is notable for an elevated jugular venous pressure, an S_3, and some bibasilar crackles. The neurologic examination shows some marked proximal muscle weakness in the deltoids and biceps and the hip flexors. Distal muscle strength is normal. Sensory examination and reflexes are normal. Laboratories are unremarkable except for a negative antinuclear antibody screen and a creatinine kinase of 3200 IU/L. You suspect a diagnosis of polymyositis. All the following clinical conditions may occur in polymyositis *except*

A. an increased incidence of malignancy
B. interstitial lung disease
C. dilated cardiomyopathy
D. dysphagia
E. Raynaud's phenomenon

IX-11. A 64-year-old man with congestive heart failure presents to the emergency room complaining of acute onset of severe pain in his right foot. The pain began during the night and awoke him from a deep sleep. He reports the pain to be so severe that he could not wear a shoe or sock to the hospital. His current medications are furosemide, 40 mg twice daily, carvedilol, 6.25 mg twice daily, candesartan, 8 mg once daily, and aspirin, 325 mg once daily. On examination, he is febrile to 38.5°C. The first toe of the right foot is erythematous and exquisitely tender to touch. There is significant swelling and effusion of the first metatarsophalangeal joint on the right. No other joints are affected. Which of the following findings would be expected on arthrocentesis?

A. Glucose level of <25 mg/dL
B. Positive Gram stain
C. Presence of strongly negatively birefringent needle-shaped crystals under polarized light microscopy
D. Presence of weakly positively birefringent rhomboidal crystals under polarized light microscopy
E. White blood cell (WBC) count >100,000/μL

IX-12. A 32-year-old African-American woman presents to her primary care doctor complaining of fatigue, joint stiffness and pain, mouth ulcers, and hair loss. She first noticed fatigue about 6 months ago, and at that time, a complete blood count and thyroid function tests were normal. Since then, she feels like her symptoms are getting progressively worse. She now states that she sleeps ≥10 h but continues to feel fatigued. She has also developed joint stiffness and pain in her hands, wrists, and knees that is present for about 1 h upon awakening. For the past 1 month, she has had an area of hair loss on her scalp associated with a raised scaly rash. During this time, she intermittently developed painful mouth ulcerations that would spontaneously resolve. She also reports a severe "sunburn" on her face, upper neck, and back that occurred after <1 h of sun exposure and which was unusual for her. Her past medical history is positive for two spontaneous vaginal deliveries that were uncomplicated. She has not had any prior miscarriages. She is taking oral contraceptive pills and has no allergies. On physical examination, the vital signs are: temperature 36.6°C, blood pressure 136/82 mmHg, heart rate 88 beats/min, respiratory rate 12 breaths/min, Sa$_{O_2}$ 98% on room air. She has a circular raised area on her right parietal area that is 3 cm in diameter. This area has an atrophic center with hair loss and is erythematous with a hyperpigmented rim. Her conjunctiva are pink and no scleral icterus is present. The oropharynx shows a single 2-mm aphthous ulceration on the buccal mucosa. Both wrists show some slight tenderness with palpation and pain with range of motion. The patient is incapable of closing her hands tightly. In addition, there is warmth and a possible effusion in the right knee and tenderness with range of motion in the left knee. Cardiovascular, pulmonary, abdominal, and neurologic examinations are normal. Laboratory studies show the following:

White blood cell count	2300/μL
Hemoglobin	8.9 g/dL
Hematocrit	26.7%
Mean corpuscular volume	88 fL
Mean corpuscular hemoglobin count	32 g/dL
Platelet	98,000/mL

The differential is 80% polymorphonuclear cells, 12% lymphocytes, 7% monocytes, 1% eosinophils, and 1% basophils. An antinuclear antibody (ANA) is positive at a titer of 1:640. Antibodies to double-stranded DNA are negative, and anti-Smith antibodies are positive at a titer of 1:160. The rheumatoid factor level is 37 IU/L. What is the most likely diagnosis?

A. Behçet's disease
B. Discoid lupus erythematosus
C. Rheumatoid arthritis
D. Sarcoidosis
E. Systemic lupus erythematosus

IX-13. In this patient, which test should be performed next?

A. Chest radiograph
B. Echocardiogram
C. Electrocardiogram
D. Skin biopsy
E. Urinalysis

IX-14. A 35-year-old female comes to the local health clinic because for the last 6 months she has had recurrent urticarial lesions, which occasionally leave a residual discoloration. She also has had arthralgias. The sedimentation rate now is 85 mm/h. The procedure most likely to yield the correct diagnosis in this case would be

A. a battery of wheal-and-flare allergy skin tests
B. measurement of total serum IgE concentration
C. measurement of C1 esterase inhibitor activity
D. skin biopsy
E. patch testing

IX-15. A 45-year-old obese man presents to the clinic several weeks after starting a jogging regimen. He describes right-sided heel pain that has worsened over this time. The pain is worse in the morning and when the patient is barefoot. On examination, pain can be elicited with palpation of the inferior medial right heel. Which of the following is required to make a definitive diagnosis of plantar fasciitis?

A. Compatible history and provocative testing
B. History and physical examination alone
C. History, physical examination, and nuclear medicine bone scan
D. History, physical examination, and heel ultrasound showing thickening of the fascia
E. History, physical examination, and plain radiograph demonstrating heel spur

IX-16. Which of the following findings on joint aspiration is most likely to be associated with calcium pyrophosphate deposition disease (pseudogout)?

A. Fluid, clear and viscous; white blood cell count, 400/μL; crystals, rhomboidal and weakly positively birefringent
B. Fluid, cloudy and watery; white blood cell count, 8000/μL; no crystals
C. Fluid, dark brown and viscous; white blood cell count, 1200/μL; crystals, needle-like and strongly negatively birefringent
D. Fluid, cloudy and watery; white blood cell count, 12,000/μL; crystals, needle-like and strongly negatively birefringent
E. Fluid, cloudy and watery; white blood cell count, 4800/μL; crystals, rhomboidal and weakly positively birefringent

IX-17. A 45-year-old woman presents to the emergency room for evaluation of fatigue, fever, and acute onset of joint pain and swelling of the right knee, left ankle, and right second toe. She reports that she was ill with a diarrheal illness about 2 weeks ago. She did not seek evaluation as the symptoms resolved spontaneously over 48 h. She did lose about 2.3 kg, which she has been unable to regain. Three days ago, she developed a feeling of malaise with fevers and pain in her right second toe. Additional

IX-17. (Continued)
joints have become inflamed over the ensuing 72 h. She denies any prior similar episodes. She is not currently sexually active and estimates her last sexual activity to be 8 months prior to presentation. She has a history of seasonal rhinitis, but is taking no medications currently. On examination, she is febrile at 38.4°C. Her left eye has evidence of conjunctival injection. There is a superficial ulcer on the inside of her lower lip that is not painful. The right knee is warm to touch with an effusion. Passive movement results in pain. The left ankle is similarly warm and painful. The right second great toe has the appearance of a "sausage digit." There is also pain with palpation at the tendinous insertion of both Achilles tendons. There are no genital ulcers or discharge. No rash is present. Arthrocentesis is performed and is consistent with inflammatory arthritis without crystals or organisms seen on Gram stain. Cervical probes for *Neisseria gonorrhoeae* and *Chlamydia trachomatis* are negative. Reactive arthritis following *Campylobacter* infection is suspected with positive serum antibodies to *C. jejuni*. Which of the following statements is true regarding this diagnosis?

A. Chronic joint symptoms affect 15% of individuals, and recurrences of the acute syndrome may occur.
B. Presence of HLA-B27 antigen predicts individuals who are likely to have a better prognosis.
C. Reactive arthritis is self-limited and should be expected to resolve spontaneously over the next 2 weeks.
D. The causative organism has no effect on long-term outcomes following an initial episode of reactive arthritis.

IX-18. A 54-year-old female with rheumatoid arthritis is treated with infliximab for refractory disease. All the following are potential side effects of this treatment *except*

A. demyelinating disorders
B. disseminated tuberculosis
C. exacerbation of congestive heart failure
D. pancytopenia
E. pulmonary fibrosis

IX-19. A 26-year-old man presents with severe bilateral pain in his hands, ankles, knees, and elbows. He is recovering from a sore throat and has had recent fevers to 38.9°C. Social history is notable for recent unprotected receptive oral intercourse with a man ~1 week ago. Physical examination reveals a well-developed man in moderate discomfort. He is afebrile. His pharynx is erythematous with pustular exudates on his tonsils. He has tender anterior cervical lymphadenopathy. His cardiac examination is notable for a normal S_1 and S_2 and a soft ejection murmur. His lungs are clear. Abdomen is benign with no organomegaly. He has no rash, and genital examination is normal. His bilateral proximal interphalangeal joints, metacarpophalangeal joints, wrists, ankles, and metatarsophalangeal joints are red, warm, and boggy with tenderness noted with both passive and active movement. A

IX-19. *(Continued)*

complete metabolic panel and complete blood count are all within normal limits. His erythrocyte sedimentation rate is 85 mm/h and C-reactive protein is 11 mg/dL. What is the most likely diagnosis?

A. Acute HIV infection
B. Acute rheumatic fever
C. Lyme disease
D. *Neisseria gonorrhoeae* infection
E. Poststreptococcal reactive arthritis

IX-20. A 27-year-old female with SLE is in remission; current treatment consists of azathioprine 75 mg/d and prednisone 5 mg/d. Last year she had a life-threatening exacerbation of her disease. She now strongly desires to become pregnant. Which of the following is the least appropriate action to take?

A. Advise her that the risk of spontaneous abortion is high.
B. Warn her that exacerbations can occur in the first trimester and in the postpartum period.
C. Tell her it is unlikely that a newborn will have lupus.
D. Advise her that fetal loss rates are higher if anticardiolipin antibodies are detected in her serum.
E. Stop the prednisone just before she attempts to become pregnant.

IX-21. A 48-year-old male has a long-standing history of ankylosing spondylitis. His most recent spinal film shows straightening of the lumbar spine, loss of lordosis, and "squaring" of the vertebral bodies. He currently is limited by pain with ambulation that is not improved with nonsteroidal anti-inflammatory medications. Which of the following treatments has been shown to improve symptoms the best at this stage of the illness?

A. Celecoxib
B. Etanercept
C. Prednisone
D. Sulfasalazine
E. Thalidomide

IX-22. A 72-year-old woman presents to the emergency room for an episode of vision loss in her right eye. The vision loss came on abruptly and is described as a curtain falling across her visual field. She immediately called her daughter and upon arrival to the emergency room 40 min later, her vision had returned to normal. Recently she also has been experiencing dull throbbing headaches for which she is taking acetaminophen, with limited relief. She has a past medical history of hypercholesterolemia and coronary artery disease, undergoing angioplasty and stenting of the right coronary artery 8 years previously. She does not smoke currently but has a 40-pack-year history of tobacco, quitting only after her diagnosis of coronary artery disease. On review of systems, the patient recalls pain in her scalp with combing her hair, particularly on the right

IX-22. *(Continued)*

side, and occasional pain with chewing food. She has also recently noticed stiffness and pain in her hips, making it difficult to stand from seated position. On examination, she has 20/30 visual acuity in the left eye, and 20/100 visual acuity in the right eye. Funduscopic examination suggests anterior ischemic optic neuropathy. There are no carotid bruits present, but palpation of the temporal artery is painful. The neurologic examination is otherwise normal. The erythrocyte sedimentation rate (ESR) is 102 mm/h. The hemoglobin is 7.9 g/dL, and hematocrit is 25.5%. A head CT shows no acute ischemic event. Which of the following is the next most important step in the management of this patient?

A. Initiate treatment with indomethacin, 75 mg twice daily.
B. Initiate treatment with prednisone, 60 mg daily.
C. Initiate treatment with unfractionated heparin adjusted based on activated partial thromboplastin time to obtain full anticoagulation.
D. Perform magnetic resonance angiography of the brain.
E. Perform a temporal artery biopsy.

IX-23. A patient presents with 3 weeks of pain in the lower back. All the following are risk factors for serious causes of spine pathology *except*

A. age more than 50 years
B. urinary incontinence
C. duration of pain more than 2 weeks
D. bed rest without relief
E. history of intravenous drug use

IX-24. A 64-year-old man with coronary artery disease and atrial fibrillation is referred for evaluation of fevers, arthralgias, pleuritis, and malar rash. The symptoms have developed over the past 6 months. The pleuritis has responded to steroid therapy, but prednisone has been unable to be tapered off due to recurrence of symptoms at daily steroid doses <15 mg of prednisone. His medications include aspirin, procainamide, lovastatin, prednisone, and carvedilol. You suspect drug-induced lupus due to procainamide. Antibodies directed against which of the following proteins is most likely to be positive?

A. Cardiolipin
B. Double-strand DNA
C. Histone
D. Ribonucleoprotein (RNP)
E. Ribosomal P

IX-25. A 28-year-old woman seeks evaluation from her primary care doctor for recurrent episodes of hives and states that she is "allergic to cold weather." She reports that for >10 years she would develop areas of hives when exposed to cold temperatures, usually on her arms and legs. She has never sought evaluation previously and states that over the past several years the occurrence of the

IX-25. (Continued)

hives has become more frequent. Other than cold exposure, she can identify no other triggers for development of hives. She has no history of asthma or atopy. She denies food intolerance. Her only medication is oral contraceptive pills, which she has taken for 5 years. She lives in a single-family home that was built 2 years ago. On examination, she develops a linear wheal after being stroked along her forearm with a tongue depressor. Upon placing her hand in cold water, her hand becomes red and swollen. In addition, there are several areas with a wheal and flare reaction on the arm above the area of cold exposure. What is the next step in the management of this patient?

A. Assess for the presence of antithyroglobulin and antimicrosomal antibodies.
B. Check C1 inhibitor levels.
C. Discontinue the oral contraceptive pills.
D. Treat with cetirizine, 10 mg daily.
E. Treat with cyproheptadine, 8 mg daily.

IX-26. A 34-year-old man is admitted to the hospital for evaluation and treatment of renal failure and an abnormal CT of the chest. For the past 2 months, he has had fatigue, malaise, and intermittent fevers to as high as 38.2°C. About 3 weeks ago, he sought treatment from his primary provider for sinus pain and congestion with a purulent and bloody nasal discharge. He was treated for 2 weeks with ampicillin-sulbactam, but his symptoms have only minimally improved. When he returned to his physician, a basic metabolic panel was performed which showed a creatinine of 2.8 mg/dL. A urinalysis showed 1+ protein with 25 red blood cells per high-power field. Red blood cell casts were present. His chest CT is shown below. Which of the following tests would be most likely to be positive in this individual?

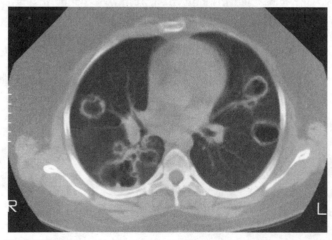

FIGURE IX-26

A. Antiglomerular basement membrane antibodies
B. Antiproteinase-3 antibodies
C. High titers of antibodies to antistreptolysin O
D. Perinuclear antineutrophil cytoplasmic antibodies
E. Positive blood cultures for *Staphylococcus aureus*

IX-27. An 18-year-old man is admitted to the hospital with acute onset of crushing substernal chest pain that began abruptly 30 min ago. He reports the pain radiating to his neck and right arm. He has otherwise been in good health. He currently plays trumpet in his high school marching band but does not participate regularly in aerobic activities. On physical examination, he is diaphoretic and tachypneic. His blood pressure is 100/48 mmHg and heart rate is 110 beats/min. His cardiovascular examination has a regular rhythm but is tachycardic. A II/VI holosystolic murmur is heard best at the apex and radiates to the axilla. His lungs have bilateral rales at the bases. The electrocardiogram demonstrates 4 mm of ST elevation in the anterior leads. On further questioning regarding his past medical history, he recalls having been told that he was hospitalized for some problem with his heart when he was 2 years old. His mother, who accompanies him, reports that he received aspirin and γ globulin as treatment. Since that time, he has required intermittent follow-up with echocardiography. What is the most likely cause of this patient's acute coronary syndrome?

A. Dissection of the aortic root and left coronary ostia
B. Presence of a myocardial bridge overlying the left anterior descending artery
C. Stenosis of a coronary artery aneurysm
D. Vasospasm following cocaine ingestion
E. Vasculitis involving the left anterior descending artery

IX-28. A 29-year-old male with episodic abdominal pain and stress-induced edema of the lips, the tongue, and occasionally the larynx is likely to have low functional or absolute levels of which of the following proteins?

A. C5A (complement cascade)
B. IgE
C. T cell receptor, α chain
D. Cyclooxygenase
E. C1 esterase inhibitor

IX-29. Which of the following joints are typically spared in osteoarthritis (OA)?

A. Ankle
B. Cervical spine
C. Distal interphalangeal joint
D. Hip
E. Knee

IX-30. A 62-year-old woman is admitted to the hospital with pneumococcal bacteremia. Her past medical history is notable for a history of pneumonia due to *Haemophilus influenzae* type B 2 years ago and hypertension. On review of systems, she reports easy bruising, peripheral paresthesias, and symptoms of carpal tunnel syndrome. On physical examination, she has ecchymoses on her face and arms. Her nails are dystrophic and she has alopecia. Her tongue has indentations on both sides. Abdominal examination shows only hepatomegaly. She takes no medications or supple-

IX-30. (*Continued*)
ments and has no significant family history. A complete blood count shows a white blood cell count of 17,000/μL, hematocrit of 30%, and platelets of 300,000/μL. Differential shows 75% neutrophils, 20% lymphocytes. Serum albumin is 3.3 mg/dL, calcium 8.0 mg/dL total protein 8.2 mg/dL, AST 32 U/L, ALT 32 U/L, total bilirubin 1.3 mg/dL, alkaline phosphatase 120 U/L. What is the most likely etiology of the patient's current infection?

A. Cyclical neutropenia
B. Functional asplenism
C. HIV infection
D. Sickle cell anemia
E. X-linked agammaglobulinemia

IX-31. Which of the following statements regarding rheumatoid arthritis is true?

A. There is an association with the class II major histocompatibility complex allele HLA-B27.
B. The earliest lesion in rheumatoid arthritis is an increase in the number of synovial lining cells with microvascular injury.
C. Females are affected three times more often than are males, and this difference is maintained throughout life.
D. Africans and African Americans most commonly have the class II major histocompatibility complex allele HLA-DR4.
E. Titers of rheumatoid factor are not predictive of the severity of rheumatoid arthritis or its extraarticular manifestations.

IX-32. Which of the following definitions best fits the term *enthesitis*?

A. Alteration of joint alignment so that articulating surfaces incompletely approximate each other
B. Inflammation at the site of tendinous or ligamentous insertion into bone
C. Inflammation of the periarticular membrane lining the joint capsule
D. Inflammation of a saclike cavity near a joint that decreases friction
E. A palpable vibratory or crackling sensation elicited with joint motion

IX-33. A 35-year-old female presents to her primary care doctor complaining of diffuse body and joint pain. When asked to describe which of her joints are most affected, she answers, "All of them." There is no associated stiffness, redness, or swelling of the joints. No Raynaud's phenomenon has been appreciated. Occasionally she notes numbness in the fingers and toes. The patient complains of chronic pain and poor sleep quality that she feels is due to her pain. She previously was seen in the clinic for chronic headaches that were felt to be tension-related. She has tried taking over-the-counter ibuprofen twice

IX-33. (*Continued*)
daily without relief of pain. She has no other medical problems. On physical examination, the patient appears comfortable. Her joints exhibit full range of motion without evidence of inflammatory arthritis. She does have pain with palpation at bilateral suboccipital muscle insertions, at C5, at the lateral epicondyle, in the upper outer quadrant of the buttock, at the medial fat pad of the knee proximal to the joint line, and unilaterally on the second right rib. The erythrocyte sedimentation rate is 12 s. Antinuclear antibodies are positive at a titer of 1:40 in a speckled pattern. The patient is HLA-B27-positive. Rheumatoid factor is negative. Radiograms of the cervical spine, hips, and elbows are normal. What is the most likely diagnosis?

A. Ankylosing spondylitis
B. Disseminated gonococcal infection
C. Fibromyalgia
D. Rheumatoid arthritis
E. Systemic lupus erythematosus

IX-34. A 42-year-old woman comes to your clinic 1 week after her primary doctor diagnosed her with fibromyalgia. She describes years of fatigue, chronic pain, poor sleep, and irritability and is unable to work due to her symptoms. A review of her physical examination confirms the presence of pain on digital palpation at 14 of 18 characteristic sites. While relieved at finally having a diagnosis, she is concerned about what treatments are available. Which of the following should be your first treatment step?

A. Improve sleep and consider tricyclics
B. Initiation of a pain diary and frequent, brief clinic visits
C. Low-dose narcotics and a long-acting benzodiazepine
D. Referral for psychotherapy with a psychologist
E. Treatment of depression with a selective serotonin reuptake inhibitor (SSRI)

IX-35. An 18-year-old man with ankylosing spondylitis (AS) is concerned about the development of disability due to his disease. Which of the following statements is true regarding the development and treatment of disability in AS?

A. Anti-TNF-α (tumor necrosis factor α) inhibitors are now first-line therapy and have been shown to limit disability while being safe for long-term therapy.
B. Despite the development of ankylosis of the spine, spinal fracture is a rare complication, affecting <10% of individuals with AS.
C. Maintenance of an exercise program to maintain posture and range of motion is important in limiting disability.
D. Nonsteroidal anti-inflammatory drugs (NSAIDs) decrease pain but have no effect on the development of disability in AS.

IX-36. A 23-year-old woman was diagnosed with systemic lupus erythematosus based upon the presence of polyarthritis, malar rash with photosensitivity, and oral ulcerations. Antibodies to double-stranded DNA, Smith protein, and antinuclear antibodies were present in high titers. A urinalysis is normal. The patient is requesting treatment for the joint symptoms as she feels they limit her activities of daily living. What is the best choice for initial therapy in this individual?

A. Hydroxychloroquine, 200–400 mg daily
B. Methotrexate, 15 mg weekly
C. Physical therapy only
D. Prednisone, 1 mg/kg daily
E. Quinacrine, 100 mg three times daily

IX-37. A 43-year-old male presents to your office complaining of weakness in the right hand for 2 days. He reports that he had been in excellent health until 2 months ago, when he was diagnosed with hypertension. Since that diagnosis, he has lost 20 lb unintentionally and complains of frequent headaches and abdominal pain that is worse after eating. He previously was an injection drug user but now is maintained on methadone. His only medications are hydrochlorothiazide 25 mg/d, methadone 70 mg/d, and lisinopril 5 mg/d. On physical examination, the patient appears well developed and without distress. Blood pressure is 148/94. He is not tachycardic. The examination is otherwise notable only for the inability to extend the right wrist and fingers against gravity. Laboratory studies show an erythrocyte sedimentation rate (ESR) of 88 mm/h, an aspartate aminotransferase (AST) of 154 IU/L, and an alanine aminotransferase (ALT) of 176 IU/L. Which of the following tests is most useful in establishing a diagnosis?

A. Hepatitis B surface antigen
B. Hepatitis C viral load
C. Anticytoplasmic neutrophil antibodies
D. Mesenteric angiography
E. Radial nerve biopsy

IX-38. A 23-year-old woman seeks evaluation for seasonal rhinitis. She reports that she develops symptoms yearly in the spring and fall. During this time, she develops rhinitis with postnasal drip and cough that disrupts her sleep. In addition, she will also note itchy and watery eyes. When the symptoms occur, she takes nonprescription loratadine, 10 mg daily, with significant improvement in her symptoms. What is the most likely allergen(s) that are causing this patient's symptoms?

A. Grass
B. Ragweed
C. Trees
D. A and B
E. B and C
F. All of the above

IX-39. A 45-year-old male has been hospitalized for several weeks in the intensive care unit for postsurgical complications after gastrojejunal bypass surgery. He is noted to have persistent fevers and on examination is found to have erythema, fluctuance, and tenderness over the posterior surface of the left elbow. Initial management of this disorder should include all the following *except*

A. incision and drainage
B. empirical antibiotics for gram-positive organisms
C. aspiration of the collection for Gram stain and culture
D. microscopic evaluation of aspirate for crystals
E. pressure-relieving devices

IX-40. A 51-year-old male presents to your office complaining of lower back pain. When he exerts himself or lifts items, he describes worsening of the pain and also pain in the left buttock that radiates down the posterior left thigh. The patient denies pain at rest and any history of trauma. You examine his lower back. Which examination maneuver is the most specific for lumbar disk herniation?

A. Right straight leg raise
B. Left straight leg raise
C. Right crossed straight leg raise
D. Left crossed straight leg raise
E. Reverse straight leg raise

IX-41. A 42-year-old woman is being treated with cyclophosphamide, 2 mg/kg daily, for Wegener's granulomatosis manifested as glomerulonephritis, tracheal stenosis, and cavitary lung disease. All of the following are potential side effects of cyclophosphamide at this dose *except*

A. alopecia
B. bone marrow suppression
C. hemorrhagic cystitis
D. infertility
E. myelodysplasia

IX-42. Which of the following statements best describes the function of proteins encoded by the human major histocompatibility complex (MHC) I and II genes?

A. Activation of the complement system
B. Binding to cell surface receptors on granulocytes and macrophages to initiate phagocytosis
C. Nonspecific binding of antigen for presentation to T cells
D. Specific antigen binding in response to B cell activation to promote neutralization and precipitation

IX-43. A 32-year-old pregnant woman presents to clinic with right thumb and wrist pain that has worsened over several weeks. She has pain when she pinches her thumb against her other fingers. On physical examination she has mild swelling and tenderness over the radial styloid process, and pain is elicited when she places her thumb in

IX-43. *(Continued)*

her palm and grasps it with her fingers. A Phalen maneuver is negative. Which condition is most likely?

A. Carpal tunnel syndrome
B. DeQuervain's tenosynovitis
C. Gouty arthritis of the first metacarpophalangeal joint
D. Palmar fasciitis
E. Rheumatoid arthritis

IX-44. A 63-year-old white female is admitted to the hospital complaining of hemoptysis and shortness of breath. She had been well until 3 months ago, when she noted vague symptoms of fatigue and a 10-lb unintentional weight loss. Past medical history is notable only for osteoporosis. Her current symptoms began on the day of presentation with the expectoration of >200 mL of red blood in the emergency department. On physical examination, the patient is in marked respiratory distress with a respiratory rate of 44 breaths per minute. Oxygen saturation is 78% on room air and 88% on nonrebreather mask. Pulse is 120 beats/min, with a blood pressure of 170/110. There are diffuse crackles throughout both lung fields, and the cardiac examination is significant only for a regular tachycardia. There are no rashes or joint swellings. Laboratory studies reveal a hemoglobin of 10.2 mg/dL with a mean corpuscular volume (MCV) of 88 μm^3 (fL). The white blood cell count is 9760/mm^3. Blood urea nitrogen (BUN) is 78 mg/dL, and creatinine is 3.2 mg/dL. The urinalysis shows 1+ proteinuria, moderate hemoglobin, 25 to 35 red blood cells (RBC) per high-power field, and occasional RBC casts. Chest computed tomography (CT) shows diffuse alveolar infiltrates consistent with alveolar hemorrhage. The antimyeloperoxidase titer is positive at 126 U/mL (normal <1.4 U/mL). What is the most likely diagnosis?

A. Goodpasture's disease
B. Wegener's granulomatosis
C. Microscopic polyangiitis
D. Polyarteritis nodosa
E. Cryoglobulinemia

IX-45. A 62-year-old white male presents with a chief complaint of right knee pain and swelling. Past medical history is significant for obesity with a body mass index (BMI) of 34 kg/m^2, diet-controlled type 2 diabetes mellitus, and hypertension. His medications include hydrochlorothiazide and acetaminophen as needed for pain. Physical examination is remarkable for a moderate-size effusion of the right knee, with range of motion limited to 90° of flexion and 160° of extension. There is minimal warmth and no redness. He has crepitus with range of motion. With weight bearing, he has outward bowing of the legs bilaterally. A radiogram of the right knee shows osteophytes and joint space narrowing. Which of the following is the most likely finding on joint fluid examination?

IX-45. *(Continued)*

A. A Gram stain showing gram-positive cocci in clusters
B. A white blood cell count of 1110/mm^3
C. A white blood cell count of 22,000/mm^3
D. Positively birefringent crystals on polarizing light microscopy
E. Negatively birefringent crystals on polarizing light microscopy

IX-46. A 25-year-old female presents with a complaint of painful mouth ulcerations. She describes these lesions as shallow ulcers that last for 1 or 2 weeks. The ulcers have been appearing for the last 6 months. For the last 2 days, the patient has had a painful red eye. She has had no genital ulcerations, arthritis, skin rashes, or photosensitivity. On physical examination, the patient appears well developed and in no distress. She has a temperature of 37.6°C (99.7°F), heart rate of 86, blood pressure of 126/72, and respiratory rate of 16. Examination of the oral mucosa reveals two shallow ulcers with a yellow base on the buccal mucosa. The ophthalmologic examination is consistent with anterior uveitis. The cardiopulmonary examination is normal. She has no arthritis, but medially on the right thigh there is a palpable cord in the saphenous vein. Laboratory studies reveal an erythrocyte sedimentation rate of 68 s. White blood cell count is 10,230/mm^3 with a differential of 68% polymorphonuclear cells, 28% lymphocytes, and 4% monocytes. The antinuclear antibody and anti-dsDNA antibody are negative. C3 is 89 mg/dL, and C4 is 24 mg/dL. What is the most likely diagnosis?

A. Behçet's syndrome
B. Systemic lupus erythematosus
C. Discoid lupus erythematosus
D. Sjögren's syndrome
E. Cicatricial pemphigoid

IX-47. What is the best initial treatment for this patient?

A. Topical glucocorticoids including ophthalmic prednisolone
B. Systemic glucocorticoids and azathioprine
C. Thalidomide
D. Colchicine
E. Intralesional interferon α

IX-48. A 42-year-old man presents to your clinic complaining of left shoulder soreness that has been bothering him for 8 months. He experiences intermittent pain that is worse at night. Active abduction of his left arm over his head causes extreme pain. He describes his pain as a dull ache in his shoulder. He cannot identify a specific trauma that led to his pain but notes that he lifts weights and plays sports on a regular basis. On physical examination, he has tenderness over the lateral aspect of the humeral head and pain with arm abduction. Which of the following is the most likely cause of his symptoms?

IX-48. (*Continued*)

A. Acromioclavicular arthritis
B. Bicipital tendonitis
C. Inflammation of the infraspinatus tendon
D. Inflammation of the supraspinatus tendon
E. Subluxation of the left humeral head

IX-49. A 42-year-old male presents with complaints of a rash and joint pain. He first noticed the rash 6 months ago. It is primarily on the hands (see Figure IX-49, Color Atlas), the extensor surfaces of the elbows, and the knees, low back, and scalp. Although he complains of the appearance of these lesions, they do not itch or hurt. The patient has not been previously evaluated for them and has recently noticed changes in the nail beds. For the last 2 weeks, the patient has had increasingly severe pain in the distal joints of the hands and feet. His hands are so painful that he is having trouble writing and holding utensils. The patient denies fevers, weight loss, fatigue, cough, shortness of breath, or changes in bowel or bladder habits. Which of the following is the most likely diagnosis?

A. Arthritis associated with inflammatory bowel disease
B. Gout
C. Osteoarthritis
D. Psoriatic arthritis
E. Rheumatoid arthritis

IX-50. Which of the following is the most common clinical manifestation of relapsing polychondritis?

A. Aortic regurgitation
B. Arthritis of weight-bearing joints
C. Auricular chondritis
D. Reduced hearing
E. Saddle-nose deformity

IX-51. A 60-year-old woman with a history of Sjögren's syndrome diagnosed 20 years ago presents to her primary care doctor complaining of facial swelling. Her xerostomia dry eye symptoms have not changed. She is known to be positive for rheumatoid factor in addition to Ro and La antibodies but is not thought to have rheumatoid arthritis. She previously had cutaneous vasculitis requiring treatment with prednisone, but she has been off steroids for 5 years without evidence of recurrence. She is currently using artificial tears and cevimeline, 30 mg three times daily. On physical examination, her right parotid gland is enlarged. It is not tender, but is firm and hard to touch. It is noted that the right parotid gland was similarly enlarged on a visit 3 months ago. She denies systemic illness or any new symptoms. What is the most likely diagnosis?

A. Adenoid cystic carcinoma
B. B cell lymphoma
C. Impacted sialolith
D. Mumps
E. Recurrent vasculitis

IX-52. A 42-year-old Turkish man presents to his physician complaining of recurring ulcers in the mouth and on his penis. He states that the ulcers are painful and last for about 2 weeks before spontaneously resolving. In addition, he intermittently gets skin lesions that he describes as painful nodules on his lower extremities. You suspect that he has Behçet's syndrome. A pathergy test is performed. What response would you expect after injecting 0.3 mL of sterile saline under the skin?

A. Development of 10 mm of induration with overlying erythema after 72 h
B. Development of a 2- to 3-mm papule at the site of insertion in 2–3 days
C. Development of granulomatous inflammation 4–6 weeks after the injection
D. Development of an urticarial reaction within 15 min
E. No reaction

IX-53. A 45-year-old African-American woman with systemic lupus erythematosus (SLE) presents to the emergency room with complaints of headache and fatigue. Her prior manifestations of SLE have been arthralgias, hemolytic anemia, malar rash, and mouth ulcers, and she is known to have high titers of antibodies to double-stranded DNA. She currently is taking prednisone, 5 mg daily, and hydroxychloroquine, 200 mg daily. On presentation, she is found to have a blood pressure of 190/110 mmHg with a heart rate of 98 beats/min. A urinalysis shows 25 red blood cells (RBCs) per high-power field with 2+ proteinuria. No RBC casts are identified. Her blood urea nitrogen is 88 mg/dL, and creatinine is 2.6 mg/dL (baseline 0.8 mg/dL). She has not previously had renal disease related to SLE and is not taking nonsteroidal anti-inflammatory drugs. She denies any recent illness, decreased oral intake, or diarrhea. What is the most appropriate next step in the management of this patient?

A. Initiate cyclophosphamide, 500 mg/m² body surface area IV, and plan to repeat monthly for 3–6 months.
B. Initiate hemodialysis.
C. Initiate high-dose steroid therapy (IV methylprednisolone, 1000 mg daily for 3 doses, followed by oral prednisone, 1 mg/kg daily) and mycophenolate mofetil, 2 g daily.
D. Initiate plasmapheresis.
E. Withhold all therapy until renal biopsy is performed.

IX-54. Which of the following statements regarding rheumatoid arthritis (RA) is true?

A. 75% of patients with RA have a first-degree relative with the disease.
B. Genetic factors explain 90% of disease susceptibility in RA.
C. Greater than 75% of patients are diagnosed in their twenties to thirties.
D. Inflammatory synovitis is the hallmark of RA.
E. The male to female ratio is 3:1.

IX-55. A 52-year-old female has poorly controlled rheumatoid arthritis on prednisone 5 mg daily and etanercept 50 mg weekly by subcutaneous injection. Despite this, she has ongoing symptoms with severe pain in the wrists, hands, feet, and ankles. She also has destructive arthritis causing swan-neck and boutonnière deformities in the hands as well as plantar subluxation of the metatarsal heads that prevents ambulation. She has subcutaneous nodules on the extensor surfaces of the arms. She presents to the emergency room complaining of fevers and dysuria. On physical examination temperature is 39.1°C (102.3°F). Heart rate is 112, and blood pressure is 122/76. The examination is unremarkable except for right costovertebral angle tenderness and splenomegaly. Laboratory studies at the time of presentation reveal a white blood cell count of 2300/mm^3 with 15% polymorphonuclear cells, 75% lymphocytes, 8% monocytes, and 2% eosinophils. She is also anemic with a hemoglobin of 9.2 mg/dL and a hematocrit of 28.7%. The mean corpuscular volume is 88 fL. The platelet count is 132,000/mm^3. A peripheral blood smear shows normocytic anemia without anisocytosis or poikilocytosis. She is found to have *Escherichia coli* bacteremia related to a urinary tract infection. She is treated with ceftriaxone and does well. However, she remains anemic and neutropenic. The patient undergoes a bone marrow biopsy that shows hypercellularity with a lack of mature neutrophils. What is the most likely diagnosis?

A. Acute myelogenous leukemia
B. B cell lymphoma
C. Disseminated *Mycobacterium tuberculosis* infection
D. Felty's syndrome
E. Idiosyncratic reaction to etanercept

IX-56. What is the most common extraarticular manifestation of ankylosing spondylitis?

A. Anterior uveitis
B. Aortic regurgitation
C. Cataracts
D. Inflammatory bowel disease
E. Third-degree heart block

IX-57. A 42-year-old female presents to the physician with 3 months of worsening dyspnea on exertion, malaise, and weakness. She reports that the symptoms have worsened gradually and are associated with low-grade fever, anorexia, and an 8-lb weight loss. She has trouble climbing stairs because of leg weakness and shortness of breath. Recently she has noticed that her arms tire while she is brushing her teeth or combing her hair. Her mother also commented that the patient seems to have difficulty rising from the couch. Her writing is normal, and she has no sensory symptoms. Physical examination is notable for a temperature of 37.8°C (100°F), bilateral lung crackles, and diminished strength in the deltoids, quadriceps, and psoas muscles. Laboratory studies are notable for an elevated creatine kinase. Chest radiography shows bilateral interstitial infiltrates, and lung volumes are reduced to

IX-57. *(Continued)*
70% of the predicted values. Which of the following autoantibodies is most likely to be present in this patient?

A. Antiglomerular basement membrane antibody
B. Antihistone antibody
C. Anti-Jo-1 antibody
D. Antimicrosomal antibody
E. Antineutrophil cytoplasmic antibody (ANCA)

IX-58. A 43-year-old man presents to your clinic complaining of bilateral knee pain. He states that the pain worsens with walking and is not present at rest. He has been experiencing knee pain for many months and has had no relief from over-the-counter analgesics. He has a history of hypertension and obesity. Which of the following represents the best initial treatment strategy for this patient?

A. Avoidance of walking for several weeks
B. Light daily walking exercises
C. Low-dose, long-acting narcotics
D. Oral steroid pulse
E. Weight loss

IX-59. A 53-year-old woman presents to your clinic complaining of fatigue and generalized pain that have worsened over 2 years. She also describes irritability and poor sleep and is concerned that she is depressed. She reveals that she was recently separated from her husband and has been stressed at work. Which of the following elements of her presentation meet American College of Rheumatology criteria for fibromyalgia?

A. Diffuse chronic pain and abnormal sleep
B. Diffuse pain without other etiology and evidence of major depression
C. Major depression, life stressor, chronic pain, and female gender
D. Major depression and pain on palpation at 6 of 18 tender point sites
E. Widespread chronic pain and pain on palpation at 11 of 18 tender point sites

IX-60. A 62-year-old female complains of aching joints. She notes intermittent stiffness and pain in the knees, hips, wrists, and hands. She also describes easy fatigability, dyspepsia, a dry cough, and itchy red eyes and also has trouble keeping her dentures in place. There is a history of diabetes but no other significant history. Medications include insulin and naproxen. She has no HIV risk factors. Examination is significant for dry mucous membranes in the oropharynx. There is no evidence of joint destruction or active inflammation. Laboratory studies show a negative antinucleolar antibody but a positive Ro/SSA autoantigen. What is the most likely diagnosis?

A. Sarcoidosis
B. Sjögren's syndrome
C. Rheumatoid arthritis
D. Psychogenic illness
E. Vitamin A deficiency

IX-61. A 46-year-old woman is referred to your clinic by her primary care physician. She describes fatigue and diffuse muscle aches that have been worsening over a period of 6 months. She also has not been sleeping well. Her primary doctor evaluated her and sent screening laboratory tests, which returned with a positive rheumatoid factor. She has read about rheumatoid arthritis on the Internet and is very concerned that she has the disease based on her symptoms and her positive test. Which of the following is true in regard to diagnosing rheumatoid arthritis (RA)?

A. 10% of healthy individuals will test positive for anti-bodies to cyclic citrullinated polypeptides (anti-CCP).
B. Erythrocyte sedimentation rate (ESR) is elevated in 70% of patients with active disease.
C. In early disease, rheumatoid factor is more accurate than anti-CCP.
D. Fewer than one-third of unselected patients with positive rheumatoid factor will have RA.
E. Radiographs should be performed in this patient to help with diagnosis.

IX-62. A 34-year-old woman is seen in the allergy clinic for complaint of chronic rhinitis. She reports that she first developed seasonal rhinitis in her early twenties, limited to the fall of the year. At that point, she would use di-phenhydramine on an as-needed basis, but she limited her use because of the sedating side effects. Since she moved into her current home 5 years ago, her symptoms have become continuous. She states her nose stays con-gested, and she has constant postnasal drip. She awakens frequently at night with a cough and complains of day-time fatigue due to inadequate sleep. She currently is tak-ing fexofenadine, 180 mg daily, but states she feels no relief from her symptoms. At night, she will occasionally take diphenhydramine because of its sedating side effects. Her past medical history is significant for eczema, for which she uses topical steroid creams, and frequent mi-graines requiring propranolol for prophylaxis. She is al-lergic to ragweed. She has no other known environmental allergens but has never had skin-prick testing. She does not smoke cigarettes or consume alcohol. She works as a librarian in a new building. Her home is a wooden single family home built in the 1930s. There is carpeting throughout the first floor of the home, including the bed-room. The basement is not finished and has been flooded in the past. She has a 1-year old cat that lives indoors. On physical examination, she has large and boggy nasal tur-binates. Her posterior oropharynx shows evidence of cobblestoning. Her lungs are clear without wheezes. Skin-prick testing demonstrates allergic responses to ragweed, grass, cat and dog dander, and dust mites. All of the fol-lowing would be appropriate initial therapy in this pa-tient *except*

A. immunotherapy for cat dander
B. intranasal mometasone furoate
C. oral montelukast

IX-62. (*Continued*)
D. removal of carpets and drapes from the bedroom
E. weekly laundry of the bedding at temperatures >54.4°C

IX-63. A 46-year-old woman presents to your clinic with multiple complaints. She describes fatigue and general malaise over 2–3 months. Her appetite has decreased. She thinks she has unintentionally lost ~5.5 kg. Lately she notes pain and stiffness in her fingers on both hands that is worse in the morning and with repetitive movement. She has a grandmother and a sister who have rheumatoid arthritis (RA), and she is very concerned that she now has it as well. Which of her complaints represents the most common manifestation of established RA?

A. Fatigue and anorexia for >2 months with concomi-tant joint pain
B. Morning joint stiffness lasting for >1 h
C. Pain in symmetric joints worsened with movement
D. Positive family history with two relatives with RA
E. Weight loss >4.5 kg during period of active disease

IX-64. A 23-year-old man seeks evaluation for low back pain. He states that when he first awakens there is a dull aching pain in his lower lumbar and gluteal region. When he first noticed the pain about 6 months ago, he thought the pain might be related to his mattress, but it has wors-ened even after buying a new mattress. Most mornings, it takes about 45–60 min to loosen up after he has awak-ened, but the pain will recur if he is idle. He is currently in law school and finds it increasingly difficult to remain in classes because of back pain. When he exercises, the pain lessens. There are occasional nights that the pain will awaken him from sleep, and he will have to move around and stretch his back to improve the pain. On physical ex-amination, there is pain with palpation at the iliac crests, ischial tuberosities, greater trochanters, and heels. With maximal inspiration, the chest expands 4 cm, and there is decreased flexion of the lumbar spine. A radiograph of the pelvis shows erosions and sclerosis of the sacroiliac joints bilaterally. Which of the following tests is most likely to be positive in this individual?

A. Alkaline phosphatase
B. Antibodies directed against cyclic citrullinated pep-tides (CCP)
C. Antinuclear antibodies
D. HLA-B27
E. Rheumatoid factor

IX-65. All the following organisms have been implicated in reactive arthritis *except*

A. *Chlamydia trachomatis*
B. *Neisseria gonorrhoeae*
C. *Salmonella enteritidis*
D. *Shigella dysenteriae*
E. *Yersinia enterocolitica*

IX-66. An 84-year-old man is seen by his primary care provider with symptoms of acute gouty arthritis in the first great toe and ankle on the left. He has a prior history of gout presenting similarly. His past medical history is significant for myelodysplasia, congestive heart failure, hypercholesterolemia, and chronic kidney disease. He is taking pravastatin, aspirin, furosemide, metolazone, lisinopril, and metoprolol XL. His baseline creatinine is 2.4 mg/dL, and uric acid level 9.3 mg/dL. His most recent complete blood count results are white blood cell count 2880/µL, hemoglobin 8.2 g/dL, hematocrit 26.2%, and platelet 68,000/µL. Which of the following medication regimens are most appropriate for the treatment of this patient?

A. Allopurinol, 100 mg once daily
B. Colchicine, 1 mg IV once, then 0.5 mg IV every 6 h until improvement
C. Indomethacin, 25 mg three times daily
D. Prednisone, 40 mg once daily
E. Probenecid, 250 mg twice daily

IX-67. A patient with primary Sjögren's syndrome that was diagnosed 6 years ago and treated with tear replacement for symptomatic relief notes continued parotid swelling for the last 3 months. She has also noted enlarging posterior cervical lymph nodes. Evaluation shows leukopenia and low C4 complement levels. What is the most likely diagnosis?

A. Chronic pancreatitis
B. Secondary Sjögren's syndrome

IX-67. (Continued)
C. HIV infection
D. Lymphoma
E. Amyloidosis

IX-68. A 19-year-old recent immigrant from Ethiopia comes to your clinic to establish primary care. She currently feels well. Her past medical history is notable for a recent admission to the hospital for new-onset atrial fibrillation. As a child in Ethiopia, she developed an illness that caused uncontrolled flailing of her limbs and tongue lasting ~1 month. She also has had three episodes of migratory large-joint arthritis during her adolescence that resolved with pills that she received from the pharmacy. She is currently taking metoprolol and warfarin and has no known drug allergies. Physical examination reveals an irregularly irregular heart beat with normal blood pressure. Her Point of Maximal Impulse (PMI) is most prominent at the mid clavicular line and is normal in size. An early diastolic rumble and 3/6 holosystolic murmur are heard at the apex. A soft early diastolic murmur is also heard at the left third intercostal space. You refer her to a cardiologist for evaluation of valve replacement and echocardiography. What other intervention might you consider at this time?

A. Glucocorticoids
B. Daily aspirin
C. Daily doxycycline
D. Monthly penicillin G injections
E. Penicillin G injections as needed for all sore throats

IX. RHEUMATOLOGY AND IMMUNOLOGY

ANSWERS

IX-1. **The answer is A.** *(Chap. 326)* Osteoarthritis (OA) represents joint failure in which pathologic changes have occurred in all structures of the affected joint. The central pathology in OA is articular cartilage loss. The components leading to the development of OA can be separated into those that contribute to joint loading and those that increase joint vulnerability. The most potent risk factor for OA, however, is aging. Approximately 70% of women >65 years have OA. A young joint has in place protective mechanisms that allow it to tolerate excessive loading without lasting damage. Gender does not play a significant role in terms of risk. Joint injury is a strong predictor of the future development of osteoarthritis. Obesity is a well-recognized risk factor in hip and knee arthritis likely due to increased loading forces. Obesity appears to play a role in OA of the hand as well, suggesting that obesity has both a mechanical and metabolic mechanism of action. The genetics of OA are not well understood. Inherited polymorphisms appear to play a role in hand and hip OA but not as much in other joints.

IX-2. **The answer is E.** *(Chap. 16)* This patient's symptoms are most consistent with abnormalities of the C8 or T1 nerve roots. The diagnosis of diabetes mellitus is possible, but his symptoms are not consistent with diabetic neuropathy, which would more commonly be symmetric in both hands. The patient does not have any other signs or symptoms of systemic vasculitis and does not describe risk factors or other findings consistent with cholesterol emboli. Cervical spondylosis is possible, but this is typically a disease process of C2–C4 nerve roots and presents with pain in the neck radiating into the back of the head, shoulders, and arms. The thoracic outlet contains the first rib, the subclavian artery and vein, the brachial plexus, the clavicle, and the lung apex. Neurogenic thoracic outlet syndrome results from compression of the lower brachial plexus. Signs may include weakness of the intrinsic muscles of the hand and diminished sensation on the palmar surface of the fourth and fifth digits. EMG testing and imaging with either contrast CT scan or magnetic resonance imaging (MRI) confirms the diagnosis. Treatment consists of surgical decompression of the brachial plexus. Other forms of thoracic outlet syndrome (TOS) include arterial TOS, which results in compression of the vasculature and subsequent thrombus formation, and disputed TOS, which is described in patients with chronic arm and shoulder pain with an unclear etiology.

IX-3. **The answer is E.** *(Chap. 319)* This patient has polyarteritis nodosa associated with hepatitis B infection. Polyarteritis nodosa (PAN) is a small- and medium-vessel vasculitis that classically involves the muscular mesenteric and renal arteries. Pulmonary arteries are spared. Classic PAN is a rare disease, but its exact prevalence is unknown because reported cases frequently also include other vasculidities such as microscopic polyangiitis. Prior to the Chapel Hill Consensus Conference of 1992, microscopic polyangiitis and PAN were considered as the same disease, but it has been recognized that these are two separate diseases with different serologic markers and vascular predilection. Clinical manifestations of PAN are commonly vague, and often patients have been ill for several months prior to diagnosis. Symptoms include fatigue, weight loss, abdominal pain, headache, and hypertension. The pathologic lesion of PAN is necrotizing inflammation of the small- and medium-sized muscular arteries, and diagnosis relies upon demonstration of this lesion on biopsy. However, in the absence of easily obtainable tissue, the presence of multiple aneurysmal dilatations on mesenteric angiogram are highly suggestive of PAN in the appropriate clinical setting. There are no serologic tests that are diagnostic of PAN. It is rare to have positive antibodies to p-ANCA or c-ANCA in PAN. Interestingly, 30% of cases of PAN are associated with active hepatitis B infection as in this patient, and it is thought that circulating immune complexes may play a role in the pathogenesis of this disease. Unlike PAN, MPA involves venules and capillaries in addition to small arteries. The histopathologic lesion of MPA is a necrotizing vasculitis that is pauci-immune with minimal deposition of immune complexes. Typical presenting features are rapidly progressive glomerulonephritis and pulmonary hemorrhage, which are distinctly uncommon features of PAN. Antimyeloperoxidase antibodies (p-ANCA) are frequently present. Mixed cryoglobulinemia is a small-vessel vasculitis most often associated with hepatitis C infection. Skin involvement with leukocytoclastic vasculitis and palpable purpura are the most common presenting features. Proliferative glomerulonephritis is present in 20–60% of individuals and is the most common cause of morbidity. Ischemic colitis typically presents with abdominal pain out of proportion to the examination as in this case, but the mesenteric angiogram would show atherosclerotic narrowing rather than aneurysmal dilatation. Hepatocellular carcinoma is not associated with vasculitis and typically presents with vague abdominal pain and obstructive jaundice.

IX-4. **The answer is A.** *(Chap. 324)* This patient presents with a multisystem illness involving the heart, kidneys, and peripheral nervous system. The physical examination is suggestive of amyloidosis with classic waxy papules in the folds of his body. The laboratories are remarkable for renal failure of unclear etiology with significant proteinuria but no cellular casts. A possible etiology of the renal failure is suggested by the elevated gamma globulin fraction and low hematocrit, bringing to mind a monoclonal gammopathy perhaps leading to renal failure through amyloid AL deposition. This could also account for the enlarged heart seen on the echocardiogram and the peripheral neuropathy. The fat pad biopsy is generally reported to be 60 to 80% sensitive for amyloid; however, it would not allow a diagnosis of this patient's likely myeloma. A right heart catheterization probably would prove that the patient has restrictive cardiomyopathy secondary to amyloid deposition; however, it too would not diagnose the underlying plasma cell dyscrasia. Renal ultrasound, although warranted to rule out obstructive uropathy, would not be diagnostic. Similarly, the electromyogram and nerve conduction studies would not be diagnostic. The bone marrow biopsy is about 50 to 60% sensitive for amyloid, but it would allow evaluation of the percent of plasma cells in the bone marrow and allow the diagnosis of multiple myeloma to be made. Multiple myeloma is associated with amyloid AL in approximately 20% of cases. Light chains most commonly deposit systemically in the heart, kidneys, liver, and nervous system, causing organ dysfunction. In these organs, biopsy would show the classic eosinophilic material that, when exposed to Congo red stain, has a characteristic apple-green birefringence.

IX-5. **The answer is E.** *(Chap. 321)* Eye inflammation (60% of cases) and arthritis (>70% of cases) can be suggestive of either rheumatoid arthritis or relapsing polychondritis. The arthritis associated with RA is typically erosive and symmetric, unlike that in relapsing polychondritis. Both conditions can present with vasculitis (15% in relapsing polychondritis). Rheumatoid factor is occasionally positive in relapsing polychondritis but is usually low titer when present. Saddle-nose deformity, which is present in 25% of patients with relapsing polychondritis, may be confused with Wegener's granulomatosis.

IX-6. **The answer is B.** *(Chap. 328)* Though the crystals suggest that the patient has active pseudogout, the more important diagnosis acutely is septic arthritis. This is highly probable based on the joint leukocyte count >100,000/µL, high percentage of PMNs, and positive Gram stain. Crystal-induced, rheumatoid, and other noninfectious causes of arthritis typically have WBC counts in the 30,000–50,000/µL range. WBC counts in indolent infections such as fungal or mycobacterial arthritis are commonly in the 10,000–30,000/µL range. The bacteria of septic arthritis usually enter the joint via hematogenous spread through synovial capillaries. Patients with rheumatoid arthritis are at high risk of a septic arthritis due to *Staphylococcus aureus* because of chronic inflammation and glucocorticoid therapy. The concurrent presence of pseudogout does not preclude the diagnosis of septic arthritis. In adults, the most common bacterial pathogens are *Neisseria gonorrhoeae* and *S. aureus*. Antibiotics, prompt surgical evaluation of possible arthroscopic drainage, and blood cultures to rule out bacteremia are all indicated. Prompt local and systemic treatment of infection can prevent destruction of cartilage, joint instability, or deformity. Direct instillation of antibiotics into the joint fluid is not necessary. If the smear shows no organisms, a third-generation cephalosporin is reasonable empirical therapy. In the presence of Gram-positive cocci in clusters, antistaphylococcal therapy should be instituted based on community prevalence of methicillin resistance or recent hospitalization (which would favor empirical vancomycin). Typically acute flairs of pseudogout can be addressed with glucocorticoids. However, this could portend a higher risk in the context of infection. Nonsteroidal anti-inflammatory agents might be a possibility depending on the patient's renal function and gastrointestinal history.

IX-7.   The answer is A. *(Chap. 331)*   Adhesive capsulitis is characterized by pain and restricted motion of the shoulder. Usually this occurs in the absence of intrinsic shoulder disease, including osteoarthritis and avascular necrosis. It is, however, more common in patients who have had bursitis or tendinitis previously as well as patients with other systemic illnesses, such as chronic pulmonary disease, ischemic heart disease, and diabetes mellitus. The etiology is not clear, but adhesive capsulitis appears to develop in the setting of prolonged immobility. Reflex sympathetic dystrophy may also occur in the setting of adhesive capsulitis. Clinically, this disorder is more commonly seen in females over age 50. Pain and stiffness develop over the course of months to years. On physical examination, the affected joint is tender to palpation, with a restricted range of motion. The gold standard for diagnosis is arthrography with limitation of the amount of injectable contrast to less than 15 mL. In most patients, adhesive capsulitis will regress spontaneously within 1 to 3 years. NSAIDs, glucocorticoid injections, physical therapy, and early mobilization of the arm are useful therapies.

IX-8.   The answer is B. *(Chap. 317)*   The patient in this vignette is presenting with severe dry eyes and mouth in the presence of autoantibodies to Ro and La (SS-A and SS-B, extractable nuclear and cytoplasmic antigens) consistent with the diagnosis of Sjögren's syndrome. This autoimmune disorder is associated with lymphocytic infiltration of exocrine glands that results in decreased tear and saliva production as the most prominent symptoms. Sjögren's syndrome affects women nine times more frequently than men and usually presents in middle age. Other autoimmune diseases often have associated xerostomia and dry eyes (secondary Sjögren's syndrome). High titers of antibodies to Ro and La are associated with longer disease duration, salivary gland enlargement, and the development of extraglandular involvement, especially cutaneous vasculitis and demyelinating syndromes. One-third of patients with Sjögren's syndrome have extraglandular involvement of the disease, most commonly in the lungs and kidneys. In this patient with acidemia and hypokalemia, the possibility of renal disease due to Sjögren's syndrome should be considered. Interstitial nephritis is a common manifestation of Sjögren's syndrome in the kidneys. Distal (type I) renal tubular acidosis is also frequent, occurring in 25% of individuals with Sjögren's syndrome. Diagnosis could be confirmed by obtaining urine electrolytes to demonstrate a positive urine anion gap. Renal biopsy is not necessary. Treatment does not require immunosuppression as the acidemia can be treated with bicarbonate replacement. Diarrhea could cause similar electrolyte abnormalities with a non-anion gap acidosis, but the patient would be symptomatic. Furthermore, gastrointestinal symptoms do not commonly occur in Sjögren's syndrome. Hypoaldosteronism is associated with a type IV renal tubular acidosis that results in hyperkalemia and a non-anion gap acidosis. Renal compensation for respiratory alkalosis should not result in hypokalemia. Purging in anorexia nervosa could result in hypokalemia and increased risk of dental caries, but it would be associated with metabolic alkalosis rather than acidosis.

IX-9.   The answer is A. *(Chap. 324)*   Patients on hemodialysis are at risk for a particular type of amyloidosis due to deposition of β_2-microglobulin ($A\beta_2M$). The protein is above the molecular weight cut-off for clearance by the dialysis membrane and is becoming less common with the advent of newer dialysis techniques. The clinical syndrome is a rheumatologic one, with joint effusions, arthropathy, and cystic bone lesions predominating. The β_2-microglobulin can be found in joint synovium, and the joint fluid is usually noninflammatory. Serum amyloid A (secondary amyloid) is associated with chronic infections or inflammatory conditions. AL (immunoglobulin light chain deposition) is the most common type of amyloidosis and is due to a clonal population of B cells. Deposition of the fibrinogen α-chain (AFib) is a familial condition associated with a systemic amyloidosis. Transthyretin is associated with a familial form of amyloidosis that is transmitted in an autosomal dominant fashion. These usually manifest in midlife with neuropathy and cardiomyopathy. One variant of transthyretin amyloid has a carrier frequency of up to 4% in African Americans and is associated with a late-onset cardiomyopathy.

IX-10. **The answer is A.** *(Chap. 383)* Polymyositis is an inflammatory myopathy that presents as symmetric, progressive muscle weakness. The patient reports difficulty with everyday tasks requiring the use of proximal muscles, such as getting up from a chair and climbing steps. Distal muscle strength is usually preserved until late in the course. In addition to the musculoskeletal findings, there are numerous extramuscular manifestations. This patient may have systemic symptoms of fever, malaise, weight loss, and Raynaud's phenomenon. There may be "overlap" features with other autoimmune diseases, such as systemic lupus erythematosus (SLE) and scleroderma. Involvement of the striated muscles and the upper esophagus may lead to dysphagia. Conduction defects, arrhythmia, and dilated cardiomyopathy may occur. Interstitial lung disease may precede myopathy or occur early in the disease, often in association with the presence of antibodies to t-RNA synthetases. Although dermatomyositis is linked with an increased incidence of cancer, polymyositis does not seem to be associated with an increased incidence.

IX-11. **The answer is C.** *(Chap. 327)* Acute gouty arthritis is frequently seen in individuals on diuretic therapy. Diuretics result in hyperuricemia through enhanced urate reabsorption in the proximal tubule of the kidney in the setting of volume depletion. Hyperuricemia remains asymptomatic in many individuals but may manifest as acute gout. Acute gout is an intensely inflammatory arthritis that frequently begins at night. While any joint may be affected, the initial presentation of gout is often in the great toe at the metatarsophalangeal joint. There is associated joint swelling, effusion, erythema, and exquisite tenderness. A typical patient will complain that the pain is so great that they are unable to wear socks or allow sheets or blankets to cover the toes. Arthrocentesis will reveal an inflammatory cloudy-appearing fluid. The diagnosis of gout is confirmed by the demonstration of monosodium urate crystals seen both extracellularly and intracellularly within neutrophils. Monosodium urate crystals appear strongly negatively birefringent under polarized light microscopy and have a typical needle- and rod-shaped appearance. The WBC count is usually <50,000/μL with values >100,000/μL being more likely to be associated with a septic arthritis. Likewise, very low glucose levels and a positive Gram stain are not manifestations of acute gout but are common in septic arthritis. Calcium pyrophosphate dihydrate crystals appear as weakly positively birefringent rhomboidal crystals and are seen in pseudogout.

IX-12 and IX-13. **The answers are E and E.** *(Chap. 313)* This patient is presenting with symptoms that are consistent with systemic lupus erythematosus (SLE). SLE can present with a wide variety of complaints affecting every organ system. The most common complaints with SLE are fatigue (95%), arthralgias (95%), photosensitivity (70%), anemia (70%), leukopenia (65%), and nonerosive polyarthritis (60%)—all of which are present in this patient. In addition, this patient has mouth ulcers, which are seen in 40%. The scalp lesion is consistent with discoid lupus erythematosus, which can be a benign condition if presenting as an isolated condition. Only 5% of individuals with isolated discoid lesions develop SLE; however, up to 20% of those with SLE will have discoid lesions. The presence of a positive ANA is sensitive, but not specific, for SLE as 98% of individuals with SLE will have a positive ANA during the course of the disease. Alternatively, persistent negative ANA results can rule out SLE. Antibodies to double-stranded DNA and to the Smith protein (nuclear U1 RNA) are both specific for SLE in high titers. Some 70% of individuals with SLE will have positive antibodies for ds-DNA, and 25% will have antibodies to the Smith protein. Individuals with anti-Sm antibodies often also have antibodies to ribonucleoprotein as well. The level of rheumatoid factor in this patient falls within the equivocal range and is not diagnostic of rheumatoid arthritis. Further, the patient's discoid rash and photosensitivity as well as positive serologies would further eliminate rheumatoid arthritis from the differential diagnosis. Behçet's disease presents with oral and genital ulcerations, and 50% will also have nonerosive arthritis. However, the skin lesions for Behçet's disease do not usually appear as discoid lesions, and Behçet's is inconsistent with the serology studies. Finally, sarcoidosis can mimic the arthritic disease of SLE. The rash associated with sarcoidosis is papular lesions along the nasolabial folds (lupus pernio) and erythema nodosum.

Nephritis is the most serious manifestation of SLE and, with infection, is the leading cause of death in the first decade following diagnosis. However, in most individuals, nephritis is clinically silent until the disease is advanced. For this reason, it is recommended that all patients suspected of having SLE undergo a urinalysis. In the presence of nephritis, the expected findings would include microscopic hematuria and proteinuria in early disease. In more severe disease, red cell casts and nephrotic range proteinuria may be seen. A skin biopsy of the discoid lesion would show hyperkeratosis and follicular plugging. A mononuclear cell infiltrate is often seen near the dermal-epidermal junction. While a biopsy would be diagnostic for discoid lupus, it would not alter management. An electrocardiogram would be indicated if the patient were complaining of pain consistent with pericarditis. Likewise, the presence of a murmur on examination may prompt an echocardiogram to assess for Libmann-Sachs valvular disease in a patient with SLE. However, these tests are not indicated in an asymptomatic patient. If sarcoidosis were being considered, chest radiography would be appropriate to assess for hilar lymphadenopathy and interstitial lung disease, but they are not indicated in this case.

IX-14.   The answer is D. *(Chap. 311)* Urticaria and angioedema are common disorders, affecting approximately 20% of the population. In acute urticarial angioedema, attacks of swelling are of less than 6 weeks' duration; chronic urticarial angioedema is by definition more long-standing. Urticaria usually is pruritic and affects the trunk and proximal extremities. Angioedema is generally less pruritic and affects the hands, feet, genitalia, and face. This female has chronic urticaria, which probably is due to a cutaneous necrotizing vasculitis. The clues to the diagnosis are the arthralgias, the presence of residual skin discoloration, and the elevated sedimentation rate, which would be uncharacteristic of other urticarial diseases. The diagnosis can be confirmed by skin biopsy. Chronic urticaria rarely has an allergic cause; hence, allergy skin tests and measurement of total IgE levels are not helpful. Measurement of C1 esterase inhibitor activity is useful in diagnosing hereditary angioedema, a disease that is not associated with urticaria. Patch tests are used to diagnose contact dermatitis.

IX-15.   The answer is B. *(Chap. 331)* The plantar fascia is a thick fibrous band that extends from the medial tuberosity of the calcaneus to insert on each of the five metatarsal heads. Plantar fasciitis is thought to be the result of repeated microtrauma to the tissue. It is a common disorder leading to foot pain and can be diagnosed on the basis of history and physical examination alone. All of the imaging modalities listed above can support the diagnosis, but by themselves are neither sufficient nor necessary for diagnosis. Management includes stretching and orthotics in addition to reducing activities that elicit pain. Local glucocorticoid injections have also been shown effective but may have a risk of plantar fascia rupture. The differential diagnosis includes calcaneal stress fracture, spondyloarthropathy, rheumatoid arthritis, gout, neoplastic or infiltrative bone processes, and nerve entrapment/compression syndromes.

IX-16.   The answer is E. *(Chaps. 325 and 328; Baker, N Engl J Med 329:1013–1020, 1993.)* The analysis of synovial fluid begins at the bedside. When fluid is withdrawn from a joint into a syringe, its clarity and color should be assessed. Cloudiness or turbidity is caused by the scattering of light as it is reflected off particles in the fluid; these particles are usually white blood cells, although crystals may also be present. The viscosity of synovial fluid is due to its hyaluronate content. In patients with inflammatory joint disease, synovial fluid contains enzymes that break down hyaluronate and reduce fluid viscosity. In contrast, synovial fluid taken from a joint in a person with a degenerative joint disease, a noninflammatory condition, would be expected to be clear and have good viscosity. The color of the fluid can indicate recent or old hemorrhage into the joint space. Pigmented villonodular synovitis is associated with noninflammatory fluid that is dark brown in color ("crankcase oil") as a result of repeated hemorrhage into the joint. Gout and calcium pyrophosphate deposition disease produce inflammatory synovial effusions, which are cloudy and watery. In addition, these disorders may be diagnosed by identification of crystals in the fluid: Sodium urate crystals of gout are needle-like and strongly negatively birefringent, whereas calcium pyrophosphate crystals are rhomboidal and weakly positively birefringent.

IX-17. The answer is A. *(Chap. 318)* Reactive arthritis is an acute inflammatory arthritis that occurs in the context of an infection elsewhere in the body. The most common causes of reactive arthritis are diarrhea and urethritis. Individuals with reactive arthritis typically present with asymmetric polyarthritis with associated fever, fatigue, and weight loss. Most often these symptoms begin 1–4 weeks after an antecedent illness. The arthritis usually begins with a single joint affected, but additional joints become inflamed over the next 1–2 weeks. The arthritis is painful with frequent effusions present. The most commonly affected joints are those of the lower extremities. Dactylitis presenting as a "sausage digit" with diffuse swelling of a single toe or finger may occur. Pain at tendinous insertion, known as *enthesitis*, is also a feature of reactive arthritis. Extraarticular manifestations of reactive arthritis include urethritis, prostatitis, uveitis, and oral ulcers. In rare instances, life-threatening systemic manifestations can occur including cardiac conduction defects, aortic insufficiency, pulmonary infiltrates, and central nervous system disease. The arthritis typically persists for 3–5 months and can be present for up to a year. Fifteen percent of individuals will develop chronic joint symptoms, and relapses with recurrence of acute arthritis may occur. Risk factors for a worse outcome include presence of HLA-B27 antigen and epidemic shigellosis.

IX-18. The answer is E. *(Chap. 318)* Anti-TNF-α therapy for rheumatoid arthritis has been used since 2000. Two agents are currently used. Infliximab is a chimeric human-mouse anti-TNF-α monoclonal antibody, and etanercept is a soluble p75 TNF-α monoclonal antibody. These agents are potent immunosuppressants, and six types of common side effects have been described. Serious infections are most frequently seen, with a marked increase in disseminated tuberculosis. Other side effects include pancytopenia, demyelinating disorders, exacerbations of congestive heart failure, hypersensitivity to the infusion or injection, and the development of drug-induced systemic lupus erythematosus. An increased incidence of malignancy is of theoretical concern, but this has not been borne out in the limited follow-up of patients treated with these drugs. Pulmonary fibrosis has not been reported.

IX-19. The answer is E. *(Chap. 315)* This patient has a small-joint, symmetric polyarthritis in the setting of a very recent sore throat. Although acute HIV commonly presents with a sore throat, other common features, such as rash, are missing. Moreover, the incubation period between this patient's high-risk sexual encounter and clinical syndrome would be too short for acute HIV infection. Certainly, this patient should be screened for HIV infection. The patient meets clinical criteria for group A *Streptococcus* throat infection given his recent fever, pustular exudates on examination, tender cervical lymph nodes, and lack of cough. His syndrome is consistent with a reactive arthritis, given the symmetric small-joint involvement and very short incubation period. Acute rheumatic fever is also seen with streptococcal throat infections but is very uncommon in the developed world. One would expect to see a latency period ranging between 1 and 5 weeks between resolution of sore throat and arthritis; asymmetric large-joint involvement; and possibly evidence of carditis, chorea, erythema marginatum, or subcutaneous nodules to suspect a diagnosis of acute rheumatic fever. Gonococcal infection can cause pharyngitis but is more commonly associated with single large-joint infection or enthesopathy, but not small-joint polyarthritis. Lyme disease is a clinical diagnosis contingent upon tick exposure, a classic target lesion rash, and, if present, a migratory large-joint arthritis.

IX-20. The answer is E. *(Chap. 313)* Although most clinicians believe that females with SLE should not become pregnant if they have active disease or advanced renal or cardiac disease, the presence of SLE itself is not an absolute contraindication to pregnancy. The outcome of pregnancy is best for females who are in remission at the time of conception. Even in females with quiescent disease, exacerbations may occur (usually in the first trimester and the immediate postpartum period), and 25 to 40% of these pregnancies end in spontaneous abortion. Fetal loss rates are higher in patients with lupus anticoagulant or anticardiolipin antibodies. Flare-ups should be anticipated and vigorously treated with steroids. Steroids given throughout pregnancy also usually have no adverse effects on the child. In this case, the fact that the female had a life-threatening bout of disease a year ago would argue against stopping her drugs at this time. Neonatal lupus, which is manifested by thrombocytopenia, rash, and heart block, is rare but can occur when mothers have anti-Ro antibodies.

IX-21. The answer is B. *(Chap. 318)* Before the introduction of anti-tumor necrosis factor (TNF) α therapy, the mainstay of treatment for ankylosing spondylitis was nonsteroidal anti-inflammatory drugs (NSAIDs) and exercise therapy. In 2000, infliximab and etanercept were introduced and since that time have been shown to confer a rapid, profound, and sustained reduction in all clinical and laboratory measures of disease activity. Even patients with long-standing disease and ankylosis show significant improvement in spinal mobility and pain relief. MRI findings in patients treated with these agents also show marked improvement in marrow edema, enthesitis, and joint effusions. The long-term effects of these agents are not known.

Other treatments for AS can be used, including NSAIDs and COX-2 inhibitors, to decrease pain, especially in mild cases. An ongoing exercise program is encouraged to maintain posture and range of motion. In patients with more severe pain, sulfasalazine or methotrexate may be added with modest benefit, especially in those with peripheral arthritis. Diverse other agents have been tried, including thalidomide, bisphosphonates, and radium-224. Glucocorticoids have no role in the treatment of this disease.

IX-22. The answer is B. *(Chap. 319)* This patient is presenting with amaurosis fugax with evidence of decreased visual acuity and anterior ischemic optic neuropathy in the setting of a compatible clinical history of giant cell arteritis (temporal arteritis). In an individual >50 years, this clinical history should prompt immediate initiation of glucocorticoids in order to prevent the development of monocular blindness. Giant cell arteritis is exquisitely sensitive to steroid therapy, and initiation of prednisone, 40–60 mg daily, is usually effective at managing the symptoms. If ocular symptoms recur, prednisone may be increased further. Once symptoms are controlled, gradual tapering of the steroid dose should occur. Most patients do require prolonged courses of steroid, usually for >2 years. The elevation in ESR can be a useful marker of disease activity during a steroid taper. Aspirin is often used in combination with glucocorticoids as it has been shown to decrease ischemic complications of giant cell arteritis. Indomethacin is not frequently used and should not be used alone in a patient presenting with symptoms of ischemic optic neuropathy. There is no role for anticoagulation in the treatment of giant cell arteritis. Definitive diagnosis of giant cell arteritis is confirmed by temporal artery biopsy, which should be performed in this patient. However, treatment should not be withheld for performance of the biopsy as sudden and irreversible blindness may occur. Ultrasonography of the temporal artery may also be a suggestive. While the patient's age and history of coronary artery disease raise the suspicion of a transient ischemic attack, the patient's other symptoms in this case make giant cell arteritis more likely. These symptoms are chronic, occurring over the several weeks to months prior to presentation. The symptoms include new-onset headache, jaw claudication, scalp pain, and symptoms of polymyalgia rheumatica. In this clinical setting, performance of magnetic resonance angiography would not be indicated.

IX-23. The answer is C. *(Chap. 16)* Acute low back pain is defined as pain of less than 3 months' duration. Most patients with back pain have symptoms that are "mechanical," such as pain that is worsened by activity and relieved by rest. Initial assessment of all these patients must evaluate for serious causes of spine pathology, such as infection, malignant disease, and trauma. Risk factors include age over 50 years, prior diagnosis of cancer, intravenous drug use, chronic infection such as cystitis or pneumonia, a history of spine trauma, bed rest without relief, duration of pain of more than 1 month, urinary incontinence or nocturia, focal leg weakness or numbness, pain radiating into the leg or legs from the back, pain that increases with standing and is relieved by sitting, and chronic steroid use. Examination findings that raise concern for serious underlying disease include fever, weight loss, a positive straight leg raise, an abdominal or rectal mass, and neurologic examination abnormalities, either motor or sensory.

IX-24. **The answer is C.** *(Chap. 313)* Drug-induced lupus can occur with a variety of medications and should be considered when individuals present atypically. Individuals with drug-induced lupus are more likely to be male and of Caucasian race. Drug-induced lupus usually presents with fever, malaise, intense arthralgias/myalgias, serositis, and rash. The brain and kidneys are rarely involved. Discontinuation of the medication usually leads to resolution of the symptoms over a period of weeks, although anti-inflammatory medications may need to be utilized to control symptoms until the inflammation subsides. Common drugs that cause lupus include procainamide, propafenone, hydralazine, propylthiouracil, lithium, phenytoin, carbamazepine, sulfasalazine, and minocycline. Beta blockers, angiotensin-converting enzyme inhibitors, lovastatin, and simvastatin have also been reported to cause drug-induced lupus. Antibody testing usually reveals a positive antinuclear antibody and antihistone antibodies. Antibodies to ds-DNA are rare. Anticardiolipin antibodies are seen in antiphospholipid antibody syndrome, which would present with arterial and venous thromboembolic disease. Anti-RNP antibodies are seen with mixed connective tissue disease that usually presents with features of lupus, rheumatoid arthritis, and/or scleroderma. Anti-ribosomal P antibodies are associated with depression and psychosis with central nervous system involvement of SLE.

IX-25. **The answer is D.** *(Chap. 311)* This patient presents with symptoms of cold urticaria, an IgE-dependent urticarial reaction to cold exposure. After exposure to cold, urticarial lesions appear in exposed areas and usually last for <2 h. Histologic examination of the urticarial lesion would demonstrate mast cell degranulation with edema of the dermis and subcutaneous tissues. In experimental exposure to a cold challenge such as an ice water bath, elevated levels of histamine in venous blood may be demonstrated if assessed in the extremity exposed to a cold environment, whereas the histamine levels would be normal in a nonexposed extremity. The appearance of a linear wheal after a firm stroke is indicative of dermatographism. This condition can be seen in 1–4% of the population and is often found in individuals with cold urticaria. In general, cold urticaria is a localized process without adverse consequences. However, vascular collapse may occur if an individual is submerged in cold water. Many individuals request treatment because they are embarrassed by their condition or are symptomatic from the recurrent urticaria and pruritus. Treatment with H_1 histamine receptor blockers is usually adequate for symptom control. Cyproheptadine or hydroxyzine can be added to therapy if H_1 antihistamines are inadequate. In this patient, there is a clear precipitant for developing urticaria—cold exposure. Thus, no other evaluation is necessary. In the evaluation and management of chronic urticaria, identification and elimination of precipitating factors are important. Possible etiologic factors include foods, pollens, molds, and medications. In this case the urticaria predates the use of oral contraceptive medications; thus, stopping oral contraceptives would be unlikely to be helpful. Assessment of antithyroglobulin and antimicrosomal antibodies can be helpful in individuals with chronic urticaria in whom a cause is not otherwise identified. Deficiency of C1 or the presence of a C1 inhibitor presents as recurrent angioedema rather than urticaria.

IX-26. **The answer is B.** *(Chap. 319)* The presenting symptoms of this patient include rapidly progressive renal failure, sinusitis, and cavitary lung disease. These symptoms are consistent with the diagnosis of Wegener's granulomatosis (WG). WG is characterized by granulomatous vasculitis of small vessels that primarily manifests in the airways and kidneys. An uncommon disease, WG has an estimated prevalence of 3 per 100,000 population. The male-to-female ratio is equal. The upper airway is involved in 95% of patients and, in this setting, the disease often presents as chronic sinusitis unresponsive to antibiotic therapy. Facial pain and bloody nasal discharge are commonly present. Untreated disease can progress to complete cartilaginous destruction with nasal septal perforation and saddle-nose deformity. The lungs are the second most commonly affected organ in about 85% of individuals with WG. The spectrum of lung disease may vary widely from asymptomatic pulmonary infiltrates to massive hemoptysis. In this patient, there are characteristic cavitary lung lesions that help to differentiate WG from microscopic polyangiitis, as no cavitary disease is seen in microscopic polyangiitis. Rapidly progressive glomerulonephritis is present in 77% of patients and is responsible for the majority of deaths in WG. Nonspecific symptoms are also present when the disease is active including fatigue, weight loss, and fevers. Diagnosis of WG is made by demonstration of necrotizing vasculitis on tissue biopsy of an affected organ. Serologic testing can offer supporting evidence for the diagnosis of WG. Ninety percent of individuals with WG will demonstrate antibodies to cytoplasmic antineutrophil cytoplasmic antibodies (c-ANCA). The specific c-ANCA target in WG is proteinase-3. Rapid initiation of therapy is important. Prior to the use of cyclophosphamide, WG was almost universally fatal within 5 years, even with the use of glucocorticoids. With the combined use of glucocorticoids and cyclophosphamide, survival is now 75–80% at 5 years. Perinuclear antineutrophil cytoplasmic antibodies (p-ANCA) are usually directed against myeloperoxidase. The p-ANCA are seen in a minority of patients with WG but are more commonly present in microscopic polyangiitis. Antistreptolysin O antibodies are seen with poststreptococcal glomerulonephritis. This patient's prior upper respiratory symptoms were primarily sinusitis and not associated with pharyngitis, and the CT scan of the chest would not be expected to be abnormal.

Antiglomerular basement membrane (anti-GBM) antibodies are present in Goodpasture's syndrome. This pulmonary-renal syndrome frequently presents with rapidly progressive glomerulonephritis and respiratory failure. Diffuse alveolar hemorrhage is common. The CT of the chest in Goodpasture's syndrome would not be expected to show cavitary lung lesions. Endocarditis due to *S. aureus* may cause a similar CT appearance with multiple septic emboli causing cavitary lung disease. However, the constellation of findings with sinusitis and glomerulonephritis would not be expected.

IX-27.   **The answer is C.** *(Chap. 319; JW Newberger et al: Circulation 110:2747, 2004.)* The most likely cause of the acute coronary syndrome in this patient is thrombosis of a coronary artery aneurysm in an individual with a past history of Kawasaki disease. Kawasaki disease is an acute multisystem disease that primarily presents in children <5 years of age. The clinical manifestations in childhood are nonsuppurative cervical lymphadenitis; desquamation of the fingertips; and erythema of the oral cavity, lips, and palms. Approximately 25% of cases are associated with coronary artery aneurysms that occur late in illness in the convalescent stage. Early treatment (within 7–10 days of onset) with IV immunoglobulin and high-dose aspirin decreases the risk of developing coronary aneurysms to about 5%. Even if coronary artery aneurysms develop, most regress over the course of the first year if the size is <6 mm. Aneurysms >8 mm, however, are unlikely to regress. Complications of persistent coronary artery aneurysms include rupture, thrombosis and recanalization, and stenosis at the outflow area. Dissection of the aortic root and coronary ostia is a common cause of death in Marfan's syndrome and can also be seen with aortitis due to Takayasu's arteritis. In this patient, there is no history of hypertension, limb ischemia, or systemic symptoms that would suggest an active vasculitis. In addition, there are no other ischemic symptoms that would be expected in Takayasu's arteritis. Myocardial bridging overlying a coronary artery is seen frequently at autopsy but is an unusual cause of ischemia. The possibility of cocaine use as a cause of myocardial ischemia in a young individual must be considered, but given the clinical history, it is a less likely cause of ischemia in this case.

IX-28.   **The answer is E.** *(Chap. 308; Frank, N Engl J Med 316:1525–1530, 1987.)* Complement activity, which results from the sequential interaction of a large number of plasma and cell-membrane proteins, plays an important role in the inflammatory response. The classic pathway of complement activation is initiated by an antibody-antigen interaction.

The first complement component (C1, a complex composed of three proteins) binds to immune complexes with activation mediated by C1q. Active C1 then initiates the cleavage and concomitant activation of components C4 and C2. The activated C1 is destroyed by a plasma protease inhibitor termed *C1 esterase inhibitor*. This molecule also regulates clotting factor XI and kallikrein. Patients with a deficiency of C1 esterase inhibitor may develop angioedema, sometimes leading to death by asphyxia. Attacks may be precipitated by stress or trauma. In addition to low antigenic or functional levels of C1 esterase inhibitor, patients with this autosomal dominant condition may have normal levels of C1 and C3 but low levels of C4 and C2. Danazol therapy produces a striking increase in the level of this important inhibitor and alleviates the symptoms in many patients. An acquired form of angioedema caused by a deficiency of C1 esterase inhibitor has been described in patients with autoimmune or malignant disease.

IX-29. **The answer is A.** *(Chap. 326)* OA is the most common type of arthritis. Roughly 12% of the United States population above the age of 60 has evidence of OA of the knee. OA in the hands may affect 10% of the elderly. Commonly affected sites include the cervical and lumbosacral spine, hip, and the knee. In the hands, both the proximal and distal interphalangeal joints are frequently affected. The wrist, elbow, and ankle are typically spared. The ankle joint's articular cartilage may be the reason it is less susceptible to OA, but this remains unclear. There is a notable difference between affected joints in osteoarthritis in comparison to rheumatoid arthritis (RA); the lumbar spine and distal interphalangeal joints are rarely affected in RA, and the wrist joints are almost always involved.

IX-30. **The answer is B.** *(Chap. 324)* Recurrent infections due to encapsulated organisms strongly suggests asplenism. Functional asplenism along with easy bruising, neuropathy, and macroglossia suggests amyloidosis. Other findings that argue for amyloidosis are alopecia, dystrophic nails, and the elevated globulin fraction. The functional asplenism of amyloidosis is due to direct involvement of the spleen, although hypersplenism may be present. HIV-infected patients are more likely to have recurrent infections but without splenomegaly, and they are not more susceptible to encapsulated organisms than other patients. A new diagnosis of sickle cell anemia is unlikely given the patient's demographic. Cyclical neutropenia usually occurs in children, although there are also adult forms. The cycle of cyclical neutropenia is usually 3 weeks. X-linked agammaglobulinemia is a rare congenital disorder of males whose B cells do not mature. Patients with this disorder do not make immunoglobulins and develop severe upper respiratory infections, often with encapsulated organisms.

IX-31. **The answer is B.** *(Chap. 314)* The prevalence of rheumatoid arthritis (RA) is 0.8%, and females are three times more likely to be affected than are males. However, as the population ages, the prevalence increases and the sex difference diminishes. RA is found throughout the world and affects people of all races. Age of onset is most commonly 35 to 50 years. Family studies show a clear genetic predisposition. First-degree relatives have approximately four times the expected rate of RA. Other risk factors for RA include the class II major histocompatibility antigen HLA-DR4. Approximately 70% of patients with RA have HLA-DR4. However, this association is not true in Africans or African Americans, among whom 75% do not show this allele. The role of this allele in the pathogenesis of RA remains unknown because the cause of RA is unknown. The earliest lesion in RA is microvascular injury with an increase in the number of synovial lining cells. Increased numbers of mononuclear cells are seen in the synovial lining, and this is thought to be under the control of CD4+ T lymphocytes. As the inflammation continues, the articular matrix is degraded by collagenases and cathepsins produced by the inflammatory cells. Other cytokines produced by the inflammatory cells include IL-1 and TNF-α. Over time, bone and cartilage are destroyed, leading to the end-stage clinical manifestations. Rheumatoid factor (RF) is an IgM molecule directed against the Fc portion of IgG and is found in two-thirds of patients with RA. However, this molecule is found in approximately 5% of healthy persons and more than 10% of persons older than age 60. It is not known to have a role in the pathogenesis of the disease, but titers of RF are shown to be predictive of the severity of clinical manifestations or the presence of extraarticular manifestations.

IX-32. **The answer is B.** *(Chap. 318)* *Enthesopathy* or *enthesitis* is the term used to describe inflammation at the site of tendinous or ligamentous insertion into bone. This type of inflammation is seen most frequently in patients with seronegative spondyloarthropathies and various infections, especially viral infections. The other definitions apply to other terms used in the orthopedic and rheumatic examination. *Subluxation* is the alteration of joint alignment so that articulating surfaces incompletely approximate each other. *Synovitis* refers to inflammation at the site of tendinous or ligamentous insertion into bone. Inflammation of a saclike cavity near a joint that decreases friction is the definition of *bursitis*. Finally, *crepitus* is a palpable vibratory or crackling sensation elicited with joint motion.

IX-33. **The answer is C.** *(Chaps. 318 and 329)* This patient complains of symptoms consistent with a diagnosis of fibromyalgia. These patients frequently complain of diffuse body pain, stiffness, paresthesias, disturbed sleep, easy fatigability, and headache. The prevalence of fibromyalgia is approximately 3.4% of females and 0.5% of males. This disorder is thought to represent a disturbance of pain perception. Disturbed sleep with a loss of stage 4 sleep has been implicated as a factor in the pathogenesis of the disease. Serotonin levels in the cerebrospinal fluid have also commonly been seen and may play a role in the pathogenesis. A diagnosis of fibromyalgia is based on the American College of Rheumatology criteria, which combine symptoms and physical examination. The patient must exhibit diffuse pain in all areas of the body with tenderness to palpation at 11 of 18 designated tender point sites. These sites include the occiput, trapezius, cervical spine, lateral epicondyles, supraspinatus muscle, second rib, gluteus, greater trochanter, and knee. Digital palpation should be performed with a moderate degree of pressure. Examination of the joints shows no evidence of inflammatory arthropathy. There are no laboratory tests that are specific for the diagnosis. Positive antinuclear antibodies may be seen, but at the same frequency as in the normal population. HLA-B27 is found in 7% of the white population, but only 1 to 6% of people with HLA-B27 will develop ankylosing spondylitis. Radiograms are normal in these patients.

IX-34. **The answer is A.** *(Chap. 329)* The first step in the treatment of fibromyalgia is to improve the quality of the patient's sleep. This has been shown to improve quality of life and reduce symptoms. Improving sleep hygiene through nonpharmacologic methods should be encouraged, though tricyclic antidepressants are also recommended. Tricyclic antidepressants improve stage 4 sleep, resulting in clinical improvement. Other treatments that have shown improvement in sleep or symptoms independent of depressive disorder include trazodone, zolpidem, and duloxetine. All patients should be reassured that their condition is not degenerative nor life-threatening, and that a variety of treatments are available. Mind-body therapies such as acupuncture, meditation, and yoga have shown benefit in some patients with fibromyalgia and should also be considered.

IX-35. **The answer is C.** *(Chap. 318)* Ankylosing spondylitis is a chronic disease that progresses to complete ankylosis over the course of several decades in a minority of individuals with this disease. Poor prognostic factors that are associated with an increased risk of progression include earlier onset of disease, male sex, and involvement of the hip joints. Spinal fracture is the most serious complication, with even minor trauma increasing the risk of fracture in the rigid spine. Spinal cord injury is a dreaded complication of spinal fracture. The estimate lifetime risk of spinal fracture in AS is >10%. An important component to prevent disability is to maintain a healthy weight and an exercise program with the goal of maintaining posture and range of motion in the spine. In addition to an exercise program, use of NSAIDs reduces pain and tenderness and increases mobility. When individuals who used NSAIDs daily regardless of pain symptoms were compared to a group of individuals who used NSAIDs only when pain was more severe, those with daily use of NSAIDs had less radiographic progression of their disease. Anti-TNF-α therapy (infliximab, etanercept, adalimumab) has a rapid and dramatic effect in AS, but these drugs are not first-line therapy at the present time because the effects of long-term use are unknown. However, there can be remarkable improvement in mobility and bone mineral density once TNF-α inhibitors are initiated.

IX-36.   **The answer is A.** *(Chap. 313)* SLE is a chronic disease that has relapses and remissions, but is without cure. In individuals without major organ involvement, therapy can be directed at suppression of symptoms. This patient's limiting symptoms are due to articular involvement of SLE. Hydroxychloroquine was developed as an antimalarial drug and has been demonstrated to result in significant improvement in arthritis, dermatitis, and fatigue in SLE. Further, there is evidence that hydroxychloroquine reduces the number of disease flares, and this drug is often first-line therapy for treatment of joint and skin symptoms in SLE. Acetaminophen may be prescribed to control joint pain but is often less effective. While nonsteroidal anti-inflammatory drugs (NSAIDs) are often effective, caution should be used when prescribing these medications because there is an increased risk of NSAID-induced aseptic meningitis in SLE patients. Further, NSAIDs may also worsen hypertension and cause renal disease. Quinacrine is another antimalarial drug that may be substituted for hydroxychloroquine, but it is considered second-line therapy due to its side effect of causing diffuse yellowish skin discoloration. Physical therapy may be appropriate in combination with anti-inflammatory medications but is not expected to significantly improve the patient's functioning without control of the underlying disease. Prednisone is a potent anti-inflammatory medication that would be effective in suppressing the patient's symptoms. However, high-dose therapy (0.5–1.0 mg/kg daily) is not indicated in mild disease unless the patient is refractory to conservative therapies or develops major organ involvement, as the benefits in this situation would not outweigh the side effects. Methotrexate is often useful for joint symptoms as well as systemic manifestations, if prednisone therapy cannot be safely decreased or if the patient develops intolerable side effects of less toxic medications.

IX-37.   **The answer is E.** *(Chap. 319)* This patient most likely has polyarteritis nodosa with a symptom complex consisting of abdominal pain, weight loss, hypertension, and mononeuritis. Polyarteritis nodosa (PAN) is an uncommon vasculitis that affects primarily medium-size arteries without the involvement of venules. There are no diagnostic serologic tests for PAN. Up to 30% of patients with PAN are positive for hepatitis B surface antigen. In cases of PAN associated with hepatitis B, the virus, IgM, and complement can be demonstrated in vessel walls on biopsy. In light of the patient's past history of injection drug use, the presence of hepatitis B should be evaluated. However, demonstration of hepatitis B surface antigen is not diagnostic of PAN. ANCA is rarely positive in PAN patients, and hepatitis C is associated with cryoglobulinemic vasculitis but not with PAN. With the patient's abdominal pain that is worsened with eating, mesenteric ischemia caused by vasculitis should be considered. On mesenteric angiography, one would expect to find aneurysmal dilatation of the arteries. Again, however, this is not pathognomonic for PAN. The most definitive way to diagnose PAN is by finding vasculitis on a biopsy of the affected nerve. Therefore, a radial nerve biopsy should be pursued.

IX-38.   **The answer is E.** *(Chap. 311)* Allergic rhinitis is a common problem in the United States and North America. It is estimated that ~1 in 5 individuals experiences allergic rhinitis. The incidence is greatest in childhood and adolescence, and the symptoms tend to regress with aging. Complete remissions, however, are uncommon. Many individuals experience seasonal symptoms only. These symptoms are due to pollen production by weeds, grasses, and trees that are dependent upon wind currents, rather than insects, for cross-pollination. The timing of the pollination events predicts seasonal severity of symptoms and varies little from year to year within a particular locale. Based on this pattern, one is able to predict which allergens are most likely responsible for a patient's symptoms. In the temperate regions of North America, trees pollinate in the spring, and ragweed pollinates in the fall. Grasses are responsible for seasonal allergic symptoms in the summer months. Mold allergens can have a variable pattern of symptoms, depending upon climactic conditions that allow them to sporulate. Perennial rhinitis does not have a seasonal pattern and is more continually present. Allergens that cause perennial rhinitis include animal dander, dust, and cockroach-derived proteins.

IX-39.   **The answer is A.** *(Chap. 331)* This patient has a classic presentation for olecranon bursitis, with warmth, swelling, fluctuance, and tenderness over the posterior aspect of the elbow. Most often this is due to repeated trauma or pressure to the area that can occur through leaning on the elbow or through immobility with continuous pressure. Alternatively, infections, generally with gram-positive organisms, can cause olecranon bursitis, and crystalline disease, especially monosodium urate, can cause this picture. Initial evaluation involves aspiration of the fluid for Gram stain, culture, cell count and differential, and crystal evaluation. Empirical antibiotics would be warranted in this patient because of concern for infection with fevers and systemic illness. Incision and drainage should be reserved for bursitis of infectious etiology that is not responding to antibiotics and repeated aspirations.

IX-40.   The answer is C. *(Chap. 16)* In a patient with back pain, any symptoms of pain at rest or pain not associated with specific postures should raise suspicion for a serious underlying cause, such as fracture, infection, or spinal tumors. The examination includes inspection of the lower spine, the surrounding musculature, and both hips. Straight leg raising is performed with the patient lying flat with passive flexion of the extended leg at the hip, which stretches L5, S1, and the sciatic nerve. Flexion of up to 80° is normal. A positive maneuver occurs if the patient's usual pain is reproduced. This maneuver may also be performed in the sitting position to determine if the pain is indeed reproducible. The crossed straight leg raising sign is positive when flexion of one leg reproduces the pain in the opposite leg or buttocks. This sign is less sensitive than straight leg raising, but it is more specific for disk herniation. The nerve or nerve root lesion is always on the side of the pain. The reverse straight leg raising maneuver is performed by having the patient stand next to the examination table and passively extend each leg. This stretches the L2–L4 nerve roots and the femoral nerve.

IX-41.   The answer is A. *(Chap. 319)* Cyclophosphamide in combination with glucocorticoids has increased the survival in Wegener's granulomatosis from 5% at 5 years to >70%. However, cyclophosphamide is a cytotoxic alkylating agent that has serious side effects that limit its long-term use. The incidence of cystitis at doses of 2 mg/kg daily is at least 30%, with a concomitant incidence of bladder cancer of at least 6%. For this reason, patients are instructed to take cyclophosphamide in the morning with large volumes of water. Frequent urinalyses are performed to assess for development of microscopic hematuria. In addition, there are significant bone marrow effects, including bone marrow suppression and development of chromosomal abnormalities, that may lead to myelodysplasia. Most clinicians monitor complete blood counts at least monthly. Infertility with gonadal suppression may occur during treatment, and the effects of cyclophosphamide can result in permanent infertility in both men and women. Other side effects of cyclophosphamide at the usual doses for vasculitis include gastrointestinal intolerance, hypogammaglobulinemia, pulmonary fibrosis, and oncogenesis. Alopecia, however, is unusual at the doses for chronic administration.

IX-42.   The answer is C. *(Chap. 309)* The human major histocompatibility complex genes are located on a 4-megabase region on chromosome 6. The major function of the MHC complex genes is to produce proteins that are important in developing immunologic specificity through their role in binding antigen for presentation to T cells. This process is nonspecific, and the ability of an HLA molecule to bind to a particular protein depends upon the molecular fit between the amino acid sequence of a particular protein and the corresponding domain on the MCH molecule. Once a peptide has bound, the MHC-peptide complex binds to the T cell receptor, after which the T cell must determine if an immune response should be generated. If an antigen is similar to an endogenous protein, the potential antigen will be recognized as a self-peptide and tolerance to the antigen will be continued. The MHC I and II complexes have been implicated in the development of many autoimmune diseases, which occur when T cells fail to recognize a peptide as a self-peptide and an immune response is allowed to develop. MHC I and II genes also play a major role in tissue compatibility for transplantation and are important in generating immune-mediated rejection. The other options listed as answers refer to functions of immunoglobulins. The variable region of the immunoglobulin is a B cell–specific response to an antigen to promote neutralization of the antigen through agglutination and precipitation. The constant region of the immunoglobulin is able to nonspecifically activate the immune system through complement activation and promotion of phagocytosis by neutrophils and macrophages.

IX-43. **The answer is B.** *(Chap. 331)* Inflammation of the abductor pollicis longus and the extensor pollicis brevis at the radial styloid process tendon sheath is known as DeQuervain's tenosynovitis. Repetitive twisting of the wrist can lead to this condition. Pain occurs when grasping with the thumb and can extend radially along the wrist to the radial styloid process. Mothers often develop this tenosynovitis by holding their babies with the thumb outstretched. The Finkelstein sign is positive in DeQuervain's tenosynovitis. It is positive if the patient develops pain by placing the thumb in the palm, closing the fingers around the thumb and deviating the wrist in the ulnar direction. Management of DeQuervain's tenosynovitis includes nonsteroidal anti-inflammatory drugs and splinting. Glucocorticoid injections can be effective. A Phalen maneuver is used to diagnose carpal tunnel syndrome and does not elicit pain. The wrists are flexed for 60 s to compress the median nerve to elicit numbness, burning, or tingling. Gouty arthritis will present with an acutely inflamed joint with crystal-laden fluid. Rheumatoid arthritis is a systemic illness with characteristic joint synovitis and radiographic features.

IX-44. **The answer is C.** *(Chap. 319)* Microscopic polyangiitis (MPA) is a small-vessel vasculitis associated with antineutrophil cytoplasmic antibodies (ANCAs) of the perinuclear type. MPA was recognized as a discrete entity in 1992, when it was distinguished from polyarteritis nodosa because of the involvement primarily of small vessels. Twelve percent of cases present primarily with diffuse alveolar hemorrhage. MPA is distinct from Wegener's granulomatosis because it does not induce granulomatous inflammation. The glomerulonephritis associated with MPA is pauci-immune, showing a lack of immunoglobulin deposition. p-ANCA staining is positive in 75% of patients with MPA, with anti-myeloperoxidase antibodies being the target of the immunofluorescent staining pattern of the p-ANCA. Therapy begins with high-dose steroids and often requires the addition of cytotoxic therapy with cyclophosphamide. The 5-year survival rate is 74%; however, the disease tends to be chronic, with at least a 34% relapse rate.

IX-45. **The answer is B.** *(Chap. 325)* This patient has degenerative arthritis. His obesity predisposes him to degenerative joint disease that will be worse in the large weight-bearing joints. The physical examination findings of decreased range of motion, crepitus, and varus deformity that is exacerbated on weight bearing are consistent with this diagnosis. The radiogram of the knee demonstrates narrowing of the joint space with osteophyte formation. Occasional effusions may be seen, especially after overuse injuries. The joint fluid analysis in patients with degenerative disease reveals a clear, viscous fluid with a white blood cell count less than 2000/µL. Positively birefringent crystals on polarizing light microscopy will be seen in pseudogout that most commonly affects the knee, whereas negatively birefringent crystals are characteristic of gout. Joint fluid in these inflammatory conditions would generally have a white blood cell count of less than 50,000/mm^3 and is yellow and turbid in character. Septic arthritis presents with fevers and a very warm and tender joint. The joint fluid can have the appearance of frank pus and is opaque. The white blood cell count is usually higher than 50,000/mm^3 and can have a positive Gram stain for organisms.

IX-46 and IX-47. **The answers are A and B.** *(Chap. 320)* Behçet's syndrome is a multisystem disorder of uncertain cause that is marked by oral and genital ulcerations and ocular involvement. This disorder affects males and females equally and is more common in persons of Mediterranean, Middle Eastern, and Far Eastern descent. Approximately 50% of these persons have circulating autoantibodies to human oral mucosa. The clinical features are quite varied. The presence of recurrent aphthous ulcerations is essential for the diagnosis. Most of these patients have primarily oral ulcerations, although genital ulcerations are more specific for the diagnosis. The ulcers are generally painful, can be shallow or deep, and last for 1 or 2 weeks. Other skin involvement may occur, including folliculitis, erythema nodosum, and vasculitis. Eye involvement is the most dreaded complication because it may progress rapidly to blindness. It often presents as panuveitis, iritis, retinal vessel occlusion, or optic neuritis. This patient also presents with superficial venous thrombosis. Superficial and deep venous thromboses are present in one-fourth of these patients. Neurologic involvement occurs in up to 10%. Laboratory findings are nonspecific with elevations in the erythrocyte sedimentation rate and the white blood cell count. Treatment varies with the extent of the disease. Patients with mucous membrane involvement alone may respond to topical steroids. In more serious or refractory cases, thalidomide is effective. Other options for mucocutaneous disease include colchicines and intralesional interferon α. Ophthalmologic or neurologic involvement requires systemic glucocorticoids and azathioprine or cyclosporine. Life span is usually normal unless neurologic disease is present. Ophthalmic disease frequently progresses to blindness.

IX-48. **The answer is D.** *(Chap. 331)* Rotator cuff tendonitis is the most common cause of shoulder pain. The rotator cuff consists of the tendons of the supraspinatus, infraspinatus, subscapularis, and teres minor muscles. It inserts on the humeral tuberosities. The supraspinatus tendon is most frequently involved, likely due to the impingement that can occur between the humeral head and the acromion and coracoacromial ligament. Abduction of the arm causes a decrease in blood supply to this tendon, likely increasing the supraspinatus tendon's susceptibility to inflammation as well. Patients over 40 are particularly susceptible to rotator cuff injury, and pain is often worse at night. Nonsteroidal anti-inflammatory drugs, glucocorticoid injection, and physical therapy are all first-line management strategies for rotator cuff tendonitis. Bicipital tendonitis is produced by friction on the tendon of the long head of the biceps as it passes through the bicipital groove. Patients experience anterior shoulder pain that radiates down the biceps to the forearm. The bicipital groove is painful to palpation.

IX-49. **The answer is D.** *(Chap. 318)* This patient shows the typical features of psoriatic arthritis. Five to 10% of patients with psoriasis will develop an arthritis associated with the rash. In 60 to 70% of cases, the rash precedes the diagnosis. However, another 15 to 20% of patients will have joint complaints as the presenting symptom of their psoriasis. The disease typically begins in the fourth or fifth decade of life. Psoriatic arthritis has varied joint presentations with five commonly described patterns of joint involvement: (1) arthritis of the distal interphalangeal (DIP) joints, (2) asymmetric oligoarthritis, (3) symmetric polyarthritis similar to rheumatoid arthritis (RA), (4) axial involvement, and (5) arthritis mutilans with the typical "pencil in cup" deformity seen on hand radiography. Erosive joint disease ultimately develops in almost all these patients, and most of them become disabled. Nail changes are prominent in 90% of patients with psoriatic arthritis. Changes that are frequently seen include pitting, horizontal ridging, onycholysis, yellowish discoloration of the nail margins, and dystrophic hyperkeratosis. The diagnosis of psoriatic arthritis is primarily clinical. Thus, in patients with joint symptoms that precede the onset of rash, the diagnosis is frequently missed until dermatologic or nail changes develop. A family history of psoriasis is important to ascertain in any patient with an undiagnosed inflammatory polyarthropathy. The differential diagnosis of DIP arthritis is short; only osteoarthritis and gout are commonly seen in these joints. Radiography may show typical changes, particularly in patients with arthritis mutilans. Treatment is directed at both the rash and the joint disease simultaneously. Anti-TNF-α therapy has recently been shown to be helpful for both dermatologic and joint manifestations of disease. Other treatments include methotrexate, sulfasalazine, cyclosporine, retinoic acid derivatives, and psoralen plus ultraviolet light.

IX-50. **The answer is C.** *(Chap. 321)* Relapsing polychondritis is frequently a disease of abrupt onset with inflammation of one or more cartilaginous sites. Systemic symptoms such as fever and fatigue may precede the overt inflammation. The peak age of onset is in the forties to fifties, but it may occur at all ages. Approximately 30% of patients will have another rheumatologic disorder, most commonly systemic vasculitis. Auricular chondritis is the most common clinical manifestation of relapsing polychondritis, occurring 43% of the time as the presenting complaint, and with 89% cumulative frequency. Reduced hearing can occur in up to 40% of patients. Arthritis is a presenting complaint in 32% of patients. Saddle-nose deformity, perhaps a well-known, or "classic," sign associated with relapsing polychondritis, is a presenting complaint of only 11% of patients and has a cumulative frequency of 25%. Aortic regurgitation, due to dilation of the aortic ring or destruction of the cusps, is an uncommon finding in this illness, occurring in ≤5% of cases. The diagnosis of relapsing polychondritis is based on recognition of the characteristic clinical features, including two or more separate sites of cartilaginous inflammation that responded to treatment with prednisone or dapsone. Biopsy can confirm the diagnosis but may not be necessary if the clinical features are typical.

IX-51. **The answer is B.** *(Chap. 317)* Sjögren's syndrome is associated with a lifetime risk of non-Hodgkin's lymphoma of 5% that usually presents later in the illness. The primary non-Hodgkin's lymphoma associated with Sjögren's syndrome is a low-grade, marginal zone B cell lymphoma that usually presents extranodally. Many instances are found incidentally on labial biopsy. Persistent parotid enlargement, leukopenia, cryoglobulinemia, and presence of rheumatoid factor should prompt evaluation for possible lymphoma. Treatment for Sjögren's syndrome should be same as that for other B cell non-Hodgkin's lymphomas. Factors that influence survival include size >7 cm, presence of B symptoms, and high or intermediate histologic grade. Adenoid cystic carcinoma is the second most common malignant tumor of the salivary glands after mucoepidermoid carcinoma, but it does not occur more commonly in Sjögren's syndrome. An impacted sialolith could cause unilateral enlargement of the parotid gland but should present with pain with palpation. A sialolith may be complicated by bacterial sialadenitis. Pain is worse with eating or the anticipation of eating, which would stimulate saliva production. Mumps is unusual in the United States today due to immunization. Mumps most commonly presents with associated fever and systemic symptoms. Recurrent vasculitis would also be likely to present with systemic symptoms. Salivary glands are unlikely to be affected by vasculitis.

IX-52. **The answer is B.** *(Chap. 320)* Behçet's syndrome is a multisystem inflammatory disease of unknown etiology that presents with recurrent oral and genital ulcerations. The ulcerations are generally painful, occur in groups, and subside spontaneously in 1–2 weeks without leaving scars. Diagnosis of Behçet's syndrome is made based on clinical characteristics. The diagnosis requires the presence of recurrent oral ulcers plus two of the following criteria: recurrent genital ulcers, eye lesions, skin lesions (including erythema nodosum), or positive pathergy test. A pathergy test is considered positive when nonspecific skin inflammation develops 2–3 days after a scratch or injection of sterile saline. This is manifested as a small 2- to 3-mm papule at the site of injection. Other clinical manifestations of Behçet's syndrome include nonerosive arthritis, gastrointestinal ulcerations, and neurologic involvement. In addition, individuals with Behçet's syndrome are at increased risk of venous thromboembolic disease. The cause of Behçet's syndrome is unknown. It is more common in individuals from the Mediterranean region, Middle East, and Far East. In advanced disease, antibodies to α-enolase of endothelial cells and *Saccharomyces cerevisiae* have been shown. The pathologic lesion is perivasculitis with neutrophilic infiltration, endothelial swelling, and fibrinoid necrosis. Oral and genital lesions can usually be treated with topical glucocorticoids alone. Other treatments that are effective include thalidomide, colchicine, and systemic glucocorticoids. For central nervous system disease, azathioprine is added to systemic glucocorticoids. The severity of the disease tends to abate over time, and lifespan in Behçet's disease is normal. Development of 10 mm of dermal induration with overlying erythema occurring 49–72 h after injection of an antigenic protein is typical of a type IV hypersensitivity reaction. The most common use of this reaction is to assess for infection with tuberculosis after injection of a purified protein derivative to *Mycobacterium tuberculosis*. The Kveim reaction refers to the development of granulomatous inflammation 4–6 weeks after injection of a protein derived from the lesion of sarcoidosis. An urticarial reaction demonstrates immediate hypersensitivity reaction and is typical of allergy phenomena.

IX-53. **The answer is C.** *(Chap. 313)* This patient is presenting with acute lupus nephritis with evidence of hematuria, proteinuria, and an acute rise in creatinine. Together with infection, nephritis is the most common cause of mortality in the first decade after diagnosis of SLE and warrants prompt immunosuppressive therapy. It is important to assess for other potentially reversible causes of acute renal insufficiency, but this patient is not otherwise acutely ill and is taking no medications that would cause renal failure. The urinalysis shows evidence of active nephritis with hematuria and proteinuria. Even in the absence of RBC casts, therapy should not be withheld to await biopsy results in someone with a known diagnosis of SLE with consistent clinical presentation and urinary findings. This patient also has other risk factors known to predict the development of lupus nephritis, including high titers of anti-dsDNA and African-American race. The mainstay of treatment for any life-threatening or organ-threatening manifestation of SLE is high-dose systemic glucocorticoids. Addition of cytotoxic or other immunosuppressive agents (cyclophosphamide, azathioprine, mycophenolate mofetil) is recommended to treat serious complications of SLE, but their effects are delayed for 3–6 weeks after initiation of therapy, whereas the effects of glucocorticoids begin within 24 h. Thus, these agents alone should not be used to treat acute serious manifestations of SLE. The choice of cytotoxic agent is at the discretion of the treating physician. Cyclophosphamide in combination with steroid therapy has been demonstrated to prevent development of end-stage renal disease better than steroids alone. Likewise, mycophenolate also prevents development of end-stage renal disease in combination with glucocorticoids, and some studies suggest that African Americans have a greater response to mycophenolate than to cyclophosphamide. Plasmapheresis is not indicated in the treatment of lupus nephritis but is useful in cases of severe hemolytic anemia or thrombotic thrombocytopenic purpura associated with SLE. Finally, this patient has no acute indication for hemodialysis and, with treatment, may recover renal function.

IX-54. The answer is D. *(Chap. 314)* Rheumatoid arthritis (RA) is a multisystem disease without a known etiology. Genetic factors appear to explain ~60% of disease susceptibility. The hallmark, or characteristic feature, of RA is persistent, inflammatory synovitis. The prevalence of RA is 0.8% in the general population, and women are affected three times more often than men. About 10% of patients will have a first-degree relative with the disease. 80% of patients will develop the disease between the ages of 35 and 50. The disease course can be variable between patients; some patients experience minimal joint damage, while others have a relentless and debilitating polyarthritis.

IX-55. The answer is D. *(Chap. 314)* Felty's syndrome is a syndrome of chronic RA, splenomegaly, and neutropenia. Anemia and thrombocytopenia are also sometimes related. Patients who develop Felty's syndrome most commonly have more active disease with high titers of rheumatoid factor, subcutaneous nodules, and other systemic manifestations of disease. However, Felty's syndrome can develop when joint inflammation has regressed. The leukopenia is a selective neutropenia with polymorphonuclear leukocytes below 1500/mm^3. Bone marrow biopsy reveals hypercellularity with a lack of mature neutrophils. Hypersplenism has been proposed as a cause of Felty's syndrome, but splenectomy does not consistently correct the abnormality. Excessive margination of granulocytes caused by antibodies to these cells, complement activation, or binding of immune complexes may contribute to neutropenia.

IX-56. The answer is A. *(Chap. 318)* Anterior uveitis occurs in up to 30% of AS patients and may antedate the onset of the spondylitis. Attacks usually occur unilaterally with pain, photophobia, and blurred vision. Recurrent attacks are common, and ultimately cataracts may result. Other commonly seen problems include inflammation in the colon and ileum in up to 60% of AS patients, but only rarely do these patients develop inflammatory bowel disease. Cardiac disease is present in only a few percent of these patients and most commonly presents as aortic regurgitation. Other cardiac manifestations include complete heart block and congestive heart failure. Rare complications are upper lobe pulmonary fibrosis and retroperitoneal fibrosis.

IX-57. The answer is C. *(Chap. 383)* This patient presents with the classic symptoms, signs, and laboratory findings of polymyositis (PM) with antisynthetase antibodies. The differential diagnosis for a patient with proximal muscle weakness includes inclusion-body myositis, viral infections, denervating conditions such as amyotrophic lateral sclerosis (ALS), metabolic myopathies such as acid maltase deficiency, endocrine myopathies such as hypothyroidism, paraneoplastic myopathy, and drug-induced myopathies such as D-penicillamine, procainamide, statins, and glucocorticoids. PM is associated with an elevated creatine kinase, electromyography (EMG) showing irritability, and biopsy showing T cell infiltrates primarily in the muscle fascicles. Many patients with PM have autoantibodies targeted against the ribonucleoproteins involved in protein synthesis (antisynthetases). The antibody directed against histidyl-transfer RNA synthetase or anti-Jo-1 identifies a group of patients with PM who have a high likelihood (80%) of having interstitial lung disease. Antiglomerular antibodies are found in patients with Goodpasture's syndrome, antihistone antibodies in those with drug-induced lupus, and antimicrosomal antibodies in those with autoimmune hepatitis.

IX-58. **The answer is E.** *(Chap. 326)* Osteoarthritis (OA) is a disease of joint failure due to joint stress and vulnerability. As the primary driving force of the disease is mechanical, first-line therapy should be nonpharmacologic. Avoiding activities that cause pain and overload the joint, strengthening and conditioning the adjacent muscle groups, and supporting or unloading the joint with a brace or crutch are all examples of fundamental treatments aimed at reversing the pathophysiology of OA. In the case above, weight loss should be the primary goal of therapy. Each pound of weight increases loading across a weight-bearing joint three- to six-fold. This patient would benefit from a daily minimal-weight-bearing exercise regimen combined with nutritional goals aimed at slow, consistent weight loss. Avoidance of walking is impractical; a cane or supportive device to lessen the joint load can be offered. Steroids and narcotics are not indicated in this case.

IX-59. **The answer is E.** *(Chap. 329)* Fibromyalgia is characterized by chronic widespread musculoskeletal pain, stiffness, paresthesia, disturbed sleep, and easy fatigability. It occurs in a 9:1 female to male ratio. It is not confined to any particular region, ethnicity, or climate. While the pathogenesis is not clear, there are associations with disturbed sleep (disruption of stage 4 sleep) and abnormal pain perception. Fibromyalgia is diagnosed by the presence of widespread pain, a history of widespread musculoskeletal pain that has been present for >3 months, and pain on palpation at 11 of 18 tender point sites. Besides pain on palpation, the neurologic and musculoskeletal examinations are normal in patients with fibromyalgia. Psychiatric illnesses, particularly depression and anxiety disorders, are common comorbidities in these patients but do not help satisfy any diagnostic criteria.

IX-60. **The answer is B.** *(Chap. 317)* Sjögren's syndrome may present in patients as a primary disease or as a secondary disease in association with other autoimmune disorders, such as rheumatoid arthritis, systemic lupus erythematosus, scleroderma, mixed connective tissue disease, and primary biliary cirrhosis. This patient is typical in that most persons affected by this disorder are middle-aged females with a female-to-male ratio of 9:1. Symptoms are related to diminished lacrimal and salivary gland function. Oral dryness, or xerostomia, is very common. Parotid enlargement occurs in 66% of these patients. Ocular involvement resulting in symptoms of a sandy or gritty feeling under the eyelids, burning, redness, itching, decreased tearing, and photosensitivity is due to destruction of corneal and bulbar conjunctival epithelium, defined as keratoconjunctivitis sicca. Diagnostic evaluation includes the measurement of tear flow by Schirmer's test. Slit-lamp examination of the cornea after rose Bengal staining may show punctate corneal ulcerations and attached filaments of corneal epithelium. The most common extranodal manifestation of Sjögren's syndrome is arthralgias or arthritis (up to 60% of patients). Autoantibodies to Ro/SSA or La/SSB are very suggestive of this syndrome and are part of the classification criteria. Rheumatoid arthritis may be considered; however, the examination did not demonstrate inflammation, and the diffuse joint complaints without persistent morning stiffness make this less likely. Vitamin A deficiency may lead to dry eye but does not explain the patient's other symptoms.

IX-61. **The answer is D.** *(Chap. 314)* There are no blood tests that are specific for diagnosing rheumatoid arthritis (RA). Rheumatoid factors, which are autoantibodies to the Fc portion of IgG, have been used to help with diagnosis, and can be found in two-thirds of patients with RA. In the general population, rheumatoid factors become more prevalent with age, and 10–20% of patients older than 65 will have them. In unselected individuals, the predictive value of a positive rheumatoid factor is poor; no more than one-third of those with rheumatoid factors will have RA. False-positive results can occur in patients with systemic lupus erythematosus, Sjögren's syndrome, chronic liver disease, sarcoidosis, hepatitis B, mononucleosis, tuberculosis, malaria, and a host of other conditions. Recently, antibodies to cyclic citrullinated polypeptides (anti-CCP) have been shown to be helpful in diagnosing RA. In early RA, anti-CCP has been shown to be more predictive of disease than rheumatoid factor. Anti-CCP is felt to be a more specific test, and is positive in 1.5% of healthy individuals. The ESR has been used for decades as a nonspecific marker of inflammation. It is elevated in virtually all patients with active RA. In the patient above, radiographs would not add anything to the diagnostic evaluation. In early disease they are no more revealing of active synovitis than a careful physical examination.

TABLE IX-61   The 1987 Revised Criteria for the Classification of RA

1. Guidelines for classification
   a. Four of seven criteria are required to classify a patient as having rheumatoid arthritis (RA).
   b. Patients with two or more clinical diagnoses are not excluded.
2. Criteria[a]
   a. Morning stiffness: Stiffness in and around the joints lasting 1 h before maximal improvement.
   b. Arthritis of three or more joint areas: At least three joint areas, observed by a physician simultaneously, have soft tissue swelling or joint effusions, not just bony overgrowth. The 14 possible joint areas involved are right or left proximal interphalangeal, metacarpophalangeal, wrist, elbow, knee, ankle, and metatarsophalangeal joints.
   c. Arthritis of hand joints: Arthritis of wrist, metacarpophalangeal joint, or proximal interphalangeal joint.
   d. Symmetric arthritis: Simultaneous involvement of the same joint areas on both sides of the body.
   e. Rheumatoid nodules: Subcutaneous nodules over bony prominences, extensor surfaces, or juxtaarticular regions observed by a physician.
   f. Serum rheumatoid factor: Demonstration of abnormal amounts of serum rheumatoid factor by any method for which the result has been positive in less than 5% of normal control subjects.
   g. Radiographic changes: Typical changes of RA on posteroanterior hand and wrist radiographs that must include erosions or unequivocal bony decalcification localized in or most marked adjacent to the involved joints.

[a]Criteria a–d must be present for at least 6 weeks. Criteria b–e must be observed by a physician.
Source: From Arnett et al.

IX-62. **The answer is A.** *(Chap. 311)* This patient presents with perennial allergic rhinitis with multiple factors that are likely contributing to the persistent symptoms. Her skin testing shows multiple sensitivities including ragweed, grass, pet dander, and dust mites. The initial step in the treatment of chronic perennial rhinitis is avoidance of the offending allergens. This should include removal of the pet from the home, which is often difficult given the emotional attachment to the pet. In this instance, the first approach to the patient's sensitivity to cat dander is to discuss potentially removing the pet from the home. In addition, multiple other interventions are available that might decrease her symptoms. Other avoidance strategies that would decrease her exposure to offending allergens include removal of carpet and drapes from the bedroom, weekly laundering of the bedding and clothes at high temperatures, use of a filter-equipped vacuum, and plastic-lined covers for the mattress, pillows, and comforters. In addition, air-filtration devices can decrease the concentration of air-borne allergens. The medical therapy of perennial rhinitis should include use of H_1 antihistamines, which the patient is currently prescribed. α-Adrenergic agents can also be utilized for short periods to decrease congestion, but their use is limited by the development of rebound vasodilatation and worsening nasal congestion. Intranasal glucocorticoids are the most potent drugs for alleviating the symptoms of allergic rhinitis and should be considered in this case. Other agents with efficacy in treating perennial rhinitis include montelukast and intranasal cromolyn sodium. Immunotherapy may be considered if these interventions fail to work. Immunotherapy (previously called hyposensitization) involves weekly subcutaneous injections of gradually increasing concentrations of the suspected offending allergen. Studies have demonstrated partial relief of symptoms, but the injections must be continued for 3–5 years. Immunotherapy is also considered contraindicated in this patient because of the use of beta blockers, which could interfere with treatment of anaphylaxis, a rare side effect of immunotherapy.

IX-63. **The answer is C.** *(Chap. 314)* Rheumatoid arthritis is chronic, symmetric inflammatory polyarthritis. In two-thirds of patients, an initial clinical presentation of fatigue, anorexia, and weakness precedes joint complaints. In established RA (i.e., in a patient known to be diagnosed with this disorder), the most common manifestation is pain in affected joints that is worsened by movement. Morning stiffness of an hour or more is very frequent in these patients as well, but it is worth noting that this clinical finding does not allow differentiation between inflammatory and noninflammatory arthritides. Arthritic pain comes from the joint capsule itself, which is innervated and very sensitive to distention. 10% of patients with RA will have a first-degree relative with the disease. Weight loss is a nonspecific symptom and is not definitively associated with active disease.

IX-64. **The answer is D.** *(Chap. 318)* This patient presents with low back pain with morning stiffness and evidence of sacroiliitis on plain radiograph. The most likely diagnosis is ankylosing spondylitis (AS). Some 90% of individuals diagnosed with AS are HLA-B27 positive. However, HLA-B27 is present in 7% of North American Caucasian individuals and thus is not specific for the diagnosis of AS. Only 1–6% of individuals with HLA-B27 antigen will develop AS. AS is a spondyloarthropathy that usually presents with a dull low back and gluteal pain. There is a male predominance (2–3:1) with a median age at presentation of 23 years. The main joints involved are those of the axial skeleton. About 20–30% will have arthritis of the hips or shoulders, and asymmetric polyarthritis of the small joints occurs in 25–35%. On physical examination, pain with palpation is present over the affected joints. There is decrease flexion and extension of the spine, and decreased chest expansion (<5 cm) may be seen with inspiration. Radiographically, sacroiliitis is demonstrated by blurring of the cortical margins of the subchondral bone with progression to bony erosions and sclerosis. In the lumbar spine, there is progressive loss of lumbar lordosis. Laboratory testing frequently shows HLA-B27 positivity as stated previously. C-reactive protein and erythrocyte sedimentation rate may be elevated. Anemia is also common. An elevation in alkaline phosphatase may be seen in severe disease, but this is not common. Anti-CCP antibodies, antinuclear antibodies, and rheumatoid factor are largely absent unless caused by a coexistent disease.

IX-65. **The answer is B.** *(Chap. 318)* The presence of arthritis after episodes of infectious diarrhea or urethritis has been recognized for centuries, with the symptoms of diarrhea or dysuria occurring 1 to 4 weeks before the onset of the arthritis. The most common organisms that are implicated are bacteria that cause acute infectious diarrhea. All four *Shigella* species have been reported to cause reactive arthritis, although *S. flexneri* is only rarely implicated. Other bacteria that have been identified as triggers include several *Salmonella* species, *Yersinia enterocolitica,* and *Campylobacter jejuni.* In addition, some organisms that cause urethritis are also causative; these include *Chlamydia trachomatis* and *Ureaplasma urealyticum.* Arthritis associated with disseminated gonococcal infection is directly related to an infectious cause and responds to antibiotics, unlike reactive arthritis.

IX-66. **The answer is D.** *(Chap. 327)* In acute gouty arthritis, the initial therapy is directed against the intense inflammatory response. Typical agents include colchicine, nonsteroidal anti-inflammatory drugs (NSAIDs), and oral glucocorticoids. The choice of agent should be made in the context of the patient's comorbid conditions and medications as well as potential side effects of the medication. Oral glucocorticoids are the treatment of choice for this patient. These medications, such as prednisone, are highly effective, and there are no contraindications to the use of prednisone. Colchicine may be poorly tolerated in the elderly. In addition, renal disease and blood dyscrasias are relative contraindications to the use of the colchicine. Colchicine is usually administered orally as 0.6-mg tablets, which may be taken every 6 h until the appearance of intolerance or gastrointestinal side effects. Intravenous colchicine is rarely used except in hospitalized individuals who are unable to take oral medications. Sudden death with IV administration has been reported as well as marked bone marrow suppression, and thus this medication should not be used in this individual. NSAIDs, such as indomethacin in full anti-inflammatory doses, are effective in ~90% of individuals with acute gout, with resolution of symptoms in 5–8 days. The most effective drugs are indomethacin, ibuprofen, or diclofenac. However, given the degree of renal impairment in this patient, NSAIDs should not be used. Hypouricemic agents such as allopurinol and probenecid should not be used in acute gouty arthritis as they may worsen the acute attack. Probenecid is a uricosuric agent that is also contraindicated in this patient because of the underlying renal disease.

IX-67. The answer is D. *(Chap. 317)* Lymphoma is well known to develop specifically in the late stage of Sjögren's syndrome. Common manifestations of this malignant condition include persistent parotid gland enlargement, purpura, leukopenia, cryoglobulinemia, and low C4 complement levels. Most of the lymphomas are extranodal, marginal zone B cell, and low-grade. Low-grade lymphomas may be detected incidentally during a labial biopsy. Mortality is higher in patients with concurrent B symptoms (fevers, night sweats, and weight loss), a lymph node mass >7 cm, and a high or intermediate histologic grade.

IX-68. The answer is D. *(Chap. 315)* This patient has a history very suggestive of recurrent bouts of acute rheumatic fever (ARF) with evidence of mitral regurgitation, mitral stenosis, and aortic regurgitation on physical examination. This and the presence of atrial fibrillation imply severe rheumatic heart disease. Risk factors for this condition include poverty and crowded living conditions. As a result, ARF is considerably more common in the developing world. Daily aspirin is the treatment of choice for the migratory large-joint arthritis and fever that are common manifestations of ARF. Practitioners sometimes use steroids during acute bouts of carditis to quell inflammation, though this remains a controversial practice and has no role between flares of ARF. Secondary prophylaxis with either daily oral penicillin or, preferably, monthly IM injections is considered the best method to prevent further episodes of ARF, and therefore prevent further valvular damage. Primary prophylaxis with penicillin on an as-needed basis is equally effective for preventing further bouts of carditis. However, most episodes of sore throat are too minor for patients to present to a physician. Therefore, secondary prophylaxis is considered preferable in patients who already have severe valvular disease. Doxycycline is not a first-line agent for group A *Streptococcus*, the pathogen that incites ARF.

X. ENDOCRINOLOGY AND METABOLISM

QUESTIONS

DIRECTIONS: Choose the **one best** response to each question.

X-1. What is the most common cause of hypothyroidism worldwide?

A. Autoimmune disease
B. Graves' disease
C. Iatrogenic causes
D. Iodine deficiency
E. Medication side effects

X-2. A 23-year-old woman presents to clinic complaining of months of weight gain, fatigue, amenorrhea, and worsening acne. She cannot identify when her symptoms began precisely, but she reports that without a change in her diet she has noted a 12.3-kg weight gain over the past 6 months. She has been amenorrheic for several months. On examination she is noted to have truncal obesity with bilateral purplish striae across both flanks. Cushing's syndrome is suspected. Which of the following tests should be used to make the diagnosis?

A. 24-h urine free cortisol
B. Basal adrenocorticotropic hormone (ACTH)
C. Corticotropin-releasing hormone (CRH) level at 8 A.M.
D. Inferior petrosal venous sampling
E. Overnight 1 mg dexamethasone suppression test

X-3. Secretion of gonadotropin releasing-hormone (GnRH) normally stimulates release of luteinizing hormone (LH) and follicle-stimulating hormone (FSH) which promote production and release of testosterone and estrogen. Which mechanism below best explains how long-acting gonadotropin-releasing hormone agonists (e.g., leuprolide) decrease testosterone levels in the management of prostate cancer?

A. GnRH agonists also promote production of sex hormone–binding globulin, which decreases the availability of testosterone
B. Negative feedback loop between GnRH and LH/FSH
C. Sensitivity of LH and FSH to pulse frequency of GnRH
D. Translocation of the cytoplasmic nuclear receptor into the nucleus with constitutive activation of GnRH

X-4. A 44-year-old woman seeks evaluation for irregular menstrual cycles with heavy menstrual bleeding. She reports that her menses had been regular with 28-day cycles since her early twenties. However, for the past 6 months, her cycles have been 22–25 days with heavy associated bleeding that is unusual for her. She has had rare hot flashes and sleep disturbance. She is requesting assistance in controlling these symptoms. You suspect she is perimenopausal, and hormonal testing on day 2 of her menses confirms this suspicion. You are considering treatment with oral contraceptives for control of her symptoms and to protect against unintended pregnancy. All of the following would be considered contraindications to use of oral contraceptive pills *except*

A. breast cancer
B. cigarette smoking
C. kidney disease
D. liver disease
E. prior history of deep venous thrombosis

X-5. All the following are risk factors for the development of osteoporotic fractures *except*

A. African-American race
B. current cigarette smoking
C. female sex
D. low body weight
E. physical inactivity

X-6. All the following drugs are associated with an increased risk of osteoporosis in adults *except*

A. cyclosporine
B. dilantin
C. heparin
D. prednisone
E. ranitidine

X-7. A 34-year-old woman presents to your clinic with a variety of complaints that have been worsening over the past year or so. She notes fatigue, amenorrhea, and weight gain. She states that her primary physician diagnosed her

X-7. *(Continued)*

with hypothyroidism several months ago, and she has been faithfully taking thyroid hormone replacement. Her thyroid-stimulating hormone (TSH) has been in the normal range over the last two laboratory checks. When her symptoms did not improve on synthroid, she was sent to your clinic for further evaluation. A diagnosis of panhypopituitarism is considered. All of the following are consistent with normal pituitary function *except*

A.   basal elevation of follicle-stimulating hormone (FSH) and luteinizing hormone (LH) in a postmenopausal woman
B.   elevation of aldosterone after infusion of cosyntropin
C.   elevation of growth hormone after ingestion of a glucose load
D.   elevation of cortisol after injection of regular insulin
E.   elevation of TSH after infusion of thyrotropin-releasing hormone (TRH)

X-8. A 33-year-old male with end-stage renal disease who is on hemodialysis complains of decreased libido, inability to maintain erections, increasing fatigue, and mild weakness. He has been on a stable hemodialysis regimen for 8 years, and all his electrolytes are normal. Further evaluation reveals a reduced serum testosterone level. Measurement of which of the following will distinguish primary from secondary hypogonadism?

A.   Aldosterone
B.   Cortisol
C.   Estradiol
D.   Luteinizing hormone
E.   Thyroid-stimulating hormone

X-9. A 42-year-old woman is brought to the emergency room by ambulance for altered mental status. The glucose level by fingerstick monitoring was below the measurement capabilities of the monitor (<40 mg/dL). After 2 ampules of 50% dextrose, the patient's fingerstick glucose remains at 42 mg/dL. She remains unconscious and had a 1-min seizure while in transport. She has no history of diabetes mellitus. Her family denies that she has been recently ill, but recently she has been depressed. She works as a registered nurse on a medical floor of the hospital. Which of the following tests would confirm an overdose of exogenous insulin?

A.   Plasma glucose <55 mg/dL, plasma insulin >18 pmol/L, and plasma C-peptide levels undetectable
B.   Plasma glucose <55 mg/dL, plasma insulin >18 pmol/L, and plasma C-peptide levels >0.6 ng/mL
C.   Plasma glucose <55 mg/dL, plasma insulin <18 pmol/L, and plasma glucagon <12 pmol/L
D.   Plasma glucose <55 mg/dL, plasma insulin <18 pmol/L, and C-peptide levels undetectable

X-10. A 44-year-old male is involved in a motor vehicle collision. He sustains multiple injuries to the face, chest, and

X-10. *(Continued)*

pelvis. He is unresponsive in the field and is intubated for airway protection. An intravenous line is placed. The patient is admitted to the intensive care unit (ICU) with multiple orthopedic injuries. He is stabilized medically and on hospital day 2 undergoes successful open reduction and internal fixation of the right femur and right humerus. After his return to the ICU, you review his laboratory values. TSH is 0.3 mU/L, and the total T_4 level is normal. T_3 is 0.6 µg/dL. What is the most appropriate next management step?

A.   Initiation of levothyroxine
B.   A radioiodine uptake scan
C.   A thyroid ultrasound
D.   Observation
E.   Initiation of prednisone

X-11. All the following biochemical markers are a measure of bone resorption *except*

A.   serum alkaline phosphatase
B.   serum cross-linked N-telopeptide
C.   serum cross-linked C-telopeptide
D.   urine hydroxyproline
E.   urine total free deoxypyridinoline

X-12. A 54-year-old woman is referred to endocrinology for evaluation of osteoporosis after a recent evaluation of back pain revealed a compression fracture of the T4 vertebral body. She is perimenopausal with irregular menstrual periods and frequent hot flashes. She does not smoke. She otherwise is well and healthy. Her weight is 70 kg, and height is 168 cm. A bone mineral density scan shows a T-score of −3.5 SD and a Z-score of −2.5 SD. All of the following tests are indicated for the evaluation of osteoporosis in this patient *except*

A.   24-h urine calcium
B.   follicle-stimulating hormone and luteinizing hormone levels
C.   serum calcium
D.   renal function panel
E.   vitamin D levels (25-hydroxyvitamin D)

X-13. A 67-year-old woman presents to clinic after a fall on the ice a week ago. She visited the local emergency room immediately after the fall, where hip radiographs were performed and were negative for fracture or dislocation. They did reveal fusion of the sacroiliac joints and coarse trabeculations in the ilium, consistent with Paget disease. A comprehensive metabolic panel was also sent at that visit and is remarkable for an alkaline phosphatase of 157 U/L, with normal serum calcium and phosphate levels. She was discharged with analgesics and told to follow up with her primary care doctor for further management of her radiographic findings. She is recovering from her fall and denies any long-standing pain or immobility of her hip joints. She states that her father

X-13. *(Continued)*

suffered from a bone disease that caused him headaches and hearing loss near the end of his life. She is very concerned about the radiographs and wants to know what they mean. Which of the following is the best treatment strategy at this point?

A. Initiate physical therapy and non-weight bearing exercises to strengthen the hip.
B. No treatment; she is asymptomatic. Follow radiographs and laboratory findings every 6 months.
C. Prescribe vitamin D and calcium.
D. Start an oral bisphosphonate.
E. Start high-dose prednisone with rapid taper over 1 week.

X-14. A 26-year-old woman presents with 2 weeks of nausea, vomiting, and jaundice. She has been previously healthy and has no past medical history. On examination, a palpable liver edge is appreciated. Ocular findings are presented in Figure X-14 (Color Atlas). Her transaminases and total bilirubin are elevated. Which of the following tests will lead to a definitive diagnosis in this patient?

A. Anti-smooth-muscle antibody
B. Hepatitis B surface antigen
C. Liver biopsy with quantitative copper assay
D. Serum ceruloplasmin
E. Total iron-binding capacity and ferritin

X-15. A 29-year-old woman presents to your clinic complaining of difficulty swallowing, sore throat, and tender swelling in her neck. She has also noted fevers intermittently over the past week. Several weeks prior to her current symptoms she experienced symptoms of an upper respiratory tract infection. She has no past medical history. On physical examination, she is noted to have a small goiter that is painful to the touch. Her oropharynx is clear. Laboratory studies are sent, and reveal a white blood cell count of 14,100 cells/μL with a normal differential, erythrocyte sedimentation rate (ESR) of 53 mm/h, and a thyroid-stimulating hormone (TSH) of 21 μIU/mL. Thyroid antibodies are negative. What is the most likely diagnosis?

A. Autoimmune hypothyroidism
B. Cat-scratch fever
C. Graves' disease
D. Ludwig's angina
E. Subacute thyroiditis

X-16. What is the most appropriate treatment for the patient described above?

A. Iodine ablation of the thyroid
B. Large doses of aspirin
C. Local radiation therapy
D. No treatment necessary
E. Propylthiouracil

X-17. The Diabetes Control and Complications Trial (DCCT) provided definitive proof that reduction in chronic hyperglycemia

A. improves microvascular complications in type 1 diabetes mellitus
B. improves macrovascular complications in type 1 diabetes mellitus
C. improves microvascular complications in type 2 diabetes mellitus
D. improves macrovascular complications in type 2 diabetes mellitus
E. improves both microvascular and macrovascular complications in type 2 diabetes mellitus

X-18. A 54-year-old woman undergoes thyroidectomy for follicular carcinoma of the thyroid. About 6 h after surgery, the patient complains of tingling around her mouth. She subsequently develops a pins-and-needles sensation in the fingers and toes. The nurse calls the physician to the bedside to evaluate the patient after she has severe hand cramps when her blood pressure is taken. Upon evaluation, the patient is still complaining of intermittent cramping of her hands. Since surgery, she has received morphine sulfate, 2 mg, for pain and compazine, 5 mg, for nausea. She has had no change in her vital signs and is afebrile. Tapping on the inferior portion of the zygomatic arch 2 cm anterior to the ear produces twitching at the corner of the mouth. An electrocardiogram (ECG) shows a QT interval of 575 ms. What is the next step in evaluation and treatment of this patient?

A. Administration of benztropine, 2 mg IV
B. Administration of calcium gluconate, 2 g IV
C. Administration of magnesium sulphate, 4 g IV
D. Measurement of calcium, magnesium, phosphate, and potassium levels
E. Measurement of forced vital capacity

X-19. A 49-year-old male is brought to the hospital by his family because of confusion and dehydration. The family reports that for the last 3 weeks he has had persistent copious watery diarrhea that has not abated with the use of over-the-counter medications. The diarrhea has been unrelated to food intake and has persisted during fasting. The stool does not appear fatty and is not malodorous. The patient works as an attorney, is a vegetarian, and has not traveled recently. No one in the household has had similar symptoms. Before the onset of diarrhea, he had mild anorexia and a 5-lb weight loss. Since the diarrhea began, he has lost at least 10 pounds. The physical examination is notable for blood pressure of 100/70, heart rate of 110/min, and temperature of 36.8°C (98.2°F). Other than poor skin turgor, confusion, and diffuse muscle weakness, the physical examination is unremarkable. Laboratory studies are notable for a normal complete blood count and the following chemistry results:

X-19. *(Continued)*

Na$^+$	146 meq/L
K$^+$	3.0 meq/L
Cl$^-$	96 meq/L
HCO$_3^-$	36 meq/L
BUN	32 mg/dL
Creatinine	1.2 mg/dL

A 24-h stool collection yields 3 L of tea-colored stool. Stool sodium is 50 meq/L, potassium is 25 meq/L, and stool osmolality is 170 mosmol/L. Which of the following diagnostic tests is most likely to yield the correct diagnosis?

A.   Serum cortisol
B   Serum TSH
C.   Serum VIP
D.   Urinary 5-HIAA
E.   Urinary metanephrine

X-20. A 68-year-old woman with stage IIIB squamous cell carcinoma of the lung is admitted to the hospital because of altered mental status and dehydration. Upon admission, she is found to have a calcium level of 19.6 mg/dL and phosphate of 1.8 mg/dL. Concomitant measurement of parathyroid hormone was 0.1 pg/mL (normal 10–65 pg/mL), and a screen for parathyroid hormone–related peptide was positive. Over the first 24 h, the patient receives 4 L of normal saline with furosemide diuresis. The next morning, the patient's calcium is now 17.6 mg/dL and phosphate is 2.2 mg/dL. She continues to have delirium. What is the best approach for ongoing treatment of this patient's hypercalcemia?

A.   Continue therapy with large-volume fluid administration and forced diuresis with furosemide.
B.   Continue therapy with large-volume fluid administration, but stop furosemide and treat with hydrochlorothiazide.
C.   Initiate therapy with calcitonin alone.
D.   Initiate therapy with pamidronate alone.
E.   Initiate therapy with calcitonin and pamidronate.

X-21. Differentiating primary dysmenorrhea from other causes of chronic cyclical pelvic pain is important because there is a specific treatment for primary dysmenorrhea. What is the pathophysiology/treatment for primary dysmenorrhea?

A.   Ectopic endometrium/oral contraceptives
B.   History of sexual abuse/counseling
C.   Increased stores of prostaglandin precursors/anti-inflammatory medication
D.   Ruptured graafian follicle/oral contraceptives

X-22. A 25-year-old female notes increasing facial hair and acne for the last 4 months. She has noticed some deepening of her voice but denies changes in her libido or genitalia. She weighs 94 kg and is 5 feet 5 inches tall. Blood pressure is 126/70 mmHg. Examination is notable for moderate obesity. There is no evidence of abdominal

X-22. *(Continued)*

striae or bruising. All the following would be important initial steps in the clinical assessment of this patient *except*

A.   medication history
B.   family history
C.   serum testosterone level
D.   serum dehydroepiandrosterone sulfate (DHEAS) level
E.   abdominal ultrasound

X-23. A patient visited a local emergency room 1 week ago with a headache. She received a head MRI, which did not reveal a cause for her symptoms, but the final report states "an empty sella is noted. Advise clinical correlation." The patient was discharged from the emergency room with instructions to follow-up with her primary care physician as soon as possible. Her headache has resolved, and the patient has no complaints; however, she comes to your office 1 day later very concerned about this unexpected MRI finding. What should be the next step in her management?

A.   Diagnose her with subclinical pan-hypopituitarism, and initiate low-dose hormone replacement.
B.   Reassure her and follow laboratory results closely.
C.   Reassure her and repeat MRI in 6 months.
D.   This may represent early endocrine malignancy—whole-body positron-emission tomography/CT is indicated.
E.   This MRI finding likely represents the presence of a benign adenoma—refer to neurosurgery for resection.

X-24. A 16-year-old previously healthy teenage boy presents to the local emergency room with a headache that has been worsening over the course of 2 months. His parents note that "he just hasn't seemed like himself," and over the past 2 weeks has been complaining of double vision. He experienced profuse vomiting this afternoon, which prompted his visit. He also describes weight gain over the same 2 month time period and has not been sleeping well. On examination, he is drowsy, and funduscopic examination reveals papilledema. He has no fever, neck stiffness, or elevated white blood cell count. Which of the following is the most likely cause?

A.   Carney syndrome
B.   Congenital pan-hypopituitarism
C.   Craniopharyngioma
D.   McCune-Albright syndrome
E.   Meningioma

X-25. At the midpoint of the menstrual cycle, a luteinizing hormone (LH) surge occurs via an estrogen-mediated pathway. Though chronic low levels of estrogen are inhibitory to LH release, gradually rising estrogen levels stimulate LH secretion. This relationship between estrogen and LH is an example of which endocrine regulatory system?

A.   Autocrine regulation
B.   Negative feedback control

X-25. *(Continued)*

    C. Paracrine regulation

    D. Positive feedback control

X-26. Which of the following is the most common site for a fracture associated with osteoporosis?

    A. Femur

    B. Hip

    C. Radius

    D. Vertebra

    E. Wrist

X-27. Postmenopausal estrogen therapy has been shown to increase a female's risk of all the following clinical outcomes *except*

    A. breast cancer

    B. hip fracture

    C. myocardial infarction

    D. stroke

    E. venous thromboembolism

X-28. All the following therapies have been shown to reduce the risk of hip fractures in postmenopausal women with osteoporosis *except*

    A. alendronate

    B. estrogen

    C. parathyroid hormone

    D. raloxifene

    E. risedronate

    F. vitamin D plus calcium

X-29. A 45-year-old man is diagnosed with pheochromocytoma after presentation with confusion, marked hypertension to 250/140 mmHg, tachycardia, headaches, and flushing. His fractionated plasma metanephrines show a normetanephrine level of 560 pg/mL and a metanephrine level of 198 pg/mL (normal values: normetanephrine: 18–111 pg/mL; metanephrine: 12–60 pg/mL). CT scanning of the abdomen with IV contrast demonstrates a 3-cm mass in the right adrenal gland. A brain MRI with gadolinium shows edema of the white matter near the parietooccipital junction consistent with reversible posterior leukoencephalopathy. You are asked to consult regarding management. Which of the following statements is true regarding management of pheochromocytoma is this individual?

    A. Beta-blockade is absolutely contraindicated for tachycardia even after adequate alpha-blockade has been attained.

    B. Immediate surgical removal of the mass is indicated, because the patient presented with hypertensive crisis with encephalopathy.

    C. Salt and fluid intake should be restricted to prevent further exacerbation of the patient's hypertension.

    D. Treatment with phenoxybenzamine should be started at a high dose (20–30 mg three times daily) to rap-

X-29. *(Continued)*

idly control blood pressure, and surgery can be undertaken within 24–48 h.

    E. Treatment with IV phentolamine is indicated for treatment of the hypertensive crisis. Phenoxybenzamine should be started at a low dose and titrated to the maximum tolerated dose over 2–3 weeks. Surgery should not be planned until the blood pressure is consistently below 160/100 mmHg.

X-30. Inhibition of renin activity is a contemporary target mechanism for treatment of hypertension. All of the following physiologic alterations will cause an increase in renin secretion *except*

    A. decreased effective circulating blood volume

    B. high-potassium diet

    C. increased sympathetic activity

    D. low solute delivery to the distal convoluted tubules

    E. upright posture

X-31. Which of the following represents the likelihood of finding a pituitary microadenoma at autopsy in the general population?

    A. 0.1%

    B. 2%

    C. 5%

    D. 11%

    E. 25%

X-32. A 33-year-old woman presents to the emergency room complaining of headache, palpitations, sweating, and anxiety. These feelings began abruptly about 30 min ago, and she reports intermittent symptoms similar to these that occur perhaps once per month. She has previously been diagnosed with panic attacks and has been prescribed paroxetine 20 mg daily. Her symptoms have not improved since initiation of this drug, and she believes that her episodes of palpitations and anxiety have worsened since this time. Her past medical history includes a diagnosis of hypertension, but treatment with amlodipine has recently been discontinued because her blood pressure was 88/50 mmHg with symptomatic orthostasis at her last visit with her primary care provider. Her only other medical history is headaches for the past year for which she has been prescribed ibuprofen, 600 mg as needed. She believes the headaches accompany her episodes and last for several hours after the sweating has subsided. On physical examination, the patient appears flushed and diaphoretic. Her blood pressure while lying down is 170/100 mmHg with a heart rate of 90 beats/min. Upon standing her blood pressure falls to 132/74 mmHg with a heart rate of 112 beats/min. Her respiratory rate is 22 beats/min, and her temperature is 37.4°C. Her examination is otherwise normal. There is no papilledema. Which of the following is most likely to correctly diagnose this patient?

    A. 24-h urine collection for 5-hydroxyindoleacetic acid (5-HIAA)

X-32. *(Continued)*

    B.   24-h urine collection for fractionated metanephrines

    C.   CT scan of the abdomen with intravenous contrast

    D. ^{131}I-metaiodobenzylguanidine scan (MIBG)

    E.   No testing is necessary; the patient is suffering from a panic attack

X-33. The mineralocorticoid receptor in the renal tubule is responsible for the sodium retention and potassium wasting that is seen in mineralocorticoid excess states such as aldosterone-secreting tumors. However, states of glucocorticoid excess (e.g., Cushing's syndrome) can also present with sodium retention and hypokalemia. What characteristic of the mineralocorticoid-glucocorticoid pathways explain this finding?

    A.   Higher affinity of the mineralocorticoid receptor for glucocorticoids

    B.   Oversaturation of the glucocorticoid degradation pathway in states of glucocorticoid excess

    C.   Similar, but distinct, DNA binding sites producing the same metabolic effect

    D.   Upregulation of the mineralocorticoid-binding protein in states of glucocorticoid excess

X-34. A 40-year-old female with Graves' disease was recently started on methimazole. One month later she comes to the clinic for a routine follow-up. She notes some low-grade fevers, arthralgias, and general malaise. Laboratories are notable for a mild transaminitis and a glucose of 150 mg/dL. All the following are known side effects of methimazole *except*

    A.   agranulocytosis

    B.   rash

    C.   arthralgia

    D.   hepatitis

    E.   insulin resistance

X-35. A 60-year-old woman is referred to your office for evaluation of hypercalcemia of 12.9 mg/dL. This was found incidentally on a chemistry panel that was drawn during a hospitalization for cervical spondylosis. Despite fluid administration in the hospital, her serum calcium at discharge was 11.8 mg/dL. The patient is asymptomatic. She is otherwise in good health and has had her recommended age-appropriate cancer screening. She denies constipation or bone pain and is now 8 weeks out from her spinal surgery. Today, her serum calcium level is 12.4 mg/dL, and phosphate is 2.3 mg/dL. Her hematocrit and all other chemistries including creatinine were normal. What is the most likely diagnosis?

    A.   Breast cancer

    B.   Hyperparathyroidism

    C.   Hyperthyroidism

    D.   Multiple myeloma

    E.   Vitamin D intoxication

X-36. A 62-year-old man presents to a local emergency room complaining of chest pressure and feeling "like my heart is fluttering inside my chest." He experienced similar symptoms 1 month ago that resolved spontaneously. He did not seek medical attention at that time. He has no significant past medical history. On review of systems he notes some recent weight loss and excessive sweating. He feels as though his appetite has increased lately. His wife adds that he has recently taken some time off work due to fatigue; despite his time off he has not been able to relax and has not been sleeping well. On physical examination his heart rate is irregular at 140–150 beats/minute. Blood pressure is 134/55 mmHg. He is admitted to the hospital and screening tests reveal an undetectable thyroid-stimulating hormone level. Which of the following statements is true?

    A.   50% of hyperthyroid patients will convert from atrial fibrillation to normal sinus rhythm with thyroid management alone.

    B.   A firm, small thyroid on physical examination would be compatible with a diagnosis of Graves' disease.

    C.   Atrial fibrillation is the most common cardiac manifestation of hyperthyroidism.

    D.   His excessive sweating is likely not related to hyperthyroidism.

    E.   Hyperthyroidism leads to a high-output state for the heart, and narrowing pulse pressure.

X-37. The patient described above is started on atenolol and his heart rate slows to 80 beats/min. Which of the following additional therapies is indicated?

    A.   Diltiazem

    B.   Itraconazole

    C.   Liothyronine

    D.   Methimazole

    E.   Phenoxybenzamine

X-38. A patient presents to his primary care physician complaining of fatigue and hair loss. He has gained 6.4 kg since his last clinic visit 6 months ago but notes markedly decreased appetite. On review of systems, he reports that he is not sleeping well and feels cold all the time. He is still able to enjoy his hobbies and spending time with his family, and does not believe that he is depressed. His examination reveals diffuse alopecia and slowed deep tendon reflex relaxation. Hypothyroidism is high on the differential for this patient. Which of the statements regarding that diagnosis is correct?

    A.   A normal thyroid-stimulating hormone (TSH) excludes secondary, but not primary hypothyroidism.

    B. T_3 measurement is not indicated to make the diagnosis.

    C.   The T_3/T_4 ratio is important for determining response to therapy.

    D.   Thyroid peroxidase antibodies distinguish between primary and secondary hypothyroidism.

    E.   Unbound T_4 is a better screening test than TSH for subclinical hypothyroidism.

X-39. Which of the following statements regarding autoimmune hypothyroidism is true?

A. 10% of 40- to 60-year-old adults have subclinical hypothyroidism.

B. Absence of a goiter makes autoimmune hypothyroidism unlikely.

C. Family history of autoimmune disorders does not significantly increase risk.

D. It is more common in the Pacific Rim where diets are lower in iodine.

E. Viral thyroiditis does not induce subsequent autoimmune thyroiditis.

X-40. You are researching a cell line with an altered membrane structure that makes the cell membrane impermeable to extracellular molecules of all size and charge. You then expose the cell line to varying concentrations of various hormones. Of the following hormones, which one should no longer exert an effect on this cell line?

A. Dopamine

B. Gonadotropin-releasing hormone

C. Insulin

D. Vitamin D

X-41. In regard to Graves' disease, which of the following is true?

A. It accounts for >90% of all causes of thyrotoxicosis.

B. It occurs in 2% of women.

C. It typically occurs in patients between 50 and 60 years of age.

D. Populations with a low iodine intake have an increased prevalence.

E. There is an equal male-to-female prevalence.

X-42. The parents of a 14-year-old boy want your opinion about treatment of their child's lipid disorder. The family emigrated from South Africa to the United States recently. The child has had cutaneous xanthomas on the hands, elbows, heels, and buttocks since childhood. In South Africa, he underwent thoracotomy for a problem with his aortic valve 3 years ago. He currently experiences exertional dyspnea, and his diet consists mostly of unhealthy, fatty foods. On examination, you appreciate bruits in the femoral arteries and abdominal aorta. His most recent lipid profile shows a total cholesterol of 734 mg/dL and a low-density lipoprotein (LDL) of 376 mg/dL. What is the most appropriate step in this patient's evaluation?

A. Genetic test for familial defective apoB100

B. Rule out congenital syphilis

C. Rule out hypothyroidism

D. Screen the parents for Münchhausen-by-proxy syndrome

X-43. A 16-year-old male is brought to your clinic by his parents due to concern about his weight. He has not seen a physician for many years. He states that he has gained

X-43. *(Continued)*

weight due to inactivity and that he is less active because of exertional chest pain. He takes no medications. He was adopted and his parents do not know the medical history of his biologic parents. Physical examination is notable for Stage 1 hypertension and body mass index of 30 kg/m². He has xanthomas on his hands, heels, and buttocks. Laboratory testing shows a low-density lipoprotein (LDL) of 210 mg/dL, creatinine of 0.7 mg/dL, total bilirubin of 3.1 mg/dL, haptoglobin <6 mg/dL, and a glycosylated hemoglobin of 6.7%. You suspect a hereditary lipoproteinemia due to the clinical and laboratory findings. Which test would be diagnostic of the primary lipoprotein disorder in this patient?

A. Congo red staining of xanthoma biopsy

B. CT scan of the liver

C. Family pedigree analysis

D. Gas chromatography

E. LDL receptor function in skin biopsy

X-44. A 35 year-old woman presents with amenorrhea over the past 4 months. She has been trying to get pregnant without success. She complains of a thin milky discharge from her nipples and over the past several days has noted some blurry vision. On laboratory testing, her prolactin level is 110 µg/L (normal: 5–20 µg/L). A head MRI is performed and reveals an 11-mm pituitary macroadenoma. What is the next step in management?

A. Follow visual fields; if worse in 1 month, refer for surgery.

B. Reassure the patient and follow-up closely.

C. Refer for urgent neurosurgery.

D. Repeat MRI in 4 months.

E. Do visual field testing and initiate a dopamine agonist.

X-45. A patient is asked to undergo a testing protocol to assess adrenocortical function. After 5 days of severe sodium restriction (10 mmol/day), blood is drawn for analysis. Which hormone abnormality may be detected using this protocol?

A. Hypercorticolism

B. Glucocorticoid deficiency

C. Mineralocorticoid deficiency

D. Mineralocorticoid excess

E. Vasopressin excess

X-46. A 38-year-old woman presents to her primary care doctor complaining of fatigue and irritability. She thinks these symptoms have been worsening over a period of several months. She has a history of mild intermittent asthma and hypertriglyceridemia. Physical examination reveals a resting heart rate of 105 beats/min, blood pressure of 136/72 mmHg, bilateral proptosis and warm, moist skin. Screening tests are sent and reveal a thyroid-stimulating hormone (TSH) level that is undetectable and a normal unbound T₄. What should be the next step in diagnosis?

X-46. *(Continued)*
- A. Radionuclide scan of the thyroid
- B. Thyroid-stimulating antibody screen
- C. Thyroid peroxidase (TPO) antibody screen
- D. Total T_4
- E. Unbound T_3

X-47. A 24-year-old female patient returns to your office to review her recent laboratory data. On her last clinic visit, you began an evaluation for secondary amenorrhea. Her vital signs are normal and her body mass index (BMI) is 20 kg/m^2. Her β-human chorionic gonadotropin is negative. Serum follicle-stimulation hormone (FSH) is below the lower limit of normal. Serum testosterone is within normal limits. Morning cortisol is 24 mg/dL. Urinalysis is unremarkable and there is no glucose in the urine. Thyroid-stimulating hormone is 3.7 mU/L. Serum prolactin is elevated. What is the most likely cause of this patient's secondary amenorrhea?

- A. Ectopic pregnancy
- B. Pituitary tumor
- C. Primary ovarian failure
- D. Uterine outflow obstruction
- E. Malnutrition

X-48. A couple seeks advice regarding infertility. The female partner is 35 years old. She has never been pregnant and was taking oral contraceptive pills from age 20 until age 34. It is now 16 months since she discontinued her oral contraceptives. She is having menstrual cycles approximately once every 35 days, but occasionally will go as long as 60 days between cycles. Most months, she develops breast tenderness about 2–3 weeks after the start of her menstrual cycle. When she was in college, she was treated for *Neisseria gonorrhoeae* that was diagnosed when she presented to the student health center with a fever and pelvic pain. She otherwise has no medical history. She works about 60 h weekly as a corporate attorney and exercises daily. She drinks coffee daily and alcohol at social occasions only. Her body mass index (BMI) is 19.8 kg/m^2. Her husband, who is 39 years old, accompanies her to the evaluation. He also has never had children. He was married previously from the ages of 24–28. He and his prior wife attempted to conceive for about 15 months, but were unsuccessful. At that time, he was smoking marijuana on a daily basis and attributed their lack of success to his drug use. He has now been completely free of drugs for 9 years. He suffers from hypertension and is treated with lisinopril, 10 mg daily. He is not obese (BMI, 23.7 kg/m^2). They request evaluation for their infertility and request help with conception. Which of the following statements is true in regards to their infertility and likelihood of success in conception?

- A. Determination of ovulation is not necessary in the female partner as most of her cycles occur regularly, and she develops breast tenderness mid-cycle indicative of ovulation

X-48. *(Continued)*
- B. Lisinopril should be discontinued immediately because of the risk of birth defects associated with its use
- C. The female partner should be assessed for tubal patency by a hysterosalpingogram. If significant scarring is found, in vitro fertilization should be strongly considered to decrease the risk of ectopic pregnancy.
- D. The prolonged use of oral contraceptives for >10 years has increased the risk of anovulation and infertility
- E. The use of marijuana by the male partner is directly toxic to sperm motility, and this is the likely cause of their infertility.

X-49. A 22-year-old male seeks evaluation from his primary care doctor for gynecomastia that has developed over the past 2 years. He states he did not enter puberty until much later than his friends and has only had sparse growth of facial and axillary hair. He continues to have poor libido and rarely desires sexual intercourse, even though he has been in a monogamous relationship for the past 8 months. His girlfriend is increasingly frustrated by his lack of sexual desire and also urged him to seek medical evaluation. He has no other medical history and was born prematurely at 34 weeks' gestation. His birth weight was 2400 g (50th percentile). His early development was normal. During elementary school, he was held back in third grade because of learning difficulties and thereafter was in special educational classes to assist him with reading and mathematics. He is taking no medications. On physical examination, he is 188 cm tall and has eunuchoid features. His facial, axillary, and genital hair is sparse. Gynecomastia is present. The testes are small, measuring 2.8 cm in length. What is the most likely diagnosis in this patient?

- A. Androgen insensitivity syndrome (testicular feminization)
- B. Klinefelter syndrome
- C. Mixed gonadal dysgenesis (45,X/46,XY mosaicism)
- D. Testicular dysgenesis
- E. True hermaphroditism

X-50. All the following drugs may interfere with testicular function *except*

- A. cyclophosphamide
- B. ketoconazole
- C. metoprolol
- D. prednisone
- E. spironolactone

X-51. A 65-year-old man with a central left upper lobe lung mass presents with renal stones and generalized bone pain. He is found to have a calcium level of 16.4 mg/dL with a phosphate level of 1.2 mg/dL. A bone scan is normal. Which of the following laboratory tests is most likely to establish a diagnosis?

X-51. *(Continued)*

- A. Adrenocorticotropic hormone (ACTH)
- B. Cortisol
- C. Magnesium level
- D. Parathyroid hormone (intact PTH or PTHi)
- E. Parathyroid hormone–related peptide (PTHrp)

X-52. A biopsy of the lung mass in the patient in Question X-51 will most likely show:

- A. Bronchoalveolar lung carcinoma
- B. Bronchial carcinoid
- C. Poorly differentiated adenocarcinoma
- D. Small cell carcinoma
- E. Squamous cell carcinoma

X-53. All the following are direct actions of parathyroid hormone (PTH) *except*

- A. increased calcium resorption from bone
- B. increased calcium resorption from the kidney
- C. increased calcium resorption from the gastrointestinal tract
- D. increased synthesis of 1,25 dihydroxyvitamin D
- E. decreased phosphate resorption from the kidney

X-54. A 45-year-old Caucasian woman seeks advice from her primary care physician regarding her risk for osteoporosis and the need for bone density screening. She is a lifelong nonsmoker and drinks alcohol only socially. She has a history of moderate-persistent asthma since age 12. She is currently on fluticasone, 44 mg/puff twice daily, with good control currently. She last required oral prednisone therapy about 6 months ago when she had influenza that was complicated by an asthma flare. She took prednisone for a total of 14 days. She has had three pregnancies and two live births at ages 39 and 41. She currently has irregular periods occurring approximately every 42 days. Her follicle-stimulating hormone level is 25 mIU/L and 17β-estradiol level is 115 pg/mL on day 12 of her menstrual cycle. Her mother and maternal aunt both have been diagnosed with osteoporosis. Her mother also has rheumatoid arthritis and requires prednisone therapy, 5 mg daily. Her mother developed a compression fracture of the lumbar spine at age 68. On physical examination, the patient appears well and healthy. Her height is 168 cm. Her weight is 66.4 kg. The chest, cardiac, abdominal, muscular, and neurologic examinations are normal. What do you tell the patient about the need for bone density screening?

- A. As she is currently perimenopausal, she should have a bone density screen every other year until she completes menopause and then have bone densitometry measured yearly thereafter.
- B. Because of her family history, she should initiate bone density screening yearly beginning now.
- C. Bone densitometry screening is not recommended until after completion of menopause.

X-54. *(Continued)*

- D. Delayed childbearing until the fourth and fifth decade decreases her risk of developing osteoporosis
- E. Her use of low-dose inhaled glucocorticoids increases her risk of osteoporosis threefold, and she should undergo yearly bone density screening.

X-55. A 62-year-old woman presents to your clinic complaining of fatigue and lethargy over a period of 6 months. She cannot recall exactly when these symptoms started, but feels that they are worsening with time. She describes dry skin and has noted that she is losing hair. On examination she is mildly bradycardic at 52 beats/min with normal blood pressure and has dry, coarse skin. There are areas of alopecia and mild lower extremity edema is noted. Which of the following is the most likely clinical diagnosis and which test would be indicated for screening for the diagnosis?

- A. Hyperthyroidism: thyroid-stimulating hormone (TSH)
- B. Hyperthyroidism: unbound T_4
- C. Hypothyroidism: TSH
- D. Hypothyroidism: unbound T_4

X-56. A 55-year-old male is admitted to the intensive care unit with 1 week of fever and cough. He was well until 1 week before admission, when he noted progressive shortness of breath, cough, and productive sputum. On the day of admission the patient was noted by his wife to be lethargic and unresponsive. 911 was called, and the patient was intubated in the field and then brought to the emergency department. His medications include insulin. The past medical history is notable for alcohol abuse, diabetes mellitus, and chronic renal insufficiency. Temperature is 38.9°C (102°F). He is hypotensive with a blood pressure of 76/40 mmHg. Oxygen saturation is 86% on room air. On examination, the patient is sedated and intubated. Jugular venous pressure is normal. There are decreased breath sounds at the right lung base with egophony. Heart sounds are normal. The abdomen is soft. There is no peripheral edema. Chest radiography shows a right lower lobe infiltrate with a moderate pleural effusion. An electrocardiogram is normal. Sputum Gram stain shows gram-positive diplococci. White blood cell count is $23 \times 10^3/\mu L$, with 70% polymorphonuclear cells and 6% bands. Blood urea nitrogen is 80 mg/dL, and creatinine is 6.1 mg/dL. Plasma glucose is 425 mg/dL. He is started on broad-spectrum antibiotics, intravenous fluids, omeprazole, and an insulin drip. A nasogastric tube is inserted, and tube feedings are started. On hospital day 2 plasma phosphate is 1.0 mg/dL. All of following are causes of hypophosphatemia *except*

- A. sepsis
- B. renal failure
- C. insulin
- D. alcoholism
- E. malnutrition

X-57. A 50-year-old male presents to the clinic for a routine health examination. A comprehensive metabolic panel shows a serum calcium level of 11.2 mg/dL. Serum phosphate is 3.0 mg/dL. Serum creatinine is normal. He denies bone pain, lethargy, weakness, or weight loss. What is the most common cause of hypercalcemia in outpatients?

A. Malignancy
B. Medications
C. Milk-alkali syndrome
D. Primary hyperparathyroidism
E. Granulomatous disease

X-58. All of the following would be indicated in the workup of infertility *except*

A. endometrial biopsy
B. hysterosalpingogram
C. measurement of testosterone and dehydroepiandosterone in the female partner
D. measurement of testosterone, follicle-stimulating hormone (FSH) and luteinizing hormone (LH) in the male partner
E. semen analysis

X-59. You are asked to see a 15-year-old African-American girl because of anovulation. She has never experienced menarche, and her mother is concerned since most women in her family experience menarche around 13 years of age. The patient has prominent nipples and the areola are part of the breast. Pubic hair is dark, curly, and coarse and is abundant in the pubic area and inner thigh. There is no facial hair, and muscular development is age and sex appropriate. She does have cyclical pelvic pain. What is the next step in her evaluation?

A. Examination with a speculum
B. MRI of the abdomen and pelvis
C. Serum follicle-stimulating hormone (FSH)
D. Serum prolactin

X-60. A 21-year-old patient presents to the emergency room with several days of severe nausea and vomiting. His roommate noted that he hadn't been able to keep down solid foods and that his eyes and skin have taken on a "yellow" appearance. The patient has no past medical history and denies alcohol or substance abuse. He takes no medications. He is admitted to the hospital for further management. On examination he is ill-appearing and jaundiced. The liver edge is palpable and he has mild abdominal tenderness. He has a normal neurologic examination. His total bilirubin is 2.0 mg/dL (normal range 0.1–1.2 mg/dL) and AST is 86 U/L (normal range 0–37 U/L). His prothrombin time is normal. Viral hepatitis serologies are all negative. A liver biopsy and quantitative copper assay are performed and the patient is subsequently diagnosed with Wilson disease. Which of the following is the most appropriate treatment for this patient?

A. Dimercaprol
B. Immediate liver transplant
C. Penicillamine

X-60. *(Continued)*
D. Trientine and liver transplant evaluation
E. Zinc

X-61. The World Health Organization (WHO) recently defined osteoporosis operationally as

A. a patient with a bone density less than the mean of age-, race-, and gender-matched controls
B. a patient with a bone density less than 1.0 standard deviation (SD) below the mean of race-and gender-matched controls
C. a patient with a bone density less than 1.0 SD below the mean of age-, race-, and gender-matched controls
D. a patient with a bone density less than 2.5 SD below the mean of race-and gender-matched controls
E. a patient with a bone density less than 2.5 SD below the mean of age-, race-, and gender-matched controls

X-62. A 54-year-old man has been hospitalized following a myocardial infarction. He has a history of hypertension, hypertriglyceridemia, obesity, mild renal insufficiency and diet-controlled diabetes. His condition is improving, and on the third day of admission his serum urate is elevated at 8.8 mg/dL. He denies any joint complaints and cannot recall ever having symptoms compatible with gout. His serum creatinine is 1.5 mg/dL, which is close to his baseline over the past 3 years. In regard to this patient's hyperuricemia, which of the following is true?

A. >70% of hospitalized patients will have increased serum urate levels.
B. His hyperuricemia is unrelated to his heart disease.
C. His renal disease is likely caused by his increased serum urate levels.
D. No treatment is needed.
E. This patient should be discharged on low-dose allopurinol.

X-63. A 25-year-old female visits her primary care physician after 3 years of intermittent abdominal pain, peripheral neuropathy, and increasing episodes of anxiety and hallucinations. The physician suspects acute intermittent porphyria. She can make this diagnosis by doing which of the following tests?

A. Sunlight administration with observation for rash
B. Urine porphobilinogen (PBG) level during an attack
C. Peripheral blood testing for an HFE C282Y mutation
D. Urine PBG level when the patient is well
E. Hypoglycemic provocation testing

X-64. All the following are side effects of HMG-CoA reductase inhibitors (statins) *except*

A. hepatitis
B. myopathy
C. dyspepsia
D. headache
E. pulmonary fibrosis

X-65. Which of the following is consistent with a diagnosis of subacute thyroiditis?

A. A 38-year-old female with a 2-week history of a painful thyroid, elevated T_4, elevated T_3, low TSH, and an elevated radioactive iodine uptake scan

B. A 42-year-old male with a history of a painful thyroid 4 months ago, fatigue, malaise, low free T_4, low T_3, and elevated TSH.

C. A 31-year-old female with a painless enlarged thyroid, low TSH, elevated T_4, elevated free T_4, and an elevated radioiodine uptake scan

D. A 50-year-old male with a painful thyroid, slightly elevated T_4, normal TSH, and an ultrasound showing a mass

E. A 46-year-old female with 3 weeks of fatigue, low T_4, low T_3, and low TSH

X-66. All of the following statements regarding hypoglycemia in diabetes mellitus are true *except*

A. Individuals with type 2 diabetes mellitus experience less hypoglycemia than those with type 1 diabetes mellitus.

B. Recurrent episodes of hypoglycemia predispose to the development of autonomic failure with defective glucose counterregulation and hypoglycemia unawareness.

C. The average person with type 1 diabetes mellitus has two episodes of symptomatic hypoglycemia weekly.

D. Thiazolidinediones and metformin cause hypoglycemia more frequently than sulfonylureas.

E. From 2–4% of deaths in type 1 diabetes mellitus are directly attributable to hypoglycemia.

X-67. Which of the following forms of contraception have theoretical efficacy of >90%?

A. Condoms
B. Intrauterine devices
C. Oral contraceptives
D. Spermicides
E. All of the above

X-68. A patient is seen in the clinic for follow-up of type 2 diabetes mellitus. Her hemoglobin A_{1C} has been poorly controlled at 9.4% recently. The patient can be counseled to expect all the following improvements with improved glycemic control *except*

A. decreased microalbuminuria
B. decreased risk of nephropathy
C. decreased risk of neuropathy
D. decreased risk of peripheral vascular disease
E. decreased risk of retinopathy

X-69. A healthy 53-year-old man comes to your office for an annual physical examination. He has no complaints and has no significant medical history. He is taking an over-the-counter multivitamin and no other medicines. On physical examination he is noted to have a nontender

X-69. *(Continued)*

thyroid nodule. His thyroid-stimulating hormone (TSH) level is checked and is found to be low. What is the next step in his evaluation?

A. Close follow-up and measure TSH in 6 months
B. Fine-needle aspiration
C. Low-dose thyroid replacement
D. Positron emission tomography followed by surgery
E. Radionuclide thyroid scan

X-70. During a routine checkup, a 67-year-old male is found to have a level of serum alkaline phosphatase three times the upper limit of normal. Serum calcium and phosphorus concentrations and liver function test results are normal. He is asymptomatic. The most likely diagnosis is

A. metastatic bone disease
B. primary hyperparathyroidism
C. occult plasmacytoma
D. Paget's disease of bone
E. osteomalacia

X-71. A 78-year-old man presents to your clinic and describes headaches and back pain. These have been chronic complaints, and he thinks they are getting worse despite conservative management. His wife believes he is experiencing some hearing loss. She describes how over the past several months he needs to turn up the volume on the television and has a difficult time talking to his children on the telephone. Physical examination is largely unremarkable; straight leg raise is normal. Based on Rinne and Weber tests, the patient appears to have some mild sensorineural hearing loss on the right side. A comprehensive chemistry panel shows an elevated alkaline phosphatase of 170 U/L. Paget disease is now high on the differential. Which of the following is true regarding this diagnosis?

A. Family history is not predictive.
B. Hearing loss is the most common symptom.
C. Nuclear medicine bone scan is required for diagnosis.
D. Serum calcium and phosphate are usually abnormal.
E. The pelvis, skull, and vertebrae are most commonly affected.

X-72. Which of the following is the most common sign of Cushing's syndrome?

A. Amenorrhea
B. Hirsutism
C. Obesity
D. Purple skin striae
E. Skin hyperpigmentation

X-73. A patient receives CT of the head as part of a "virtual wellness physical exam" he received as a gift certificate from his family. A 7-mm sellar mass "most consistent with a pituitary adenoma" is reported, and he comes to your office very concerned that he has a life-threatening brain tumor. A full panel of endocrine laboratory mea-

X-73. *(Continued)*

surements reveals no abnormalities, and besides his anxiety he reports feeling quite healthy. What is the next step in management?

A. Perform positron emission tomography/CT (PET-CT) to evaluate for metabolic activity.

B. Reassure the patient that this finding is common and benign; take no action.

C. Reassure and repeat laboratory measurements in 6 months.

D. Reassure and repeat head imaging in 1 year.

E. Refer to neurosurgery.

X-74. Which of the following statements regarding hormone release from the anterior pituitary is true?

A. All hormones are released in a pulsatile manner.

B. Follicle-stimulating hormone (FSH) and luteinizing hormone (LH) release are suppressed prior to puberty and after menopause.

C. Somatostatin acts in a feedback loop to inhibit adrenocorticotropin hormone (ACTH) release.

D. Thyroid-stimulating hormone (TSH) is released primarily at night.

E. With the exception of prolactin, none of the anterior pituitary hormones are present in a fetus until week 28 of gestation.

X-75. All the following are features of lipoprotein lipase deficiency *except*

A. low levels of plasma chylomicrons

B. acute pancreatitis

C. hepatosplenomegaly

D. xanthomas

E. autosomal recessive inheritance

X-76. A 21-year-old female with a history of type 1 diabetes mellitus is brought to the emergency room with nausea, vomiting, lethargy, and dehydration. Her mother notes that she stopped taking insulin 1 day before presentation. She is lethargic, has dry mucous membranes, and is obtunded. Blood pressure is 80/40 mmHg, and heart rate is 112 beats/min. Heart sounds are normal. Lungs are clear. The abdomen is soft, and there is no organomegaly. She is responsive and oriented × 3 but diffusely weak. Serum sodium is 126 meq/L, potassium is 4.3 meq/L, magnesium is 1.2 meq/L, blood urea nitrogen is 76 mg/dL, creatinine is 2.2 mg/dL, bicarbonate is 10 meq/L, and chloride is 88 meq/L. Serum glucose is 720 mg/dL. All the following are appropriate management steps *except*

A. arterial blood gas

B. intravenous insulin

C. intravenous potassium

D. 3% sodium solution

E. intravenous fluids

X-77. All the following are effects of hypercalcemia *except*

A. diarrhea

B. confusion

C. polyuria

D. a shortened QT interval

E. nephrolithiasis

X-78. All of the following are actions of parathyroid hormone *except*

A. direct stimulation of osteoblasts to increase bone formation

B. direct stimulation of osteoclasts to increase bone resorption

C. increased reabsorption of calcium from the distal tubule of the kidney

D. inhibition of phosphate reabsorption in the proximal tubule of the kidney

E. stimulation of renal 1-α-hydroxylase to produce 1,25-hydroxycholecalciferol

X-79. Which of the following statements regarding hypothyroidism is true?

A. Hashimoto's thyroiditis is the most common cause of hypothyroidism worldwide.

B. The annual risk of developing overt clinical hypothyroidism from subclinical hypothyroidism in patients with positive thyroid peroxidase (TPO) antibodies is 20%.

C. Histologically, Hashimoto's thyroiditis is characterized by marked infiltration of the thyroid with activated T cells and B cells.

D. A low TSH level excludes the diagnosis of hypothyroidism.

E. Thyroid peroxidase antibodies are present in less than 50% of patients with autoimmune hypothyroidism.

X-80. You are evaluating a patient for secondary causes of hypertension. The patient is a 39-year-old woman who has hypertension despite using four different classes of antihypertensive medications, including a diuretic at therapeutic doses. She mainly has diastolic hypertension and has been found to have hypokalemia on several routine blood chemistry analyses. You hold her diuretics and provide her with potassium supplementation for 14 days, after which you find the serum potassium is in the normal range. She denies licorice ingestion. Plasma renin activity is low. After days of saline loading, aldosterone levels are elevated. A CT scan of the adrenal glands reveal no masses. An overnight dexamethasone suppression test shows no aldosterone suppression. What is the most likely diagnosis?

A. Conn's syndrome

B. Cortical nodular hyperplasia

C. Glucocorticoid remediable aldosteronism

D. Liddle's syndrome

E. Renin-secreting tumor

X-81. A 17-year-old woman is evaluated in your office for primary amenorrhea. She does not feel as if she has entered puberty in that she has never had a menstrual period and has sparse axillary and pubic hair growth. On examination, she is noted to be 150 cm tall. She has a low hairline and slight webbing of her neck. Her follicle-stimulating hormone level is 75 mIU/mL, luteinizing hormone is 20 mIU/mL, and estradiol level 2 pg/mL. You suspect Turner syndrome. All of the following tests are indicated in this individual *except*

A. buccal smear for nuclear heterochromatin (Barr body)
B. echocardiogram
C. karyotype analysis
D. renal ultrasound
E. thyroid-stimulating hormone (TSH)

X-82. A 30-year-old male, the father of three children, has had progressive breast enlargement during the last 6 months. He does not use any drugs. Laboratory evaluation reveals that both LH and testosterone are low. Further evaluation of this patient should include which of the following?

A. Blood sampling for serum glutamic-oxaloacetic transaminase (SGOT) and serum alkaline phosphatase and bilirubin levels
B. Measurement of estradiol and human chorionic gonadotropin (hCG) levels
C. A 24-h urine collection for the measurement of 17 ketosteroids
D. Karyotype analysis to exclude Klinefelter syndrome
E. Breast biopsy

X-83. Obesity is associated with an increased incidence of all the following *except*

A. diabetes mellitus
B. cancer
C. hypertension
D. biliary disease
E. chronic obstructive lung disease

X-84. Which of the following statements regarding Paget disease is true?

A. 1% of patients over the age of 50 have evidence of Paget disease.
B. A majority of patients with disease will experience symptoms at the time of diagnosis.
C. The disease frequency has decreased over the past 20 years.
D. There is a significant female predominance.
E. While prevalent worldwide, Paget disease is most common in Asia.

X-85. Which of the following statements is true about familial hypocalciuric hypercalcemia (FHH)?

X-85. *(Continued)*
A. It is inherited in an autosomal recessive pattern.
B. The cause is a defect in the parathyroid hormone receptor.
C. Clinical symptoms first manifest in the third and fourth decades of life.
D. Treatment is rarely necessary.
E. Renal calcium reabsorption is more than 99%.

X-86. Which of the following is true of Wilson disease?

A. Early diagnosis is crucial as highly effective therapy is available.
B. It is inherited in an autosomal dominant pattern.
C. Serum copper levels are usually two to three times above normal.
D. The frequency of disease in the general population is ~1%.
E. The liver and pancreas are the most commonly affected organs.

X-87. A 48-year-old female is undergoing evaluation for flushing and diarrhea. Physical examination is normal except for nodular hepatomegaly. A CT scan of the abdomen demonstrates multiple nodules in both lobes of the liver consistent with metastases in the liver and a 2-cm mass in the ileum. The 24-h urinary 5-HIAA excretion is markedly elevated. All the following treatments are appropriate *except*

A. diphenhydramine
B. interferon-α
C. octreotide
D. odansetron
E. phenoxybenzamine

X-88. While undergoing a physical examination during medical student clinical skills, this patient develops severe flushing, wheezing, nausea, and light-headedness. Vital signs are notable for a blood pressure of 70/30 mmHg and a heart rate of 135/min. Which of the following is the most appropriate therapy?

A. Albuterol
B. Atropine
C. Epinephrine
D. Hydrocortisone
E. Octreotide

X-89. A 66-year-old Asian woman seeks treatment for osteoporosis. She fell and fractured her right hip, requiring a surgical intervention 3 months ago. She was told while hospitalized that she had osteoporosis but had not previously been evaluated for this. During the hospitalization, she developed a deep venous thrombosis (DVT) with pulmonary embolus, for which she is currently taking warfarin. She completed menopause at age 52. She is a former smoker, quitting about 6 years ago. She has always been thin, and her current body mass index (BMI) is 19.2 kg/m^2. Her labora-

X-89. *(Continued)*

tory studies show a calcium of 8.7 mg/dL, phosphate 3 mg/dL, creatinine 0.8 mg/dL, and 25-hydroxyvitamin D levels of 18 ng/mL (normal >30 ng/mL). A dual-energy x-ray absorptiometry scan of bone mineral density has a T-score of −3.0. What is the best initial therapy for this patient?

A. Calcitonin, 200 IU intranasally daily
B. Calcium carbonate, 1200 mg, and vitamin D 400 IU daily
C. Ethinyl estradiol, 5 μg, and medroxyprogesterone acetate 625 mg daily
D. Raloxifene, 60 mg daily
E. Risedronate, 35 mg once weekly

X-90. All of the following would be expected to increase prolactin levels *except*

A. chest wall trauma
B. hyperthyroidism
C. pregnancy
D. renal failure
E. sexual orgasm

X-91. A 35-year-old male is referred to your clinic for evaluation of hypercalcemia noted during a health insurance medical screening. He has noted some fatigue, malaise, and a 4-lb weight loss over the last 2 months. He also has noted constipation and "heartburn." He is occasionally nauseated after large meals and has water brash and a sour taste in his mouth. The patient denies vomiting, dysphagia, or odynophagia. He also notes decreased libido and a depressed mood. Vital signs are unremarkable. Physical examination is notable for a clear oropharynx, no evidence of a thyroid mass, and no lymphadenopathy. Jugular venous pressure is normal. Heart sounds are regular with no murmurs or gallops. The chest is clear. The abdomen is soft with some mild epigastric tenderness. There is no rebound or organomegaly. Stool is guaiac-positive. Neurologic examination is nonfocal. Laboratory values are notable for a normal complete blood count. Calcium is 11.2 mg/dL, phosphate is 2.1 mg/dL, and magnesium is 1.8 meq/dL. Albumin is 3.7 g/dL, and total protein is 7.0 g/dL. TSH is 3 μIU/mL, prolactin is 250 μg/L, testosterone is 620 ng/dL, and serum insulin-like growth factor 1 (IGF-1) is normal. Serum intact parathyroid hormone level is 135 pg/dL. In light of the patient's abdominal discomfort and heme-positive stool, you perform an abdominal computed tomography (CT) scan that shows a lesion measuring 2 cm by 2 cm in the head of the pancreas. What is the diagnosis?

A. Multiple endocrine neoplasia (MEN) type 1
B. MEN type 2a
C. MEN type 2b
D. Polyglandular autoimmune syndrome
E. Von–Hippel Lindau (VHL) syndrome

X-92. Your 60-year-old patient with a monoclonal gammopathy of unclear significance presents for a follow-

X-92. *(Continued)*

up visit and to review recent laboratory data. His creatinine is newly elevated to 2.0 mg/dL, potassium is 3.7 mg/dL, calcium is 12.2 mg/dL, low-density lipoprotein (LDL) is 202 mg/dL and triglycerides are 209 mg/dL. On further questioning he reports 3 months of swelling around the eyes and "foamy" urine. On examination, he has anasarca. Concerned for multiple myeloma and nephrotic syndrome, you order a urine protein/creatinine ratio, which returns at 14:1. Which treatment option would be most appropriate to treat his lipid abnormalities?

A. Cholesterol ester transfer protein inhibitor
B. Dietary management
C. HMG-CoA reductase inhibitors
D. Lipid apheresis
E. Niacin and fibrates

X-93. All of the following statements regarding asymptomatic adrenal masses (incidentalomas) are true *except*

A. All patients with incidentalomas should be screened for pheochromocytoma.
B. Fine-needle aspiration may distinguish between benign and malignant primary adrenal tumors.
C. In patients with a history of malignancy, the likelihood the mass is a metastasis is ~50%.
D. The majority of adrenal incidentalomas are nonsecretory.
E. The vast majority of adrenal incidentalomas are benign.

X-94. Which of the following studies is most sensitive for detecting diabetic nephropathy?

A. Serum creatinine level
B. Creatinine clearance
C. Urine albumin
D. Glucose tolerance test
E. Ultrasonography

X-95. A 28-year-old woman seeks counseling before getting pregnant. She had a brother who died at age 9 of the Lesch-Nyhan syndrome, and she is a known carrier of the genetic defect. She has no significant past medical history, and her husband has no significant family history. Which of the following statements is true?

A. Her children have no risk of disease since she is not symptomatic.
B. Her husband should be screened for carrying the genetic defect of Lesch-Nyhan syndrome.
C. If she has a daughter, the child has a 50% chance of being a carrier.
D. If she has an affected son, starting him on allopurinol from birth will prevent clinical manifestations of disease.
E. She should start taking allopurinol to decrease her risk of gout and urate nephropathy.

X. ENDOCRINOLOGY AND METABOLISM

ANSWERS

X-1. The answer is D. *(Chap. 335)* The thyroid produces two related hormones, T_3 and T_4. These hormones act on nuclear receptors inside cells to regulate differentiation during development and maintain metabolic homeostasis in virtually all human cells. T_4 is secreted in excess of T_3 from the thyroid and both are protein-bound in the plasma. Protein binding delays hormone clearance. Unbound protein appears to be more biologically active. T_4 is converted to more active T_3 in peripheral tissues. Two thyroid hormone receptors are bound to specific DNA sequences; when activated by thyroid hormone, these receptors can act to up-regulate or down-regulate gene transcription. Iodide uptake by the thyroid is the critical first step of thyroid hormone synthesis. Dietary iodine deficiency leads to decreased production of thyroid hormone and represents the most common cause of hypothyroidism worldwide. In areas of iodine sufficiency, autoimmune disease such as Hashimoto's thyroiditis and iatrogenic causes are the most common etiologies for hypothyroidism. Paradoxically, chronic iodine excess can also cause goiter and hypothyroidism via unclear mechanisms. This is the mechanism for the hypothyroidism that occurs in up to 13% of patients taking amiodarone. Graves' disease leads to hyperthyroidism.

X-2. The answer is A. *(Chap. 333)* The diagnosis of Cushing's syndrome relies on documentation of endogenous hypercortisolism. Of the list above, the most cost-effective and precise test is the 24-h urine free cortisol. Failure to suppress plasma A.M. cortisol after overnight suppression with 1 mg dexamethasone is an alternative. Most ACTH-secreting pituitary adenomas are <5 mm in diameter and approximately half are not detected even with sensitive MRI. Further, because incidental microadenomas are common in the pituitary, the presence of a small pituitary abnormality on MRI may not establish the source of ACTH production. Basal plasma ACTH levels are used to distinguish between ACTH-independent (adrenal or exogenous glucocorticoid) and ACTH-dependent (pituitary, ectopic ACTH) sources of hypercortisolism. Mean basal ACTH levels are higher in patients with ectopic ACTH production than in patients with pituitary ACTH adenomas. There is significant overlap in ACTH levels, however, and this test should not be used as an initial diagnostic test. Rarely, patients have Cushing's syndrome and elevated ACTH due to a CRH-releasing tumor. In this case, CRH levels are elevated. Inferior petrosal venous sampling can be used to identify a pituitary source of ACTH secretion when imaging modalities do not reveal a source.

X-3. The answer is C. *(Chap. 332)* Intermittent pulses of GnRH are necessary to maintain pituitary sensitivity to the hormone. Continuous exposure to GnRH causes pituitary gonadotrope desensitization, which ultimately leads to decreased levels of testosterone. The relationship between GnRH and LH/FSH is a positive feedback loop where GnRH causes secretion of LH and FSH. Receptor translocation from the cytoplasm into the nucleus occurs with certain hormones (e.g., glucocorticoid); however, this receptor phenomenon is not specific to any regulatory mechanism. GnRH does not promote production of sex hormone binding globulin. Moreover, although binding globulins can decrease the amount of bound hormone measured in the serum, abnormal levels of binding globulins usually do not have any clinical significance because the free hormone levels usually increase.

X-4. **The answer is C.** *(Chap. 342)* Perimenopause refers to the time period prior to menopause during which menstrual cycles become increasingly irregular and fertility wanes. This period usually lasts for 2–8 years before final menses and menopause. In perimenopause, the interval between menses typically declines by about 3 days because of acceleration of the follicular phase of the menstrual cycle. Measurement of hormone levels in the perimenopausal period can be difficult to interpret because hormone levels are "irregularly irregular." Measurement of follicle-stimulating hormone during the early follicular phase (days 2–5) of the menstrual cycle can rule out perimenopause if the levels are very low, while high levels are suggestive of the perimenopausal state. Perimenopause is generally a hyperestrogenic state, and there is an increased risk of endometrial carcinoma, uterine polyps, and leiomyoma during this period. Because of these risks, low-dose oral contraceptive pills are commonly used during perimenopause. Use of oral contraceptives is also important because the risk of unintended pregnancy in this period rivals that of adolescence. However, the risks of oral contraceptives need to be weighed against the increased risk of thrombosis and breast cancer. Contraindications to the use of oral contraceptives are breast cancer, cigarette smoking, liver disease, history of thromboembolic or cardiovascular disease, or unexplained vaginal bleeding.

X-5 and X-6. **The answers are A and E.** *(Chap. 348)* Osteporosis is a significant public health problem in the United States affecting 8 million women and 2 million men. An additional 18 million individuals are at risk for development of osteoporosis as measured by low bone density (osteopenia). Most of these individuals are unaware of the presence of osteopenia or osteoporosis. In the United States and Europe, fractures related to osteoporosis are much more common in women than men, although this is not seen in all races. Nonmodifiable risk factors for the development of osteoporosis include a personal history of fracture or a history of fracture in a first-degree relative, female sex, advanced age, and white race. African Americans have approximately one-half the risk of osteoporotic fractures as whites. Diseases that increase the risk of falls or frailty, such as dementia and Parkinson's disease, also increase fracture risk. Cigarette smoking, low body weight, low calcium intake, alcoholism, and lack of physical activity are all associated with increased bone loss and fractures. Multiple drugs are associated with an increased risk of osteoporosis. In addition to those listed, other anticonvulsants, cytotoxic drugs, excessive thyroxine, aluminum, gonadotropin-releasing hormone agonists, and lithium are associated with decreased bone mass and osteoporosis. Histamine antagonists are not associated with osteoporosis.

X-7. **The answer is C.** *(Chap. 333)* Osteoporosis is a significant public health problem in the United States affecting 8 million women and 2 million men. An additional 18 million individuals are at risk for development of osteoporosis as measured by low bone density (osteopenia). Most of these individuals are unaware of the presence of osteopenia or osteoporosis. In the United States and Europe, fractures related to osteoporosis are much more common in women than men, although this is not seen in all races. Diagnosis of pituitary insufficiency is made by biochemical demonstration of low levels of trophic hormones in the setting of low target hormone levels. Thus, in a postmenopausal woman, a low FSH and LH would suggest hypopituitarism. Provocative tests may also be used to test reduced pituitary reserve. Growth hormone should elevate during hypoglycemic stress, not during hyperglycemia. Elevation of aldosterone (or cortisol) after cosyntropin, cortisol after insulin-induced hypoglycemia, or TSH after TRH are consistent with intact pituitary function. A summary of tests of pituitary insufficiency is shown in the following table.

TABLE X-7 Tests of Pituitary Sufficiency

Hormone	Test	Blood Samples	Interpretation
Growth hormone	Insulin tolerance test: Regular insulin (0.05–0.15 U/kg IV)	–30, 0, 30, 60, 120 min for glucose and GH	Glucose < 40 mg/dL; GH should be >3 µg/L
	GHRH test: 1 µg/kg IV	0, 15, 30, 45, 60, 120 min for GH	Normal response is GH >3 µg/L
	L-Arginine test: 30 g IV over 30 min	0, 30, 60, 120 min for GH	Normal response is GH >3 µg/L
	L-dopa test: 500 mg PO	0, 30, 60, 120 min for GH	Normal response is GH >3 µg/L
Prolactin	TRH test: 200–500 µg IV	0, 20, and 60 min for TSH and PRL	Normal prolactin is >2 µg/L and increase >200% of baseline
ACTH	Insulin tolerance test: Regular insulin (0.05–0.15 U/kg IV)	–30, 0, 30, 60, 90 min for glucose and cortisol	Glucose <40 mg/dL Cortisol should increase by >7 µg/dL or to >20 µg/dL
	CRH test: 1 µg/kg ovine CRH IV at 0800 h	0, 15, 30, 60, 90, 120 min for ACTH and cortisol	Basal ACTH increases 2- to 4-fold and peaks at 20–100 pg/mL Cortisol levels >20–25 µg/dL
	Metyrapone test: Metyrapone (30 mg/kg) at midnight	Plasma 11-deoxycortisol and cortisol at 8 A.M.; ACTH can also be measured	Plasma cortisol should be <4 µg/dL to assure an adequate response Normal response is 11-deoxycortisol >7.5 µg/dL or ACTH >75 pg/mL
	Standard ACTH stimulation test: ACTH 1-24 (Cosyntropin), 0.25 mg IM or IV	0, 30, 60 min for cortisol and aldosterone	Normal response is cortisol >21 µg/dL and aldosterone response of >4 ng/dL above baseline
	Low-dose ACTH test: ACTH 1-24 (Cosyntropin), 1 µg IV	0, 30, 60 min for cortisol	Cortisol should be >21 µg/dL
	3-day ACTH stimulation test consists of 0.25 mg ACTH 1-24 given IV over 8 h each day		Cortisol >21 µg/dL
TSH	Basal thyroid function tests: T₄, T₃, TSH	Basal tests	Low free thyroid hormone levels in the setting of TSH levels that are not appropriately increased
	TRH test: 200–500 µg IV	0, 20, 60 min for TSH and PRL[a]	TSH should increase by >5 mU/L unless thyroid hormone levels are increased
LH, FSH	LH, FSH, testosterone, estrogen	Basal tests	Basal LH and FSH should be increased in postmenopausal women Low testosterone levels in the setting of low LH and FSH
	GnRH test: GnRH (100 µg) IV	0, 30, 60 min for LH and FSH	In most adults, LH should increase by 10 IU/L and FSH by 2 IU/L Normal responses are variable
Multiple hormones	Combined anterior pituitary test: GHRH (1 µg/kg), CRH (1 µg/kg), GnRH (100 µg), TRH (200 µg) are given IV	–30, 0, 15, 30, 60, 90, 120 min for GH, ACTH, cortisol, LH, FSH, and TSH	Combined or individual releasing hormone responses must be elevated in the context of basal target gland hormone values and may not be uniformly diagnostic (see text)

[a]Evoked PRL response indicates lactotrope integrity.
Note: For abbreviations, see HPIM, 17e.

X-8. **The answer is D.** *(Chap. 325)* Measurement of luteinizing hormone (LH) or follicle-stimulating hormone (FSH) will distinguish primary from secondary hypogonadism in men with reduced serum testosterone levels. Elevations in LH and FSH suggest primary gonadal dysfunction, whereas normal or reduced LH and FSH suggest a central hypothalamic pituitary defect. Patients with chronic illness such as HIV, end-stage renal disease, COPD, and cancer and patients receiving chronic corticosteroids have a high frequency of hypogonadism that is associated with muscle wasting. There are some reports of reversal of hypogonadism in patients with end-stage renal disease on hemodialysis after a renal transplant.

X-9. The answer is A. *(Chap. 339)* When an individual presents with profound hypoglycemia and no history of diabetes mellitus, one must determine the cause expediently and treat accordingly. Immediate treatment of this patient should include ongoing glucose administration while attempting to determine the cause. The initial step for diagnosing this patient is to determine the plasma glucose, insulin, and C-peptide levels. When the plasma glucose level is <55 mg/dL, the plasma insulin levels should be low. If the insulin levels are inappropriately high (≥18 pmol/L or ≥3 μU/mL), the C-peptide level should be assessed simultaneously. C-peptide is the protein fragment that remains after proinsulin is cleaved to insulin. C-peptide would be high (≥0.6 ng/mL) in individuals with an endogenous source of hyperinsulinemia such as insulinoma. However, C-peptide levels are low or undetectable when the source of insulin is exogenous, such as in surreptitious insulin intake or insulin overdose. One exception to consider in this individual is surreptitious intake or overdose of a sulfonylurea, an insulin secretagogue. In this case, insulin and C-peptide levels would both be elevated, and a sulfonylurea screen is also appropriate in this patient.

X-10. The answer is D. *(Chap. 335)* Sick-euthyroid syndrome can occur in the setting of any acute, severe illness. Abnormalities in the levels of circulating TSH and thyroid hormone are thought to result from the release of cytokines in response to severe stress. Multiple abnormalities may occur. The most common hormone pattern is a decrease in total and unbound T_3 levels as peripheral conversion of T_4 to T_3 is impaired. Teleologically, the fall in T_3, the most active thyroid hormone, is thought to limit catabolism in starved or ill patients. TSH levels may vary dramatically, from 0.1 to >20 mU/L, depending on when they are measured during the course of illness. Very sick patients may have a decrease in T_4 levels. This patient undoubtedly has abnormal thyroid function tests as a result of his injuries from the motor vehicle accident. There is no indication for obtaining further imaging in this case. Steroids have no role. The most appropriate management consists of simple observation. Over the course of weeks to months, as the patient recovers, thyroid function will return to normal.

X-11. The answer is A. *(Chap. 348)* A number of biochemical tests are used to assess the rate of bone remodeling. Bone remodeling is related to the rate of formation and resorption. Remodeling markers do not predict bone loss well enough to be applied clinically. However, measures of bone resorption may help in the prediction of risk of fracture in older patients. In women over 65 years old, even in the presence of normal bone density, a high index of bone resorption should prompt consideration for treatment. Measures of bone resorption fall quickly after the initiation of antiresorptive therapy (bisphosphonates, estrogen, raloxifene, calcitonin) and provide an earlier measure of response than does bone densitometry. Serum alkaline phosphatase is a measure of bone formation, not resorption, as are serum osteocalcin and serum propeptide of type I procollagen.

Biochemical Markers of Bone Metabolism in Clinical Use

Bone formation
  Serum bone-specific alkaline phosphatase
  Serum osteocalcin
  Serum propeptide of type I procollagen
Bone resorption
  Urine and serum cross-linked N-telopeptide
  Urine and serum cross-linked C-telopeptide
  Urine total free deoxypyridinoline
  Urine hydroxyproline
  Serum tartrate-resistant acid phosphatase
  Serum bone sialoprotein
  Urine hydroxylysine glycosides

X-12. **The answer is B.** *(Chap. 348)* Osteoporosis is a common disease affecting 8 million women and 2 million men in the United States. It is most common in postmenopausal women, but the incidence is also increasing in men. Estrogen loss probably causes bone loss by activation of bone remodeling sites and exaggeration of the imbalance between bone formation and resorption. Osteoporosis is diagnosed by bone mineral density scan. Dual-energy x-ray absorptiometry (DXA) is the most accurate test for measuring bone mineral density. Clinical determinations of bone density are most commonly measured at the lumbar spine and hip. In the DXA technique, two x-ray energies are used to measure the area of the mineralized tissues and compared to gender- and race-matched normative values. The T-score compares an individual's results to a young population, whereas the Z-score compared the individual's results to an age-matched population. Osteoporosis is diagnosed when the T-score is –2.5 SD in the lumbar spine, femoral neck, or total hip. An evaluation for secondary causes of osteoporosis should be considered in individuals presenting with osteoporotic fractures at a young age and those who have very low Z-scores. Initial evaluation should include serum and 24-h urine calcium levels, renal function panel, hepatic function panel, serum phosphorous level, and vitamin D levels. Other endocrine abnormalities including hyperthyroidism and hyperparathyroidism should be evaluated, and urinary cortisol levels should be checked if there is a clinical suspicion for Cushing's syndrome. Follicle-stimulating hormone and luteinizing hormone levels would be elevated but are not useful in this individual as she presents with a known perimenopausal state.

X-13. **The answer is D.** *(Chap. 349)* Despite her lack of symptoms, this patient has enough evidence to diagnose her with Paget disease. Her radiographs show characteristic changes of active disease in the pelvis, one of the most common areas for Paget disease to present. Her elevated alkaline phosphatase provides further evidence of active bone turnover. The normal serum calcium and phosphate levels are characteristic for Paget disease. Management of asymptomatic Paget disease has changed since effective treatments have become available. Treatment should be initiated in all symptomatic patients and in asymptomatic patients who have evidence of active disease (high alkaline phosphatase or urine hydroxyproline) or disease adjacent to weight-bearing structures, vertebrae, or the skull. Second-generation oral bisphosphonates such as tiludronate, alendronate, and risedronate are excellent choices due to their ability to decrease bone turnover. The major side effect from these agents is esophageal ulceration and reflux. They should be taken in the morning, on an empty stomach, sitting upright to minimize the risk of reflux. Duration of use depends upon the clinical response; typically 3–6 months are needed to see the alkaline phosphatase begin to normalize. IV zoledronate and pamidronate are adequate alternatives to oral bisphosphonates. While their IV administration avoids the risk of reflux, there is a potential of developing a flulike syndrome within 24 h of use. The presence of this side effect does not require drug discontinuation. The same time to response can be expected from these agents.

X-14. **The answer is C.** *(Chap. 354)* This patient is suspected to have Wilson disease, based on clinical presentation and the visible Kayser-Fleischer ring seen in this image. The "gold-standard" for diagnosis is liver biopsy with quantitative copper assays. Kayser-Fleischer rings can be diagnosed definitively only with a slit-lamp examination and are highly specific for the disease: they are present in >99% of patients who have concomitant neuropsychiatric manifestations of copper toxicity and in 30–50% of patients with liver involvement alone or who are presymptomatic. They do not cause visual impairment. Serum ceruloplasmin levels are an unreliable marker of illness and should not be used for diagnosis; they are normal in 10% of affected patients. Ceruloplasmin is a liver-derived acute-phase reactant that may be elevated in systemic inflammatory states, even in patients with Wilson disease. A 24-h urine copper test can be helpful, particularly in patients who are already experiencing symptoms. Anti-smooth-muscle antibodies are often present in autoimmune hepatitis. Total iron-binding capacity and ferritin will be abnormal in hemochromatosis.

X-15 and X-16. **The answers are E and B.** *(Chap. 335)* Subacute thyroiditis, also known as de Quervain's thyroiditis, granulomatous thyroiditis, or viral thyroiditis, is a multiphase illness three times more frequent in women than men. Multiple viruses have been implicated, but none have been definitively identified as the trigger for subacute thyroiditis. The diagnosis can be overlooked in patients as the symptoms mimic pharyngitis, and it frequently has a similarly benign course. In this patient, Graves' disease is unlikely given her elevated TSH and negative antibody panel. Autoimmune hypothyroidism should be considered; however, the tempo of her illness, the tenderness of the thyroid on examination, and her preceding viral illness make this diagnosis less likely. Ludwig's angina is a potentially life-threatening bacterial infection of the retropharyngeal and submandibular spaces, often caused by preceding dental infection. Cat-scratch fever is a usually benign illness that presents with lymphadenopathy, fever, and malaise. It is caused by *Bartonella henselae* and is frequently transmitted from cat scratches that penetrate the epidermis. It will not cause an elevated TSH. Subacute thyroiditis can present with hypothyroidism, thyrotoxicosis, or neither. In the first phase of the disease, thyroid inflammation leads to follicle destruction and release of thyroid hormone. Thyrotoxicosis ensues. In the second phase, the thyroid is depleted of hormone and hypothyroidism results. A recovery phase typically follows in which decreased inflammation allows the follicles to heal and regenerate hormone.

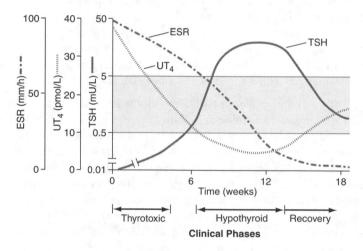

FIGURE X-15/16 Clinical course of subacute thyroiditis. The release of thyroid hormones is initially associated with a thyrotoxic phase and suppressed thyroid-stimulating hormone (TSH). A hypothyroid phase then ensues, with low T_4 and TSH levels that are initially low but gradually increase. During the recovery phase, increased TSH levels combined with resolution of thyroid follicular injury leads to normalization of thyroid function, often several months after the beginning of the illness. ESR, erythrocyte sedimentation rate; UT_4, unbound T_4.

Large doses of aspirin (such as 600 mg by mouth every 4–6 h) or nonsteroidal anti-inflammatory drugs are often sufficient for what is usually a self-limited illness. A glucocorticoid taper can be used if symptoms are severe. Thyroid function should be monitored closely; some patients may require low-dose thyroid hormone replacement.

X-17.   The answer is A. *(Chap. 338)* The DCCT found definitive proof that reduction in chronic hyperglycemia can prevent many of the complications of type 1 DM. This multicenter randomized trial enrolled over 1400 patients with type 1 DM to either intensive or conventional diabetes management and prospectively evaluated the development of retinopathy, nephropathy, and neuropathy. The intensive group received multiple administrations of insulin daily along with education and psychological counseling. The intensive group achieved a mean hemoglobin A_{1C} of 7.3% versus 9.1% in the conventional group. Improvement in glycemic control resulted in a 47% reduction in retinopathy, a 54% reduction in nephropathy, and a 60% reduction in neuropathy. There was a nonsignificant trend toward improvement in macrovascular complications. The results of the DCCT showed that individuals in the intensive group would attain up to 7 more years of intact vision and up to 5 more years free from lower limb amputation. Later, the United Kingdom Prospective Diabetes Study (UKPDS) studied over 5000 individuals with type 2 DM. Individuals receiving intensive glycemic control had a reduction in microvascular events but no significant change in macrovascular complications. These two trials were pivotal in showing a benefit of glycemic control in reducing microvascular complications in patients with type 1 and type 2 DM, respectively. Another result from the UKPDS was that strict blood pressure control resulted in an improvement in macrovascular complications.

X-18.   The answer is B. *(Chap. 347)* Hypocalcemia can be a life-threatening consequence of thyroidectomy if the parathyroid glands are inadvertently removed during the surgery, as the four parathyroid glands are located immediately posterior to the thyroid gland. This is an infrequent occurrence currently as the parathyroid glands are better able to be identified both before and during surgery. However, hypoparathyroidism may occur even if the parathyroid glands are not removed by thyroidectomy due to devascularization or trauma to the parathyroid glands. Hypocalcemia following removal of the parathyroid glands may begin any time during the first 24–72 h, and monitoring of serial calcium levels is recommended for the first 72 h. The earliest symptoms of hypocalcemia are typically circumoral paresthesias and paresthesias with a "pins-and needles" sensation in the fingers and toes. The development of carpal spasms upon inflation of the blood pressure cuff is a classic sign of hypocalcemia and is known as Trousseau sign. Chvostek sign is the other classic sign of hypocalcemia and is elicited by tapping the facial nerve in the preauricular area causing spasm of the facial muscles. A prolongation of the QT interval on the ECG suggests life-threatening hypocalcemia that may progress to fatal arrhythmia, and treatment should not be delayed for serum testing to occur in a patient with a known cause of hypocalcemia. Immediate treatment with IV calcium should be initiated. Maintenance therapy with calcitriol and vitamin D is necessary for ongoing treatment of acquired hypoparathyroidism. Alternatively, surgeons may implant parathyroid tissue into the soft tissue of the forearm, if it is thought that the parathyroid glands will be removed. Hypomagnesemia can cause hypocalcemia by suppressing parathyroid hormone release despite the presence of hypocalcemia. However, in this patient, hypomagnesemia is not suspected after thyroidectomy, and magnesium administration is not indicated. Benztropine is a centrally acting anticholinergic medication that is used in the treatment of dystonic reactions that can occur after taking centrally acting antiemetic medications with dopaminergic activity, such as metoclopramide or compazine. Dystonic reactions involve focal spasms of the face, neck, and extremities. While this patient has taken a medication that can cause a dystonic reaction, the spasms that she is experiencing are more consistent with tetanic contractions of hypocalcemia than dystonic reaction. Finally, measurement of forced vital capacity is most commonly used as a measurement of disease severity in myasthenia gravis or Guillain-Barré syndrome. Muscle weakness is a typical presenting feature but not paresthesias.

X-19.   **The answer is C.**   *(Chap. 344)*   This patient presents with the classic findings of a VIPoma, including large-volume watery diarrhea, hypokalemia, dehydration, and hypochlorhydria (WDHA, or Verner-Morrison, syndrome). Abdominal pain is unusual. The presence of a secretory diarrhea is confirmed by a stool osmolal gap [2(stool Na + stool K) – (stool osmolality)] <35 and persistence during fasting. In osmotic or laxative-induced diarrhea, the stool osmolal gap is over 100. In adults, over 80% of VIPomas are solitary pancreatic masses that usually are larger than 3 cm at diagnosis. Metastases to the liver are common and preclude curative surgical resection. The differential diagnosis includes gastrinoma, laxative abuse, carcinoid syndrome, and systemic mastocytosis. Diagnosis requires the demonstration of large-volume secretory diarrhea (over 700 mL/d) and elevated serum VIP. CT scan of the abdomen will often demonstrate the pancreatic mass and liver metastases.

X-20.   **The answer is E.**   *(Chap. 347)*   Malignancy can cause hypercalcemia by several different mechanisms, including metastasis to bone, cytokine stimulation of bone turnover, and production of a protein structurally similar to parathyroid hormone by the tumor. This protein is called parathyroid hormone–related peptide (PTHrp) and acts at the same receptors as parathyroid hormone (PTH). Squamous cell carcinoma of the lung is the most common tumor associated with the production of PTHrp. Serum calcium levels can become quite high in malignancy because of unregulated production of PTHrp that is outside of the negative feedback control that normally results in the setting of hypercalcemia. PTH hormone levels should be quite low or undetectable in this setting. When hypercalcemia is severe (>15 mg/dL), symptoms frequently include dehydration and altered mental status. The electrocardiogram may show a shortened QTc interval. Initial therapy includes large-volume fluid administration to reverse the dehydration that results from hypercalciuria. In addition, furosemide is also added to promote further calciuria. If the calcium remains elevated, as in this patient, additional measures should be undertaken to decrease the serum calcium. Calcitonin has a rapid onset of action with a decrease in serum calcium seen within hours. However, tachyphylaxis develops, and the duration of benefit is limited. Pamidronate is a bisphosphonate that is useful for the hypercalcemia of malignancy. It decreases serum calcium by preventing bone resorption and release of calcium from the bone. After IV administration, the onset of action of pamidronate is 1–2 days with a duration of action of at least 2 weeks. Thus, in this patient with ongoing severe symptomatic hypercalcemia, addition of both calcitonin and pamidronate is the best treatment. The patient should continue to receive IV fluids and furosemide. The addition of a thiazide diuretic is contraindicated because thiazides cause increased calcium resorption in the kidney and would worsen hypercalcemia.

X-21. **The answer is C.** *(Chap. 51)* Dysmenorrhea refers to the crampy lower abdominal discomfort that begins with the onset of menstrual bleeding and gradually decreases over 12–72 h. Primary dysmenorrhea results from increased stores and subsequent release of prostaglandin precursors. Nonsteroidal anti-inflammatory medications are effective in >80% of cases. Secondary dysmenorrhea is caused by underlying pelvic pathology, the causes of which are many. The differential diagnosis includes endometriosis (ectopic endometrium), mittelschmerz (ruptured graafian follicle), adenomyosis (ectopic endometrial glands within the myometrium), and cervical stenosis. A history of sexual abuse correlates with dyspareunia more often than dysmenorrhea.

X-22. **The answer is E.** *(Chap. 50)* Hirsutism is defined as excessive male-pattern hair growth. It may represent a variation on the norm or be a prelude to a more serious underlying condition. Virilization refers to the state in which androgen levels are elevated enough to cause signs and symptoms of changes in voice, enlargement of genitalia, and increased libido. Virilization is a concerning sign for an ovarian or adrenal cause of excess androgen production. This patient's change in voice and body habitus heightens one's concern about a virilizing process. A thorough medication history is indicated because drugs such as phenytoin, minoxidil, and cyclosporine have been associated with androgen-dependent hair growth. Family history is critical as some families have a higher incidence of hirsutism than others do. Congenital conditions such as congenital adrenal hyperplasia can show distinct patterns of inheritance. Androgens are secreted by both the ovaries and the adrenal glands. An elevation in plasma total testosterone above 12 nmol/L usually indicates a virilizing tumor. A basal DHEAS level above 18.5 μmol/L suggests an adrenal source. Therefore, checking both levels is a useful initial hormonal screen in evaluating virilization. Although polycystic ovarian syndrome is by far the most common cause of ovarian androgen excess, initial screening with ultrasound is not recommended. Polycystic ovaries may be found in females without any evidence of excess androgen secretion. Likewise, females may have an ovarian source of androgen secretion with only slightly enlarged ovaries on ultrasound. Therefore, ultrasound is an insensitive and nonspecic test.

X-23. **The answer is B.** *(Chap. 333)* The identification of an empty sella is often the result of an incidental MRI finding. Typically these patients will have normal pituitary function and should be reassured. It is likely that the surrounding rim of pituitary tissue is functioning normally. An empty sella may signal the insidious onset of hypopituitarism, and laboratory results should be followed closely. Unless her clinical situation changes, repeat MRI is not indicated. Endocrine malignancy is unlikely, and surgery is not part of the management of an empty sella.

X-24. **The answer is C.** *(Chap. 333)* Craniopharyngiomas are benign suprasellar cystic masses that typically present with headaches, visual field deficits, and hypopituitarism. They arise near the pituitary stalk and extend into the suprasellar cistern. They are most common in children and often present with signs of increased intracranial pressure. More than half present before the age of 20. Weight gain, cognitive changes, sleep disorders, and visual field defects are common. Hypopituitarism is present in 90% of cases, and diabetes insipidus in 10% of cases. MRI is the test of choice for evaluation. Definitive management includes transcranial or transsphenoidal surgical resection followed by radiation. Meningioma should appear on the differential of the patient above; epidemiologically, these tumors are more common in women than men, and tend to occur between the ages of 40 and 70. Congenital pan-hypopituitarism would not explain his acute worsening nor his increased intracranial pressure. McCune-Albright syndrome consists of polyostotic fibrous dysplasia, pigmented skin patches, and a variety of endocrine disorders including adenomas and pituitary tumors. Carney syndrome consists of myxomas; endocrine tumors including adrenal, testicular, and pituitary adenomas; and skin pigmentation.

X-25. **The answer is D.** *(Chap. 332)* Positive feedback control is the least understood of the endocrine regulatory systems. The estrogen-LH relationship is a classic example of rising levels of a hormone having a positive effect on the release of another. Paracrine regulation refers to factors released by one cell that act on adjacent cells in the same tissue (e.g., somatostatin released from pancreatic δ cells inhibits secretion of insulin from adjacent β cells). Insulin-like growth factor I released from chondrocytes acts on the cells that produce it, which is an example of autocrine regulation. Negative feedback control is the classic model of an endocrine regulatory system (e.g., high levels of thyroxine inhibit further release of thyroid-stimulating hormone).

X-26. **The answer is D.** *(Chap. 348)* The epidemiology of fractures follows trends similar to those for loss of bone density. Fractures of the radius increase until age 50 and then plateau by age 60. There are approximately 250,000 wrist fractures each year in the United States. However, there are approximately 300,000 hip fractures annually, with incidence rates doubling every 5 years after age 70. The shift from arm and wrist fractures to hip fractures may be related to the way elderly people fall, with less frequent landing on the hands and more frequent direct hip trauma with increasing age. There are approximately 700,000 vertebral fractures each year in the United States. Most are clinically silent and rarely require hospitalization. They may lead to height loss, kyphosis, and pain secondary to altered biomechanics.

X-27. **The answer is B.** *(Chap. 348)* The Women's Health Initiative (WHI) demonstrated that estrogen-progestin therapy can reduce the risk of hip fractures by 34%. Other clinical trials have shown a decrease in all osteoporotic fractures, including vertebral compression fractures. The beneficial effect of estrogen appears to be maximal in those who start therapy early and continue taking the medication. The benefit declines after discontinuation, and there is no net benefit by 10 years after discontinuation. These effects are present for oral and transdermal formulations. However, the WHI also demonstrated that estrogens are associated with a 30% increase in myocardial infarction, a 40% increase in stroke, a 100% increase in venous thromboembolism, and a 25% increase in breast cancer. In the WHI study there was no overall effect of estrogen-progestin therapy on mortality, probably because of the balance between the detrimental cardiovascular effects and the beneficial effects (in addition to fractures, there was a beneficial effect on the development of colon cancer).

X-28. **The answer is D.** *(Chap. 348)* The selective estrogen receptor modulators (SERMs) tamoxifen and raloxifene act in a fashion similar to that of estrogen in decreasing bone turnover and bone loss in postmenopausal women. These agents have been shown to decrease the risk of invasive breast cancer. Raloxifene, which is approved for the prevention of osteoporosis, reduces the risk of vertebral fractures by 30 to 50%. There are no data confirming a similar effect on nonvertebral fractures. Optimal calcium intake reduces bone loss and suppresses bone turnover. Vitamin D plus calcium supplements have been shown to reduce the risk of hip fractures by 20 to 30%. The bisphosphonates alendronate and risedronate are structurally related to pyrophosphate and are incorporated into bone matrix. They reduce the number of osteoclasts and impair the function of those already present. Both have been shown to reduce the risk of vertebral and hip fractures by 40 to 50%. One trial found that risedronate reduced hip fractures in osteoporotic women in their seventies but not in older women without osteoporosis. Risedronate may be administered weekly. The newer bisphosphonates zoledronate and ibandronate may be dosed yearly or monthly. A daily injection of exogenous parathyroid hormone analogue superimposed on estrogen therapy produced increases in bone mass and decreased vertebral and nonvertebral fractures by 45 to 65%. There are no published studies of combinations of parathyroid hormone and SERMs or bisphosphonates.

X-29. **The answer is E.** *(Chap. 337)* Complete removal of the pheochromocytoma is the only therapy that leads to a long-term cure, although 90% of tumors are benign. However, preoperative control of hypertension is necessary to prevent surgical complications and lower mortality. This patient is presenting with encephalopathy in a hypertensive crisis. The hypertension should be managed initially with IV medications to lower the mean arterial pressure by ~20% over the initial 24-h period. Medications that can be used for hypertensive crisis in pheochromocytoma include nitroprusside, nicardipine, and phentolamine. Once the acute hypertensive crisis has resolved, transition to oral α-adrenergic blockers is indicated. Phenoxybenzamine is the most commonly used drug and is started at low doses (5–10 mg three times daily) and titrated to the maximum tolerated dose (usually 20–30 mg daily). Once alpha blockers have been initiated, beta blockade can safely be utilized and is particularly indicated for ongoing tachycardia. Liberal salt and fluid intake helps expand plasma volume and treat orthostatic hypotension. Once blood pressure is maintained below 160/100 mmHg with moderate orthostasis, it is safe to proceed to surgery. If blood pressure remains elevated despite treatment with alpha blockade, addition of calcium channel blockers, angiotensin receptor blockers, or angiotensin-converting enzyme inhibitors should be considered. Diuretics should be avoided as they will exacerbate orthostasis.

X-30.   The answer is B.   *(Chap. 336)*   Control of renin release involves the independent actions of four factors: the juxtaglomerular cells, macula densa cells, the sympathetic nervous system, and circulating factors such as potassium concentration and atrial natriuretic peptide concentration. When effective circulating volume is low, cells in the juxtaglomerular apparatus (JGA) perceive this as a decreased stretch exerted on the afferent arteriole wall, and renin secretion is augmented. Macula densa cells may function as chemoreceptors monitoring the sodium and chloride load delivered to the distal tubule. Under conditions of low solute load delivered to the distal tubule, a signal is conveyed to increase juxtaglomerular release of renin. Increased sympathetic activity stimulates the JGA to release renin when upright posture is assumed. Increased potassium intake and release of atrial natriuretic peptide both decrease renin release.

X-31.   The answer is E.   *(Chap. 333)*   Pituitary adenomas are very common and are the most likely cause of pituitary hormone excess or deficiency states in adults. They make up 10% of all intracranial neoplasms. Pituitary microadenomas are present in ~25% of all autopsies, independent of ante-mortem clinical disease, and are usually unsuspected. 10% of the general population will have a microadenoma on head imaging. The clinical and biochemical phenotype of pituitary adenomas depend on the cell type from which they arise. They may cause hypersecretion or hyposecretion syndromes.

X-32.   The answer is B.   *(Chap. 337)*   This patient has the classic triad of symptoms for pheochromocytoma: headaches, palpitations, and profuse sweating. When this triad of symptoms is found in association with hypertension, pheochromocytoma is the most likely diagnosis. Differential diagnosis for pheochromocytoma includes panic disorder, essential hypertension, cocaine or methamphetamine abuse, carcinoid syndrome, intracranial mass, clonidine withdrawal, and factitious disorder. While episode hypertension is classically described in association with pheochromocytoma, many patients have sustained hypertension that may be difficult to treat. In addition, 5–15% of individuals may present with normal blood pressure (*WM Manger: J Clin Hypertens 4: 62, 2002*). The patient also exhibits significant orthostatic changes in blood pressure which is a common finding in pheochromocytoma. Interestingly, there is a case report of treatment with paroxetine unmasking symptoms of pheochromocytoma (*MA Seeler et al: Ann Intern Med 126: 333, 1997*). The cornerstone of diagnosis of pheochromocytoma is the documentation of elevated levels of urine and plasma catecholamines. The usual diagnostic algorithm includes the measurement of vanillylmandelic acid, catecholamines, and fractionated metanephrines in a 24-h urine collection or plasma sample. These tests should be greater than two to three times the upper limit of normal. If metanephrines are elevated, a CT scan or MRI of the chest, abdomen, and pelvis is performed with contrast to localize the site of the pheochromocytoma. Nuclear imaging with ^{123}I or ^{131}I-metaiodobenzylguanidine (MIBG) can also be utilized for localization of the pheochromocytoma after biochemical testing has confirmed elevated levels of catecholamines. Given the classic symptoms of this patient, panic attack is a diagnosis of exclusion because the missed diagnosis of pheochromocytoma increases the risk of adverse outcomes, including death and stroke. Carcinoid syndrome is diagnosed with 24-h urine testing for 5-HIAA, but is unlikely in this patient because carcinoid syndrome is not associated with hypertension.

X-33.   The answer is B. *(Chap. 332)* With few exceptions, hormone binding is highly specific for a single type of nuclear receptor. The mineralocorticoid-glucocorticoid hormones are a notable exception because the mineralocorticoid receptor also has a high, but not greater, affinity for glucocorticoid. An enzyme (11 β-hydroxysteroid dehydrogenase) located in renal tubules inactivates glucocorticoid, allowing selective responses to mineralocorticoid. When there is glucocorticoid excess, the enzyme becomes oversaturated and glucocorticoid can exhibit mineralocorticoid effects. This effect is in contrast to the estrogen receptor, where different compounds confer unique transcription machinery. Mineralocorticoid hormones do not have serum-binding proteins. Examples of hormones that circulate with serum-binding proteins are: T_4, T_3, cortisol, estrogen, and growth hormone. Most binding protein abnormalities have little clinical consequence because the free concentrations of the hormone often remain normal.

X-34.   The answer is E. *(Chap. 335)* The thionamides propylthiouracil (PTU), carbimazole, and methimazole are the main antithyroid medications used for the treatment of hyperthyroidism. They all inhibit the function of thyroid peroxidase, reducing oxidation and organification of iodide. PTU also inhibits the deiodination of T_4 to T_3. PTU has a half-life much shorter than that of methimazole. Rash, urticaria, fever, and arthralgias are common side effects, occurring in up to 5% of these patients. They may resolve spontaneously. Major side effects are rare but include hepatitis, agranulocytosis, and a systemic lupus erythematosus (SLE)-like syndrome. If major side effects are noted, it is essential that antithyroid medications be stopped.

X-35.   The answer is B. *(Chap. 347)* Hyperparathyroidism is the most common cause of hypercalcemia and is the most likely cause in an adult who is asymptomatic. Cancer is the second most common cause of hypercalcemia but usually is associated with symptomatic hypercalcemia. In addition, there are frequently symptoms from the malignancy itself that dominate the clinical picture. Primary hyperparathyroidism results from autonomous secretion of parathyroid hormone (PTH) that is no longer regulated by serum calcium levels, usually related to development of parathyroid adenomas. Most patients are asymptomatic or have minimal symptoms at the time of diagnosis. When present, symptoms include recurrent nephrolithiasis, peptic ulcers, dehydration, constipation, and altered mental status. Laboratory studies show elevated serum calcium with decreased serum phosphate. Diagnosis can be confirmed with measurement of parathyroid hormone levels. Surgical removal of autonomous adenomas is generally curative, but not all patients need to be treated surgically. It is recommended that individuals <50 undergo primary surgical resection. However, in those >50 years, a cautious approach with frequent laboratory monitoring is often used. Surgery can then be undertaken if a patient develops symptomatic or worsening hypercalcemia or complications such as osteopenia. Breast cancer is a frequent cause of hypercalcemia because of metastatic disease to the bone. In this patient who has received routine mammography as part of age-appropriate cancer screening and is asymptomatic, this would be unlikely. Multiple myeloma is another malignancy frequently associated with hypercalcemia that is thought to be due to production of cytokines and humoral mediators by the tumor. Multiple myeloma should not present with isolated hypercalcemia and is associated with anemia and elevations in creatinine.

Approximately 20% of individuals with hyperthyroidism develop hypercalcemia related to increased bone turnover. This patient exhibits no signs or symptoms of hyperthyroidism, making the diagnosis unlikely. Vitamin D intoxication is a rare cause of hypercalcemia. An individual must ingest 40–100 times the recommended daily amount in order to develop hypercalcemia. Because vitamin D acts to increase both calcium and phosphate absorption from the intestine, serum levels of both minerals would be elevated, which is not seen in this case.

X-36.   The answer is A. *(Chap. 335)* Thyrotoxicosis presents with a characteristic set of signs and symptoms. Common signs include tachycardia and atrial fibrillation, tremor, goiter, and warm, moist skin. Common symptoms include hyperactivity, dysphoria, irritability, heat intolerance, excessive sweating, and fatigue. Weight loss occurs frequently; however, some patients will gain weight as they typically have a marked increase in appetite. The most common cardiac abnormality of thyrotoxicosis is sinus tachycardia. In older patients atrial fibrillation is frequently seen. These arrhythmias are a manifestation of a high-output state, which frequently leads to a widened pulse pressure and a systolic murmur. This can exacerbate underlying heart failure or coronary disease. Up to 50% of patients with atrial fibrillation related to untreated thyrotoxicosis will convert to normal sinus rhythm with management of their thyroid condition.

X-37. **The answer is D.** *(Chap. 335)* Hyperthyroidism is treated by reducing thyroid hormone synthesis, using antithyroid drugs, reducing the amount of thyroid tissue with radioactive iodine, or by thyroidectomy. Antithyroid drugs are used more frequently in Japan and Europe, whereas radioactive thyroid is used more frequently in North America. Propthiouracil and methimazole are the most commonly used antithyroid drugs and act by inhibiting the function of thyroid peroxidase. In Graves' disease, they also reduce thyroid antibody levels. Thyroid function tests and clinical manifestations are reviewed every 3–4 weeks with dose titrated based on unbound T_4 levels. Euthyroidism usually takes 6–8 weeks with this regimen. Agranulocytosis occurs in <1% of patients. Since radioactive iodine is contraindicated in pregnancy, propthiouracil may be used carefully since blocking doses may cause fetal hypothyroidism. Diltiazem may be used to slow heart rate in atrial fibrillation; however, beta blockers are effective in hyperthyroidism to control adrenergic symptoms. Itraconazole is an antifungal agent. Phenoxybenzamine is an α-adrenergic blocker often used to control blood pressure in patients with pheochromocytoma. Liothyronine is the oral form of triiodothyronine (T_3) and would not be used in hyperthyroidism. Levothyroxine has been used in combination with antithyroid drugs (block-replace regimen) to avoid drug-induced hypothyroidism.

X-38. **The answer is B.** *(Chap. 335)* While hypothyroidism may be strongly suspected from history and physical examination findings, it is definitively diagnosed with serum laboratory measurements. TSH should be the first test sent. A normal TSH level excludes primary, but not secondary, hypothyroidism. Primary hypothyroidism refers to disease caused by hypofunction of the thyroid gland itself. Secondary hypothyroidism typically arises from disease of the anterior pituitary. If the TSH is low or normal and pituitary disease is suspected, a free T_4 should be sent. If this test is low, the differential includes anterior pituitary dysfunction, sick euthyroid syndrome, and drug effects. TSH, not unbound T_4, is the test of choice for diagnosing subclinical hypothyroidism. In these cases, TSH is elevated and T_4 is normal. Thyroid peroxidase antibodies are present in >90% of patients with autoimmune hypothyroidism; this test helps distinguish autoimmune causes of hypothyroidism from other possibilities. Circulating T_3 levels are normal in ~25% of patients with clinical hypothyroidism and are not indicated for diagnosis. A T_3/T_4 ratio is not helpful for diagnosis or prognosis.

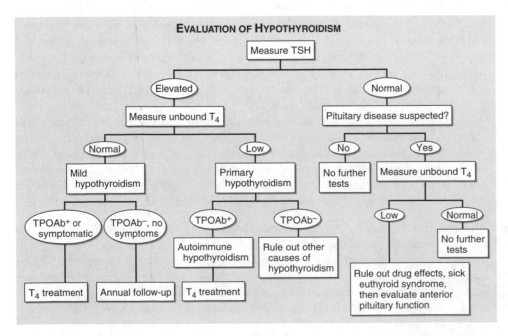

FIGURE X-38 Evaluation of hypothyroidism. TPOAb+, thyroid peroxidase antibodies present; TPOAb−, thyroid peroxidase antibodies not present; TSH, thyroid-stimulating hormone.

X. ENDOCRINOLOGY AND METABOLISM — *ANSWERS*

X-39. **The answer is E.** *(Chap. 335)* Autoimmune hypothyroidism is a common diagnosis, present in 4 per 1000 women and 1 per 1000 men. The mean age of diagnosis is 60 years. It is more prevalent in locations with chronic exposure to a high-iodine diet, such as Japan. Subclinical hypothyroidism (elevated thyroid-stimulating hormone, normal unbound T_4) is present in 6–8% of women and 3% of men. It is present in up to 10% of adults >60 years of age. There is an association between autoimmune hypothyroidism and other autoimmune conditions, and there appears to be a heritable familial risk of developing disease. There are likely environmental triggers other than heavy iodine exposure that predispose to the disease phenotype in susceptible individuals, but these have not been identified. Autoimmune thyroiditis may present with or without a goiter. When a goiter is present, it is termed *Hashimoto's thyroiditis*. The goiter is due to lymphocytic infiltration of the thyroid. Eventually atrophy of thyroid follicles leads to shrinkage of the gland. Atrophic thyroiditis likely represents the end stage of Hashimoto's thyroiditis. There is no evidence that viral thyroiditis induces subsequent autoimmune thyroiditis.

X-40. **The answer is D.** *(Chap. 332)* Hormones can be broadly divided into five classes: amino acid derivatives, small neuropeptides, large proteins, steroid hormones, and vitamin derivatives. As a rule, amino acid derivatives and peptide hormones interact with cell-surface proteins while steroids, thyroid hormone, vitamin D, and retinoids interact with intracellular nuclear receptors. In a cell line impermeable to passage by extracellular molecules, steroids, thyroid hormone, vitamin D, and retinoids would not be able to exert their effect on the nuclear receptors. Hormones that interact with cell-surface membrane receptors would still be able to initiate their signaling. Dopamine is an amino acid derivative. Gonadotropin-releasing hormone is a small neuropeptide. Insulin is a large protein.

X-41. **The answer is B.** *(Chap. 335)* Thyrotoxicosis is a state of hormone excess. It is not synonymous with hyperthyroidism, which is the result of excessive thyroid function. Graves' disease accounts for 60–80% of thyrotoxicosis. Graves' disease is caused by the presence of thyroid-stimulating antibodies, which autonomously activate the thyroid-stimulating hormone receptor and cause overproduction of thyroid hormone. Other common causes of thyrotoxicosis include toxic multinodular goiter and toxic thyroid adenoma. Thyrotoxicosis without hyperthyroidism may occur in subacute thyroiditis, thyroid destruction from amiodarone or radiation, or ingestion of excess thyroid hormone. Graves' disease is common among populations with high iodine intake and occurs in up to 2% of women. It is one-tenth as frequent in men. It rarely presents in adolescence, and is most prevalent in patients between the ages of 20 and 50 years.

X-42. **The answer is C.** *(Chap. 350)* The child exhibits clinical and laboratory manifestations of homozygous familial hypercholesterolemia (FH). The presence of childhood xanthomas including hands, wrists, elbows, knees, and buttocks with evidence of premature atherosclerosis is characteristic. The atherosclerosis often develops initially in the aortic root, causing valvular or supravalvular stenosis. Drug therapy is often ineffective, and LDL apheresis is usually the necessary therapy. Before initiating therapy to reduce his LDL, it is necessary to rule out hypothyroidism, nephrotic syndrome, and obstructive liver disease. Although parental control of the patient's diet is also partly to blame, deliberate or unintentional ingestion of a poor diet is less likely to be responsible than a genetic disorder. Familial defective apoB100 is a dominantly inherited disorder that may be confused with heterozygous FH, but not homozygous. These patients usually present with cardiovascular disease in adulthood. Syphilis can cause aortitis; however, it does not cause premature coronary artery disease.

X-43. **The answer is D.** *(Chap. 350)* This patient has signs and symptoms of familial hypercholesterolemia (FH) with elevated plasma LDL, normal triglycerides, tendon xanthomas, and premature coronary artery disease. FH is an autosomal codominant lipoprotein disorder that is the most common of these syndromes caused by a single gene disorder. It has a higher prevalence in Afrikaners, Christian Lebanese, and French Canadians. There is no definitive diagnostic test for FH. FH may be diagnosed with a skin biopsy that shows reduced LDL receptor activity in cultured fibroblasts (although there is considerable overlap with normals). FH is predominantly a clinical diagnosis, although molecular diagnostics are being developed. Hemolysis is not a feature of FH. Sitosterolemia is distinguished from FH by episodes of hemolysis. It is a rare autosomal recessive disorder that causes a marked increase in the dietary absorption of plant sterols. Hemolysis is due to incorporation of plant sterols into the red blood cell membrane. Sitosterolemia is confirmed by demonstrating an increase in the plasma levels of sitosterol using gas chromatography. CT scanning of the liver does not sufficiently differentiate between the hyperlipoproteinemias. Many of the primary lipoproteinemias, including sitosterolemia, are inherited in an autosomal recessive pattern, and thus, a pedigree analysis would not be likely to isolate the disorder.

X-44. **The answer is E.** *(Chap. 333)* Oral dopamine agonists, cabergoline or bromocriptine, are the mainstay of treatment for prolactinomas, regardless of their size. Patients with macroadenomas (>1 cm in diameter) should undergo visual field testing before starting therapy. MRI and visual field testing should be assessed at 6- to 12-month intervals to evaluate for shrinkage of the mass. Indications for surgery include dopamine agonist resistance or intolerance, invasive tumor or lack of improvement on visual field testing.

X-45. **The answer is C.** *(Chap. 336)* Plasma and urine assessment of steroid levels may be misleading due to improper collection or altered metabolism. Moreover, the plasma level depends on the secretion rate and the rate at which the hormone is metabolized. As such, stimulation tests are used to diagnose hormone deficiency states, while suppression tests document hypersecretion of adrenal hormones. One protocol for assessing mineralocorticoid deficiency involves severe sodium restriction, which is a potent stimulator of mineralocorticoid release. Rates of aldosterone secretion should increase two- to threefold. When dietary sodium intake is normal, stimulation testing of mineralocorticoid deficiency may be achieved by injection of a potent diuretic (e.g., 40–80 mg of furosemide) followed by 2–3 h of upright posture. The normal response is a two- to fourfold increase in plasma aldosterone levels.

X-46. **The answer is E.** *(Chap. 335)* This patient has signs and symptoms of Graves' disease. In patients with thyrotoxicosis due to Graves' disease, the TSH level is low and total and unbound thyroid hormone levels are increased. In 2–5% of patients, only the T_3 levels will be increased. In this patient, with a high pre-test probability of Graves' disease, a suppressed TSH and normal T_4 supports Graves'; however, testing of T_3 should be per-

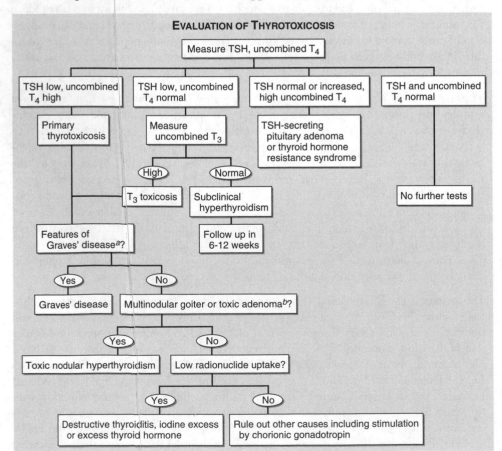

FIGURE X-46 Evaluation of thyrotoxicosis. [a]Diffuse goiter, positive TPO antibodies, ophthalmopathy, dermopathy; [b]can be confirmed by radionuclide scan. TSH, thyroid-stimulating hormone.

formed to definitively make the diagnosis. A total T_4 level would not provide definitive evidence of Graves' disease. Radionuclide scan of the thyroid is used to evaluate for toxic multinodular goiter and toxic adenoma. Measurement of thyroid-stimulating antibodies and thyroid peroxidase antibodies will help confirm the diagnosis of Graves' but are not routinely used since the diagnosis may be made with a consistent clinical picture combined with supportive TSH and thyroid hormone results.

X-47. **The answer is B.** *(Chap. 51)* Pregnancy, whether intrauterine or ectopic, is the most common cause of secondary amenorrhea and should be ruled out early in the evaluation of such patients. In a patient with secondary amenorrhea, uterine outflow tract obstruction is uncommon unless there has been curettage for pregnancy complications or, in an endemic region, genital tuberculosis. Primary ovarian failure is ruled out by the low levels of FSH in that FSH levels should be very elevated if anovulation is caused by ovarian pathology. Malnutrition or extreme weight loss (BMI <18) may cause secondary amenorrhea, but these are not likely in this case. An MRI is indicated in this patient with secondary amenorrhea because she is not pregnant, does not have evidence of primary ovarian failure, has an elevated prolactin levels and a normal thyroid-stimulating hormone levels. These results suggest the possibility of central nervous system pathology.

X-48. **The answer is C.** *(Chap. 341)* Evaluation of infertility should include evaluation of common male and female factors that could be contributing. Abnormalities of menstrual function are the most common cause of female infertility, and initial evaluation of infertility should include evaluation of ovulation and assessment of tubal and uterine patency. The female partner reports an episode of gonococcal infection with symptoms of pelvic inflammatory disease, which would increase her risk of infertility due to tubal scarring and occlusion. A hysterosalpingogram is indicated. If there is evidence of tubal abnormalities, many experts recommend in vitro fertilization for conception as these women are at increased risk of ectopic pregnancy if conception occurs. The female partner reports some irregularity of her menses, suggesting anovulatory cycles, and thus, evidence of ovulation should be determined by assessing hormonal levels. There is no evidence that prolonged use of oral contraceptives affects fertility adversely (A Farrow, et al: *Hum Reprod* 17: 2754, 2002). Angiotensin-converting enzyme inhibitors, including lisinopril, are known teratogens when taken by women, but have no effects on chromosomal abnormalities in men. Recent marijuana use may be associated with increased risk of infertility, and in vitro studies of human sperm exposed to a cannabinoid derivative showed decreased motility (LB Whan, et al: *Fertil Steril* 85: 653, 2006). However, no studies have shown long-term decreased fertility in men who previously used marijuana.

X-49. **The answer is B.** *(Chap. 343)* Disorders of sexual differentiation involve both chromosomal disorders as well as gonadal and phenotypic disorders. Klinefelter syndrome classically is associated with a 47,XXY karyotype resulting from meiotic nondisjunction. Clinically, individuals with Klinefelter syndrome present in young adulthood with poor virilization and eunuchoid proportions noted by tall height with long leg length. Secondary sexual development is poor, with decreased facial and axillary hair and low sexual drive. Gynecomastia is frequently present, and the testes have a median length of 2.5 cm with almost all <3.5 cm. It is noted that the testes seem particularly small given the degree of androgenization present. A testicular biopsy would show hyalinization of the seminiferous tubules and azoospermia. Learning difficulties are frequently associated. Individuals with Klinefelter syndrome are also at increased risk of thromboembolic disease, diabetes mellitus, breast tumors, and obesity. Laboratory tests would reveal elevated follicle-stimulating hormone and luteinizing hormone with low plasma testosterone consistent with primary testicular failure. Increased concentrations of estradiol are also commonly encountered and are responsible for the development of gynecomastia. Treatment of the disorder primarily is androgen supplementation. Severe gynecomastia may require surgical reduction of breast tissue.

Androgen insensitivity syndrome (AIS) was previously known as testicular feminization and is a disorder caused by a mutation in the androgen receptor. Complete AIS is characterized by a female phenotype in XY individuals with normal breast development. However, there is no uterus, the vagina is short, and there is minimal axillary and pubic hair development.

Mixed gonadal dysgenesis results from a 45,X/46,XY mosaicism. Phenotype can be either male or female, and most individuals have ambiguous genitalia at birth. If the primary phenotype is male, hypospadias are common, and dysgenetic gonads lead to an increased risk of gonadoblastomas and other malignancies.

Testicular dysgenesis is also known as Swyer syndrome. These individuals have a complete absence of androgenization, and external genitalia is usually female or ambiguous.

True hermaphroditism is now known as ovotesticular DSD (disorder of sexual development). Both ova and testes are found in a single individual, and sometimes this is manifest as an ovotestis. The karyotype is most frequently 46,XX.

X-50.   The answer is C.   *(Chap. 340)*   Many drugs may interfere with testicular function through a variety of mechanisms. Cyclophosphamide damages the seminiferous tubules in a dose- and time-dependent fashion and causes azoospermia within a few weeks of initiation. This effect is reversible in approximately half these patients. Ketoconazole inhibits testosterone synthesis. Spironolactone causes a blockade of androgen action. Glucocorticoids lead to hypogonadism predominantly through inhibition of hypothalamic-pituitary function. Sexual dysfunction has been described as a side effect of therapy with beta blockers. However, there is no evidence of an effect on testicular function. Most reports of sexual dysfunction were in patients receiving older beta blockers such as propranolol and timolol.

X-51 and X-52.   The answer is E for both.   *(Chaps. 347 and 85)*   Malignancy may cause hypercalcemia by metastasizing to bone or producing ectopic PTHrp. Bone scan is a sensitive test for bone metastasis, making ectopic hormone production more likely in this case. PTHrp is a tumor-associated protein that is most often seen in squamous cell tumors of the lung. There are high concentrations in human breast milk, although the physiologic significance is unknown. At the cellular level it behaves like PTHi binding to receptors on bone and kidney to increase calcium resorption and stimulate synthesis of 1,25 vitamin D. Elevations of PTHrp and PTHi cause an elevated calcium and low phosphate. While primary hyperparathyroidism is the most common cause of hypercalcemia, in the presence of a lung mass, PTHrp is more likely. Serum magnesium is usually normal in primary hyperparathyroidism or in PTHrp-related hypercalcemia. Small cell carcinoma of the lung may secrete ACTH, causing Cushing's syndrome, but this would not present with isolated hypercalcemia. It also may secrete antidiuretic hormone, causing syndrome of inappropriate antidiuretic hormone. Bronchial carcinoids may produce peptide hormones including serotonin, bradykinin, ACTH, or somatostatin. Adenocarcinomas cause hypercalcemia by metastasizing to bone, which would cause an abnormal bone scan. Bronchoalveolar carcinomas do not usually cause ectopic hormone production or metastasize to bone.

X-53.   The answer is C.   *(Chap. 347)*   The four parathyroid glands are located posterior to the thyroid gland. Parathyroid hormone is the primary regulator of calcium. PTH acts directly on bone and the kidney and indirectly, through the action of vitamin D, on the GI tract. Calcium induces calcium absorption from the kidney and bone. It stimulates hydroxylation of 25-hydroxyvitamin D, resulting in the more active form. Vitamin D stimulates calcium resorption from the GI tract. Calcium and vitamin D are part of a feedback loop that inhibits PTH release and synthesis. PTH prevents resorption of phosphate from the kidney.

X-54.   The answer is C.   *(Chap. 348)*   Determination of when to initiate screening for osteoporosis with bone densitometry testing can be complicated by multiple factors. In general, most women do not require screening for osteoporosis until after completion of menopause unless there have been unexplained fractures or other risk factors that would suggest osteoporosis. There is no benefit to initiating screening for osteoporosis in the perimenopausal period. Indeed most expert recommendations do not recommend routine screening for osteoporosis until age 65 or older unless risk factors are present. Risk factors for osteoporosis include advanced age, cigarette smoking, low body weight (<57.7 kg), family history of hip fracture, and long-term glucocorticoid use. Inhaled glucocorticoids may cause increased loss of bone density, but as this patient is on a low dose of inhaled fluticasone and is not estrogen-deficient, bone mineral densitometry cannot be recommended at this time. The risk of osteoporosis related to inhaled glucocorticoids is not well-defined, but most studies suggest that the risk is relatively low, and inhaled glucocorticoids do not confer a threefold greater risk of osteoporosis. Delaying childbearing until the fourth and fifth decade does increase the risk of osteoporosis but does not cause early onset of osteoporosis prior to completion of menopause. The patient's family history of menopause likewise does not require early screening for osteoporosis.

X-55. **The answer is C.** *(Chap. 335)* The main clinical symptoms of hypothyroidism include tiredness, weakness, dry skin, feeling cold, hair loss, difficulty concentrating, constipation with poor appetite, dyspnea, and hoarse voice. Menorrhagia, amenorrhea, paresthesias, and impaired hearing may also occur. Signs of hypothyroidism include dry coarse skin, puffy hands/face/feet (myxedema), diffuse alopecia, bradycardia, peripheral edema, delayed tendon reflex relaxation, carpal tunnel syndrome, and serous cavity effusions. The symptoms of hyperthyroidism include hyperactivity, irritability, dysphoria, heat intolerance, sweating, palpitations, fatigue and weakness, weight loss with increased appetite, diarrhea, loss of libido, polyuria, and oligomenorrhea. Signs include tachycardia, atrial fibrillation (particularly in the elderly), tremor, goiter, warm moist skin, proximal myopathy, lid lag, and gynecomastia. Exophthalmous is specific for Graves' disease. TSH is the most effective screening test for hypothyroidism. If elevated, an unbound T_4 is necessary to confirm clinical hypothyroidism. Testing of unbound T_4 will not detect subclinical hypothyroidism. Subclinical hypothyroidism is present when the TSH is elevated and unbound T_4 is normal. Patients may have minor or early symptoms of hypothyroidism in this stage.

X-56. **The answer is B.** *(Chap. 346)* Hypophosphatemia results from one of three mechanisms: inadequate intestinal phosphate absorption, excessive renal phosphate excretion, and rapid redistribution of phosphate from the extracellular space into bone or soft tissue. Inadequate intestinal absorption is rare. Malnutrition from fasting or starvation may result in depletion of phosphate, causing hypophosphatemia during refeeding. In hospitalized patients, redistribution is the main cause. Insulin drives phosphate into cells. Sepsis may cause destruction of cells and metabolic acidosis, resulting in a net shift of phosphate from the extracellular space into cells. Renal failure is associated with hyperphosphatemia, not hypophosphatemia.

X-57. **The answer is D.** *(Chap. 347)* Primary hyperparathyroidism and malignancy account for over 90% of cases of hypercalcemia. In asymptomatic patients, primary hyperparathyroidism is the most common cause. In patients admitted to the hospital with symptomatic hypercalcemia, malignancy is the most common cause. Calcium is regulated in bone, the gastrointestinal tract, and the kidney. Other causes of increased bone turnover include Paget's disease, immobilization, hyperthyroidism, hypervitaminosis A, and adrenal insufficiency. Causes of increased GI absorption include vitamin D intoxication and milk-alkali syndrome. Hypercalcemia from thiazide diuretics and familial hypocalciuric hypercalcemia result from disordered regulation of calcium in the kidney.

X-58. **The answer is A.** *(Chap. 341)* Infertility is defined as the inability to conceive after 12 months of unprotected sexual intercourse and affects 14% of couples in the United States. Infertility is attributable to female causes in 58% of cases, male causes in 25% of cases, and 17% remain unexplained after evaluation. Initial evaluation of the infertile couple includes counseling regarding the appropriate timing of intercourse and discussion of modifiable risk factors for infertility, including drug and alcohol use, cigarette smoking, caffeine, and obesity. A semen analysis is performed to determine sperm count, and if the sperm count is low on repeated analysis, measurement of serum testosterone, FSH, and LH are indicated to determine if hypogonadism is contributing to infertility. In the female partner, it is important to confirm ovulation and assess tubal patency. This evaluation includes testing of FSH, LH, prolactin, and estradiol levels in many individuals. A mid-cycle progesterone level may also be useful to document that the mid-cycle LH surge has occurred. Polycystic ovarian syndrome can be found in 30% of women who have anovulatory cycle and is associated with androgen excess. If polycystic ovarian syndrome is suspected, the female partner should have levels of testosterone and dehydroepiandosterone assessed. Determination of patency of the uterine outflow tract and Fallopian tubes is also recommended through performance of a hysterosalpingogram. Endometrial biopsy was once a frequent component of the evaluation of infertility to exclude luteal-phase insufficiency, which would affect fetal implantation.

However, prior research has a high degree of intraobserver variability in the dating criteria used to assess endometrial biopsies (*TC Li, et al: Fertil Steril 51: 759, 1989*). Moreover, out-of-phase biopsies are seen on a single endometrial sample in >30–50% of fertile women and in sequential samples in 7–27% (*OK Davis, et al: Fertil Steril 51: 582, 1989*).

X-59.   The answer is A. *(Chap. 51)* This patient describes primary amenorrhea. It is important to rule out disorders of the uterus or outflow tract before initiating an exhaustive workup for hormonal causes. On examination, one may find obstruction of the transverse vaginal septum or an imperforate hymen, which should be treated surgically. An MRI may further delineate an abnormal genital tract but should not be performed prior to a physical examination. In a nonpregnant woman with primary amenorrhea, an elevated FSH would suggest primary ovarian failure. An elevated prolactin in such a patient should direct your evaluation towards a neuroanatomic abnormality or hypogonadotrophic hypogonadism.

X-60.   The answer is E. *(Chap. 354)* The management strategy for Wilson disease is dependent on the clinical status of the patient. Patients who are presymptomatic or who have hepatitis but no evidence of liver decompensation should be treated with zinc. This nontoxic therapy acts to block copper uptake in the gastrointestinal tract and sequesters copper in the body by inducing hepatic metallothionein synthesis. Patients with mild to moderate hepatic decompensation should receive both zinc and trientine, a copper-chelating agent that has replaced penicillamine because of its superior side-effect profile. Those with severe hepatic decompensation are candidates for liver transplantation. Tetrathiomolybdate combined with zinc are first-line for patients with neuropsychiatric symptoms. Treatment is life-long for all patients. Dimercaprol is used in lead poisoning and has no role in Wilson disease.

X-61.   The answer is D. *(Chap. 348)* Osteoporosis is defined as a reduction of bone mass or density or the presence of a fragility fracture. Operationally, the WHO defines osteoporosis as a bone density more than 2.5 SD less than the mean for young healthy adults of the same race and sex. Dual-energy x-ray absorptiometry (DXA) is the most widely used study to determine bone density. Bone density is expressed as a *t*-score, that is, the SD below the mean of young adults of the same race and gender. A *t*-score higher than 2.5 characterizes osteoporosis, and a *t*-score less than 1 identifies patients at risk of osteoporosis. The *z*-score compares individuals with those in an age-, race-, and gender- matched population. The figure shows the relationship between *z*-scores and *t*-scores.

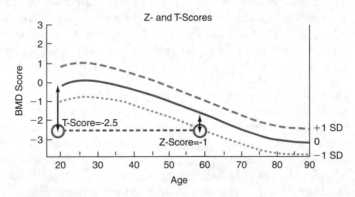

FIGURE X-61

X-62.   The answer is D. *(Chap. 353)* Hyperuricemia is present in 5% of the population and in up to 25% of hospitalized patients. The vast majority are at no clinical risk. Hyperuricemia is considered a component of metabolic syndrome; however, this is not an indication to treat elevated urate levels. Instead, an aggressive management strategy to improve lipid levels, diabetic control, and other cardiovascular risk factors should be implemented. This patient has multiple reasons for renal insufficiency. His asymptomatic hyperuricemia is not one of them; structural kidney damage and stone formation only occur with symptomatic hyperuricemia. Treating his urate level will not improve his kidney function nor prevent future stone formation. It is important to remember that hyperuricemia alone does not represent a disease and is not by itself an indication for treatment.

X-63.   The answer is B.   *(Chap. 352)*   Acute intermittent porphyria (AIP) is one of a collection of disorders characterized by enzyme dysfunction in the heme biosynthetic pathway. Heme is synthesized in the bone marrow and liver, and mutations in the gene generally affect one organ system or the other. For instance, the erythropoietic porphyrias, including porphyria cutanea tarda (PCT), have primarily dermatologic manifestations, whereas AIP is a hepatic porphyria that presents with intermittent abdominal pain, peripheral neuropathy caused by axonal degeneration, and psychiatric symptoms that include paranoia, depression, anxiety, and hallucinations. During an attack of AIP, the precursors to heme build up. The diagnosis is made by demonstrating elevated levels of these precursors, most commonly porphobilinogen, during the episode. The porphobilinogen level will drop in the recovery phase and can be normal when the patient is well. These patients often have triggers of attacks, including menstruation, steroids, calorie restriction, alcohol, and numerous drugs. PCT, in contrast, is triggered by sunlight, with the development of the classic vesicular rash in exposed areas. PCT is closely associated with mild iron overload, and many of these patients also have hemochromatosis-causing mutations such as HFE C282Y. This mutation, however, is not associated with AIP.

X-64.   The answer is E.   *(Chap. 335)*   Statins have emerged over the last decade as one of the most clinically important classes of medications. Numerous studies have indicated important benefits in both primary and secondary prevention of cardiovascular disease. Statins act by inhibiting HMG-CoA reductase, the rate-limiting step in cholesterol biosynthesis. Statins are generally well tolerated, with an excellent safety profile over the years. However, attention must be paid to the side effects, which may be severe. Dyspepsia, headache, fatigue, and myalgias may occur and are generally well tolerated. Myopathy and rhabdomyolysis are rare but serious side effects. The risk of myopathy is increased in the presence of renal insufficiency and with concomitant use of certain medications, including some antibiotics, antifungal agents, some immunosuppressive drugs, and fibric acid derivatives. Hepatitis is another side effect. Liver transaminases should be checked before therapy is started and 4 to 8 weeks afterward. Elevations more than three times the normal range may mandate stopping therapy.

X-65.   The answer is B.   *(Chap. 335)*   Subacute thyroiditis, also known as de Quervain's thyroiditis, granulomatous thyroiditis, and viral thyroiditis, is characterized clinically by fever, constitutional symptoms, and a painful enlarged thyroid. The etiology is thought to be a viral infection. The peak incidence is between 30 and 50 years of age, and women are affected more frequently than are men. The symptoms depend on the phase of the illness. During the initial phase of follicular destruction, there is a release of thyroglobulin and thyroid hormones. As a result, there is increased circulating T_4 and T_3, with concomitant suppression of TSH. Symptoms of thyrotoxicosis predominate at this point. Radioiodine uptake is low or undetectable. After several weeks, thyroid hormone is depleted and a phase of hypothyroidism ensues, with low unbound T_4 levels and moderate elevations of TSH. Radioiodine uptake returns to normal. Finally, after 4 to 6 months, thyroid hormone and TSH levels return to normal as the disease subsides. Patient A is consistent with the thyrotoxic phase of subacute thyroiditis except for the increased radioiodine uptake scan. Patient C is more consistent with Graves' disease with suppression of TSH, an elevated uptake scan, and elevated thyroid hormones as a result of stimulating immunoglobulin. Patient D is consistent with a neoplasm. Patient E is consistent with central hypothyroidism.

X-66.   The answer is D.   *(Chap. 339)*   The most common cause of hypoglycemia is related to the treatment of diabetes mellitus. Individuals with type 1 diabetes mellitus (T1DM) have more symptomatic hypoglycemia than individuals with type 2 diabetes mellitus (T2DM). On average, those with T1DM experience two episodes of symptomatic hypoglycemia weekly; and at least once yearly, individuals with T1DM will have a severe episode of hypoglycemia that is at least temporarily disabling. It is estimated that 2–4% of individuals with T1DM will die from hypoglycemia. In addition, recurrent episodes of hypoglycemia in T1DM contribute to the development of hypoglycemia-associated autonomic failure. Clinically, this is manifested as hypoglycemia unawareness and defective glucose counterregulation, with lack of glucagon and epinephrine secretion as glucose levels fall. Individuals with T2DM are less likely to develop hypoglycemia. Medications that are associated with hypoglycemia in T2DM are insulin and insulin secretagogues, such as sulfonylureas. Metformin, thiazolidinediones, α-glucosidase inhibitors, glucagon-like peptide-1 receptor agonists, and dipeptidyl peptidase-IV inhibitors do not cause hypoglycemia.

X-67. **The answer is E.** *(Chap. 341)* All of the choices have a theoretical efficacy in preventing pregnancy of >90%. However, the actual effectiveness can vary widely. Spermicides have the greatest failure rate of 21%. Barrier methods (condoms, cervical cap, diaphragm) have an actual efficacy between 82 and 88%. Oral contraceptives and intrauterine devices perform similarly, with 97% efficacy in preventing pregnancy in clinical practice.

X-68. **The answer is D.** *(Chap. 338)* Tight glycemic control with a hemoglobin A_{1C} of 7% or less has been shown in the Diabetes Control and Complications Trial (DCCT) in type 1 diabetic patients and the United Kingdom Prospective Diabetes Study (UKPDS) in type 2 diabetic patients to lead to improvements in microvascular disease. Notably, a decreased incidence of neuropathy, retinopathy, microalbuminuria, and nephropathy was shown in individuals with tight glycemic control. Interestingly, glycemic control had no effect on macrovascular outcomes. Instead, it was blood pressure control to at least moderate goals (142/88 mmHg) in the UKPDS that resulted in a decreased incidence of macrovascular outcomes, namely, DM-related death, stroke, and heart failure. Improved blood pressure control also resulted in improved microvascular outcomes.

X-69. **The answer is E.** *(Chap. 335)* Thyroid nodules are found in 5% of patients. Nodules are more common with age, in women, and in iodine-deficient areas. Given their prevalence, the cost of screening, and the generally benign course of most nodules, the choice and order of screening tests have been very contentious. A small percentage of incidentally discovered nodules will represent thyroid cancer, however. A TSH should be the first test to check after detection of a thyroid nodule. A majority of patients will have normal thyroid function tests. In the case of a normal TSH, fine-needle aspiration or ultrasound-guided biopsy can be pursued. If the TSH is low, a radionuclide scan should be performed to determine if the nodule is the source of thyroid hyperfunction (a "hot" nodule). In the case above, this is the best course of action. "Hot" nodules can be treated medically, resected, or ablated with radioactive iodine. "Cold" nodules should be further evaluated with a fine-needle aspiration. 4% of nodules undergoing biopsy will be malignant, 10% are suspicious for malignancy and 86% are indeterminate or benign.

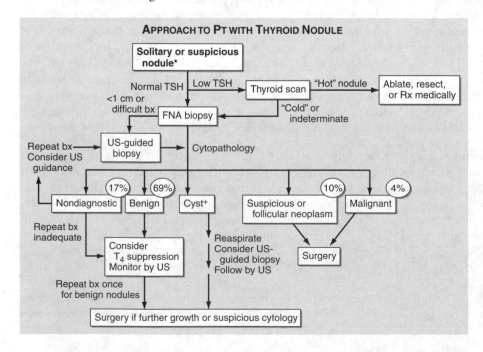

FIGURE X-69 Approach to the patient with a thyroid nodule. See text and references for details. *About one-third of nodules are cystic or mixed solid-cystic. US, ultrasound; TSH, thyroid-stimulating hormone; FNA, fine-needle aspiration.

X-70. **The answer is D.** *(Chap. 349)* Paget's disease of bone is relatively common, and the incidence increases with age. An estimated prevalence of 3% in persons over age 40 years is a generally accepted figure. Most frequently, the disease is asymptomatic and is diagnosed only when the typical sclerotic bones are incidentally detected on x-ray examinations done for other reasons or when increased alkaline phosphatase activity is recognized during routine laboratory measurements. The etiology is unknown, but increased bone resorption followed by intensive bone repair is thought to be the mechanism that causes increased bone density and increased serum alkaline phosphatase activity as a marker of osteoblast activity. Because increased mineralization of bone takes place (although in an abnormal pattern), hypercalcemia is not present unless a severely affected patient becomes immobilized. Hypercalcemia in fact would be an expected finding in a patient with primary hyperparathyroidism, bone metastases, or plasmacytoma, with plasmacytoma typically producing no increase in alkaline phosphatase activity. Osteomalacia resulting from vitamin D deficiency is associated with bone pain and hypophosphatemia; normal or decreased serum calcium concentration produces secondary hyperparathyroidism, further aggravating the defective bone mineralization.

X-71. **The answer is E.** *(Chap. 349)* Paget's disease, a disorder characterized by increased osteoclastic activity and subsequent bony remodeling with structurally unsound woven bone, is often diagnosed incidentally when screening tests reveal an increased alkaline phosphatase or when a radiograph displays characteristic abnormalities. Serum calcium and phosphate levels are normal in Paget's disease. Rarely, immobilization in a patient with Paget's disease may cause hypercalcemia. The most common symptom of Paget's disease is pain. Hearing loss is very frequent, usually due to bony compression of the eighth cranial nerve. The most commonly affected areas include the pelvis, the skull, and the vertebral bodies. Diagnosis does not require nuclear bone scan. Physical findings of bony deformity such as frontal bossing of the skull or bowing of an extremity, an elevated alkaline phosphatase level, or characteristic findings on plain radiographs, such as cortical thickening, lytic and sclerotic changes suffice. Increased osteoclastic activity, possibly initiated by viral infection and likely modulated by genetic factors, drives the pathogenesis of Paget's disease. The disease tends to run in families, with a positive family history in 15–25% of patients.

X-72. **The answer is C.** *(Chap. 333)* Cushing's syndrome is caused by hypercortisolism, typically from an adrenocorticotropic hormone (ACTH)-secreting adenoma, ectopic tumor ACTH production, or iatrogenic ingestion of cortisol. Iatrogenic hypercortisolism is the most common cause of cushingoid features. ACTH-secreting adenomas account for 10–15% of all pituitary tumors. Ectopic ACTH-secreting tumors include bronchial and abdominal carcinoids, small cell lung cancer, and thymoma. In patients with Cushing's syndrome, the frequency of obesity is 80%. Thin skin is also very common and present in up to 80% of patients. Purple skin striae and hirsutism occur 65% of the time in these patients, and amenorrhea about 60% of the time. Skin hyperpigmentation occurs in about 20% of patients. Patients with Cushing's syndrome may also develop hyperglycemia, osteoporosis, proximal muscle weakness, acne, hirsutism, leukocytosis, lymphopenia, and eosinopenia. Patients die of cardiovascular disease, infections, and suicide.

X-73. **The answer is D.** *(Chap. 333)* Pituitary adenomas, often called "incidentalomas," are commonly discovered on head MRI or CT. At autopsy, unsuspected microadenomas are present in up to 25% of cases. In the absence of symptoms or endocrine laboratory abnormalities, adenomas <1 cm in diameter can be safely monitored with annual MRI. PET-CT is not indicated; laboratory testing is used to evaluate for functional activity. Surgery is not indicated for microadenomas (<1 cm). About one-third of macroadenomas (>1 cm) will become invasive or exert mass effect; surgery should be considered for incidental macroadenomas.

X-74. **The answer is A.** *(Chap. 333)* The anterior pituitary produces six major hormones: prolactin, growth hormone (GH), ACTH, luteinizing hormone, follicle-stimulating hormone, and TSH. These hormones are all released in a pulsatile manner from the pituitary. GH and ACTH are present in the fetus at 6 and 8 weeks, respectively; the remainder of the anterior pituitary hormones appear by week 12 of gestation. All of the hormones have inhibitors that act in a negative feedback loop to regulate their production and release. Somatostatin, along with insulin-like growth factor I, inhibits GH. ACTH is suppressed by glucocorticoids.

X-75. **The answer is A.** *(Chap. 335)* Lipoprotein lipase (LPL) and its cofactor apo CII are required for the hydrolysis of triglycerides in chylomicrons and very low density lipoproteins (VLDLs). A genetic deficiency of either protein impairs lipolysis and results in an elevation in plasma chylomicrons. VLDL is also elevated. The triglyceride-rich proteins persist for days in the circulation, causing fasting levels higher than 1000 mg/dL. The inheritance pattern is autosomal recessive. Heterozygotes have normal or mildly elevated plasma triglyceride levels. Clinically, these patients may have repeated episodes of pancreatitis secondary to hypertriglyceridemia. Eruptive xanthomas may appear on the back, the buttocks, and the extensor surfaces of the arms and legs. Hepatosplenomegaly may result from the uptake of circulating chylomicrons by the reticuloendothelial cells. The diagnosis is made by assaying triglyceride lipolytic activity in plasma. Dietary fat restriction is the treatment of choice.

X-76. **The answer is D.** *(Chap. 338)* Diabetic ketoacidosis is an acute complication of diabetes mellitus. It results from a relative or absolute deficiency of insulin combined with a counterregulatory hormone excess. In particular, a decrease in the ratio of insulin to glucagons promotes gluconeogenesis, glycogenolysis, and the formation of ketone bodies in the liver. Ketosis results from an increase in the release of free fatty acids from adipocytes, with a resultant shift toward ketone body synthesis in the liver. This is mediated by the relationship between insulin and the enzyme carnitine palmitoyltransferase I. At physiologic pH, ketone bodies exist as ketoacids, which are neutralized by bicarbonate. As bicarbonate stores are depleted, acidosis develops. Clinically, these patients have nausea, vomiting, and abdominal pain. They are dehydrated and may be hypotensive. Lethargy and severe central nervous system depression may occur. The treatment centers on replacement of the body's insulin, which will result in cessation of the formation of ketoacids and improvement of the acidotic state. Assessment of the level of acidosis may be done with an arterial blood gas. These patients have an anion gap acidosis and often a concomitant metabolic alkalosis resulting from volume depletion. Volume resuscitation with intravenous fluids is critical. Many electrolyte abnormalities may occur. Patients are total body sodium-, potassium-, and magnesium-depleted. As a result of the acidosis, intracellular potassium may shift out of cells and cause a normal or even elevated potassium level. However, with improvement in the acidosis, the serum potassium rapidly falls. Therefore, potassium repletion is critical despite the presence of a "normal" level. Because of the osmolar effects of glucose, fluid is drawn into the intravascular space. This results in a drop in the measured serum sodium. There is a drop of 1.6 meq/L in serum sodium for each rise of 100 mg/dL in serum glucose. In this case, the serum sodium will improve with hydration alone. The use of 3% saline is not indicated because the patient has no neurologic deficits, and the expectation is for rapid resolution with intravenous fluids alone.

X-77. **The answer is A.** *(Chap. 347)* Hypercalcemia manifests in a variety of ways. "Stones, bones, groans, and psychiatric overtones" often is used on rounds as a way to remember the clinical symptoms and signs. Neurologic changes may range from depression to confusion and frank coma. These patients often are constipated and may have nausea, vomiting, and abdominal pain. Increased calcium may affect the genitourinary tract with nephrolithiasis, renal tubular acidosis, and polyuria. A shortened QT interval may result in cardiac arrhythmias.

X-78. **The answer is B.** *(Chap. 347)* Parathyroid hormone (PTH) is produced by the four small parathyroid glands that lie posterior to the thyroid gland and is the primary hormone responsible for regulating serum calcium and phosphate balance. PTH secretion is tightly regulated with negative feedback to the parathyroid glands by serum calcium and vitamin D levels. PTH primarily affects serum calcium and phosphate levels through its action in the bone and the kidney. In the bone, PTH increases bone remodeling through its actions on the osteoblasts and osteoclasts. It directly stimulates osteoblasts to increase bone formation, and this action of PTH has been utilized in the treatment of osteoporosis. Its action on osteoclasts, however, is indirect and likely is mediated through its actions on the osteoblasts. The osteoclast has no receptors for PTH. It has been hypothesized that cytokines produced by osteoblasts are responsible for increased osteoclastic activity that is seen after PTH administration, as PTH fails to have an effect on osteoclasts in the absence of osteoblasts. The net effect of PTH on the bone is to increase bone remodeling. Ultimately, this leads to an increase in serum calcium, an effect that can be seen within hours of drug administration. In the kidney, PTH acts to increase calcium reabsorption while increasing phosphate excretion. At the proximal tubule, PTH acts to decrease phosphate transport, thus facilitating its excretion. Calcium reabsorption is increased by the action of PTH on the distal tubule. A final action of PTH in the kidney is to increase the production of 1,25-hydroxycholecalciferol, the activated form of vitamin D, through stimulation of 1-α-hydroxylase. Activated vitamin D then helps to increase calcium levels by increasing intestinal absorption of both calcium and phosphate.

X-79. **The answer is C.** *(Chap. 335)* Iodine deficiency is the most common worldwide cause of hypothyroidism. Autoimmune, or Hashimoto's, thyroiditis is a common cause in developed countries with dietary iodine supplementation. Histologically, it is characterized by lymphocytic infiltration of the thyroid with activated T cells and B cells. Thyroid cell destruction is thought to be mediated by cytotoxic CD8+ T lymphocytes. Primary hypothyroidism is characterized by an elevation in TSH as the feedback inhibition of the anterior pituitary is diminished. However, patients with hypothyroidism may have low TSH in the setting of secondary hypothyroidism. In this case, a clinical and radiologic evaluation of the pituitary is required. Subclinical hypothyroidism is characterized by abnormalities in the serum levels of TSH but minimal symptoms and often minimal change in the free T_4 level. The rate of development of overt, symptomatic hypothyroidism is about 4% per year, especially in the case of positive TPO antibodies, which are present in 90 to 95% of patients with autoimmune hypothyroidism.

X-80. **The answer is B.** *(Chap. 336)* Primary hyperaldosteronism is suggested by diastolic hypertension without edema, hyposecretion of renin that fails to increase appropriately during volume depletion, and hypersecretion of aldosterone that fails to suppress in response to volume expansion. When signs of hyperaldosteronism are present without a solitary adenoma, these patients have bilateral cortical nodular hyperplasia or nodular hyperplasia. One distinguishing feature between these two conditions is the lack of severe hypokalemia in patients with cortical nodular hyperplasia. After potassium supplementation, patients with cortical nodular hyperplasia, but not patients with primary hyperaldosteronism, may have normal potassium levels. A low-renin state is characteristic of hyperaldosteronism. Conn's syndrome is defined by an aldosterone-secreting adrenal adenoma. Liddle's syndrome resembles hyperaldosteronism clinically and biochemically except that aldosterone levels are low or normal in patients with Liddle's syndrome. The defect in Liddle's syndrome is due to dysregulation of an epithelial Na^+ channel. A rare form of hyperaldosteronism, glucocorticoid-remediable aldosteronism, resembles cortical nodular hyperplasia. Whereas dexamethasone suppression does not affect aldosterone levels in patients with cortical nodular hyperplasia, profound suppression is seen in patients with glucocorticoid-remediable aldosteronism.

X-81. **The answer is A.** *(Chap. 343)* Turner syndrome most frequently results from a 45,X karyotype, but mosaicism (45,X/46,XX) also can result in this disorder. Clinically, Turner syndrome manifests as short stature and primary amenorrhea if presenting in young adulthood. In addition, chronic lymphedema of the hands and feet, nuchal folds, a low hairline, and high arched palate are also common features. To diagnose Turner syndrome, karyotype analysis should be performed. A Barr body results from inactivation of one of the X chromosomes in women and is not seen in males. In Turner syndrome, the Barr body should be absent, but only 50% of individuals with Turner syndrome have the 45,X karyotype. Thus, the diagnosis could be missed in those with mosaicism or other structural abnormalities of the X chromosome.

Multiple comorbid conditions are found in individuals with Turner syndrome, and appropriate screening is recommended. Congenital heart defects affect 30% of women with Turner syndrome, including bicuspid aortic valve, coarctation of the aorta, and aortic root dilatation. An echocardiogram should be performed, and the individual should be assessed with blood pressures in the arms and legs. Hypertension can also be associated with structural abnormalities of the kidney and urinary tract, most commonly horseshoe kidney. A renal ultrasound is also recommended. Autoimmune thyroid disease affects 15–30% of women with Turner syndrome and should be assessed by screening TSH. Other comorbidities that may occur include sensorineural hearing loss, elevated liver function enzymes, osteoporosis, and celiac disease.

X-82. **The answer is B.** *(Chap. 341)* Pathologic gynecomastia develops when the effective ratio of testosterone to estrogen ratio is decreased owing to diminished testosterone production (as in primary testicular failure) or increased estrogen production. The latter may arise from direct estradiol secretion by a testis stimulated by LH or hCG or from an increase in peripheral aromatization of precursor steroids, most notably androstenedione. Elevated androstenedione levels may result from increased secretion by an adrenal tumor (leading to an elevated level of urinary 17-ketosteroids) or decreased hepatic clearance in patients with chronic liver disease. A variety of drugs, including diethylstilbestrol, heroin, digitalis, spironolactone, cimetidine, isoniazid, and tricyclic antidepressants, also can cause gynecomastia. In this patient, the history of paternity and the otherwise normal physical examination indicate that a karyotype is unnecessary, and the bilateral breast enlargement essentially excludes the presence of carcinoma and thus the need for biopsy. The presence of a low LH and testosterone suggests either estrogen or hCG production. Because of the normal testicular examination, a primary testicular tumor is not suspected. Carcinoma of the lung and germ cell tumors both can produce hCG, causing gynecomastia.

X-83. **The answer is E.** *(Chap. 74)* Obesity leads to a major increase in morbidity and mortality. Individuals who are more than 150% of their ideal body weight have as much as a 12-fold increase in mortality. Insulin resistance leading to diabetes mellitus is one of the most prominent features of obesity. The vast majority of patients with type 2 diabetes are obese. Weight loss to a moderate degree may be associated with improvements in insulin sensitivity. Obesity is an independent risk factor for cardiovascular disease. Obesity is associated with hypertension. The impact of obesity on cardiovascular mortality may be seen in persons with BMIs above 25. Obesity is associated with an increased incidence of cholesterol stones. Periodic fasting may increase the supersaturation of bile by decreasing the phospholipid component. Multiple studies have indicated increased mortality from cancer in obese individuals. Some of this increase may result from the increased conversion of androstenedione to estrone in adipose tissue. Obesity decreases chest wall compliance. Restrictive lung defects may occur in these individuals. Sleep apnea and obesity hypoventilation syndrome may occur. Although obesity may be associated with obstructive sleep apnea, it is not typically associated with other forms of chronic obstructive lung disease (COPD).

X-84. **The answer is C.** *(Chap. 349)* Paget disease is a disorder of bone remodeling that affects multiple areas of the skeleton. The prevalence increases with age, and it is more common in men than women. There is wide variation in global prevalence; Western Europe and North America are disproportionately and heavily affected. In autopsy series, 3% of those over the age of 40 have evidence of disease. For reasons that are not clear, the frequency of disease appears to be declining over the past 20 years. A majority of patients with Paget disease are asymptomatic. The etiology of the disease is unknown, though both genetic and environmental factors have been implicated. The central pathophysiology is driven by overactive and overabundant osteoclasts, which erode bone. Accelerated bone formation from recruited osteoblasts leads to woven, poorly structured bone that is prone to fracture and bowing. A viral etiology has been postulated, based on findings of viral inclusion bodies and viral mRNA in osteoclasts of patients with Paget disease. To date no full-length viral genes have been recovered, and virus has never been cultured from Pagetic bone.

X-85.   The answer is D.   *(Chap. 347)*   FHH is inherited as an autosomal dominant trait. It results from a defect in serum calcium sensing by the parathyroid gland and renal tubule, causing inappropriate secretion of PTH and excessive renal reabsorption of calcium. The calcium-sensing receptor is sensitive to extracellular calcium concentration, suppressing PTH secretion and therefore resulting in negative-feedback regulation. Many different mutations in the calcium-sensing receptor have been described in patients with FHH. These mutations lower the ability of the sensor to bind calcium, resulting in excessive secretion of PTH and subsequent hypercalcemia. Urinary excretion of calcium is very low, with reabsorption more than 99%. The hypercalcemia is often detected in the first decade of life. This contrasts with primary hyperparathyroidism, which rarely occurs before age 10. Few clinical signs or symptoms are present in patients with FHH. These patients have excellent outcomes, and surgery or medical therapy is rarely necessary. Jansen's disease refers to mutations in the PTH receptor.

X-86.   The answer is A.   *(Chap. 354)*   Wilson disease is an autosomal recessive disorder caused by mutations in the *ATP7B* gene, which leads to copper accumulation and toxicity. The *ATP7B* gene encodes a membrane-bound copper-transporting ATPase. Deficiency of this protein leads to decreased biliary copper excretion and resultant buildup of copper in the tissues. The two most affected organs are the liver and the brain. Patients may present with hepatitis, cirrhosis, hepatic failure, movement disorders, or psychiatric disorders. Serum copper levels are usually lower than normal due to low blood ceruloplasmin, which usually binds serum copper. About 1% of the population are carriers of an *ATP7B* mutation; the disease is present in 1 in 30,000–40,000. The disease is close to 100% penetrant and requires treatment in almost all cases. DNA haplotype analysis can be used to genotype siblings of an affected patient. Patients are treated with zinc, which induces a negative copper balance by blocking intestinal absorption; trientine, which acts as a potent copper chelator; or both. Severe hepatic decompensation may require liver transplantation.

X-87 and X-88.   The answers are E and E.   *(Chap. 344)*   In patients with a nonmetastatic carcinoid, surgery is the only potentially curative therapy. The extent of surgical resection depends on the size of the primary tumor because the risk of metastasis is related to the size of the tumor. Symptomatic treatment is aimed at decreasing the amount and effect of circulating substances. Drugs that inhibit the serotonin 5-HT$_1$ and 5-HT$_2$ receptors (methysergide, cyproheptadine, ketanserin) may control diarrhea but not flushing. 5-HT$_3$ receptor antagonists (odansetron, tropisetron, alosetron) control nausea and diarrhea in up to 100% of these patients and may alleviate flushing. A combination of histamine H$_1$ and H$_2$ receptor antagonists may control flushing, particularly in patients with foregut carcinoid tumors. Somatostatin analogues (octreotide, lanreotide) are the most effective and widely used agents to control the symptoms of carcinoid syndrome, decreasing urinary 5-HIAA excretion and symptoms in 70 to 80% of patients. Interferon α, alone or combined with hepatic artery embolization, controls flushing and diarrhea in 40 to 85% of these patients. Phenoxybenzamine is an α$_1$-adrenergic receptor blocker that is used in the treatment of pheochromocytoma.

Carcinoid crisis is a life-threatening complication of carcinoid syndrome. It is most common in patients with intense symptoms from foregut tumors or markedly high levels of urinary 5-HIAA. The crisis may be provoked by surgery, stress, anesthesia, chemotherapy, or physical trauma to the tumor (biopsy or, in this case, physical compression of liver lesions). These patients develop severe typical symptoms plus systemic symptoms such as hypotension and hypertension with tachycardia. Synthetic analogues of somatostatin (octreotide, lanreotide) are the treatment of choice for carcinoid crisis. They are also effective in preventing crises when administered before a known inciting event. Octreotide 150 to 250 μg subcutaneously every 6 to 8 h should be started 24 to 48 h before a procedure that is likely to precipitate a carcinoid crisis.

X-89.   The answer is E.   *(Chap. 348)*   Multiple treatment choices are available to prevent fractures and reverse bone loss in osteoporosis, and the side-effect profiles should be carefully considered when making the appropriate choice for this patient. Risedronate belongs to a family of drugs called bisphosphonates. Bisphosphonates act to inhibit osteoclast activity to decrease bone resorption and increase bone mass. Alendronate, risedronate, and ibandronate are approved for treatment of postmenopausal osteoporosis, and alendronate and risedronate are also approved for the treatment of steroid-induced osteoporosis and osteoporosis in men. In clinical trials, risedronate decreases risk of hip and vertebral fracture by 40–50% over 3 years. However, risedronate is not effective in decreasing hip fracture in women over the age of 80. The major side effect of bisphosphonate compounds taken orally is esophagitis. These drugs should be taken with a full glass of water, and the patient should remain upright for 30 min after taking the drug. Estrogens are also effective in preventing and treating osteoporosis. Epidemiologic data indicate that women taking estrogen have a 50% decreased risk of hip fracture. Raloxifene is a selective estrogen receptor modulator (SERM). The effect of raloxifene on bone density is somewhat less than that of estrogen, but it does decrease the risk of vertebral fracture by 30–50%. However, both drugs are contraindicated in this patient because of the recent occurrence of venous thromboembolic disease. Both estrogen and SERMs increase the risk of DVT and pulmonary embolus several-fold. If estrogen is to be used, it should be used in combination with a progestin compound in women with an intact uterus to decrease the risk of uterine cancer associated with unopposed estrogen stimulation. Calcium and vitamin D supplementation are recommended, but given the degree of osteoporosis are inadequate alone. Calcitonin is available as an intranasal spray a1nd produces small increases in bone density, but it has no proven effectiveness on prevention of fractures.

X-90.   The answer is B. *(Chap. 333)* Hyperprolactinemia is the most common pituitary hormone secretion syndrome in men and women. Prolactin-secreting pituitary adenomas (prolactinomas) are the most common cause of high prolactin levels. Hyperprolactinemia has a wide array of etiologies. Pregnancy and lactation are physiologic causes of increased prolactin levels. Chronic renal failure increases prolactin levels by decreasing clearance. Nipple stimulation and sexual orgasm both can increase prolactin release into the blood. Chest wall trauma, including surgery and herpes zoster infection, can induce prolactin secretion likely by activating a reflex suckling arc. Primary hypothyroidism can cause mild hyperprolactinemia due to compensatory thyrotropin-releasing hormone secretion. Many drugs including dopamine receptor blockers (phenothiazines, haloperidol, metoclopramide), opiates, H_2 blockers, serotonin reuptake inhibitors (fluoxetine), verapamil, estrogens, and antiestrogens are associated with prolactin hypersecretion. Hyperthyroidism is not associated with increased prolactin levels.

X-91.   The answer is A. *(Chap. 345)* This patient's clinical scenario is most consistent with MEN 1, or the "3 Ps": parathyroid, pituitary, and pancreas. MEN 1 is an autosomal dominant genetic syndrome characterized by neoplasia of the parathyroid, pituitary, and pancreatic islet cells. Hyperparathyroidism is the most common manifestation of MEN 1. The neoplastic changes affect multiple parathyroid glands, making surgical care difficult. Pancreatic islet cell neoplasia is the second most common manifestation of MEN 1. Increased pancreatic islet cell hormones include pancreatic polypeptide, gastrin, insulin, vasoactive intestinal peptide, glucagons, and somatostatin. Pancreatic tumors may be multicentric, and up to 30% are malignant, with the liver being the first site of metastases. The symptoms depend on the type of hormone secreted. Elevations of gastrin result in the Zollinger-Ellison syndrome (ZES). Gastrin levels are elevated, resulting in an ulcer diathesis. Conservative therapy is often unsuccessful. Insulinoma results in documented hypoglycemia with elevated insulin and C-peptide levels. Glucagonoma results in hyperglycemia, skin rash, anorexia, glossitis, and diarrhea. Elevations in vasoactive intestinal peptide result in profuse watery diarrhea. Pituitary tumors occur in up to half of patients with MEN 1. Prolactinomas are the most common. The multicentricity of the tumors makes resection difficult. Growth hormone–secreting tumors are the next most common, with ACTH- and corticotropin-releasing hormone (CRH)-secreting tumors being more rare. Carcinoid tumors may also occur in the thymus, lung, stomach, and duodenum.

X-92. **The answer is C.** *(Chap. 350)* This patient has nephrotic syndrome, which is likely a result of multiple myeloma. The hyperlipidemia of nephrotic syndrome appears to be due to a combination of increased hepatic production and decreased clearance of very low density lipoproteins, with increased LDL production. It is usually mixed but can manifest as hypercholesterolemia or hypertriglyceridemia. Effective treatment of the underlying renal disease normalizes the lipid profile. Of the choices presented, HMG-CoA reductase inhibitors would be the most effective to reduce this patient's LDL. Dietary management is an important component of lifestyle modification but seldom results in a >10% fall in LDL. Niacin and fibrates would be indicated if the triglycerides were higher, but the LDL is the more important lipid abnormality to address at this time. Lipid apheresis is reserved for patients who cannot tolerate the lipid-lowering drugs or who have a genetic lipid disorder refractory to medication. Cholesterol ester transfer protein inhibitors have been shown to raise high-density lipoprotein levels and their role in the treatment of lipoproteinemias is still under investigation.

X-93. **The answer is B.** *(Chap. 336)* Incidental adrenal masses are often discovered during radiographic testing for another condition and are found in ~6% of adult subjects at autopsy. Fifty percent of patients with a history of malignancy and a newly discovered adrenal mass will actually have an adrenal metastasis. Fine-needle aspiration of a suspected metastatic malignancy will often be diagnostic. In the absence of a suspected nonadrenal malignancy, most adrenal incidentalomas are benign. Primary adrenal malignancies are uncommon (<0.01%), and fine-needle aspiration is not useful to distinguish between benign and malignant primary adrenal tumors. Although 90% of these masses are nonsecretory, patients with an incidentaloma should be screened for pheochromocytoma and hypercortisolism with plasma free metanephrines and an overnight dexamethasone suppression test, respectively. When radiographic features suggest a benign neoplasm (<3 cm), scanning should be repeated in 3–6 months. When masses are >6 cm, surgical removal (if more likely primary adrenal malignancy) or fine-needle aspiration (if more likely metastatic malignancy) is preferred.

X-94. **The answer is C.** *(Chap. 338; Nathan, N Engl J Med 328:1676–1685, 1993.)* Nephropathy is a leading cause of death in diabetic patients. Diabetic nephropathy may be functionally silent for 10 to 15 years. Clinically detectable diabetic nephropathy begins with the development of microalbuminuria (30 to 300 mg of albumin per 24 h). The glomerular filtration rate actually may be elevated at this stage. Only after the passage of additional time will the proteinuria be overt enough (0.5 g/L) to be detectable on standard urine dipsticks. Microalbuminuria precedes nephropathy in patients with both non-insulin-dependent and insulin-dependent diabetes. An increase in kidney size also may accompany the initial hyperfiltration stage. Once the proteinuria becomes significant enough to be detected by dipstick, a steady decline in renal function occurs, with the glomerular filtration rate falling an average of 1 mL/min per month. Therefore, azotemia begins about 12 years after the diagnosis of diabetes. Hypertension clearly is an exacerbating factor for diabetic nephropathy.

X-95. **The answer is C.** *(Chap. 353)* Lesch-Nyhan syndrome is characterized by complete absence of the enzyme hypoxanthine phosphoribosyltransferase (HPRT), a component of purine metabolism that is related to purine recycling into guanosine monophosphate and inosine monophosphate. Hyperuricemia develops from urate overproduction. The gene for HPRT is located on the X-chromosome, so Lesch-Nyhan disease is transmitted as an X-linked disorder. Homozygous males have the disease, and heterozygous carrier females are asymptomatic. Therefore, the daughter of a carrier has a 50% chance of being a carrier and a son has a 50% chance of having the disease. Carrier females do not have an increased risk of gout or urate nephropathy. Lesch-Nyhan syndrome is characterized by hyperuricemia, gouty arthritis, nephrolithiasis, self-mutilative behavior, choreoathetosis, and mental retardation. Treatment of affected patients with allopurinol will eliminate or prevent the problems related to hyperuricemia but will not have any beneficial effect on the behavioral or neurologic manifestations. Since it is an X-linked disorder, screening the husband has no value.

XI. NEUROLOGIC DISORDERS

QUESTIONS

DIRECTIONS: Choose the **one best** response to each question.

XI-1. Delirium, an acute confusional state, is a common disorder that remains a major cause of morbidity and mortality in the United States. Which patient is at the highest risk for developing delirium?

A. A 36-year-old man admitted to the medical ward with a deep venous thrombosis
B. A 55-year-old man postoperative day 2 from a total colectomy
C. A 68-year-old woman admitted to the intensive care unit (ICU) with esophageal rupture
D. A 74-year-old woman in the preoperative clinic before hip surgery
E. An 84-year-old man living in an assisted living facility

XI-2. A 46-year-old man presents for evaluation of severe unilateral headache. He states that he has had episodes of intermittent headache for the past 3 years. He describes the headaches as a stabbing pain located near his right temple. They occur abruptly and last up to 3 h at a time, during which he feels incapacitated, rating the pain as a 10 out of 10. Most of the time, the headaches begin in the early morning hours. When they occur, he finds it impossible to sleep. He feels that rubbing his head improves the pain but has noticed no other factors that relieve the pain. Specifically, he has had no improvement with acetaminophen, naprosyn, or oxycodone. When the headaches occur, he develops nasal congestion and tearing on the side of the pain. He believes the headaches occur in cycles. He will have the headaches almost daily for up to 2 weeks at a time, but then have no headaches at all for as long as 3 months. He has decided to seek medical advice because he is worried about the possibility of a brain tumor because of the severity of the headaches. He takes no medicines regularly. His vital signs and physical examination are normal. What is the best approach to treatment of these headaches?

A. Fluticasone nasal spray and loratadine, 10 mg orally
B. Indomethacin, 25 mg three times daily
C. Oxygen at 10–12 L/min by nasal cannula at the onset of an attack

XI-2. *(Continued)*
D. Sumatriptan, 50 mg orally, at the onset of an attack
E. Surgical consultation for microvascular decompression of the trigeminal nerve

XI-3. You are seeing your patient with polymyositis in follow-up. He has been taking prednisone at high doses for 2 months, and you initiated mycophenolate mofetil at the last clinic visit for a steroid-sparing effect. He began a steroid taper 2 weeks ago. His symptoms were predominantly in the lower extremities and face, and he has improved considerably. He no longer needs a cane and his voice has returned to normal. Laboratory data show a creatine kinase (CK) of 1300 U/L, which is unchanged from 2 months ago. What is the most appropriate next step in this patient's management?

A. Continue current management
B. Continue high-dose steroids with no taper
C. Switch mycophenolate to methotrexate
D. Repeat muscle biopsy

XI-4. A patient complains of numbness in his neck. Over months, the numbness has become more pronounced and involves a dense area bilaterally from the sternal notch to the area behind the ear. On examination, scalp sensation, cranial nerve function, and upper extremity motor examination are normal. The patient has decreased pain and temperature sensation in the distribution of C4. Vibration sense is normal. Cranial and caudal to the affected area, sensation is intact. Bladder and anal sphincter function are also normal. What is the most likely cause of this patient's neurologic disorder?

A. Amyotrophic lateral sclerosis
B. Disc herniation
C. Intramedullary tumor
D. Knife or bullet injury
E. Neurosyphilis

XI-5. A 56-year-old male is admitted to the intensive care unit with a hypertensive crisis after cocaine use. Initial blood pressure is 245/132. On physical examination the patient is

XI-5. *(Continued)*

unresponsive except to painful stimuli. He has been intubated for airway protection and is being mechanically ventilated, with a respiratory rate of 14. His pupils are reactive to light, and there are normal corneal, cough, and gag reflexes. The patient has a dense left hemiparesis. When presented with painful stimuli, the patient responds with flexure posturing on the right side. Computed tomography (CT) reveals a large area of intracranial bleeding in the right frontoparietal area. Over the next several hours the patient deteriorates. The most recent examination reveals a blood pressure of 189/100. The patient now has a dilated pupil on the right side. The patient continues to have corneal reflexes. You suspect rising intracranial pressure related to the intracranial bleed. All but which of the following can be done to decrease the patient's intracranial pressure?

A. Administer intravenous mannitol at a dose of 1 g/kg body weight.
B. Administer hypertonic fluids to achieve a goal sodium level of 155 to 160 meq/L.
C. Consult neurosurgery for an urgent ventriculostomy.
D. Initiate intravenous nitroprusside to decrease the mean arterial pressure to a goal of 100 mmHg.
E. Increase the respiratory rate to 30.

XI-6. What percentage of cigarette smokers will die prematurely if they are unable to quit?

A. 2%
B. 10%
C. 40%
D. 70%

XI-7. For the last 5 weeks a 35-year-old female has had episodes of intense vertigo that last several hours. Each episode is associated with tinnitus and a sense of fullness in the right ear; during the attacks she prefers to lie on the left side. Examination during an attack shows that she has fine rotary nystagmus that is maximal on gaze to the left. There are no ocular palsies, cranial nerve signs, or long-tract signs. An audiogram shows high-tone hearing loss in the right ear, with recruitment but no tone decay. The most likely diagnosis in this case is

A. labyrinthitis
B. Ménière's disease
C. vertebral-basilar insufficiency
D. acoustic neuroma
E. multiple sclerosis

XI-8. Lumbar puncture should be preceded by CT or MRI in all of the following subsets of patients suspected of having meningitis *except* those with:

A. depressed consciousness
B. focal neurologic abnormality
C. known central nervous system (CNS) mass lesion
D. positive Kernig's sign
E. recent head trauma

XI-9. You are a physician practicing in a small community in the Rocky Mountains near Aspen, Colorado. A 33-year-old female comes to your office for evaluation of a bilateral tingling sensation in the fingertips. She describes the sensation as affecting all the fingers on both hands. She has no medical problems and takes no medications. She is a vegetarian and is visiting the area from San Diego, California. She denies any other symptoms, including headache, nausea, vomiting, shortness of breath, and urinary frequency. On physical examination the patient has a normal sensory examination, including reaction to light touch and pinprick and vibratory sensation. She is able to stand normally with the arms extended and the eyes closed. A cerebellar examination reveals normal finger-to-nose testing and no dysdiadochokinesis. Her gait is normal, including tandem gait, toe walking, and heel walking. What would you recommend as the next step?

A. Blood tests for serum vitamin B_{12}
B. Fasting blood glucose level
C. Reassurance
D. Serologic testing for syphilis
E. Treatment with acetazolamide for altitude sickness

XI-10. You are doing rounds and see a patient admitted with weakness. He is a 46-year-old man who noticed the acute onset of facial weakness and slurred speech 1 day prior to presentation. At the onset of his symptoms, he also complained of right arm weakness and double vision. He went to bed and woke up the next morning without any residual neurologic deficits. He came to the emergency department for evaluation. On examination of the patient on evening rounds, you note 3/5 weakness in the upper and lower extremities, with increasing weakness with exertion. He has intact phonation and mental status, but you also note a disconjugate gaze. He denies any pain. Sensation is intact. What is the most likely location of his neurologic disease?

A. Brainstem
B. Muscle
C. Neuromuscular junction
D. Peripheral nerve
E. Spinal root

XI-11. A 34-year-old female complains of lower extremity weakness for the last 3 days. She has noted progressive weakness in the lower extremities with loss of sensation "below the belly button" and incontinence. She had had some low-grade fevers for the last week. She denies recent travel. Past medical history is unremarkable. Physical examination is notable for a sensory level at the level of the umbilicus. The lower extremities show +3/5 strength bilaterally proximally and distally. Reflexes, cerebellar examination, and mental status are normal. All the following are appropriate steps in evaluating this patient *except*

A. antinuclear antibodies
B. electromyography
C. lumbar puncture

XI-11. (*Continued*)

D. MRI of the spine

E. viral serologies

XI-12. Which clinical signs would you expect in a 53-year-old man with gait ataxia and these MRI findings (see Figure XI-12)?

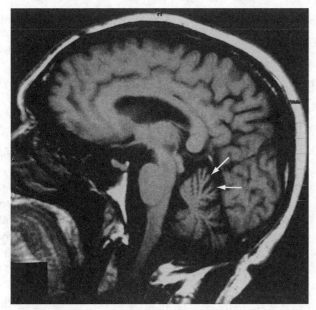

FIGURE XI-12

A. Gait instability, urinary incontinence, dementia

B. Hypertension, tachycardia, diaphoresis

C. Migraine headache, limb weakness, breathing difficulties

D. Scanning speech, oscillatory tremor of the head, nystagmus

XI-13. A 17-year-old adolescent is seen in clinic several weeks after he suffered a concussion during a high-school football game. At the time of the event, paramedics reported that he experienced no loss of consciousness but was confused for a period of about 10 min. Head imaging was normal. He describes a generalized headache that is present all the time since his trauma, and he occasionally feels dizzy. His mother is concerned that he is having a hard time concentrating in school and seems depressed to her lately; she describes him as very energetic prior to his concussion. The patient's physical examination is entirely normal except for a somewhat flattened affect. Which of the following statements regarding his condition is true?

A. He has an excellent prognosis.

B. He meets criteria for postconcussive syndrome and should improve over 1–2 months.

C. He should avoid contact sports for the next month.

D. He is most likely malingering.

E. Low-dose narcotics should be started for headache.

XI-14. Variant Creutzfeldt-Jakob disease (vCJD) has been diagnosed in which of the following populations?

XI-14. (*Continued*)

A. Family members with well-defined germ-line mutations leading to autosomal dominant inheritance of a fatal neurodegenerative disease

B. New Guinea natives practicing cannibalism

C. Patients accidentally inoculated with infected material during surgical procedures

D. Worldwide, in sporadic cases mostly during the fifth and sixth decades of life

E. Young adults in Europe thought to have been exposed to tainted beef products

XI-15. A 44-year-old man with a history of hypertension and Paget's disease has had lower back pain for the past 3 months. The pain is worse with standing and improves with sitting. Walking does not necessarily exacerbate his symptoms. He has no leg or buttock pain. On examination, he has mild weakness on the right at the hip flexors, knee extenders, and knee flexors and more distally to the same degree. Reflexes are diminished in the right lower extremity. He has no sensory findings in the lower extremities or in the perineum. What is the most likely diagnosis?

A. Intervertebral disk herniation

B. Lumbar spinal stenosis

C. Metastatic malignancy

D. Occlusive aortoiliac atherosclerosis

E. Tethered cord syndrome

XI-16. On the neurologic consultation service, you are asked to evaluate a patient with mesial temporal lobe epilepsy syndrome. The patient has a history of intractable complex partial seizures that rarely generalize. Her seizures often begin with an aura and commonly manifest as behavioral arrests, complex automatisms, and unilateral posturing. MRI findings include small temporal lobes and a small hippocampus with increased signal on T2-weighted sequences. Which of these additional historic factors are also likely to be present in this patient?

A. History of febrile seizures

B. Hypothyroidism

C. Neurofibromas

D. Recurring genital ulcers

E. Type 2 diabetes mellitus

XI-17. The patient in the preceding scenario was admitted with refractory seizures. You are asked to see the patient and offer treatment options. What treatment option will be the most efficacious in a patient with mesial temporal lobe epilepsy (MTLE) syndrome?

A. Acyclovir

B. Amygdalohippocampectomy

C. Levetiracetam

D. Primidone

E. Vagus nerve stimulation

XI-18. The deep tendon reflex requires all of the following structures to be functional *except*

XI-18. *(Continued)*

A. α motor neurons
B. γ motor neurons
C. pyramidal neurons
D. spindle afferent neurons

XI-19. The most common presenting finding or symptom of multiple sclerosis is

A. internuclear ophthalmoplegia
B. transverse myelitis
C. cerebellar ataxia
D. optic neuritis
E. urinary retention

XI-20. You are evaluating a patient with neck pain and you suspect cervical degenerative disk disease based on the history. Based on the most common findings with cervical disk disease, which finding do you expect when you examine this patient?

A. Biceps weakness
B. Decreased light touch sensation in the axilla and medial arm
C. Decreased pin-prick sensation over the lateral deltoid
D. Weak finger flexors

XI-21. A 64-year-old woman is brought to the emergency department by her family complaining of weakness. The patient reports difficulty walking and frequent falls. She also has blurry vision bilaterally. She denies light headedness or vertigo. These symptoms have been present for at least the past 9 months and are getting progressively worse. She has great difficulty walking from the waiting room to the examination room but is not dizzy while doing so. On further questioning she denies numbness or tingling. On physical examination, her cranial nerves are intact, and strength examination shows 5 out of 5 strength in both upper and lower extremities. Reflexes are normal throughout. Light touch sensation is normal, and she is not orthostatic. You order a noncontrast head CT and it is read as normal. Which test is most likely to reveal the correct diagnosis?

A. Cerebrospinal fluid viral polymerase chain reaction
B. Lithium level
C. Rapid plasma reagent (RPR)
D. Serum alcohol level
E. Vitamin B_{12} deficiency

XI-22. A 78-year-old female with a long history of vascular disease presents after an embolic cerebrovascular accident (CVA) with severe and unrelenting pain on the right side. She describes the pain as burning as if she had been bathed in acid. Where is the most likely site of the recent embolic CVA?

A. Frontal lobe
B. Hypothalamus
C. Pons
D. Temporal lobe
E. Thalamus

XI-23. You are counseling your patient on the need to quit smoking cigarettes. She has been smoking for over two decades and wants to quit in order to avoid the harmful physical effects of smoking. Wanting to take "baby steps," she has switched to low-tar, low-nicotine cigarettes. Which of the following statements is true about the potential benefit of switching to these low-yield cigarettes?

A. Fewer smoking-drug interactions are found among smokers of low-yield cigarettes.
B. Most smokers inhale the same amount of nicotine and tar even if they switch to low-yield cigarettes.
C. Smoking low-yield cigarettes decreases the harmful cardiovascular effects of cigarette smoking.
D. Smoking low-yield cigarettes is a reasonable alternative to complete smoking cessation for chronic smokers.

XI-24. A 34-year-old man complains of 1 week of dizziness, vertigo, tinnitus, and right-sided gait ataxia. Electronystagmography (calorics) with sequential administration of warm and cold water into the ear canal is performed. On the left, cold water causes right-beating nystagmus and warm water causes left-beating nystagmus. On the right ear, there is no response to the cold caloric. What is the cause of this patient's dizziness and vertigo?

A. Acoustic neuroma
B. Aminoglycoside antibiotics
C. Cerebellar ischemia
D. Otoconia (ear otoliths)

XI-25. A 49-year-old man is admitted to the hospital with a seizure. He does not have a history of seizures and he currently takes no medications. He has AIDS and is not under any care at this time. His physical examination is most notable for small, shoddy lymphadenopathy in the cervical region. A head CT shows a ring-enhancing lesion in the right temporal lobe, with edema but no mass effect. A lumbar puncture shows no white or red blood cells, and the Gram stain is negative. His serum *Toxoplasma* IgG is positive. Which of the following is the best course of action for this patient at this time?

A. Biopsy of the central nervous system (CNS) lesion
B. Dexamethasone
C. Search for systemic malignancy
D. Treatment for CNS toxoplasmosis
E. Whole-brain radiation therapy

XI-26. The patient in the preceding scenario returns for reevaluation after 2 weeks of appropriate therapy. The CNS lesion has not changed in size, and he has not had any more seizures. All microbiologic cultures and viral studies, including Epstein-Barr virus DNA from the cerebrospinal fluid are negative. What is the best course of action for this patient at this time?

A. Continue treatment for CNS toxoplasmosis
B. Dexamethasone
C. Intravenous acyclovir

XI-26. *(Continued)*

   D.   Stereotactic brain biopsy
   E.   Whole-brain radiation therapy

XI-27. Which of the following statements about syringomyelia is true?

   A.   More than half the cases are associated with Chiari
        malformations.
   B.   Symptoms typically begin in middle age.
   C.   Vibration and position sensation are usually dimin-
        ished.
   D.   Syrinx cavities are always congenital.
   E.   Neurosurgical decompression is usually effective in
        relieving the symptoms.

XI-28. A 34-year-old female complains of weakness and
double vision for the last 3 weeks. She has also noted a
change in her speech, and her friends tell her that she is
"more nasal." She has noticed decreased exercise tolerance and difficulty lifting objects and getting out of a
chair. The patient denies pain. The symptoms are worse
at the end of the day and with repeated muscle use. You
suspect myasthenia gravis. All the following are useful in
the diagnosis of myasthenia gravis *except*

   A.   acetylcholine receptor (AChR) antibodies
   B.   edrophonium
   C.   electrodiagnostic testing
   D.   muscle-specific kinase (MuSK) antibodies
   E.   voltage-gated calcium channel antibodies

XI-29. A 49-year-old woman presents for a second opinion
regarding symptoms of tremors, difficulty with ambulation, and periodic flushing. Her symptoms originally began
~3 years ago. At that time, she was hospitalized for a syncopal episode, after which she was told to increase her salt intake. Since then, she has had progressive motor difficulties
including bilateral tremors and a stiff slow gait. She also has
had several more episodes of syncope. She states that she
knows when these syncopal events will occur because she
feels faint and weak. She has never had an injury from syncope. A final recent symptom has been periodic flushing
and sweating. A neurologist previously diagnosed her with
Parkinson's disease and prescribed therapy with ropinirole.
Despite increasing doses, she does not feel improved, but
rather has recently noticed uncontrollable movements that
she describes at tics of her face. Her only other medical history is recent recurrent urinary tract infections. Her medications are ropinirole, 24 mg daily, and nitrofurantoin, 100
mg daily. She reports no history of drug use. On physical
examination, her blood pressure is 130/70 mmHg with a
heart rate of 78 beats/min while sitting. Upon standing, her
blood pressure drops to 90/50 mmHg with a heart rate of
110 beats/min. Her ocular movements are full and intact.
She has recurrent motor movements of the right side of her
face. Her neurologic examination shows increased muscle
tone in the lower extremities with bilateral 4-Hz tremor.
Deep tendon reflexes are brisk and 3+ in upper and lower

XI-29. *(Continued)*

extremities. Three beats of myoclonus is present at the ankles bilaterally. She walks with a spastic gait. Strength is
normal. What is the most likely diagnosis?

   A.   Corticobasal degeneration
   B.   Diffuse Lewy body dementia
   C.   Drug-induced Parkinson's disease
   D.   Multiple systems atrophy with parkinsonian fea-
        tures (Shy-Drager syndrome)
   E.   Parkinson's disease with inadequate treatment

XI-30. A 68-year-old man is brought to clinic for evaluation by his wife. She has noticed that over past 2–3
months he's had increasingly slowed thinking and a
change in his personality in that he's become very withdrawn. His only complaint is a mild, but persistent, diffuse headache. There is no history of head trauma, prior
neurologic or psychiatric disease, or family history of dementia. Physical examination is only notable for a moderate cognitive deficit with a mini-mental examination of
19/30. His head CT is shown in Figure XI-30. What is the
most likely diagnosis?

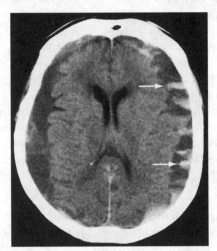

FIGURE XI-30

   A.   Acute epidural hematoma
   B.   Acute subarachnoid hemorrhage
   C.   Alzheimer's disease
   D.   Chronic subdural hematoma
   E.   Normal-pressure hydrocephalus

XI-31. You are evaluating a patient who complains of vertigo. The patient complains of seeing the room spin and
feeling faint with certain head movements to the left. In
your office, you perform provocative maneuvers to differentiate the cause of this patient's vertigo. He has been diagnosed with benign paroxysmal positional vertigo
(BPPV), but symptoms have remained for many months.
Which of the following findings would be suggestive of a
central positional vertigo?

   A.   Disappearance of the symptoms with maintenance
        of the offending position

XI-31. *(Continued)*

B.   Immediate vertigo and nystagmus with head turning to the affected side

C.   Lessening of symptoms with repeated trials

D.   Increased severity of symptoms with provocative testing

XI-32. A 65-year-old man presents to your office complaining of a tremor and progressive gait abnormalities. He states that he first noticed a slowing of his gait ~6 months ago. He has difficulty rising to a standing position and states that he shuffles when he walks. In addition, he states that his right hand shakes more so than his left, and he is right-handed. He believes it to be worse when not moving but states there are times when he spills his morning coffee because of the tremors. He has retired but states he is not able to play tennis and golf any longer because of his motor symptoms. He denies syncope or presyncope, difficulty swallowing, changes to his voice, or memory difficulties. His past medical history is significant for hypertension and hypercholesterolemia. His medications are hydrochlorothiazide, 25 mg daily, ezetimibe, 10 mg daily, and lovastatin, 40 mg daily. He drinks a glass of wine with dinner daily and is a lifelong nonsmoker. On physical examination, he has masked facies. His gait shows decreased arm swing with slow shuffling steps. He turns en bloc. A pill-rolling tremor is present on the right side. There is cogwheel rigidity bilaterally. Eye movements are full and intact. There is no orthostatic hypotension. A brain MRI with gadolinium shows no evidence of mass lesions, hydrocephalus, or vascular disease. You diagnose the patient with Parkinson's disease. The patient asks about his prognosis and likelihood of disability. Which of the following is correct about the clinical course and treatment of Parkinson's disease?

A.   Early initiation of therapy with levodopa predisposes an individual to a higher likelihood of dyskinesias early in the disease.

B.   Early therapy with bilateral deep-brain stimulation of the subthalamic nuclei slows progression of Parkinson's disease.

C.   Initial treatment with a dopamine agonist such as pramipexole is likely to be effective in controlling his motor symptoms for 1–3 years before the addition of levodopa or another agent is necessary.

D.   Levodopa should be started immediately to prevent development of disabling rigidity.

E.   Monotherapy with selegiline, a monoamine oxydase (MAO) inhibitor, causes a marked improvement in tremors in most individuals with Parkinson's disease.

XI-33. A 74-year-old woman comes to clinic complaining of muscle weakness. She has bilateral deltoid weakness, which has been present for 4 months. She has myalgias as well throughout the day. Her symptoms are exacerbated by activity and when she initially lays down to sleep. Neu-

XI-33. *(Continued)*

rologic examination shows intact cranial nerves II through XII, except for poor vision due to cataracts. She has hyperesthesia in her arms in the area of her deltoids, but otherwise sensation is normal. Deep tendon reflexes are normal. Strength examination shows weakness initially, but it improves with encouragement. Creatine kinase, erythrocyte sedimentation rate, and C-reactive protein are within normal limits. An MRI of the deltoid muscles shows joint degeneration and a partial rotator cuff tear on the left. You are considering a muscle biopsy. What is the biopsy most likely to show?

A.   Endomysial deposits of amyloid

B.   Necrotic muscle

C.   Normal muscle

D.   Scattered inflammatory foci surrounding muscle fibers

XI-34. Which of the following criteria suggests the diagnosis of trigeminal neuralgia?

A.   Deep-seated steady facial pain

B.   Elevated erythrocyte sedimentation rate (ESR)

C.   Known metastatic brain tumor

D.   Objective signs of sensory loss on physical examination

E.   Response to gabapentin therapy

F.   None of the above

XI-35. CT scanning is superior to MRI of the back in which setting?

A.   Delineation of the extent of a syrinx

B.   Evaluation of old lumbar-spine fracture

C.   Evaluation of paraspinal mass

D.   Imaging of the lateral recesses of the spinal canal

XI-36. All the following cause primarily a sensory neuropathy *except*

A.   acromegaly

B.   critical illness

C.   HIV infection

D.   hypothyroidism

E.   vitamin B_{12} deficiency

XI-37. A 45-year-old woman presents for evaluation of a tingling sensation in her feet that has become more apparent over the past 5 months. She states that it currently is causing a painful sensation and is interfering with her sleep at night. On physical examination, you identify decreased sensation to pinprick and light touch in her feet extending to her mid-calf area. All of the following laboratory tests may be useful in determining the cause of her peripheral neuropathy *except*

A.   blood lead level

B.   fasting blood glucose

C.   hemoglobin A1C

D.   rapid plasma reagin for syphilis

E.   red blood cell folate levels

XI-38. A young man with a history of a low-grade astrocytoma comes into your office complaining of weight gain and low energy. He is status post resection of his low-grade astrocytoma and had a course of whole-brain radiation therapy (WBRT) 1 year ago. A laboratory workup reveals a decreased morning cortisol level of 1.9 µg/dL. In addition to depressed adrenocorticotropic hormone (ACTH) function, which of the following hormones is most sensitive to damage from whole-brain radiation therapy?

A. Growth hormone
B. Follicle stimulating hormone
C. Prolactin
D. Thyroid stimulating hormone

XI-39. A 29-year-old man being treated for lung cancer comes into your office for an acute visit. He has had backache for a few weeks that has improved with ibuprofen but has developed right lower abdominal pain and inguinal pain. On physical examination, he has tenderness over the lower thoracic spinous processes and hyperesthesia in the T11 distribution on the right. Strength is normal in the upper extremities, but he has symmetric weakness in the lower extremities with hyperreflexia. He also has decreased sensation below the T11 distribution symmetrically. What is the next step in the management of this patient?

A. Add gabapentin to his pain regimen.
B. Order a paraneoplastic antibody panel.
C. Start treatment with glucocorticoids.
D. Order thoracic and lumbar radiographs.

XI-40. A 50-year-old man complains of weakness. His symptoms began as difficulty with buttoning his shirt and using keys to open doors about 2 years ago. He was treated empirically with nonsteroidal anti-inflammatory medications for arthritis, but responded only minimally. His symptoms have slowly progressed to the point where he has weakness in both hands and feet. He avoids going outside because of frequent falls. On examination, he has weakness and atrophy of the foot extensor and finger flexors. Proximal muscle strength is normal. Reflexes are normal, and sensation is intact. He is able to rise out of a chair, but the Romberg test is not able to be performed due to weakness once standing. Cranial nerves are intact. Serum creatine kinase is 600 U/L. Complete blood count, differential, electrolytes, and thyroid-stimulating hormone (TSH) are normal. Based on the clinical presentation, what is the most likely diagnosis?

A. Dermatomyositis
B. Eosinophilic myofasciitis
C. Inclusion body myositis
D. Polymyositis
E. Hyperthyroidism

XI-41. You are conducting research on a cellular model of myasthenia gravis in which you measure features of the acetylcholine (ACh) neuromuscular junction and its mi-

XI-41. *(Continued)*
croenvironment. In a patient with untreated myasthenia gravis, which of the following do you expect to find at the neuromuscular junction after release of ACh from the presynaptic neuron?

A. Decreased levels of ACh-esterase
B. Decreased numbers of available ACh receptors
C. Decreased released of ACh from the presynaptic neuron
D. High numbers of mitochondria in the postsynaptic neuron

XI-42. You have just admitted a young man with a prior history of seizure disorder who was witnessed to have a seizure. His family's description suggests a simple partial seizure involving the left hand that spread to involve the entire arm. He did not lose consciousness. He was brought in 2 h after symptom onset and is currently awake, alert, and oriented. He has not had any further seizures but has been unable to move his left hand since his seizure. His electrolytes and complete blood count are within normal limits. A noncontrast CT scan of his head is unremarkable. On examination, sensation is intact in the affected limb but his strength is 0 out of 5 in the musculature of the left hand. What is the best course of action at this time?

A. Cerebral angiogram
B. Lumbar puncture
C. Magnetic resonance angiogram
D. Psychiatric evaluation
E. Reassess in a few hours

XI-43. A 78-year-old man with diabetes mellitus presents with fever, headache and altered sensorium. On physical exam his temperature is 40.2°C, heart rate is 103 beats/min, blood pressure is 84/52 mmHg. His neck is stiff and he has photophobia. His cerebrospinal fluid (CSF) examination shows 2100 cells/µL, with 100% neutrophils, glucose 10 mg/dL, and protein 78 mg/dL. CSF gram stain is negative. Empirical therapy should include which of the following?

A. Amphotericin
B. Dexamethasone after antibiotics
C. Dexamethasone prior to antibiotics
D. Doxycycline
E. Piperacillin/tazobactam

XI-44. A 24-year-old woman seeks evaluation for headaches. She first began having recurrent headaches her senior year of high school. The headaches increased in frequency during college, and she has always attributed her headaches to tension. The headaches would be more prominent during times of sleep loss, stress, and in the perimenstrual period. She states that she expected her headaches to improve now that she has finished college and has a more regular schedule. She works as a financial counselor for a university in the human resources department and denies a large degree of stress in her job. She has had this job for 2 years, but the

XI-44. *(Continued)*

headaches continue to disrupt her life. She states the headaches occur about seven times monthly. She estimates that the headaches occur >90% of the time on the right side and have a throbbing nature. She has no aura before the onset of a headache but describes occasional visual disturbance and photophobia during the headache. She also states that she frequently develops sensitivity of her scalp on the side of the headache with associated paresthesias. She rates the pain as about 7 to 8 out of 10 for a usual headache. On two occasions over the past 6 months, she has developed severe vertigo that resolved over the course of several hours in association with a mild headache. She has never had to miss work because of headache, but feels like her productivity is limited when she feels unwell. Other triggers for her headaches include red wine and aged cheese, which she has restricted from her diet for this reason. Ibuprofen, acetaminophen, and naprosyn sodium have no effect on the duration of her headaches. She is otherwise healthy and denies associated rhinorrhea or lacrimation. Her only medication is oral contraceptive pills. Her family history is significant for a maternal aunt with classic migraine headaches with aura. The physical examination is normal without any evidence of neurologic deficits and normal blood pressure. What is the most appropriate next step in evaluation and management of this patient?

A. Ask the subject to keep a headache diary for the next 2 months to assess the frequency and severity of headaches and assess for specific triggers.

B. Encourage the patient to keep a regular routine including consistent sleep-wake cycle and regular exercise such as yoga.

C. Initiate therapy with rizatriptan, 10 mg orally, at onset of attacks.

D. Perform an MRI of the brain.

E. A, B, and C

F. All of the above

XI-45. Which of the following cranial nerve physical examination techniques represents the correct approach to the patient with suspected neurologic disease?

A. Olfactory nerve: With eyes closed, ask the patient to sniff a pungent stimulus such as ammonia or alcohol.

B. Optic nerve: Check visual acuity in both eyes using a Snellen chart without having the patient use their corrective lenses.

C. Trigeminal nerve: Examine the motor territories on each side of the face by testing jaw clench, eyebrow elevation and forehead wrinkling.

D. Accessory nerve: Check shoulder shrug and head rotation on each side against resistance.

XI-46. You are going on morning rounds to see a 38-year-old woman who presented the prior day with weakness and double vision. It is reported that on examination at that time she had pronounced weakness in cranial nerves VII

XI-46. *(Continued)*

and XII. She also had weakness in the extraocular muscles, which is described to you as "googly eyes" with repeat examinations. The patient reports that she has profound double vision almost exclusively when she watches television in the evening. On your examination, you find no neurologic abnormalities. A head CT is unremarkable. The patient denies any other past medical history and has a mini-mental status examination score of 30/30. What is the next appropriate step in the management of this patient?

A. Formal psychiatric evaluation

B. MRI of the brain

C. Serum anti-acetylcholine receptor antibodies

D. Serum lead level

E. Slit-lamp examination

XI-47. A 37-year-old man is witnessed by his family to have a generalized tonic-clonic seizure at a party. He does not have a known seizure disorder. There is no history of head trauma, stroke, or tumor. The patient is unemployed, married, and takes no medication. Physical examination shows no skin abnormalities and no stigmata of chronic liver or renal disease. The patient is postictal. His neck is difficult to maneuver due to stiffness. His white blood cell count is 19,000/μL, hematocrit 36%, and platelets 200,000/μL. Glucose is 102 mg/dL, sodium 136 meq/dL, calcium 9.5 mg/dL, magnesium 2.2 mg/dL, SGOT 18 U/L, blood-urea nitrogen 7 mg/dL, and creatinine 0.8 mg/dL. Urine toxicology screen is positive for cocaine metabolites. Which next step is most appropriate in this patient's management?

A. Electroencephalogram (EEG)

B. Intravenous loading with antiepileptic medication

C. Lumbar puncture

D. Magnetic resonance imaging

E. Substance abuse counseling

XI-48. All of the following myopathies would be inherited from the female parent *except*

A. Becker muscular dystrophy

B. Duchenne muscular dystrophy

C. Kearns-Sayre syndrome

D. limb-girdle muscular dystrophy

E. myoclonic epilepsy with ragged red fibers (MERFF)

XI-49. A patient is brought to the emergency room after a head-on motor vehicle collision. The patient is unresponsive even to painful stimuli and is apneic; however, he does have a pulse. Which of the following clinical findings would exclude a diagnosis of brain death?

A. Bilateral positive Babinski signs

B. Constricted pupils

C. Invariant pulse rate

D. Positive deep tendon reflexes

E. Presence of diabetes insipidus

XI-50. A 45-year-old male presents with a daily headache. He describes two attacks per day over the last 3 weeks. Each attack lasts about an hour and awakens the patient from sleep. The patient has noted associated tearing and reddening of the right eye as well as nasal stuffiness. The pain is deep, excruciating, and limited to the right side of the head. The neurologic examination is nonfocal. The most likely diagnosis of this patient's headache is

A. migraine headache
B. cluster headache
C. tension headache
D. brain tumor
E. giant cell arteritis

XI-51. A 72-year-old woman presents with recurrent episodes of incapacitating facial pain lasting from second to minutes and then dissipating. The episodes occur usually twice per day, usually without warning, but are also occasionally provoked by brushing of her teeth. On physical examination, she appears well with normal vital signs. Detailed cranial nerve examination reveals no sensory or motor abnormalities. The remainder of her neurologic examination is normal. What is the next step in her management?

A. Brain MRI
B. Brain MRI plus carbamazepine therapy
C. Carbamazepine therapy
D. Glucocorticoid therapy
E. Referral to Otolaryngology for surgical cure

XI-52. A 26-year-old man presents to the emergency room complaining of weakness and difficulty breathing. He first noticed a feeling of weakness in his legs with difficulty climbing the stairs to his third-floor apartment 5 days ago. Over the ensuing days, his weakness has progressed such that he feels like he is tripping when he walks on flat surfaces and was unable to climb to his apartment yesterday. In addition, he now states that he is having difficulty lifting his arms above his head to comb his hair and twice dropped a bottle of soda on the floor due to a feeling of weakness in his arms. He also states that he feels short of breath, especially if lying flat. He complains of a tingling in his hands and feet. His past medical history is notable for sickle cell trait. Three weeks ago, he was treated for dehydration in the emergency room for food poisoning with diarrhea, abdominal pain, and low-grade fevers. This resolved within 2 days, and he had been feeling in his usual state of health prior to the onset of the current symptoms. He is on no medication and has no history of illicit drug use. He has no recent travel and has not eaten shellfish, honey, or home-canned foods. On physical examination, he appears breathless, has difficulty completing sentences, and is using accessory muscles of respiration. His vital signs show a respiratory rate of 32 breaths/min, a heart rate of 95 beats/min, a blood pressure of 112/76 mmHg, and a temperature of 37.6°C. His weight is 80 kg. His ocular movements are full. There is no papillary dilatation. On pulmonary examination, his breath sounds are clear. There is paradoxical motion of the abdomen with inspiration. Neu-

XI-52. *(Continued)*
rologic examination shows 3/5 strength symmetrically in the upper and lower extremities with absent deep tendon reflexes. Cardiovascular, gastrointestinal, and skin examinations are normal. Arterial blood gases show a pH of 7.55, a Pa_{CO_2} of 28 mmHg, and a Pa_{O_2} of 84 mmHg while breathing room air. His vital capacity is 800 mL. What is the most appropriate treatment for this individual?

A. Botulinum antitoxin
B. Intravenous immunoglobulin (IVIg)
C. IVIg and mechanical ventilation
D. IVIg, mechanical ventilation, and ciprofloxacin
E. Plasmapheresis and glucocorticoids

XI-53. The most common cause of a cerebral embolism is

A. cardiac prosthetic valves
B. rheumatic heart disease
C. dilated cardiomyopathy
D. endocarditis
E. atrial fibrillation

XI-54. When evaluating a patient for low back pain, which statement is true regarding the utility of the straight leg raise test?

A. Passive dorsiflexion of the foot during the maneuver will elicit pain from the contralateral nerve root.
B. The crossed straight leg raise is more specific for disk herniation than the straight leg raise.
C. The reverse straight leg raise is indicative of back pain referred from visceral organs.
D. The straight leg raise test is positive if there is restricted range of motion of the affected limb.

XI-55. A 37-year-old woman complains of headache and blurry vision that have been present for a year and are slowly getting worse. As part of her evaluation an MRI is obtained and shown below:

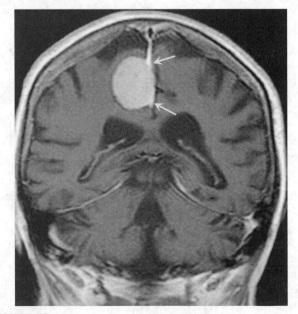

FIGURE XI-55

XI-55. *(Continued)*
What is the most likely diagnosis in this patient?

A. Brain abscess
B. Glioblastoma
C. Low-grade astrocytoma
D. Meningioma
E. Oligodendroglioma

XI-56. All but which of the following statements regarding epilepsy are true?

A. The incidence of suicide is higher in epileptic patients than it is in the general population.
B. Mortality is no different in patients with epilepsy than it is in age-matched controls.
C. A majority of patients with epilepsy that is completely controlled with medication eventually will be able to discontinue therapy and remain seizure free.
D. Surgery for mesial temporal lobe epilepsy (MTLE) decreases the number of seizures in over 70% of patients.
E. Tricyclic antidepressants lower the seizure threshold and may precipitate seizures.

XI-57. A 54-year-old male is referred to your clinic for evaluation of atrial fibrillation. He first noted the irregular heartbeat 2 weeks ago and presented to his primary care physician. He denies chest pain, shortness of breath, nausea, or gastrointestinal symptoms. Past medical history is unremarkable. There is no history of hypertension, diabetes, or tobacco use. His medications include metoprolol. The examination is notable for a blood pressure of 126/74 mmHg and a pulse of 64 beats/min. The jugular venous pressure is not elevated. His heart is irregularly irregular, with normal S_1 and S_2. The lungs are clear, and there is no peripheral edema. An echocardiogram shows a left atrial size of 3.6 cm. Left ventricular ejection fraction is 60%. There are no valvular or structural abnormalities. Which of the following statements regarding his atrial fibrillation and stroke risk is true?

A. He requires no antiplatelet therapy or anticoagulation because the risk of embolism is low.
B. Lifetime warfarin therapy is indicated for atrial fibrillation in this situation to reduce the risk of stroke.
C. He should be admitted to the hospital for intravenous heparin and undergo electrical cardioversion; afterward there is no need for anticoagulation.
D. His risk of an embolic stroke is less than 1%, and he should take a daily aspirin.
E. He should be started on subcutaneous low-molecular-weight heparin and transitioned to warfarin.

XI-58. A 34-year-old woman seeks evaluation for weakness. She has noted tripping when walking, particularly in her left foot, for the past 2 years. She recently also began to drop things, once allowing a full cup of coffee to spill onto her legs. In this setting, she also feels as if the

XI-58. *(Continued)*
appearance of her face has changed over the course of many years, stating that she feels as if her face is becoming more hollow and elongated although she hasn't lost any weight recently. She has not seen a physician in many years and has no past medical history. Her only medications are a multivitamin and calcium with vitamin D. Her family history is significant for similar symptoms of weakness in her brother who is 2 years older. Her mother, who is 58 years old, was diagnosed with mild weakness after her brother was evaluated, but is not symptomatic. On physical examination, the patient's face appears long and narrow with wasting of the temporalis and masseter muscles. Her speech is mildly dysarthric, and the palate is high and arched. Strength is 4/5 in the intrinsic muscles of the hand, wrist extensors, and ankle dorsiflexors. After testing handgrip strength, you notice that there is a delayed relaxation of the muscles of the hand. What is the most likely diagnosis?

A. Acid maltase deficiency (Pompe's disease)
B. Becker muscular dystrophy
C. Duchenne muscular dystrophy
D. Myotonic dystrophy
E. Nemaline myopathy

XI-59. A 20-year-old woman is brought to the emergency department after a witnessed generalized tonic-clonic seizure. She has no identifying information, and her past medical history is unknown. What is the most likely cause of her seizure?

A. Amyloid angiopathy
B. Fever
C. Genetic disorder
D. Illicit drug use
E. Uremia

XI-60. The presence of startle myoclonus in a 60-year-old man with rapidly progressive deficits in cortical dysfunction is which one of the following?

A. Neither sensitive nor specific for Creutzfeldt-Jacob disease (CJD) but does represent grounds to explore further for this condition with an electroencephalogram (EEG)
B. Neither sensitive nor specific for CJD but does represent grounds to explore further for this condition with an EEG and brain MRI
C. Sensitive but not specific for CJD and is not enough to prompt a further workup for this condition unless other clinical criteria are met
D. Specific but not sensitive for CJD and should therefore prompt immediate referral for brain biopsy to confirm the diagnosis
E. Virtually diagnostic for CJD, and further workup including EEG, brain MRI, and perhaps brain biopsy serves only a prognostic purpose

XI-61. Which nerve functions are spared in a patient with ventral cord syndrome due to an anterior spinal cord infarct?

A. Bladder sphincter control
B. Motor strength
C. Pain sensation
D. Proprioception
E. Tendon reflexes

XI-62. A 33-year-old woman complains of a rash on her chest. She has had a nonpruritic red rash on the upper chest for 4 weeks associated with a raised erythematous rash on her hands. She does not wear V-neck shirts, but the chest rash is in a V-neck distribution. Her hands have a scaly reddish-purple eruption, and her finger pads have become thicker and rougher (see Figure XI-62, Color Atlas). She also has a slight red hue on the upper eyelids.

What other findings are likely to be present in this patient?

A. Delayed relaxation phase of deep tendon reflexes
B. Hepatosplenomegaly
C. Muscle weakness
D. Situs inversus
E. Subcutaneous nodules on the back of the forearm

XI-63. A 65-year-old male presents with severe right-sided eye and facial pain, nausea, vomiting, colored halos around lights, and loss of visual acuity. His right eye is quite red, and that pupil is dilated and fixed. Which of the following diagnostic tests would confirm the diagnosis?

A. CT of the head
B. MRI of the head
C. Cerebral angiography
D. Tonometry
E. Slit-lamp examination

XI-64. A 21-year-old man presents to your clinic complaining of progressive weakness in the feet for the last 2 years. He describes slowly progressive difficulty in lifting his feet off the ground when walking. The legs have "gotten smaller" in bulk. Past medical history is unremarkable. The family history is significant for his father, brother, and paternal grandmother all having similar "weaknesses." The examination is notable for distal atrophy below the mid-calves and for prominent high arches. There is obvious footdrop, and dorsiflexion of the foot is severely diminished bilaterally. You suspect a form of Charcot-Marie-Tooth disease and order nerve conduction studies. Which of the following statements about CMT disease is true?

A. CMT disease is usually a motor neuropathy; sensory features are rare and should prompt an alternative diagnosis.
B. Immunotherapy with intravenous immune globulin and/or plasmapheresis may slow the progression of CMT disease.
C. CMT disease affects approximately 1 in 100,000 individuals.

XI-64. *(Continued)*
D. Transmission is most commonly autosomal dominant but may be autosomal recessive or X-linked.
E. The age of this patient at presentation is atypical; patients usually present in the fourth and fifth decades of life.

XI-65. A 45-year-old African-American man presents to the emergency room complaining of facial weakness. He first noticed a slight weakness of the left side of his face the day previously, and upon awakening today, had no movement on the left side of his face. Over the next several hours, the right side of his face also develops significant weakness as well. He denies any recent fevers, chills, rashes, or night sweats. His weight is 90 kg and is stable. He lives in an urban area of North Carolina and does not have any pets. He works as an accountant. He is married and is monogamous. He has hypertension treated with isradipine, 5 mg twice daily. On physical examination, he has complete paralysis of the left face with marked weakness of the right face. He is unable to lift his eyebrows on the left but can minimally do so on the right. A chest radiograph on admission shows bilateral hilar adenopathy and increased interstitial markings that are most prominent in the lung apices. An MRI scan with gadolinium shows bilateral enhancement of the seventh cranial nerves with mild meningeal enhancement. A lumbar puncture is performed with the following results: opening pressure 12 cmH$_2$O, red blood cell count 0/μL, white blood cell count 21/μL (differential 78% lymphocytes, 22% neutrophils), protein 80 mg/dL, and glucose 62 mg/dL. No organisms are seen on smear. What is the most likely diagnosis?

A. Lyme disease
B. Multiple sclerosis
C. Sarcoidosis
D. Tuberculosis
E. Viral meningitis

XI-66. Which of the following groups of patients should receive empirical antibiotic therapy that includes coverage of *Listeria monocytogenes* in cases of presumed meningitis?

A. Immunocompromised patients
B. Elderly patients
C. Infants
D. All of the above

XI-67. Which of the following neurologic phenomena is classically associated with herniation of the brain through the foramen magnum?

A. Third-nerve compression and ipsilateral papillary dilation
B. Catatonia
C. "Locked-in" state
D. Miotic pupils
E. Respiratory arrest

XI-68. A 72-year-old female presents with brief, intermittent excruciating episodes of lancinating pain in the lips, gums, and cheek. These intense spasms of pain may be initiated by touching the lips or moving the tongue. The results of a physical examination are normal. MRI of the head is also normal. The most likely cause of this patient's pain is

A. acoustic neuroma
B. meningioma
C. temporal lobe epilepsy
D. trigeminal neuralgia
E. facial nerve palsy

XI-69. A 38-year-old female patient with facial and ocular weakness has just been diagnosed with myasthenia gravis. You intend to initiate therapy with anticholinesterase medications and glucocorticoids. All of the following tests are necessary before instituting this therapy *except*

A. MRI of mediastinum
B. purified protein derivative skin test
C. lumbar puncture
D. pulmonary function tests
E. thyroid-stimulating hormone

XI-70. A 76-year-old nursing home resident is brought to the local emergency room after falling out of bed. The fall was not witnessed; however, she was suspected to have hit her head. She is not responsive to verbal or light tactile stimuli. At baseline she is able to converse but is frequently disoriented to place and time. She has a medical history that includes stable coronary disease, mild emphysema, and multi-infarct dementia. Immediately after triage she is taken for a CT scan of the head. Which of the following is true regarding head injury and hematomas?

A. More than 80% of patients with subdural hematomas will experience a lucid interval prior to loss of consciousness.
B. Epidural hematomas generally arise from venous sources.
C. Epidural hematomas are common among the elderly with minor head trauma.
D. Most patients presenting with epidural hematomas are unconscious.
E. Subdural hematomas lead to rapid increases in intracranial pressure and can require arterial ligation.

XI-71. A 45-year-old male complains of severe right arm pain. He gives a history of having slipped on the ice and severely contusing his right shoulder approximately 1 month ago. At this time he has sharp knifelike pain in the right arm and forearm. Physical examination reveals a right arm that is more moist and hairy than the left arm. There is no specific weakness or sensory change. However, the right arm is clearly more edematous than the left, and the skin appears somewhat atrophic in the affected limb. The patient's pain most likely is due to

XI-71. (Continued)
A. subclavian vein thrombosis
B. brachial plexus injury
C. reflex sympathetic dystrophy
D. acromioclavicular separation
E. cervical radiculopathy

XI-72. Which of the following statements regarding the long-term outcomes in individuals with severe migraines is true?

A. Factors such as cigarette smoking and hypertension have no modifying risk on the development of ischemic stroke in individuals who have migraine with aura.
B. In both women and men, migraine with aura is associated with an increased risk of ischemic stroke.
C. Migraines generally persist unchanged in severity throughout life.
D. Migraine with or without aura is associated with an increased risk of subclinical posterior circulation infarction on MRI.
E. Women on oral contraceptives who have migraines without aura should discontinue these medications because of a marked increased risk of ischemic stroke.

XI-73. A 40-year-old man has recurrent bouts of tinnitus. Except for a fairly severe upper respiratory tract infection 1 year ago, he has been healthy for all of his life. In the last year he has had two self-limited episodes of tinnitus associated with dizziness and a decrement in his hearing. His symptoms are always unilateral on the same side and have required him to take off from work for a few days each time. He comes into your office at the outset of his third bout of tinnitus. He has taken meclizine at home with no relief. In your office, he has tinnitus and vertigo while seated, which is exacerbated with ambulation. His symptoms of dizziness are not reproduced with Dix-Hallpike maneuvers. Which is the best long-term treatment option for the patient at this time?

A. Diuretic
B. Glucocorticoid
C. Epley procedure
D. Metoclopramide
E. Scopolamine transdermal

XI-74. While you are working in the urgent care center, a baby-sitter brings in a 7-year-old boy who complains of visual changes. He complains of difficulty with blue-yellow color discrimination. He has no other past medical history. On examination, visual acuity in the right eye is 20/60 and in the left eye 20/80. He has blue-yellow color blindness. He has cerebellar ataxia on neurologic examination as well as ophthalmoparesis. His strength is 5 out of 5 in all major muscle groups, and all reflexes are normal except for extensor plantar responses. When the mother arrives, you find out that many relatives on the father's side of the family, including the father, have been diagnosed with cerebellar ataxia but she does not know more than that. You decide to

XI-74. *(Continued)*

perform a funduscopic examination. What do you expect to find on examination of this patient's fundi?

A. Lipemia retinalis
B. Normal examination
C. Papilledema
D. Proliferative retinopathy
E. Retinal pigmentary degeneration

XI-75. All the following have been shown to reduce the risk of atherothrombotic stroke in primary or secondary prevention *except*

A. aspirin
B. blood pressure control
C. clopidogrel
D. statin therapy
E. warfarin

XI-76. All the following are associated with a decreased sense of smell *except*

A. head trauma
B. HIV infection
C. influenza B infection
D. Kallmann syndrome
E. parainfluenza virus type 3 infection

XI-77. All the following are side effects of phenytoin *except*

A. ataxia
B. gum hyperplasia
C. hirsutism
D. leukopenia
E. lymphadenopathy

XI-78. All but which of the following statements about Becker's muscular dystrophy are true?

A. The inheritance is X-linked.
B. Serum creatinine kinase levels are elevated.
C. The underlying genetic defect is in the myosin gene.
D. Survival is better than it is in patients with Duchenne's muscular dystrophy (DMD).
E. Cardiomyopathy may occur, resulting in heart failure.

XI-79. You are following a patient who has a ruptured L4-L5 intervertebral disk with herniation. He has had left lower extremity weakness that has been constant for 6 months. He is still able to perform his daily activities. His pain is intermittent and he uses chronic narcotics on an as-needed basis. What findings would prompt you to refer this patient for surgery?

A. Absent deep tendon reflexes on the right
B. MRI shows L3-L4 herniation as well
C. Nighttime symptoms

XI-79. *(Continued)*

D. Physical examination demonstrates progressive weakness

XI-80. All of the following conditions may cause episodic generalized paresis *except*

A. carotid artery stenosis
B. hypokalemia
D. multiple sclerosis
E. myasthenia gravis
F. transient ischemic attack

XI-81. You are examining a 78-year-old patient in your clinic who is referred to you for difficulty in walking. During your motor examination with the patient lying supine, you place your hands behind one knee and rapidly raise the knee off the bed. During the maneuver, the ankle (of the same leg) is also lifted off the examining table. On repeat examination of the same leg, you find varying levels of resistance, and the ankle drags for varying distances before being lifted off the bed. The finding is not seen in the other leg nor in the upper extremities when examining the elbow/wrist. What is the significance of this finding?

A. The patient has decreased motor tone, which may be indicative of a motor neuron disease.
B. The patient has decreased motor tone related to musculoskeletal injury.
C. The patient's paratonia may be a normal reaction.
D. The patient's rigidity is a manifestation of parkinsonism.

XI-82. Which of the following medicines has been most commonly implicated in the development of noninfectious chronic meningitis?

A. Acetaminophen
B. Acyclovir
C. β-lactam antibiotics
D. Ibuprofen
E. Phenobarbital

XI-83. A 72-year-old right-handed male with a history of atrial fibrillation and chronic alcoholism is evaluated for dementia. His son gives a history of a stepwise decline in the patient's function over the last 5 years with the accumulation of mild focal neurologic deficits. On examination he is found to have a pseudobulbar affect, mildly increased muscle tone, and brisk deep tendon reflexes in the right upper extremity and an extensor plantar response on the left. The history and examination are most consistent with which of the following?

A. Binswanger's disease
B. Alzheimer's disease
C. Creutzfeldt-Jakob disease
D. Vitamin B$_{12}$ deficiency
E. Multi-infarct dementia

XI-84. A 50-year-old male complains of weakness and numbness in the hands for the last month. He describes paresthesias in the thumb and the index and middle fingers. The symptoms are worse at night. He also describes decreased grip strength bilaterally. He works as a mechanical engineer. The patient denies fevers, chills, or weight loss. The examination is notable for atrophy of the thenar eminences bilaterally and decreased sensation in a

XI-84. *(Continued)*

median nerve distribution. All the following are causes of carpal tunnel syndrome *except*

A. amyloidosis
B. chronic lymphocytic leukemia
C. diabetes mellitus
D. hypothyroidism
E. rheumatoid arthritis

XI. NEUROLOGIC DISORDERS

ANSWERS

XI-1. **The answer is C.** *(Chap. 26)* Confusion is defined as a mental and behavioral state of reduced comprehension, coherence, and capacity to reason. Delirium is used to describe an acute confusional state. Delirium often goes unrecognized despite clear evidence that it is often a cognitive manifestation of many medical and neurologic illnesses. Delirium is a clinical diagnosis that may be hyperactive (e.g., alcohol withdrawal) or hypoactive (e.g., opiate intoxication). There is often dramatic fluctuation between states. Delirium is associated with a substantial mortality with in-hospital mortality estimates ranging from 25–33%. Overall estimates of delirium in hospitalized patients range from 15–55% with higher rates in the elderly. Patients in the ICU have especially high rates of delirium, ranging from 70–87%. The clinic setting would represent the lowest risk. Postoperative patients, especially status post hip surgery, have an incidence of delirium that is somewhat higher than patients admitted to the medical wards.

XI-2. **The answer is D.** *(Chap. 15)* This patient is presenting with typical cluster headaches, one of the three recognized trigeminal autonomic cephalgias (TACs). TACs are characterized by intense episodes of head pain associated with cranial autonomic symptoms such as tearing, rhinorrhea, and conjunctival injection. Because of these associated symptoms, patients may be misdiagnosed as having sinus headache due to allergic rhinitis and treated inappropriately with antihistamine and nasal steroids. A typical presentation of cluster headaches is one of episodic severe headaches that occur at least once daily at about the same time for a period of 8–10 weeks. An attack usually lasts from 15–180 minutes, and 50% of headaches will have nocturnal onset. Between episodes of headache, the patient is generally well. The period between headache cycles typically lasts about 1 year. Men are affected three times more commonly with cluster headaches than women, and alcohol ingestion may trigger cluster headaches. A distinguishing feature between cluster headaches and migraine headaches is that individuals with cluster headaches tend to move about during attacks and frequently rub their head for relief, whereas those with migraines tend to remain motionless during attacks. Interestingly, unilateral phonophobia and photophobia can occur with cluster headaches but do not with migraines. Treatment of acute attacks of cluster headaches requires a treatment with a fast onset as the headaches reach peak intensity very quickly but are of relatively short duration. High-flow oxygen (10–12 L/min for 15–20 min) has been very effective in relieving the headaches. Alternatively, subcutaneous or intranasal delivery of sumatriptan will also halt an attack. The oral-route triptan medications are less effective because of the time to onset of effect is too great. Preventive treatment may be considered in individuals with prolonged bouts of cluster headaches or chronic cluster headaches that occur without a pain-free interval.

The other TAC syndromes are paroxysmal hemicrania and short-lasting unilateral neuralgiform headache attacks with conjunctival injection and tearing (commonly known as SUNCT). Paroxysmal hemicrania is characterized by unilateral severe headaches lasting only 2–45 min but occurring up to five times daily. There is marked autonomic symptoms, and paroxysms of headaches last <3 days. Indomethacin is very effective at preventing this syndrome. SUNCT is a rare syndrome in which the headaches last <4 min at a time. Diagnosis requires at least 20 attacks. There is no acute treatment of SUNCT because of their short duration, but preventative therapy with lamotrigine, topiramate, gabapentin, or carbamazepine may be effective.

XI-3. **The answer is A.** *(Chap. 383)* A common mistake in the management of patients with inflammatory myopathy is to "chase the CK" instead of adjusting therapy based on the clinical response. The goal of therapy is to improve strength. If that goal is being achieved, no augmentation of therapy is necessary. In this case, the plan to switch to long-term maintenance with steroid-sparing immunosuppressants should still be pursued. There have been no controlled studies comparing mycophenolate to methotrexate for the long-term use in polymyositis, and in the absence of an adverse reaction to mycophenolate, therapy should not be changed. Despite an elevated CK, patients with polymyositis who are responding to therapy do not need a repeat muscle biopsy.

XI-4. **The answer is C.** *(Chap. 23)* The central cord syndrome manifests clinically as a sensory disorder as the spinothalamic fibers in the ventral commissure of the spinal cord are disrupted. Dermatomes above and below the level of the destruction are usually spared, creating a "suspended sensory level" on physical examination. As the lesion grows, corticospinal tract or anterior horn involvement can produce weakness in the affected myotome. Common causes include syringomyelia, intramedullary tumor, and hyperextension in a patient with cervical spondylosis. Tabes dorsalis impairs proprioception and sensation and causes weakness. Disc herniation most commonly affects posterior cord function and nerve roots. A lateral hemisection syndrome (the Brown-Séquard syndrome) is classically due to penetrating trauma from a knife or bullet injury and produces ipsilateral weakness and contralateral loss of pain and temperature sensation. Amyotrophic lateral sclerosis presents with combined upper and lower motor neuron findings; sensory deficits are uncommon.

XI-5. **The answer is D.** *(Chap. 269)* This patient has evidence of increased intracranial pressure and needs to be managed urgently. A variety of maneuvers may decrease intracranial pressure acutely. Hyperventilation causes vasoconstriction, reducing cerebral blood volume and decreasing intracranial pressure. However, this can be used only for a short period as the decrease in cerebral blood flow is of limited duration. Mannitol, an osmotic diuretic, is recommended in cases of increased intracranial pressure resulting from cytotoxic edema. Hypotonic fluids should be avoided. Instead, hypertonic saline is given to elevate sodium levels and prevent worsening of edema. A more definitive treatment to decrease intracranial pressure is to have a ventriculostomy placed by which excessive pressure can be relieved by draining cerebrospinal fluid (CSF). Further decreases in mean arterial pressure may worsen the patient's clinical status. The patient already has had more than a 20% reduction in mean arterial pressure, which is the recommended reduction in cases of hypertensive emergency. In addition, the patient is exhibiting signs of increased intracranial pressure, which indicates that cerebral perfusion pressure [mean arterial pressure (MAP) – intracranial pressure (ICP)] has been lowered. Paradoxically, the patient may need a vasopressor agent to increase MAP and thus improve cerebral perfusion. Finally, in cases of increased intracranial pressure, nitroprusside is not a recommended intravenous antihypertensive agent because it causes arterial vasodilation and may decrease cerebral perfusion pressure and worsen neurologic function.

XI-6. **The answer C.** *(Chap. 390)* Cigarette smoking is associated with early mortality from a variety of causes including cardiovascular, respiratory, cerebrovascular, and oncologic causes. It is also associated with increased complications during pregnancy (premature rupture of membranes, placenta previa, abruption placenta), delay in healing of peptic ulcers, osteoporosis, cataracts, macular degeneration, cholecystis in women, and impotence in men. Children born to smoking mothers are more likely to have preterm delivery, higher perinatal mortality, higher rates of infant respiratory distress, and higher rates of sudden infant death. Moreover, 400,000 individuals die prematurely each year in the US from cigarette use, representing 1 out of every 5 deaths.

XI-7. **The answer is B.** *(Chap. 22)* The symptoms and signs described in this question are most consistent with Ménière's disease. In this disorder paroxysmal vertigo resulting from labyrinthine lesions is associated with nausea, vomiting, rotary nystagmus, tinnitus, high-tone hearing loss with recruitment, and, most characteristically, fullness in the ear.

Labyrinthitis would be an unlikely diagnosis in this case because of the hearing loss and multiple episodes. Vertebral-basilar insufficiency and multiple sclerosis typically are associated with brainstem signs. Acoustic neuroma only rarely causes vertigo as the initial symptom, and the vertigo it does cause is mild and intermittent.

XI-8. **The answer is D.** *(Chap. 376)* In a patient with suspected bacterial meningitis empirical therapy should be administered promptly to reduce mortality and morbidity. The decision to obtain an imaging study prior to lumbar puncture is based on the concern of precipitating herniation in a patient with elevated intracranial pressure or focal CNS lesions. Therefore, patients with the presence of papilledema on physical examination, history of recent head trauma, known or suspected intracranial lesions (immunosuppressed, known malignancy), focal neurologic findings, or depressed level of consciousness should have a head CT or MRI prior to lumbar puncture. Kernig's sign is elicited in a supine patient by flexing the thigh and knee. A positive sign occurs when the patient has head/neck pain when passively straightening the knee. The sensitivity and specificity of this sign (also Brudzinski's) for bacterial meningitis are unknown, but they imply meningeal irritation, not an intracranial lesion or elevated intracranial pressure. While cerebrospinal fluid cultures may be impacted by administration of antibiotics prior to lumbar puncture, stains, antigen tests, and polymerase chain reaction tests will not be affected.

XI-9. **The answer is C.** *(Chap. 25)* The patient's nonspecific dysesthesia is related to hyperventilation in response to the patient's change in altitude from sea level to a mountainous area. The normal respiratory response to decreased atmospheric oxygen tension is to increase the respiratory rate. This hyperventilation causes a mild respiratory alkalosis and is experienced as acral and periorbital dysesthesias. Acetazolamide is often given to patients who have a past history of altitude sickness manifested as headache, nausea with vomiting, and in severe cases pulmonary edema. This patient is experiencing none of those symptoms, and in fact, dysesthesias are a common side effect related to treatment with acetazolamide. No further blood testing is necessary as the symptoms are not associated with any neurologic abnormalities. Diabetes mellitus, vitamin B_{12} deficiency, and tertiary syphilis are all associated with a sensory neuropathy, which this patient does not demonstrate.

XI-10. **The answer is C.** *(Chap. 361)* This patient demonstrates increasing weakness with repeated exertion, which is characteristic of neuromuscular junction diseases such as myasthenia gravis. The course can fluctuate over the course of a day, which may explain why his symptoms appear worse at the end of the day. The absence of any sensory deficit is also characteristic of a neuromuscular junction disorder. Diseases of the muscle usually do not exhibit such a marked difference on the examination over the course of hours. Spinal root disorders are symptomatic in a nerve root distribution, and limb pain is usually a prominent component. Clues to a brainstem disease are isolated cranial nerve palsies and "crossed" weakness and sensory abnormalities of the head and limbs.

XI-11. **The answer is B.** *(Chap. 372)* This patient has a history and examination consistent with a myelopathy. The rapidity of onset and the lack of other antecedent symptoms (e.g., pain) make a noncompressive etiology most likely. An MRI is the initial test of choice and will easily identify a structural lesion such as a neoplasm or subluxation. Noncompressive myelopathies result from five basic causes: spinal cord infarction; systemic disorders such as vasculitis, systemic lupus erythematosus (SLE), and sarcoidosis; infections (particularly viral); demyelinating disease such as multiple sclerosis; and idiopathic. Therefore, serologies for antinuclear antibodies, viral serologies such as HIV and HTLV-I, and lumbar puncture are all indicated. Because the clinical scenario is consistent with a myelopathy, an electromyogram is not indicated.

XI-12. **The answer is D.** *(Chap. 368)* This MRI shows cerebellar atrophy consistent with the diagnosis of spinocerebellar ataxia (SCA). The SCAs are a group of autosomal dominant diseases. SCA1, previously known as olivopontocerebellar atrophy, is a disease of early or middle adult life. Patients develop cerebellar ataxia of the trunk and limbs with impairment of equilibrium and gait, scanning speech, nystagmus, and oscillatory tremor of the head and trunk. There may also be mild dementia. Cerebellar and brainstem atrophy are evident on MRI. Migraine headache, limb weakness, and breathing difficulties are nonspecific but may be seen in serotonin syndrome or alcohol withdrawal. Gait instability, urinary incontinence, and dementia constitute the clinical triad for normal-pressure hydrocephalus, which does not have cerebellar atrophy on MRI. Hypertension, tachycardia, and diaphoresis may be seen in a patient with an Arnold-Chiari malformation. MRI will often show abnormalities in the base of the skull.

XI-13.   The answer is A. *(Chap. 373)* Concussions result from blunt head trauma that causes anterior-posterior movement of the brain within the skull. Transient loss of consciousness is common, as are confusion and amnesia. Head imaging is typically normal. Postconcussive syndrome is a constellation of symptoms including fatigue, headache, dizziness, and difficulty concentrating that follows a concussion. The patient described above fits this diagnosis; strict diagnostic criteria do not exist. Typically patients will improve over a 6- to 12-month period. Patients who were energetic and highly functioning prior to their trauma have an excellent prognosis. Treatment is aimed at reassurance and relieving prominent symptoms. Dizziness can be treated with phenergan, which acts as a vestibular suppressant. He should avoid contact sports at least until his symptoms resolve.

XI-14.   The answer is E. *(Chap. 378)* Prions are infectious particles that cause central nervous system degeneration. The human prion diseases described to date include Creutzfeldt-Jacob disease, kuru, Gerstmann-Sträussler-Scheinker disease, and fatal insomnia. The most common prion disease is sporadic CJD (sCJD) which occurs in a seemingly random pattern in adults in their fifth and sixth decades of life. sCJD accounts for about 85% of cases of CJD and occurs in ~1 per 1 million population. Variant CJD (vCJD) results from infection from bovine exposure to tainted beef from cattle with bovine spongiform encephalopathy (BSE). Infectious CJD (iCJD) has resulted from injection of tainted human growth hormone, as well as transplant of infected dura mater grafts into humans. Familial CJD (fCJD) is due to germ-line mutations that follow an autosomal dominant inheritance. Kuru is due to infection through ritualistic cannibalism. Gerstmann-Sträussler-Scheinker disease and familial fatal insomnia (FFI) occur as dominantly inherited prion diseases. Sporadic cases of fatal insomnia (sFI) have been described.

XI-15.   The answer is B. *(Chap. 16)* Neurogenic claudication (back or leg pain induced by walking or standing and relieved by sitting) is the most common symptom of lumbar spinal stenosis. Unlike vascular claudication, symptoms are provoked by standing without walking. Symptoms are often not present, and severe findings such as paralysis and urinary incontinence are rare. Lumbar spinal stenosis can be congenital or acquired. Acquired factors that contribute to spinal stenosis include trauma, osteoporosis, hypoparathyroidism, renal osteodystrophy, and Paget's disease. Tethered cord syndrome usually presents as a cauda equina disorder (urinary incontinence, perineal anesthesia) in a young adult. Pain associated with disk herniation is differentiated from spinal stenosis when the pain is made worse with sitting. Vertebral metastases are a common cause of back pain in patients at risk of common malignancies. The pain tends to be constant, dull, unrelieved by rest, and worst at night.

XI-16.   The answer is A. *(Chap. 363)* Complex partial seizures are characterized by focal seizure activity plus impairment of the patient's ability to maintain contact with the environment. Mesial temporal lobe epilepsy is the most common syndrome associated with complex partial seizures. Patients are unable to respond to verbal or visual commands during the seizure and they often manifest complex automatisms or complex posturing. An aura is common before the seizures. There is postictal memory loss or disorientation. Patients often have a history of febrile seizures or a family history of seizures. MRI will show hippocampal sclerosis, a small temporal lobe, or enlarged temporal horn. Hypothyroidism, herpes virus infection, diabetes, and tuberous sclerosis are not associated with mesial temporal lobe epilepsy.

XI-17. **The answer is B.** *(Chap. 363)* MTLE is important to recognize because it tends to be refractory to treatment with anticonvulsants but responds extremely well to surgical intervention. Primidone is an alternative for treatment of partial and generalized tonic-clonic seizures. Levetiracetam is an alternative for simple partial, complex partial, and secondarily generalized seizures. Vagus nerve stimulation is an option for patients refractory to antiepileptic medication with seizures arising from more than one site. Herpes virus infection is not a cause of MTLE.

XI-18. **The answer is C.** *(Chap. 23)* A deep tendon reflex is elicited when a tap on a tendon stretches muscle spindles which are chronically activated by γ motor neurons. Spindle afferent neurons directly stimulate α motor neurons in the spinal cord, causing a muscle contraction. The reflex arc operates independent of upper motor neurons (pyramidal neurons); however, loss of the inhibitory input from upper motor neurons produces an exaggerated deep tendon reflex.

XI-19. **The answer is D.** *(Chap. 375)* Optic neuritis is the initial symptom in approximately 40% of persons who are eventually diagnosed with multiple sclerosis. This rapidly developing ophthalmologic disorder is associated with partial or total loss of vision, pain on motion of the involved eye, scotoma affecting macular vision, and a variety of other visual field defects. Ophthalmoscopically visible optic papillitis occurs in about half these patients.

XI-20. **The answer is A.** *(Chap. 16)* The most commonly affected nerve roots in cervical disk disease are C7 and C6. As such, common motor findings include biceps and triceps weakness. Common sensory findings include abnormal sensation in the thumb and fingers (except the little finger), radial hand, and dorsal forearm. Decreased pin-prick sensation over the lateral deltoid would be mediated by injury to the C5 nerve root. Finger flexors and sensation to the axilla and medial arm are mediated by C8 and T1.

TABLE XI-20   Cervical Radiculopathy—Neurologic Features

Cervical Nerve Roots	Examination Findings			
	Reflex	Sensory	Motor	Pain Distribution
C5	Biceps	Over lateral deltoid	Supraspinatus[a] (initial arm abduction) Infraspinatus[a] (arm external rotation) Deltoid[a] (arm abduction) Biceps (arm flexion)	Lateral arm, medial scapula
C6	Biceps	Thumb, index fingers Radial hand/forearm	Biceps (arm flexion) Pronator teres (internal forearm rotation)	Lateral forearm, thumb, index finger
C7	Triceps	Middle fingers Dorsum forearm	Triceps[a] (arm extension) Wrist extensors[a]	Posterior arm, dorsal forearm, lateral hand
C8	Finger flexors	Little finger Medial hand and forearm	Abductor pollicis brevis (abduction D1) First dorsal interosseous (abduction D2) Abductor digiti minimi (abduction D5)	4th and 5th fingers, medial forearm
T1	Finger flexors	Axilla and medial arm	Abductor pollicis brevis (abduction D1) First dorsal interosseous (abduction D2) Abductor digiti minimi (abduction D5)	Medial arm, axilla

[a]These muscles receive the majority of innervation from this root.

XI-21. **The answer is C.** *(Chap. 368)* The patient describes cerebellar ataxia, which is differentiated from ataxia associated with vestibular or labyrinthine disease by the absence of vertiginous complaints. True cerebellar ataxia is devoid of vertiginous symptoms and is clearly an unsteady gait due to imbalance. CT scanning can miss pathology in the cerebellum due to the surrounding bony structures. Alcohol intoxication, lithium toxicity, and viral cerebritis usually cause acute or subacute (days to weeks) cerebellar ataxia. Tertiary syphilis is a common cause of chronic cerebellar ataxia (months to years).

XI-22. **The answer is E.** *(Chap. 25)* Thalamic pain syndrome may follow an embolic or lacunar thalamic infarct if it affects the ventral posterolateral (VPL) nucleus or the adjacent white matter. The pain is persistent and severe, affecting only the contralateral side of the body. Other symptoms that may be associated with thalamic infarcts include hemianesthesia, hemiataxia, choreoathetoid movements, and athetoid posture. The eponym applied to this syndrome is Dejerine-Roussy syndrome.

XI-23. **The answer is B.** *(Chap. 390)* Smokers regulate their blood levels of nicotine by adjusting the frequency and intensity of their tobacco use. Smokers can compensate for the lower levels of nicotine in low-yield cigarettes by smoking more cigarettes or by adjusting their smoking technique. Therefore, smoking low-yield cigarettes is not a reasonable alternative to smoking cessation. Moreover, there is no difference in the harmful physical effects of smoking or in the potential for drug interactions.

XI-24. **The answer is A.** *(Chap. 22)* In the acute evaluation of vertigo, vestibular function tests can help to establish the side of the abnormality and differentiate between central and peripheral etiologies. When performing electronystagmography using cold and warm water sequentially, the velocity of the slow-phase of nystagmus is compared from side to side. When warm water at 44°C is infused into an ear, the normal response is nystagmus with the fast component toward the infused ear. The opposite response occurs when cold water at 30°C is infused; the normal response is nystagmus with the fast component away from the cold water–infused ear. The volume of water can be increased if no response occurs with the initial attempt. Velocity of the slow phase should be similar in patients without vestibular nerve abnormalities. An absence of response to the cold caloric indicates a labyrinth system that is "dead" and nonfunctional, such as in complete destruction of the neural input with acoustic neuroma. Otoconia are not a result of and do not cause peripheral nerve dysfunction. The caloric testing is normal in patients with otoconia. The peripheral nerve dysfunction seen with aminoglycoside antibiotics is usually bilateral. Unilateral symptoms should raise the suspicion for an anatomic as opposed to a systemic cause of the vertigo. Labyrinthine ischemia will also manifest as a "dead" labyrinth; however, the patient's age makes ischemic brainstem lesions less likely than a schwannoma.

XI-25. **The answer is D.** *(Chap. 374)* This scenario represents a common dilemma in the care of patients with HIV infection. The differential diagnosis usually falls between CNS toxoplasmosis or CNS lymphoma. The standard approach in a neurologically stable patient is to treat the patient for toxoplasmosis for 2–3 weeks then repeat neuroimaging. If the imaging shows clear improvement, continue antibiotics. If not, then a stereotactic brain biopsy is indicated. Whole-brain radiation therapy is part of the treatment for CNS lymphoma, which is not yet diagnosed in this patient, and should not be instituted empirically. In the absence of neurologic collapse, it is reasonable to treat empirically for toxoplasmosis in such a patient. The leptomeninges are a common site for metastases for patients with systemic lymphoma and those patients usually have a B cell lymphoma or leukemia. Dexamethasone is indicated for focal CNS lesions with evidence of mass effect or extensive surrounding edema.

XI-26. **The answer is D.** *(Chap. 374)* In this immunocompromised patient who has not responded to treatment for CNS toxoplasmosis, a positive CNS EBV DNA would be diagnostic of CNS lymphoma. However, in the absence of a definitive diagnosis, a biopsy should be pursued for a definitive diagnosis. If there is no response to therapy after 2 weeks, therapy does not need to be continued. Treatments directed at viral infections of the CNS or CNS lymphomas are not indicated at this time since a diagnosis is still yet to be made. In the absence of a change in neurologic status or evidence of mass effect on CT, there is no indication for dexamethasone.

XI-27. **The answer is A.** *(Chap. 372)* Syringomyelia is a developmental, slowly enlarging cavitary expansion of the cervical cord that produces a progressive myelopathy. Symptoms typically begin in adolescence or early adulthood. They may undergo spontaneous arrest after several years. More than half are associated with Chiari malformations. Acquired cavitations of the spinal cord are referred to as syrinx cavities. They may result from trauma, myelitis, infection, or tumor. The classic presentation is that of a central cord syndrome with sensory loss of pain and temperature sensation and weakness of the upper extremities. Vibration and position sensation are typically preserved. Muscle wasting in the lower neck, shoulders, arms, and hands with asymmetric or absent reflexes reflects extension of the cavity to the anterior horns. With progression, spasticity and weakness of the lower extremities and bladder and bowel dysfunction may occur. MRI scans are the diagnostic modality of choice. Surgical therapy is generally unsatisfactory. Syringomyelia associated with Chiari malformations may require extensive decompressions of the posterior fossa. Direct decompression of the cavity is of debatable benefit. Syringomyelia secondary to trauma or infection is treated with decompression and a drainage procedure, with a shunt often inserted that drains into the subarachnoid space. Although relief may occur, recurrence is common.

XI-28. **The answer is E.** *(Chap. 381)* Myasthenia gravis (MG) is a neuromuscular disorder characterized by weakness and fatigability of skeletal muscles. The primary defect is a decrease in the number of acetylcholine receptors at the neuromuscular junction secondary to autoimmune antibodies. MG is not rare, affecting at least 1 in 7500 individuals. Women are affected more frequently than are men. Women present typically in the second and third decades of life, and men present in the fifth and sixth decades. The key features of MG are weakness and fatigability. Clinical features include weakness of the cranial muscles, particularly the lids and extraocular muscles. Diplopia and ptosis are common initial complaints. Weakness in chewing is noticeable after prolonged effort. Speech may be affected secondary to weakness of the palate or tongue weakness. Swallowing may result from weakness of the palate, tongue, or pharynx. In the majority of patients the weakness becomes generalized. The diagnosis is suspected after the appearance of the characteristic symptoms and signs. Edrophonium is an acetylcholinesterase inhibitor that allows ACh to interact repeatedly with the limited number of AChRs, producing improvement in the strength of myasthenic muscles. False-positive tests may occur in patients with other neurologic diseases. Electrodiagnostic testing may show evidence of reduction in the amplitude of the evoked muscle action potentials with repeated stimulation. Testing for the specific antibodies to AChR are diagnostic. In addition to anti-AChR antibodies, antibodies to MuSK have been found in some patients with clinical MG. Antibodies to voltage-gated calcium channels are found in patients with the Lambert-Eaton syndrome.

XI-29. **The answer is D.** *(Chap. 366)* The differential diagnosis of Parkinson's disease is broad, and the disease can be difficult to diagnose, with an estimated misdiagnosis of 10–25% even by experienced physicians. This patient exhibits several atypical features that should alert the physician to search for alternative diagnoses. These include early age of onset, prominent orthostasis, autonomic symptoms of flushing and diaphoresis, and failure to respond to dopaminergic agents. In addition, recurrent urinary tract infections should prompt an evaluation for urinary retention due to autonomic dysfunction in this patient. These symptoms are most consistent with multiple systems atrophy with parkinsonian features (MSA-p). The average age of onset is 50 years, and these individuals more frequently present with bilateral, symmetric tremor and more prominent spasticity than those with Parkinson's disease. Orthostasis and autonomic symptoms are typically prominent. On MRI, one would expect to find volume loss and T2-hyperintensity in the area of the putamen, globus pallidus, and white matter. On pathologic examination, α-synuclein-positive inclusions would be seen in the affected areas. Median survival after diagnosis is 6–9 years. Dopaminergic agents are not helpful in treatment of this disorder and are usually associated with drug-induced dyskinesias of the face and neck, rather than the limbs and trunk. Corticobasal degeneration is a sporadic tauopathy that presents in the sixth to seventh decades. In contrast to Parkinson's disease, this disorder is frequently associated with myoclonic jerks and involuntary purposeful movements of a limb. Its progressive nature leads to spastic paraplegia. Diffuse Lewy body disease has prominent dementia with parkinsonian features. Neuropsychiatric complaints including paranoia, delusions, and personality changes are more common than in Parkinson's disease. Drug-induced Parkinson's disease is not seen with nitrofurantoin, and the patient has no history of illicit drugs such as MTPT, which could cause Parkinson's disease. Finally, this is unlikely to be inadequately treated Parkinson's disease because one would expect at least an initial improvement on dopaminergic agents.

XI-30.   **The answer is D.** *(Chap. 373)*   The head CT shows bilateral hypodense fluid collections in the subdural space. Acute hematomas (which would be as bright as the resolving blood shown in arrows) become hypodense in comparison with adjacent brain after ~2 months. During the isodense phase (2–6 weeks after injury), they may be difficult to discern. Chronic subdural hematoma may present without a history of trauma or injury in 20–30% of patients. Headache is common. Other symptoms may be vague as in this case, or there may be focal signs including hemiparesis mimicking stroke. Underlying cortical damage may serve as a seizure focus. In relatively asymptomatic patients with small hematomas, observation and serial imaging may be reasonable; however, surgical evacuation is often necessary for large or symptomatic chronic hematomas.

XI-31.   **The answer is B.** *(Chap 22)*   Positional vertigo is precipitated by a recumbent head position, either to the right or the left. The benign form that affects the posterior semicircular canal is the most common and is due to the accumulation of otoconia. Central positional vertigo (CPV) is due to lesions of the fourth ventricle and is much less common than BPPV. BPPV can be diagnosed and potentially treated with characteristic maneuvers (i.e., Dix-Hallpike position). With the head supine, the head is turned to the affected side (left ear down, in this case). Torsional nystagmus and vertigo will result with characteristic eye movements. In BPPV, the time from assuming head position and onset of symptoms is 3–40 s, whereas in CPV, the onset is immediate. With BPPV, symptoms will abate while the head position is maintained, and repeat trials lessen the symptoms each time and may extinguish them completely. With central causes of vertigo, symptoms are often less severe than with peripheral vertigo. Isolated horizontal nystagmus without a torsional component is also more suggestive of a central cause of vertigo.

XI-32.   **The answer is C.** *(Chap. 366)*   Therapy for Parkinson's disease should be initiated when symptoms interfere with the patient's quality of life. Choice of initial drug therapy is usually with dopamine agonists, levodopa, or MAO inhibitors. The initial choice in most individuals is a dopamine agonist (pramipexole, ropinirole), and monotherapy with dopamine agonists usually controls motor symptoms for several years before levodopa therapy becomes necessary. Over this period, escalating doses are frequently required, and side effects may be limiting. It is thought that dopamine agonists delay the onset of dyskinesias and on-off motor symptoms, such as freezing. By 5 years, over half of individuals will require levodopa to control motor symptoms. Levodopa remains the most effective therapy for the motor symptoms of Parkinson's disease, but once levodopa is started, dyskinesias and on-off motor fluctuations become more common. MAO inhibitors work by decreasing postsynaptic breakdown of dopamine. As monotherapy, these agents have only small effects and are most often used as adjuncts to levodopa. Surgical procedures such as pallidotomy and deep-brain stimulation are reserved for advanced Parkinson's disease with intractable tremor or drug-induced motor fluctuations or dyskinesias. In this setting, deep-brain stimulation can alleviate disabling symptoms.

XI-33.   **The answer is C.** *(Chap. 383)*   This patient does not have signs of an inflammatory myositis. In particular, the "give-away" weakness and improvement with encouragement suggests that this patient's "weakness" may actually be due to muscular pain. Fibrositis, polymyalgia rheumatica or fibromyalgia may present this way, although the normal erythrocyte sedimentation rate makes polymyalgia rheumatica less likely. Necrotic muscle can be seen in any of the inflammatory myopathies or necrotizing myositis. Endomysial deposits of amyloid can be seen in inclusion body myositis. Scattered inflammatory foci are seen in polymyositis.

XI-34.   **The answer is F.** *(Chap. 371)*   Trigeminal neuralgia is a clinical diagnosis based entirely on patient history. The disorder is characterized by *paroxysms* of excruciating pain in the lips, gums, cheeks, and chin that resolves over seconds to minutes. It is caused by ectopic action potentials in afferent pain fibers of the fifth cranial nerve, due either to nerve compression or other cause of demyelination. Symptoms are often, but not always, elicited by tactile stimuli on the face, tongue or lips. An elevated ESR is not part of the clinical syndrome. Elevated ESR is associated with temporal arteritis, a vasculitis associated with jaw claudication, unilateral vision loss, and symptoms of polymyalgia rheumatica. Trigeminal neuralgia is specifically notable for a lack of sensory findings on examination, unless the diagnosis comes in conjunction with another disorder such as midbrain mass lesion or aneurysm. First-line therapy is with carbamazepine followed by phenytoin, rather than gabapentin. Deep-seated facial and head pain is more a feature of migraine headache, dental pathology, or sinus disease.

XI-35. **The answer is B.** *(Chap. 16)* MRI is the radiologic test of choice for evaluation of most serious processes involving the spine. However, CT scanning is the preferred test when imaging of the bony structures is most important. In acute processes such as fracture or dislocation, MRI may reveal the edema associated with the acute inflammation, but for more chronic bony conditions, CT scanning is the test of choice. MRI is better than CT scanning for imaging the soft tissues surrounding the spine. Imaging the spinal cord itself, in the case of syringomyelia, is also better accomplished with MRI. Similarly, MRI is better than CT scanning for imaging the lateral recesses of the spinal cord; however, CT-myelography is preferred over MRI for that indication.

XI-36. **The answer is B.** *(Chap. 379)* Peripheral neuropathy is a general term indicating peripheral nerve disorders of any cause. The causes are legion, but peripheral neuropathy can be classified by a number of means: axonal versus demyelinating, mononeuropathy versus polyneuropathy versus mononeuritis multiplex, sensory versus motor, and the tempo of the onset of symptoms. Mononeuropathy typically results from local compression, trauma, or entrapment of a nerve. Polyneuropathy often results from a more systemic process. The distinction between axonal and demyelinating can often be made only with nerve conduction studies. HIV infection causes a common, distal, symmetric, mainly sensory polyneuropathy. Vitamin B_{12} deficiency typically causes a sensory neuropathy that predominantly involves the dorsal columns. Hypothyroidism and acromegaly may both cause compression and swelling of nerve fibers, resulting first in sensory symptoms and later in disease with motor symptoms. Critical illness polyneuropathy is predominantly motor in presentation. These patients may recover over the course of weeks to months. The etiology is unknown, but an association may exist with neuromuscular blockade and corticosteroids.

XI-37. **The answer is E.** *(Chap. 379)* Peripheral neuropathy is a common disorder affecting 2–8% of the adult population and increasing with age. The causes of peripheral neuropathy are myriad and can be classified by location, fiber type, histopathology, and time course. Specific features of the history and physical examination should lead the clinician towards a possible diagnosis. For example, lead toxicity is frequently associated with motor abnormalities in addition to sensory neuropathy. Laboratory examination with specific testing may be useful in assessing for a variety of etiologies of peripheral neuropathy, including diabetes mellitus, heavy metal toxicity, metabolic abnormalities, vasculitis, and infections (syphilis, Lyme disease, HIV). Of the choices listed in the question, folate deficiency is not associated with peripheral neuropathy.

XI-38. **The answer is A.** *(Chap. 374)* Endocrine dysfunction resulting in hypopituitarism frequently follows exposure of the hypothalamus or pituitary gland to therapeutic radiation. Growth hormone is the most sensitive to the damaging effects of WBRT, and thyroid-stimulating hormone is the least sensitive. ACTH, prolactin, and gonadotropins have an intermediate sensitivity. Other complications of radiation therapy to the brain include acute radiation injury manifest by headache, sleepiness, and worsening of preexisting neurologic defects. Early delayed radiation injury occurs within the first 4 months after therapy. It is associated with increased white matter signal on MRI and is steroid-responsive. Late delayed radiation injury occurs >4 months after therapy, typically 8–24 months. There may be dementia, gait apraxia, focal necrosis (after focal irradiation), or development of secondary malignancies.

XI-39. **The answer is C.** *(Chap. 374)* Spinal cord compression from solid tumor metastases usually results from growth of a bony vertebral metastasis into the epidural space. The most common primary tumors that metastasize to the bone include lung, breast, and prostate. The thoracic cord is most often involved. Back pain is a prominent symptom in 90% of patients with vertebral metastases and spinal cord compression. Concerning features of this patient's presentation include the symptoms of radicular injury as well as the signs of radicular and spinal cord impingement on physical examination. Once signs of spinal cord compression develop, they usually progress rapidly and warrant rapid therapy. Appropriate therapy includes emergent scanning with an MRI as well as immediate glucocorticoids if there are signs of spinal cord impingement. Subsequent management will depend on the extent of involvement and the primary tumor. Conservative pain management measures are not appropriate in this patient since he has very concerning neurologic findings for spinal cord compression and delay will increase the likelihood of irreversible defects. Antibody-mediated paraneoplastic neurologic syndromes are unlikely to cause focal findings such as in this patient. Radiographs may show bony metastases but will not show spinal cord damage.

XI-40.   The answer is C. *(Chap. 383)* The inflammatory myopathies (polymyositis, dermatomyositis, and inclusion body myositis) are associated with unique clinical features. Inclusion body myositis is usually seen in patients ≥50 years and initially involves the distal muscles, especially the foot extensors and finger flexors. Atrophy is seen along with weakness as this inflammatory myopathy runs a slowly progressive course, compared to polymyositis or dermatomyositis. Polymyositis is a rare disorder that usually involves the proximal not distal muscles. It is a diagnosis of exclusion after a thorough medical examination and muscle biopsy. Dermatomyositis is distinguished by the classic heliotrope rash and associated skin findings, which may precede the development of clinical muscular weakness. Eosinophilic myofasciitis is associated with myalgias, skin induration, fatigue, and eosinophilia in the peripheral blood as well as in endomysial tissue. Hyperthyroidism would cause a reduced TSH. It may cause weakness, but is generally associated with other findings such as tremor, skin changes, and irritability.

XI-41.   The answer is B. *(Chap. 381)* In myasthenia gravis, the primary defect is decreased number of available ACh receptors in the postsynaptic neuron at the neuromuscular junction (NMJ). This occurs as a result of antibody-mediated cross-linking of the ACh receptor, which causes increased turnover of ACh receptors, blockage of the active site, and damage to the postsynaptic muscle. The defect is not due to a defect in the release of ACh. Low levels of ACh-esterase would cause increased activation at the NMJ. Finally, the defect in myasthenia gravis occurs at the NMJ, not at nerve synapses.

XI-42.   The answer is E. *(Chap. 363)* Simple partial seizures cause motor, sensory, autonomic, or psychic symptoms without an obvious alteration in consciousness. The phenomenon of abnormal motor movements beginning in a restricted area then progressing to involve a larger area is termed *Jacksonian march*. The patient is describing Todd's paralysis, which may take minutes to many hours to return to normal. Although meningitis is a common cause of seizure in young patients, it is unlikely to be the cause in someone who has a known seizure disorder. If his symptoms were to persist beyond many hours, it would be reasonable to investigate a different etiology of his hand weakness with imaging studies. Overt deficits in strength are not compatible with a primary psychiatric disorder. Magnetic resonance angiogram and cerebral angiogram are useful to evaluate for cerebrovascular disorders, but there is no evidence of subarachnoid bleeding or vasculitis.

XI-43.   The answer is C. *(Chap. 376)* The release of bacterial cell wall components after killing by antibiotics may evoke a marked inflammatory cytokine response in the subarachnoid space. This inflammation may lead to increased damage of the blood brain barrier and central nervous system damage. Glucocorticoids can blunt this response by inhibiting tumor necrosis factor and interleukin-1. They work best if administered before antibiotics. Clinical trials have demonstrated that dexamethasone, 10 mg IV administered 20 min <u>before</u> antibiotics, reduced unfavorable outcomes, including death. The dexamethasone was continued for 4 days. The benefits were most striking in pneumococcal meningitis. Because this is the most common cause of meningitis in the elderly, empirical coverage should include this intervention as well. Empirical antibiotics in this case should include a third-generation cephalosporin, vancomycin, and ampicillin. However, dexamethasone may decrease vancomycin penetration into the CSF, so its use should be considered carefully in cases where the most likely organism requires vancomycin coverage.

XI-44. **The answer is E.** *(Chap. 15)* This patient has typical symptoms of migraine headaches without concerning features for an underlying disorder. Specifically, there is no report of worsening severity of headaches, fever, intractable vomiting, or abnormal neurologic examination that would be worrisome for an intracranial process. Vertigo is not an indication of a more serious intracranial process, as an estimated 33% of individuals with migraine experience vertigo both with and without accompanying headache. Therefore, imaging of the brain is unnecessary in this clinical situation. Migraine headaches are the second most common headache syndromes after tension headaches and affect 15% of women and 6% of men. The onset of headaches is usually in late adolescence, with peak prevalence of migraine occurring in the mid-thirties. Migraine headaches are typically classified as occurring with aura (previously called *classic migraine*) or without an aura. A more simplified diagnostic criterion for migraine has been adopted by the International Headache Society. Migraine is defined as repeated attacks of headache lasting 4–72 h in individuals with a normal physical examination. To be classified as a migraine, the headaches must fulfill at least two of the following symptoms: unilateral pain, throbbing quality, aggravation by movement, and moderate to severe intensity. At least one additional accompanying feature should be present, including either nausea/vomiting, phonophobia, or photophobia. Patient education and trigger avoidance are important in the management of migraine headaches. Migraines can frequently be controlled, but not eliminated, by lifestyle modifications, and it is important to understand an individual's triggers for migraine. A headache diary will help identify patterns of headaches as well as triggers. It will also provide an estimate of headache frequency and severity to aid in determining whether prophylactic medication would be required. Other nonpharmacologic treatment of migraines includes regular exercise, maintain a regular sleep-wake cycle, and stressor avoidance. Yoga, biofeedback, hypnosis, and meditation are interventions that may help alleviate stress and may have benefit in migraine treatment. Once an acute migraine is experienced, timely treatment is warranted to decrease the duration of the attack and minimize loss of productivity. If attacks are mild, analgesics such as nonsteroidal anti-inflammatory drugs or acetaminophen may be useful. However, the most effective drugs for the treatment of moderate to severe migraines are the 5-hydroxytriptamine agonists—ergotamines and the triptan drugs. Rizatriptan and almotriptan are the most efficacious of the triptan drugs. If migraine attacks occur more than five times monthly or are poorly responsive to abortive treatment, additional drug therapy for prevention is indicated.

XI-45. **The answer is D.** *(Chap. 361)* Cranial nerve XI (accessory nerve) is correctly paired with the proper examination technique. Testing cranial nerve I (olfactory nerve) should be performed with a mild stimulus (e.g., coffee or toothpaste) to eliminate any potential stimulation of pain fibers in the nasopharynx (trigeminal nerve) by noxious stimuli such as ammonia or alcohol. When testing visual acuity (cranial nerve II), corrective lenses should be worn by the patient, if necessary. This allows for testing of the neuronal aspects of vision without confounding by problems within the lens. It is also important to test each eye individually. The trigeminal (cranial nerve V) is predominantly a sensory nerve and has three sensory branches. The motor component of the trigeminal nerve predominantly innervates the masseter muscles used for chewing. Eyebrow elevation and forehead wrinkling are functions of cranial nerve VII.

XI-46. **The answer is C.** *(Chap. 381)* This patient's presentation with facial and ocular weakness in a nocturnal pattern is consistent with a typical presentation of myasthenia gravis. It is not uncommon for symptoms to be mostly nocturnal and be relatively asymptomatic in the early morning hours. Examining these patients in the evening or doing repetitive strength testing may bring out more subtle findings and requires a heightened index of suspicion. Lead poisoning would be uncommon in a woman of this age, and the findings would not be restricted to the cranial region. Psychiatric diagnoses do not correlate with myasthenia gravis, and repeat examination to corroborate the reported physical examination should be performed first. MRI of the brain is not indicated at this time as the physical examination findings point towards a serologic diagnosis. Slit-lamp examination is useful for finding abnormalities in the anterior portion of the eye, such as the iris, lens, and cornea.

XI-47. The answer is C. *(Chap. 363)*   Nuchal rigidity and an elevated white blood cell count is very concerning for meningitis as the etiology for this patient, and lumbar puncture must be performed to rule this out. In addition, acute cocaine intoxication is a plausible reason for this new-onset seizure. The figure below illustrates the evaluation of the adult patient with a seizure. MRI would be indicated if the patient had a negative metabolic and toxicologic screening. Substance abuse counseling, while indicated, is not indicated at this point

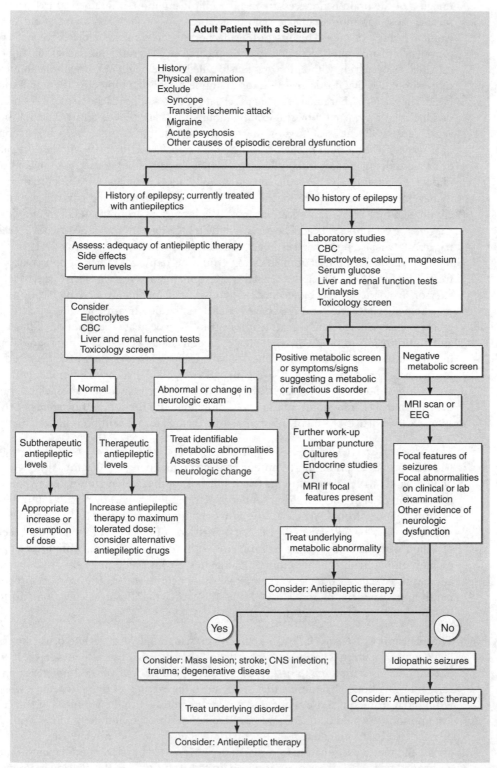

FIGURE XI-47   Evaluation of the adult patient with a seizure. CBC, complete blood count; CT, computed tomography; MRI, magnetic resonance imaging; EEG, electroencephalogram; CNS, central nervous system.

in his workup since he is postictal. The patient is not having seizures, does not have a known seizure disorder, and has not been treated for the underlying metabolic abnormality, making intravenous loading with an antiepileptic medication premature at this time.

XI-48. The answer is D. *(Chap. 382)* Becker and Duchenne muscular dystrophy are both X-linked recessive disorders associated with different mutations of the dystrophin gene located on the short arm of the X chromosome. This 2000-kb gene is among the largest identified human genes. In both Becker and Duchenne muscular dystrophy, the most common mutation is a deletion. However, deletions in Becker muscular dystrophy do not result in frame-shift mutations, yielding a delayed presentation and milder presentation of disease. Limb-girdle muscular dystrophy designates a clinical syndrome that presents as progressive weakness of pelvic and shoulder girdle muscles. There are 12 recognized limb-girdle muscular dystrophies with unique mutations. This disorder can be inherited in both an autosomal dominant or recessive fashion, depending on the mutation present. Kearns-Sayre syndrome and myoclonic epilepsy with ragged red fibers (MERFF) are mitochondrial myopathies. Each mitochondrion possesses a DNA genome unique from the nuclear genome and is inherited primarily from the oocytes, accounting for the maternal inheritance of mitochondrial disorders. Kearns-Sayre syndrome is a multisystem disorder with chronic progressive external ophthalmoplegia (CPEO). Varying degrees of proximal muscle weakness are present. MERFF presents in late childhood to adulthood with clinical features of myoclonic epilepsy, progressive weakness, and cerebellar ataxia.

XI-49. The answer is B. *(Chap. 268)* Brain death is defined by the cessation of cerebral function while somatic function is maintained by artificial means and the heart continues to pump. It is the only type of brain damage that is considered equivalent to death. The diagnosis of brain death should be confirmed with the following clinical findings: unresponsiveness to any stimuli, indicating widespread cortical destruction; brainstem damage, as evidenced by enlarged or mid-sized pupils without light reaction; absent corneal and oculovestibular reflexes; and apnea, indicating medullary destruction. The heart rate should be invariant. Because the spinal cord is intact, spinal reflexes may be present. The presence or absence of the Babinski sign does not contribute to the diagnosis of brain death. Central diabetes insipidus occurs with dysfunction of the hypothalamus or posterior pituitary. It has been described in patients with brain death but is not a component of the diagnosis.

XI-50. The answer is B. *(Chap. 15)* Cluster headaches, which can cause excruciating hemicranial pain, are notable for their occurrence during characteristic episodes. Usually attacks occur during a 4- to 8-week period in which the patient experiences one to three severe brief headaches daily. There may then be a prolonged pain-free interval before the next episode. Men between ages 20 and 50 are most commonly affected. The unilateral pain is usually associated with lacrimation, eye reddening, nasal stuffiness, ptosis, and nausea. During episodes alcohol may provoke the attacks. Even though the pain caused by brain tumors may awaken a patient from sleep, the typical history and normal neurologic examination do not mandate evaluation for a neoplasm of the central nervous system. Acute therapy for a cluster headache attack consists of oxygen inhalation, although intranasal lidocaine and subcutaneous sumatriptan may also be effective. Prophylactic therapy with prednisone, lithium, methysergide, ergotamine, or verapamil can be administered during an episode to prevent further cluster headache attacks.

XI-51. The answer is C. *(Chap. 371)* Trigeminal neuralgia is a clinical diagnosis based entirely on patient history, and as such should be treated once a patient comes with the virtually pathognomonic complaints of paroxysms of excruciating pain in the lips, gums, cheeks, and chin that resolve over seconds to minutes. Carbamazepine is first-line therapy, followed by phenytoin for the ~30–50% of patients who do not respond adequately to therapy. Surgical approaches, such as radiofrequency thermal rhizotomy, gamma-knife radiosurgery, and microvascular decompression, should be considered only when medical options fail. Steroids have no therapeutic role, as trigeminal neuralgia is not an inflammatory condition. Neuroimaging is not indicated, unless other clinical features or a focal neurologic deficit elicited on history or physical examination suggest another possible diagnosis such as intracranial mass or multiple sclerosis.

XI-52. **The answer is C.** *(Chap. 380)* The patient fulfills the diagnostic criteria for Guillain-Barré syndrome (GBS) with progressive weakness of two or more limbs, areflexia, disease course <4 weeks, and no other identifiable cause. Other characteristic features include lack of a fever, symmetric weakness, and minimal sensory symptoms. The diagnosis is further suggested by an antecedent gastrointestinal illness. In the United States, 20–30% of all cases of GBS are associated with a preceding infection with *Campylobacter jejuni*. This patient also has evidence of impending respiratory failure from neuromuscular weakness manifested by tachypnea, accessory muscle use, and paradoxical respiration. His arterial blood gas shows a respiratory alkalosis with an increase in the A – a gradient to 33 mmHg. His vital capacity is 12.5 mL/kg body weight. Laboratory findings would include normal serum chemistries with an increased cerebrospinal fluid protein without pleocytosis. Electromyography would show evidence of demyelination. Treatment for this individual should include endotracheal intubation with mechanical ventilation in addition to IVIg or plasmapheresis. IVIg is administered as five daily infusions of 2 g/kg body weight. Plasmapheresis is equally effective in treating GBS and is performed four times over the first week. Mechanical ventilation is indicated in GBS when the vital capacity <20 mL/kg *(ND Lawn et al: Arch Neurol 58(6):893, 2001)*. There is no role for glucocorticoids in the treatment of GBS. Ciprofloxacin is an effective treatment to decrease symptom duration in *C. jejuni* infection if given early in the course of the illness, but has no effect in treatment of GBS following *C. jejuni* infection. Botulism also presents as an ascending symmetric paralysis. Cranial nerves are more frequently involved than in GBS. In this patient, there is no associated risk factor for botulism such as home-canned foods or injection wounds from drug use.

XI-53. **The answer is E.** *(Chap. 364)* Cardioembolism accounts for up to 20% of all ischemic strokes. Stroke caused by heart disease is due to thrombotic material forming on the atrial or ventricular wall or the left heart valves. If the thrombus lyses quickly, only a transient ischemic attack may develop. If the arterial occlusion lasts longer, brain tissue may die and a stroke will occur. Emboli from the heart most often lodge in the middle cerebral artery (MCA), the posterior cerebral artery (PCA), or one of their branches. Atrial fibrillation is the most common cause of cerebral embolism overall. Other significant causes of cardioembolic stroke include myocardial infarction, prosthetic valves, rheumatic heart disease, and dilated cardiomyopathy. Furthermore, paradoxical embolization may occur when an atrial septal defect or a patent foramen ovale exists. This may be detected by bubble-contrast echocardiography. Bacterial endocarditis may cause septic emboli if the vegetation is on the left side of the heart or if there is a paradoxical source.

XI-54. **The answer is B.** *(Chap. 16)* The crossed straight leg raise is positive when flexion of one leg reproduces the pain in the opposite leg or buttocks. This sign is more specific for disk herniation than the straight leg raise. The nerve or nerve root lesion is always on the side of the pain. The straight leg raise test is positive if passive flexion of the leg reproduces the patient's usual back pain. The reverse straight leg raise is performed by standing the patient next to the examination table and passively extending the leg with the knee flexed. This maneuver stretches the L2-L4 nerve roots. Back pain referred from visceral organs may be palpated on abdominal examination but should not be reproduced by straight leg raise. Passive dorsiflexion of the foot during the straight leg raise will add to the stretch but does not add any more diagnostic information.

XI-55. **The answer is D.** *(Chap. 374)* This figure illustrates a mass attached to the meninges with a dural tail. Other dural tumors may appear this way, but of the options listed, the meningioma is by far the most likely to appear this way. Meningiomas derive from the cells that give rise to the arachnoid granulations. They are usually benign and attached to the dura. They rarely invade the brain. They are more frequent in women than men and have a peak incidence in middle age. Total surgical resection of a meningioma is curative. Low-grade astrocytoma and high-grade astrocytoma (glioblastoma) often infiltrate into adjacent brain and rarely have the clear margins seen in this figure. Oligodendroma comprise ~15% of all gliomas and show calcification in roughly 30% of cases. They have a more benign course and are more responsive than other gliomas to cytotoxic therapy. For low-grade oligodendromas, the median survival is 7–8 years. Brain abscess will have distinctive ring-enhancing features with a capsule, often have mass effect, and will have evidence of inflammation on MRI scanning.

XI-56. **The answer is B.** *(Chap. 363)* Optimal medical therapy for epilepsy depends on the underlying cause, type of seizure, and patient factors. The goal is to prevent seizures and minimize the side effects of therapy. The minimal effective dose is determined by trial and error. In choosing medical therapies, drug interactions are a key consideration. Certain medications, such as tricyclic antidepressants, may lower the seizure threshold and should be avoided. Patients who respond well to medical therapy and have completely controlled seizures are good candidates for the discontinuation of therapy, with about 70% of children and 60% of adults being able to discontinue therapy eventually. Patient factors that aid in this include complete medical control of seizures for 1 to 5 years, a normal neurologic examination, a normal EEG, and single seizure type. On the other end of the spectrum, about 20% of these patients are completely refractory to medical therapy and should be considered for surgical therapy. In the best examples, such as mesial temporal sclerosis, resection of the temporal lobe may result in about 70% of these patients becoming seizure free and an additional 15 to 25% having a significant reduction in the incidence of seizures. In patients with epilepsy other considerations are critical. Psychosocial sequelae such as depression, anxiety, and behavior problems may occur. Approximately 20% of epileptic patients have depression, with their suicide rate being higher than that of age-matched controls. There is an impact on the ability to drive, perform certain jobs, and function in social situations. Furthermore, there is a twofold to threefold increase in mortality for patients with epilepsy compared with age-matched controls. Although most of the increased mortality results from the underlying etiology of epilepsy, a significant number of these patients die from accidents, status epilepticus, and a syndrome known as sudden unexpected death in epileptic patients (SUDEP). The cause is unknown, but research has centered on brainstem-mediated effects of seizures on cardiopulmonary function.

XI-57. **The answer is D.** *(Chap. 364)* Nonrheumatic atrial fibrillation is the most common cause of cerebral embolism overall. The presumed stroke mechanism is thrombus formation in the fibrillating atrium or atrial appendage. The average annual risk of stroke is around 5%. However, the risk varies with certain factors: age, hypertension, left ventricular function, prior embolism, diabetes, and thyroid function. Patients younger than 60 years of age without structural heart disease or without one of these risk factors have a very low annual risk of cardioembolism: less than 0.5%. Therefore, it is recommended that these patients only take aspirin daily for stroke prevention. Older patients with numerous risk factors may have annual stroke risks of 10 to 15% and must take warfarin indefinitely. Cardioversion is indicated for symptomatic patients who want an initial opportunity to remain in sinus rhythm. However, studies have shown that there is an increased stroke risk for weeks to months after a successful cardioversion, and these patients must remain on anticoagulation for a long period. Similarly, recent studies have shown that patients who do not respond to cardioversion and do not want catheter ablation have mortality and morbidity with rate control and anticoagulation similar to those of patients who opt for cardioversion. Low-molecular-weight heparin may be used as a bridge to warfarin therapy and may facilitate outpatient anticoagulation in selected patients.

XI-58. **The answer is D.** *(Chap. 382)* There are two recognized clinical forms of myotonic dystrophy, both of which are characterized by autosomal dominant inheritance. Myotonic dystrophy 1 (DM1) is the most common form and the most likely disorder in this patient. Characteristic clinical features of this disorder include a "hatchet-faced" appearance, due to wasting of the facial muscles, and weakness of the neck muscles. In contrast to the muscular dystrophies (Becker and Duchenne), distal limb muscle weakness is more common in DM1. Palatal, pharyngeal, and tongue involvement are also common and produce the dysarthric voice that is frequently heard. The failure of relaxation after a forced hand grip is characteristic of myotonia. Myotonia can also be elicited by percussion of the thenar eminence. In most individuals, myotonia is present by age 5, but clinical symptoms of weakness that lead to diagnosis may not be present until adulthood. Cardiac conduction abnormalities and heart failure are also common in myotonic dystrophy. Diagnosis can often be made by clinical features alone in an individual with classic symptoms and a positive family history. An electromyogram would confirm myotonia. Genetic testing for DM1 would show a characteristic trinucleotide repeat on chromosome 19. Genetic anticipation occurs with an increasing number of repeats and worsening clinical disease over successive generations. Myotonic dystrophy 2 (DM2) causes proximal muscle weakness primarily and is also known by the name proximal myotonic myopathy (PROMM). Other features of the disease overlap with DM1. Acid maltase deficiency (glucosidase deficiency, or Pompe's disease) has three recognized forms, only one of which has onset in adulthood. In the adult-onset form, respiratory muscle weakness is prominent and often is the presenting symptoms. As stated previously, Becker and Duchenne muscular dystrophies present with primarily proximal muscle weakness and are X-linked recessive disorders. Becker muscular dystrophy presents at a later age than Duchenne muscular dystrophy and has a more prolonged course. Otherwise, features are similar to one another. Nemaline myopathy is a heterogeneous disorder marked by the threadlike appearance of muscle fibers on biopsy. Nemaline myopathy usually presents in childhood and has a striking facial appearance similar to myotonic dystrophy with a long, narrow face. This disease is inherited in an autosomal dominant fashion.

XI-59.   The answer is D. *(Chap. 363)*   Adolescence and early adulthood mark the period where idiopathic or genetic epilepsy syndromes become less common and seizures due to acquired CNS lesions become more common. The most common causes of seizures in the young adults are head trauma, central nervous system (CNS) infections, brain tumors, congenital CNS lesions, illicit drug use, or alcohol withdrawal. Fever rarely causes seizure in patients >12 years. Amyloid angiopathy and uremia are more common in older adults.

XI-60.   The answer is B. *(Chap. 378)*   Startle myoclonus is a worrisome sign but is not specific for CJD, though it is more so if it occurs during sleep. Lewy body dementia, Alzheimer's disease, central nervous system infections, and myoclonic epilepsy can all cause myoclonus. EEG and MRI can both help differentiate CJD from these disorders. The MRI finding of cortical ribboning and intensity in the basal ganglia on fluid-attenuated inversion recovery sequences are characteristic of CJD. EEG is useful if stereotypical periodic bursts every 1–2 s are present, but this is seen in only 60% of cases, and other findings may be less specific. Demonstration of specific immunoassays for proteolytic products of disease-causing prion proteins (PrP^{Sc}) at brain biopsy may be necessary to confirm diagnosis in some cases. However, these proteins are not uniformly distributed throughout the brain and false-negative biopsies occur. Both surgeons and pathologists must be warned to use standard precautions under these circumstances. These proteins cannot be measured from cerebrospinal fluid (CSF). CSF in CJD is usually normal except for a minimally elevated protein. Many patients with CJD have elevated CSF stress protein 14-3-3. This test alone is neither sensitive nor specific, as patients with herpes simplex virus encephalitis, multi-infarct dementia, and stroke may have similar elevations.

XI-61.   The answer is D. *(Chap. 23)*   The ventral spinal cord includes the corticospinal tracts, spinothalamic tracts, and descending autonomic tracts. Disruption of these tracts causes weakness/areflexia, loss of pain/temperature sensation, and bladder sphincter dysfunction, respectively. The dorsal columns include vibratory sense and proprioception, which are spared in the ventral cord syndrome. Other causes of the syndrome include disc herniation, radiation myelitis, and human T-lymphocyte virus 1 infection.

XI-62.   The answer is C. *(Chap. 383)*   This patient's skin findings are an example of Gottron's sign of the hands and the heliotrope facial rash of dermatomyositis. Usually the rash precedes the muscular weakness. In addition to the V-sign, as described in the scenario, one can also see the shawl sign, in which the erythematous rash is found around the shoulders and posterior neck region. In addition to the skin manifestations, skeletal muscle weakness, particularly the proximal muscles, is part of the presentation of dermatomyositis. Extramuscular manifestations include constitutional symptoms, joint contractures, dysphagia, cardiac disturbances, pulmonary dysfunction, and arthralgias. Hepatosplenomegaly is not an associated clinical finding. Situs inversus is not associated with dermatomyositis. Hypothyroidism is associated with delayed deep tendon relaxation. In hypothyroidism the skin appears swollen, dry, and coarse with a cool waxy appearance. Subcutaneous nodules on the elbows, back of the forearms, and metacarpophalangeal joints of the hands are characteristic of rheumatoid arthritis, particularly in the active phase.

XI-63.   **The answer is D.** *(Chap. 29)* This patient has acute angle-closure glaucoma resulting from obstruction of the outflow of aqueous humor at the iris. The buildup of intraocular pressure can be confirmed by measurement and requires urgent treatment with hyperosmotic agents. Permanent treatment requires laser or surgical iridotomy. Angle-closure glaucoma is less common than is primary open-angle glaucoma, which is asymptomatic and is usually detectable only through measurements of intraocular pressure at a routine eye examination.

XI-64.   **The answer is D.** *(Chap. 379)* CMT disease is a heterogeneous group of inherited peripheral neuropathies. Transmission is usually autosomal dominant but may be recessive or X-linked. Numerous genetic defects are associated with CMT disease. It is very common, affecting up to 1 in 2500 persons. Clinically, patients usually present in the first or second decade of life, but later presentations may occur. The neuropathy affects both motor and sensory nerves. Symptoms may vary, ranging from distal muscle weakness and severe atrophy and disability to only pes cavus and minimal weakness. Although sensory findings and involvement are common, these patients often do not have dominant sensory complaints. However, if patients have no evidence of sensory involvement on detailed neurologic examination or electrodiagnostic studies, an alternative diagnosis should be considered. There is no known effective therapy for CMT disease. Orthotics and physical therapy are mainstays for preserving function.

XI-65.   **The answer is C.** *(Chap. 322)* Neurologic manifestations are present in 5–10% of individuals with sarcoidosis and are the presenting complaint in up to 50% of individuals who have neurologic involvement of sarcoidosis. Any part of the systemic or central nervous system (CNS) can be affected by neurosarcoidosis. The most common manifestations are cranial nerve involvement, basilar meningitis, myelopathy, and anterior hypothalamic disease. Peripheral facial nerve palsy develops in >50% of individuals with neurosarcoidosis at some point, but may resolve spontaneously and be misdiagnosed as Bell's palsy, an idiopathic facial nerve palsy. Bilateral facial nerve palsy can occur with neurologic manifestations of sarcoidosis, but it is rare for any other disease to cause bilateral disease. In this patient, the presence of bilateral facial nerve weakness strongly suggests neurologic involvement with sarcoidosis. In addition, the presence of hilar adenopathy also strengthens the likelihood that sarcoidosis is the cause of the patient's bilateral facial nerve palsy. On MRI imaging, neurosarcoidosis shows gadolinium enhancement of the affected neurologic structures. In this case, bilateral seventh nerve enhancement and meningeal enhancement is seen. Space-occupying lesions can also be demonstrated if parenchymal disease occurs. Analysis of the cerebrospinal fluid (CSF) most often demonstrates lymphocytic meningitis with mildly increased CSF protein and normal CSF glucose levels. Identifying disease outside of the CNS is important for making the definitive diagnosis by biopsy. If the presence of noncaseating granulomas can be demonstrated by biopsy of the lungs or enlarged lymph nodes, diagnosis can be established and treatment initiated without the need for invasive diagnostic testing of the neurologic tissue involved. Treatment of neurologic involvement of sarcoidosis usually requires oral prednisone at doses of 0.5 mg/kg daily. Higher doses of glucocorticoids or additional cytotoxic therapies such as cyclophosphamide may be necessary for severe neurologic disease. Lyme disease is also a frequent cause of peripheral facial nerve paralysis. However, it is rare for Lyme disease to cause bilateral palsy, and this patient does not live in an area that is known to have prevalent Lyme disease. He lives in an urban environment and reports no exposures that would make Lyme disease more likely. In addition, Lyme disease would not explain the pulmonary abnormalities seen by chest radiograph. Multiple sclerosis does not commonly cause facial nerve palsy. Optic neuritis is a frequent presenting complaint in multiple sclerosis as well as in neurologic sarcoidosis, and it can be difficult to differentiate between the two diseases in the setting of optic neuritis. If optic neuritis is present, demonstration of disease outside the CNS is important for diagnosing sarcoidosis as the cause. While tuberculous meningitis may present with multiple cranial nerve palsies, it is unlikely in this patient who is otherwise well. Tuberculous meningitis typically presents with fevers, headache, and altered mental status. However, a protracted illness with lethargy and memory loss can be seen. The CSF evaluation is also not consistent with tuberculosis. Lymphocytic meningitis with markedly elevated protein and very low glucose would be expected. Likewise, viral meningitis should present with an acute illness with fever, headache, neck stiffness, and photophobia. While idiopathic Bell's palsy is thought to be related to herpes simples virus 1 infection, demonstration of meningeal involvement in cases of Bell's palsy is rare in this setting.

XI-66.   The answer is D.   *(Chap. 376)*   *Listeria* has become an increasingly important cause of bacterial meningitis in neonates (<1 month of age), pregnant women, individuals >60 years old, and immunocompromised individuals. Infection is acquired by eating contaminated foods such as unpasteurized dairy products, cole slaw, milk, soft cheeses, delicatessen meats, and uncooked hot dogs. Ampicillin is the agent most often added to the initial empirical regimen to cover *L. monocytogenes*.

XI-67.   The answer is E.   *(Chap. 268)*   Foraminal herniation, which forces the cerebellar tonsils into the foramen magnum, leads to compression of the medulla and subsequent respiratory arrest. Central transtentorial herniation occurs when the medial thalamus compresses the midbrain as it moves through the tentorial opening; miotic pupils and drowsiness are the classic clinical signs. A locked-in state is usually caused by infarction or hemorrhage of the ventral pons; other causes include Guillain-Barré syndrome and certain neuromuscular blocking agents. Catatonia is a semi-awake state seen most frequently as a manifestation of psychotic disorders such as schizophrenia. Third-nerve palsies arise from an uncal transtentorial herniation where the anterior medial temporal gyrus herniates into the anterior portion of the tentorial opening anterior to the adjacent midbrain. Coma may occur due to compression of the midbrain.

XI-68.   The answer is D.   *(Chap. 371)*   Brief paroxysms of severe, sharp pains in the face without demonstrable lesions in the jaw, teeth, or sinuses are called tic douloureux, or trigeminal neuralgia. The pain may be brought on by stimuli applied to the face, lips, or tongue or by certain movements of those structures. Aneurysms, neurofibromas, and meningiomas impinging on the fifth cranial nerve at any point during its course typically present with trigeminal neuropathy, which will cause sensory loss on the face, weakness of the jaw muscles, or both; neither symptom is demonstrable in this patient. The treatment for this idiopathic condition is carbamazepine or phenytoin if carbamazepine is not tolerated. When drug treatment is not successful, surgical therapy, including the commonly applied percutaneous retrogasserian rhizotomy, may be effective. A possible complication of this procedure is partial facial numbness with a risk of corneal anesthesia, which increases the potential for ulceration.

XI-69.   The answer is C.   *(Chap. 381)*   Except for lumbar puncture, all of the options listed are indicated at this time. Thymic abnormalities are present in 75% of patients with myasthenia gravis. A CT or MRI of the mediastinum may show enlargement or neoplastic changes in the thymus and is recommended upon diagnosis. Hyperthyroidism occurs in 3–8% of patients with myasthenia gravis and may aggravate weakness. Testing for rheumatoid factor and antinuclear antibodies should also be obtained because of the association of myasthenia gravis to other autoimmune diseases. Due to side effects of immunosuppressive therapy, a thorough evaluation should be undertaken to rule out latent or chronic infections such as tuberculosis. Measurements of ventilatory function are valuable as a baseline because of the frequency and seriousness of respiratory impairment in myasthenic patients, and they can be used as an objective measure of response to therapy.

XI-70.   The answer is D.   *(Chap. 373)*   Hemorrhages beneath the dural layer (subdural) or between the skull and the dura (epidural) are common sequelae of head trauma. They can be life-threatening, and prompt evaluation and management are imperative. Several clinical features allow these conditions to be distinguished from one another. Acute subdural hematomas typically arise from venous sources, often the bridging veins located immediately under the dura mater. As the brain volume decreases with age, traction on these venous structures increases and even minor head trauma in the elderly can lead to a subdural hematoma. Approximately 33% of patients with an acute subdural bleed will experience a lucid interval after the event, which is followed by obtundation. Subdural bleeding is typically slower than epidural bleeding due to their different sources. Small subdural bleeds are asymptomatic and often do not require evacuation. Epidural hematomas, on the other hand, can arise quickly and typically represent arterial bleeding. They are often caused by a lacerated middle meningeal artery from an overlying skull fracture. Rapid increase in intracranial pressure from these bleeds can necessitate arterial ligation or emergent craniotomy. Most patients with epidural bleeding are unconscious when first evaluated; a "lucid interval" can occasionally be seen.

XI-71. **The answer is C.** *(Chap. 371)* Pain, loss of function (without clear-cut sensory or motor deficits), and a localized autonomic impairment are called reflex sympathetic dystrophy (also known as shoulder-hand syndrome or causalgia). Precipitating events in this unusual syndrome include myocardial infarction, shoulder trauma, and limb paralysis. In addition to the neuropathic-type pain, autonomic dysfunction, possibly resulting from neuroadrenergic and cholinergic hypersensitivity, produces localized sweating, changes in blood flow, and abnormal hair and nail growth as well as edema or atrophy of the affected limb. Treatment is difficult; however, anticonvulsants such as phenytoin and carbamazepine may be effective, as they are in other conditions in which neuropathic pain is a major problem.

XI-72. **The answer is B.** *(Chap. 15)* The peak prevalence of migraine headaches occurs in the fourth to fifth decades of life. Many women experience decreased severity and frequency of headaches after menopause, and some individuals cease to have migraines as they age. Migraine has been demonstrated to be a risk factor for ischemic stroke in both men and women (*M Etminan et al: BMJ 330: 63, 2005; T Kurth et al: Neurology 64: 1020, 2005; JE Buring et al: Arch Neurol 52: 129, 1995*). In addition, women who have migraine with aura appear to be at greater risk of ischemic stroke if they are concurrently taking oral contraceptives. The American College of Gynecology has recommended that women who are >35 or have focal neurologic symptoms with their migraine attacks should not take oral contraceptives (*Int J Gynaecol Obstet 75: 93, 2001*), but low-dose contraceptive can otherwise be taken safely in women with migraine headaches. Any risk factors that are known to increase stroke risk such as hypertension or cigarette smoking also contribute to stroke in individuals with migraine. Interestingly, asymptomatic women with migraines have been shown to have a greater likelihood of white matter changes on MRI, and those with aura had a significant increased risk of subclinical posterior circulation infarcts (*MC Kruit et al: JAMA 291: 427, 2004*).

XI-73. **The answer is A.** *(Chap. 22)* This patient has classic symptoms and history consistent with Ménière's disease. Patients have recurrent unilateral labyrinthine dysfunction marked by hearing loss and tinnitus. The symptoms are very debilitating, and patients may be incapacitated by the tinnitus and vertigo. The severity and recurrent nature suggest Ménière's disease and argue against a central process. Ménière's disease responds to diuretic therapy and/or a low-salt diet. In addition, patients should attempt to ambulate in an attempt to induce central compensatory mechanisms. Scopolamine transdermal patches and anticholinergic medications are useful only for motion sickness. The Epley procedure attempts to reposition particulate debris within the semicircular canals such as in benign paroxysmal positional vertigo. Glucocorticoids are useful for the acute treatment of vertigo but are used only in the acute setting and have no role in the long-term treatment of Ménière's disease. Metoclopramide may be used to treat nausea but has no role in the tinnitus and vertigo of Ménière's disease.

XI-74. **The answer is E.** *(Chap. 368)* Cerebellar ataxia with a strong family history suggests one of the autosomal spinocerebellar ataxias (SCA). SCA7 is distinguished from all of the other SCAs by the presence of retinal pigmentary degeneration. The visual abnormalities first appear as blue-yellow color blindness and proceed to frank visual loss with macular degeneration. Proliferative retinopathy would be expected in someone who has poorly controlled diabetes. Lipemia retinalis is often seen in patients with hypertriglyceridemia. Papilledema is seen in increased intracranial pressure, which is not present in SCA.

XI-75.   The answer is E. *(Chap. 364)*   Numerous studies have identified key risk factors for ischemic stroke. Old age, family history, diabetes, hypertension, tobacco smoking, and cholesterol are all risk factors for atherosclerosis and therefore stroke. Hypertension is the most significant among these risk factors. All cases of hypertension must be controlled in the setting of stroke prevention. Antiplatelet therapy has been shown to reduce the risk of vascular atherothrombotic events. The overall relative risk reduction of nonfatal stroke is about 25 to 30% across most large clinical trials. The "true" absolute benefit is dependent on the individual patient's risk; therefore, patients with a low risk for stroke (e.g., younger, with minimal cardiovascular risk factors) may have a relative risk reduction with antiplatelet therapy but a meaningless "benefit." Numerous studies have shown the benefit of statin therapy in the reduction of stroke risk even in the absence of hypercholesterolemia. Although anticoagulation is the treatment of choice for atrial fibrillation and cardioembolic causes of stroke, there is no proven benefit in regard to the prevention of atherothrombotic stroke; therefore, warfarin cannot be recommended.

XI-76.   The answer is C. *(Chap. 30)*   Head trauma is the most common etiology of a decreased sense of smell in young adults and children. In most cases this is permanent, with only 10% of these patients experiencing recovery. In older adults viral infections predominate. Parainfluenza virus type 3 is the most common associated virus. Patients with HIV also frequently have a distorted sense of smell, and this is associated with HIV wasting syndrome. Although rare, genetic defects such as Kallmann syndrome and albinism are also causes of anosmia. Influenza virus is not a cause of anosmia.

XI-77.   The answer is D. *(Chap. 363)*   Phenytoin is a commonly used anticonvulsant. Its principal use is in patients with tonic-clonic seizures. It may be given either orally or intravenously. Typical dosing is about 300 to 400 mg/d in adults. The therapeutic range is between 10 and 20 µg/mL. Neurologic side effects include dizziness, ataxia, diplopia, and confusion. Systemic side effects include gum hyperplasia, hirsutism, facial coarsening, and osteomalacia. These patients may develop lymphadenopathy and Stevens-Johnson syndrome. Toxicity may be enhanced by liver disease and competition with other medications. Phenytoin alters folate metabolism and is teratogenic. Leukopenia is not a typical side effect and is seen more often with carbamazepine.

XI-78.   The answer is C. *(Chap. 382)*   The muscular dystrophies are hereditary progressive diseases. Becker's muscular dystrophy is a less severe form of X-linked recessive muscular dystrophy than Duchenne's muscular dystrophy. It occurs 10 times less frequently than DMD. The underlying defect is in the same protein, dystrophin, which is part of a large complex of sarcolemmal proteins and glycoproteins. Clinically, Becker's muscular dystrophy (BMD) shows a similar pattern of proximal muscle weakness. Weakness becomes generalized with progression of the disease. Hypertrophy of muscles, particularly the calves, is an early feature. Most patients experience the initial symptoms in the first and second decades of life, but a later onset may occur. These patients have reduced life expectancy but are significantly more functional than are patients with DMD. Mental retardation may also occur in patients with BMD, and cardiac involvement may result in congestive heart failure. Serum creatinine kinase (CK) levels are elevated, and electrodiagnostic findings are similar to those seen in DMD. The diagnosis is made by demonstrating a reduced amount of dystrophin on Western blot analysis.

XI-79.   The answer is D. *(Chap. 16)*   There are four indications for surgical repair of an intervertebral disk herniation: objective progressive motor weakness, signs of spinal cord compression (e.g., bowel or bladder incontinence), incapacitating nerve root pain despite conservative treatment, and recurrent incapacitating nerve root pain. Absent deep tendon reflexes, nighttime symptoms, and more than one level of disk herniation are not uncommon findings in patients with a disk herniation and do not mandate surgery.

XI-80. **The answer is A.** *(Chap. 23)* Episodic generalized weakness is caused by disorders of the central nervous system (CNS) or the motor unit. Weakness from CNS disorders is usually associated with altered consciousness or cognition, increased muscle tone and reflexes, and changes in sensation. Motor unit disorders include a variety of electrolyte disturbances (hypokalemia, hyperkalemia, hypercalcemia, hypernatremia, hyponatremia, hypophosphatemia, hypermagnesemia), inborn errors of metabolism (carbohydrate or fatty acid metabolism, mitochondrial function), toxins (botulism, curare), neuromuscular junction disorders (myasthenia gravis, Lambert-Eaton syndrome), and channelopathies (periodic paralysis). Transient ischemic attacks of the brainstem, but not in any other part of the brain, may also cause episodic generalized weakness. Multiple sclerosis may cause episodic generalized weakness. Atherosclerotic occlusive carotid disease may cause focal but not generalized weakness.

XI-81. **The answer is C.** *(Chap. 361)* The patient in this scenario is demonstrating *paratonia* (fluctuating changes in resistance during testing of motor tone). Paratonia may be seen in patients who have difficulty relaxing during the examination or may be evidence of aberrant frontal lobe pathways, as in some forms of dementia. The patient has increased tone, making muscle injury less likely. Dystonia, as seen in parkinsonism, manifests as cogwheel rigidity and jerky interruptions of resistance without the focality that is seen in this scenario. Motor neuron diseases, such as amyotrophic lateral sclerosis, may present with either flaccidity or spasticity. Usually patients with motor neuron disease have abnormalities that can be elicited in more than one muscle group (although asymmetry is common).

XI-82. **The answer is D.** *(Chap. 377)* Ibuprofen, isoniazid, ciprofloxacin, tolmetin, sulfa-containing medicines, and phenazopyridine have been implicated in drug hypersensitivity leading to meningitis. The cerebrospinal fluid (CSF) will typically show neutrophils, but mononuclear cells or eosinophils are occasionally present. Most causes of chronic (not recurrent) meningitis cause a predominance of mononuclear cells. The differential for chronic meningitis is broad and a diagnosis is often difficult to make. The treating physician needs to consider a diverse array of viral, fungal, bacterial, mycobacterial, helminthic, and protozoal pathogens, both common and exotic, and therefore should obtain a detailed social history and consult an expert in the field. Recurrent meningitis is often due to herpes simplex virus type 2 infection and this should be ruled out, particularly if active genital ulcers develop concurrently. Malignancy, sarcoidosis, and vasculitis are all potential causes, and history, physical examination, and appropriate further testing should dictate the degree to which these possibilities are explored. Medications are often overlooked as a cause of chronic meningitis and should always be carefully considered. When CSF neutrophils predominate after 3 weeks of illness, nocardia, actinomyces, brucella, tuberculosis (<10% of cases), fungal, and noninfectious causes of chronic meningitis should be considered.

XI-83. **The answer is E.** *(Chaps. 27 and 365)* All the choices given in the question are causes of or may be associated with dementia. Binswanger's disease, the cause of which is unknown, often occurs in patients with long-standing hypertension and/or atherosclerosis; it is associated with diffuse subcortical white matter damage and has a subacute insidious course. Alzheimer's disease, the most common cause of dementia, is also slowly progressive and can be confirmed at autopsy by the presence of amyloid plaques and neurofibrillary tangles. Creutzfeldt-Jakob disease, a prion disease, is associated with a rapidly progressive dementia, myoclonus, rigidity, a characteristic EEG pattern, and death within 1 to 2 years of onset. Vitamin B_{12} deficiency, which often is seen in the setting of chronic alcoholism, most commonly produces a myelopathy that results in loss of vibration and joint position sense and brisk deep tendon reflexes (dorsal column and lateral corticospinal tract dysfunction). This combination of pathologic abnormalities in the setting of vitamin B_{12} deficiency is also called subacute combined degeneration. Vitamin B_{12} deficiency may also lead to a subcortical type of dementia. Multi-infarct dementia, as in this case, presents with a history of sudden stepwise declines in function associated with the accumulation of bilateral focal neurologic deficits. Brain imaging demonstrates multiple areas of stroke.

XI-84.   **The answer is B.** *(Chap. 379)* Carpal tunnel syndrome is caused by entrapment of the median nerve at the wrist. Symptoms begin with paresthesias in the median nerve distribution. With worsening, atrophy and weakness may develop. This condition is most commonly caused by excessive use of the wrist. Rarely, systemic disease may result in carpal tunnel syndrome. This may be suspected when bilateral disease is apparent. Tenosynovitis with arthritis as in the case of rheumatoid arthritis and thickening of the connective tissue as in the case of amyloid or acromegaly are also causes. Other systemic diseases, such as hypothyroidism and diabetes mellitus, are also possible etiologies. Leukemia is not typically associated with carpal tunnel syndrome.

XII. DERMATOLOGY

QUESTIONS

DIRECTIONS: Choose the **one best** response to each question.

XII-1. All of the following statements regarding atopic dermatitis are true *except*

A. 80% of children with atopic dermatitis also coexpress allergic rhinitis or asthma.

B. Exacerbations and remissions are typical.

C. Patients with atopic dermatitis often have increased levels of circulating IgE.

D. The adult form of atopic dermatitis is commonly localized to the hands.

E. When one parent is affected with atopic dermatitis, there is an 80% prevalence of atopic dermatitis in the children.

XII-2. A patient with acne vulgaris is considering treatment with isotretinoin. Her acne has been refractory to oral antibiotics and topical washes. In addition to counseling regarding the teratogenic effects of this medication, which other side effect has been documented with isotretinoin for the treatment of acne vulgaris?

A. Bradycardia

B. Cutaneous lymphomas

C. Fugue state

D. Hypertriglyceridemia

E. Tooth discoloration

XII-3. A 42-year-old man recently returned from a 2-week antelope hunting/camping trip to Tanzania. Near the end of the trip, he noted a painful sore on his foot that has become worse and is pictured in the figure (Color Atlas, Figure XII-3). He is concerned about the possibility of trypanosomiasis. Which of the following is most likely to yield a diagnosis?

A. Light microscopy of fluid from the skin lesion

B. Polymerase chain reaction (PCR) from the serum

C. Serology from the serum

D. Stool analysis for parasites

E. Urinary antigen testing

XII-4. Androgen excess in women affects terminal hair growth patterns. In states of androgen excess, the upper lip, chin,

XII-4. *(Continued)*
chest, upper arms, and thighs, for example, can become hirsute. In the same person, however, hair growth on the scalp resembles male-pattern balding (androgenic alopecia). What best describes the reason for the different effects of androgens on hair growth on the scalp compared to other areas?

A. Androgen levels in the scalp are lower than they are in other parts of the body.

B. Hirsutism causes stress, which leads to male-pattern balding.

C. In the scalp, androgen excess causes hair to spend less time in the growth phase.

D. Sun-exposed areas tend to be less androgen-sensitive.

XII-5. A 22-year-old woman comes to your office concerned about sun exposure. She brings a few sun block creams into your office and wants to know which one is best for preventing wrinkling and blotchiness. She is less concerned about sunburn because she is trying to get a better tan. Blocking which ultraviolet rays will achieve her desired result?

A. UV-A

B. UV-B

C. Both UV-A and UV-B equally

D. Neither UV-A nor UV-B

XII-6. Identify this skin lesion (see Color Atlas, Figure XII-6).

A. Herpes simplex virus

B. Molluscum contagiosum

C. Scabies

D. Tinea corporis

XII-7. A 48-year-old diabetic man presents to the emergency department complaining of blistering of the skin. One week prior, he was seen by his cardiologist, where he was started on a new blood pressure medication. His major complaints are blisters on his arms, chest, and face and pruritus. On physical examination, he is afebrile. The "blisters" are actually shallow erosions associated with erythema, scale, and crust formation, Nikolsky's sign is

XII-7. *(Continued)*

present. There is no involvement of the scalp or any mucous membranes. A skin biopsy reveals IgG on the surface of keratinocytes, and there is intraepidermal vesicle formation. Much of the destruction is just beneath the stratum corneum. Basal keratinocytes, and the epidermal basement membrane are spared. Anti-Dsg1 and anti-IgG antibodies are found in the peripheral blood. Which of these statements is true regarding the disease this patient has?

A.   An endemic form of this disease is found in Latin America and Tunisia.

B.   This condition is likely to require plasmapheresis.

C.   There is high likelihood that this patient has an occult Hodgkin's lymphoma.

D.   This patient also probably has a gluten-sensitive enteropathy.

XII-8.   You are evaluating a 33-year-old woman complaining of dry hands. She is a cleaning lady who has had the slow progression of erythema and edema, which has evolved into fissuring and crusting on the palmar aspect of the hand and wrist. She has been using gloves at work, with minimal improvement, and has started using lubricating creams. Her past medical history is significant only for seasonal allergic rhinitis. The hands appear to be the only areas involved (see Color Atlas, Figure XII-8). The rest of her physical examination is normal. What is the most appropriate treatment for this patient at this time?

A.   Cephalexin 250 mg orally 4 times a day for 7–10 days

B.   High-potency topical steroids

C.   Hydroxyzine, 25 mg orally every 6 hours

D.   Oral prednisone (1 mg/kg) tapered over 2–3 weeks

E.   Topical retinoic acid

XII-9.   A 29-year-old man complains of a rash on his chest (see Color Atlas, Figure XII-9). He has no other associated symptoms and there is no pain or pruritus. It has grown slowly over the past 4 months. He is monogamous in a homosexual relationship and has never been tested for HIV infection. He smokes tobacco occasionally. He takes no medications. On physical examination, he has no other lesions and no lymphadenopathy. Which of the following conditions do you expect this patient to have?

A.   Hepatitis C infection

B.   Human herpes virus 8 (HHV-8) infection

C.   Scabies infection

D.   *Staphylococcus aureus* colonization

E.   Subacute bacterial endocarditis

XII-10.   A 28-year-old woman comes to your office because of hirsutism. She has dealt with this problem for the past 4 months mainly by the use of waxing and bleaching, but the hirsutism now involves her chest and she is rapidly developing male-pattern balding. She has no other past medical history, is unmarried, and has no children. She takes no medications. She scores 18 on the Ferriman-

XII-10. *(Continued)*

Gallwey hirsutism scale (normal <8). What is the initial step in her evaluation?

A.   Dexamethasone suppression test

B.   Measurement of total testosterone level

C.   Trial of laser phototherapy

D.   Trial of oral contraceptive pills

E.   Spironolactone

XII-11.   The patient you are evaluating has had the rash on her face shown in Figure XII-11 (Color Atlas) gradually grow over the last 6 weeks. She complains of only slight pruritus but is mostly concerned about her appearance. The lesions are not painful. Her past medical history is unremarkable and on review of systems she has dandruff. All of the following historic features are likely *except*

A.   difficulty rising from a seated position

B.   HIV infection

C.   improvement with antidandruff shampoo

D.   lesions worsen with emotional stress

E.   serum antibodies to *Malassezia furfur*

XII-12.   A 52-year-old man is concerned about changes in the appearance of his skin. He has developed thick skin on his forearms, face, and the dorsum of his hands. He occasionally develops vesicles and bullae that will rupture, leaving moist erosions that heal slowly. He has noticed increased hair growth in these areas as well. Past medical history is significant for hepatitis C infection that he cleared spontaneously 3 years ago. He takes no medications. He drinks alcohol socially. His skin lesions are shown in Figure XII-12 (see Color Atlas). What is the best treatment option for this patient?

A.   β-carotene

B.   Fluconazole

C.   Glucocorticoids

D.   Phlebotomy

E.   UV-A and UV-B protection

XII-13.   What disease is likely causing this facial rash (see Color Atlas, Figure XII-13)?

A.   Dermatomyositis

B.   Rheumatoid arthritis

C.   Sarcoid

D.   Scleroderma

E.   Systemic lupus erythematosus

XII-14.   You are evaluating a patient with a chronic rash who comes in for treatment. The patient is a 28-year-old man who complains of chronically pruritic skin with scaly, plaque-like eruptions on the knees, gluteal cleft, and scalp. He has also noticed "potholes" in his fingernails bilaterally. On review of systems, he also notes early-morning back pain, which improves with movement, and intense dandruff. The scalp lesions have significantly limited his quality of life due to the constant scaling. He has no other past

XII-14. *(Continued)*
medical history and has never been treated for this before. When considering possible treatment regimens for this disorder, all of the following may be considered *except*

A. acitretin
B. cyclosporine
C. methotrexate
D. prednisone
E. UV light therapy

XII-15. A 32-year-old woman receives amoxicillin/clavulanate for presumed bacterial sinusitis. One week later she presents with a diffuse itchy rash (see Color Atlas, Figure XII-15). Her mucus membranes are normal. Which of the following is the most likely diagnosis?

A. Morbilliform drug eruption
B. Pemphigus vulgaris
C. Stevens-Johnson syndrome
D. Toxic shock syndrome
E. Urticaria

XII-16. A patient comes into your office to see you about the intensely pruritic rash (see Color Atlas, Figure XII-16). The rash started with intense burning sensations 24 h prior to the eruptions. On examination of the skin, involved areas are mostly the extensor surfaces of the skin. Mucous membranes are spared. There are many areas of excoriation on top of the papulovesicular lesions. You make a diagnosis and initiate treatment with dapsone and advise the patient to refrain from gluten-containing foods. The patient returns to your clinic 2 months later and has improved greatly. Which other condition is this patient likely to have?

A. Ankylosing spondylitis
B. Atrophic gastritis
C. Carpal tunnel syndrome
D. Type 1 diabetes mellitus

XII-17. You have been managing a patient with a severe case of tinea pedis with oral therapy. Two weeks into the treatment course, the patient develops thickened and opacified nails on the right hand. The left hand fingernails are affected to a lesser degree. The nails have become discolored and have significant debris under the nail. Nail scrapings from the fingernails are most likely to grow which organism?

XII-17. *(Continued)*
A. *Candida* spp.
B. *Malassezia* spp.
C. *Rhizopogon* spp.
D. *Trichophyton* spp.

XII-18. A patient presents to you for evaluation of this lesion, which has been on his skin for 6 months. The lesion began as a red papule with a thick adherent scale (see Color Atlas, Figure XII-18). Since that time, it has progressed to the current pictured lesion with raised borders and scars. There has been no improvement with use of topical glucocorticoids, which the patient borrowed from a friend. What is the best course of action for this patient at this time?

A. Aminoquinoline antimalarials
B. Azathioprine
C. Systemic glucocorticoids
D. Vitamin E ointment
E. Wide surgical excision with regional lymph node dissection

XII-19. During a trip to Afghanistan, you are asked to see a young woman with the following lesion on her face (see Color Atlas, Figure XII-19). She is otherwise healthy and states that the lesion has been there for 3 weeks. Other family members have had similar lesions on their arms and feet. She has no shortness of breath, fevers, chills, or weight loss. This is the only lesion on her body. Based on local epidemiology and light microscopy of a skin biopsy, you diagnose leishmaniasis. What is the mode of transmission of this parasite?

A. Inhalation of spores
B. Mosquito bite
C. Sandfly bite
D. Tsetse fly bite
E. Undercooked pork

XII-20. Which of the following comorbid conditions is a relative contraindication for the use of oral agents for treating onychomycosis of the toenails?

A. Chronic kidney disease
B. Hepatitis
C. Leukopenia
D. Poorly controlled diabetes mellitus
E. Schizophrenia

XII. DERMATOLOGY

ANSWERS

XII-1. The answer is E. *(Chap. 53)* The clinical course of atopic dermatitis (AD) is characterized by exacerbations and remissions. Lesions are typically pruritic and appear similar to those of eczematous dermatitis. Patients with AD have increased production of IgE and increased serum levels. Delayed-type hypersensitivity reactions, however, are impaired. Most children with AD also have atopy manifested as allergic rhinitis, asthma, food allergies, or eczema. When both parents have AD, >80% of their children will have AD. When only one parent is affected, the prevalence falls to ~50%. Half of all children will continue to suffer with AD into adulthood. The distribution may be the same as in childhood, but more commonly the disease becomes localized, such as in hand eczema.

XII-2. The answer is D. *(Chap. 53)* Due to the well-known teratogenic effects of retinoic acid derivatives, all patients must be enrolled in a program designed to prevent pregnancy before initiation of a treatment regimen. Moreover, negative pregnancy tests must be obtained prior to each prescription refill. In addition, patients with a personal or family history of hypertriglyceridemia or a personal history of diabetes should be cautioned about the risks of hypertriglyceridemia and poor glucose control. Serum triglycerides should be followed during therapy. Concerns regarding a link between isotretinoin use and developing depression have not been proven. Tooth discoloration is a risk in children who receive tetracycline or related antibiotics.

XII-3. The answer is A. *(Chap. 206)* Human African trypanosomiasis (HAT) is due to infection by the flagellated protozoan *Trypanosoma brucei gambiense* (West African) or *T. brucei rhodesiense* (East African). It is transmitted by the bite of the tsetse fly. Both organisms may lead to fatal neurologic impairment (sleeping sickness) if not treated. HAT usually presents with a trypanosomal chancre that is painful and located at the site of inoculation. An acute febrile illness usually follows due to hematogenous and lymphatic dissemination. East African HAT is generally more acute than West African HAT. Central nervous system manifestations may occur within a year for East African HAT and in months to years for West African HAT. The definitive diagnosis for HAT requires identification of the parasite. Efforts should be made to examine blood, fluid from sores, lymph node aspirate, and/or cerebrospinal fluid. Fluid from the chancre may show the protozoite by direct examination or by Giemsa stain. PCR tests have been developed, but none are commercially available. Serologic tests vary in their sensitivity and specificity and are not recommended as tools to impact treatment. Stool analysis does not have a role in the diagnosis of HAT. Treatment of early-stage East African HAT is with suramin.

XII-4. The answer is C. *(Chap. 50)* There are three phases in the cycle of hair growth—the growth, involution, and rest. Androgen excess in women leads to increased hair growth in most androgen-sensitive sites. In the scalp, however, hair loss occurs because androgens cause the hair to spend less time in the growth phase. Male-pattern balding may cause stress but is primarily caused by high androgen levels. Androgen levels are equally distributed throughout the body; it is the local environment that dictates the end-organ effect. Sun-exposed areas, such as the face and arms, are as androgen-sensitive as nonexposed areas.

XII-5.　The answer is A.　*(Chap. 57)*　The UV spectrum reaching the earth is arbitrarily divided into two major segments: UV-A and UV-B. The outermost epidermal layer, the stratum corneum, is a major absorber of UV-B, and <10% of incident UV-B wavelengths penetrate through the epidermis to the dermis. In contrast, UV-A readily penetrates to the dermis. Photons in the UV-B are 1000-fold more efficient than photons in the UV-A in evoking the sunburn response. UV-B is primarily responsible for the sunburn response and for vitamin D photochemistry. UV-A is important in the pathogenesis of photoaging in human skin.

XII-6.　The answer is B.　*(Chap. e10)*　Molluscum contagiosum classically presents with umbilicated papules, as seen in this photo. A vesicular lesion with an inflammatory base is characteristic of herpes simplex. Tinea corporis presents with a circular, scaly plaque. Scabies lesions are frequently found in interdigital web spaces and usually consist of inflammatory papules.

XII-7.　The answer is C.　*(Chap. 55)*　This patient has pemphigus foliaceus (PF), an autoimmune cutaneous disorder similar to pemphigus vulgaris (PV). PF is distinguished from PV by the fact that PF is a more superficial disorder than PV. The acantholytic blisters in PF are located high in the epidermis, usually just below the stratum corneum. In PF, mucous membranes are always spared. *Fogo selvagem* is the endemic form of PF. PF is associated with several autoimmune diseases; however, its association with thymoma and/or myasthenia gravis is most notable. Patients can develop PF after exposure to drugs containing a thiol group (e.g., penicillamine, captopril, enalapril). PF usually responds to topical or systemic glucocorticoids. PV is often associated with lymphoreticular malignant diseases such as lymphoma or Hodgkin's disease.

XII-8.　The answer is B.　*(Chap. 53)*　This patient has irritant contact dermatitis. Most patients have a history of atopy. Contact dermatitis usually resolves with removal of the offending agent or with barrier protection (e.g., gloves) of the involved area. When crusting and fissuring are present, lubricating creams are helpful. Adjunctive therapies include high-potency topical steroids while the dermatitis runs its course. For patients who fail topical steroids, systemic therapy with oral prednisone will usually suffice. Hydroxyzine, an oral antihistamine, is useful when pruritus is a predominant complaint or when the lesion is thought to be due to scratching or rubbing, as in lichen simplex chronicus. Empirical antibiotics are not useful in the absence of signs of infection. Topical retinoic acid is an irritant and will worsen the skin inflammation and discomfort.

XII-9.　The answer is B.　*(Chaps. 94 and 182)*　The lesion shown is Kaposi's sarcoma (KS). The lesion is also commonly found on the extremities, face, and in the oral cavity. It typically appears as painless purple/brown macules, plaques, and nodules. They may be confused with other pigmented lesions. KS is the only sarcoma associated with a virus (HHV-8). The most common presentation is in patients infected with HIV, usually with advanced immunosuppression with CD4+ T cell counts <200/μL. Folliculitis due to *Staphylococcus aureus* causes more pain and redness. The cutaneous embolic or immunologic manifestations of bacterial endocarditis are smaller and typically found in the extremities. Hepatitis C infection may cause skin lesions due to cryoglobulinemia; however, these appear as vasculitic lesions typically on the lower extremities. There is no relation between hepatitis C infection and KS. Scabies infection will cause itchy papules and burrows.

XII-10.　The answer is B.　*(Chap. 50)*　Hirsutism is a common outpatient complaint and may be caused by hyperandrogenism, endocrine disorders, pregnancy, drugs, or congenital abnormalities. This patient has rapidly progressive virilization and concern should be present for a virilizing tumor. A number of options exist to rule out a virilizing tumor including measurement of the testosterone level or dehydroepiandrosterone sulfate (DHEAS) level. Further imaging will localize a mass, if present, in the adrenals or ovaries. Empirical therapy with an oral contraceptive or with spironolactone would be indicated if the laboratory and radiographic evaluation does not reveal a virilizing tumor. Laser therapy will be effective at removing the hair, but the long-term effects are yet to be determined. As shown in the figure, dexamethasone suppression is useful to distinguish adrenal versus ovarian causes of excess androgens and may be utilized after assessing testosterone and DHEAS.

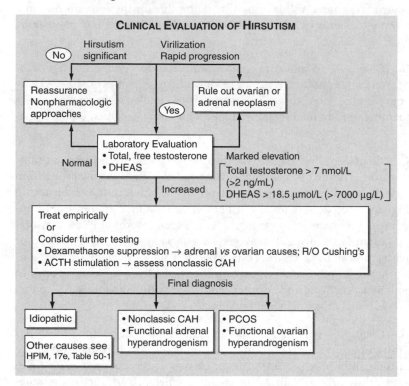

FIGURE XII-10 Algorithm for the evaluation and differential diagnosis of hirsutism. ACTH, adrenocorticotropic hormone; CAH, congenital adrenal hyperplasia; DHEAS, sulfated form of dehydroepi-androsterone; PCOS, polycystic ovarian syndrome.

XII-11. **The answer is A.** *(Chap. 53)* Seborrheic dermatitis is a common skin disorder, for which the majority of patients lack any predisposing conditions. It is characterized by greasy scales overlying erythematous plaques or patches. Induration and scale are less prominent than in psoriasis. The lesions are variably pruritic and may either improve or worsen with sunlight exposure. Pruritus is also variable. The most common location is the scalp, where it may manifest as severe dandruff. On the face, the most common locations are the eyebrows, eyelids, glabella, and nasolabial folds. Lesions typically worsen in the winter, and emotional stress also seems to exacerbate the rash. Seborrheic dermatitis is commonly seen in patients with Parkinson's disease, facial nerve palsies, and HIV infection. The pathogenesis remains unclear but the yeast *Malassezia furfur* appears to play a role. Successful treatment with topical ketoconazole and the prevalence of the disease in immunocompromised patients suggests that the yeast is pathogenic. Patients with dermatomyositis may exhibit a heliotrope rash (violaceous rash around the eyelids) and may complain of proximal muscle weakness.

XII-12. **The answer is D.** *(Chap. 57)* This patient has porphyria cutanea tarda (PCT). The description and appearance are classic for this disease, and a history of hepatitis C virus infection is an independent risk factor for PCT. Treatment consists of repeated phlebotomy to diminish excessive hepatic iron stores. β-carotene is a treatment option for erythropoietic protoporphyria which is differentiated from PCT by the acute photosensitivity, burning, and stinging that occurs after sun exposure in the former. UV protection is not specifically part of the treatment of PCT but is helpful for preventing the photoaging process. This is not an autoimmune process where glucocorticoids would potentially be of benefit. Secondary fungal infections may occur that require antifungal therapy.

XII-13. **The answer is A.** *(Chap. e10)* This image demonstrates the heliotrope rash of dermatomyositis. Lupus and sarcoid can both present with facial rashes; however, the periorbital involvement seen here is more associated with dermatomyositis. Rheumatoid arthritis and scleroderma are not distinctly associated with facial rashes.

XII-14. **The answer is D.** *(Chap. 53)* Psoriasis is a common chronic inflammatory skin disease. It is characterized by erythematous, sharply demarcated papules and rounded plaques covered by a silvery scale. The lesions are highly pruritic. Traumatized areas often develop lesions (Koebner phenomenon). Infections, stress, and medications may exacerbate psoriasis. Fingernail lesions such as pitting, onycholysis, or nail thickening or subungual hyperkeratosis are present in 50% of patients. Topical treatment options for psoriasis include mid-potency glucocorticoids, vitamin D analogues, retinoids, and ultraviolet light. Systemic therapy is reserved for severe or widespread disease. Oral glucocorticoids should not be used for the treatment of psoriasis due to the life-threatening risk of developing pustular psoriasis when therapy is discontinued. Systemic therapies approved by the U.S. Food and Drug Administration include methotrexate, retinoids, calcineurin inhibitors, and biologic agents (anti-tumor necrosis factor, anti-CD11a, anti-CD2).

XII-15. **The answer is A.** *(Chap. 56)* Morbilliform drug eruptions are the most common drug reactions. They typically begin on the trunk and consist of symmetric macules and papules that may become confluent. Moderate to severe pruritus is common. In contrast to Stevens-Johnson syndrome and toxic shock syndrome, involvement of the mucus membranes is uncommon. The principal differential diagnosis is viral exanthem, particularly in children. The rash usually develops within 1 week of initiation of therapy and resolves with discontinuation. The most common drugs that cause morbilliform eruptions include penicillin derivatives, allopurinol, sulfonamides, and nonsteroidal anti-inflammatories. Urticaria consists of superficial well-defined wheals that are pruritic. Penicillins may cause IgE-mediated urticaria. Pemphigus is an autoimmune bullous disease of the skin and mucus membranes that is rarely associated with drugs such as penicillin.

XII-16. **The answer is B.** *(Chap. 55)* The patient has classic symptoms of dermatitis herpetiformis (DH)—an intensely pruritic rash that is sometimes heralded by burning sensations 24 h prior to arrival of the rash. Biopsy of this lesion would show neutrophil-rich infiltrates in the dermal papillae. Over 90% of patients with DH express the HLA-B8/DRw3 and HLA-DQw2 haplotypes. Ankylosing spondylitis is associated with expression of HLA-B27. Patients with DH also have a high incidence of thyroid abnormalities, achlorhydria, atrophic gastritis, and antigastric parietal cell autoantibodies. There is no association with carpal tunnel syndrome or type 1 diabetes mellitus.

XII-17. **The answer is D.** *(Chap. 53)* Dermatophytes that commonly infect the skin, hair, and nails include members of the genera *Trichophyton*, *Epidermophyton*, and *Microsporum*. Tinea pedis is commonly associated with tinea manuum, unguium, or cruris (dermatophytosis of the hands, nails, or groin, respectively). Scratching the foot with the hand is a common mode of spreading the infection. *Malassezia* spp. is the pathologic agent in tinea versicolor and is thought to be pathogenic in seborrheic dermatitis. Candidal onychomycosis usually occurs only in the immunocompromised host or with chronic mucocutaneous candidiasis.

XII-18. **The answer is A.** *(Chap. 55)* The patient has discoid lupus erythematosus (DLE) or chronic cutaneous lupus erythematosus. It is characterized by discrete lesions most often on the face, scalp, or ears. The lesions are usually erythematous papules or plaques with a thick scale that occludes hair follicles. The lesions persist for years and grow slowly. Less than 10% of patients with DLE meet criteria for systemic lupus erythematosus (SLE), although skin lesions are common in patients with SLE. Chronically, the lesions evolve to look similar to the one pictured. Treatment consists of topical or intralesional glucocorticoids. If that is ineffective, systemic therapy with an aminoquinoline antimalarial may be indicated. Systemic glucocorticoids or immunosuppressives are not indicated for localized disease. Although malignant melanoma may take on myriad appearances, the location, progress, and description of this lesion is more suggestive of discoid lupus, therefore, surgical excision and lymph node dissection are not indicated at this time. Vitamin E ointment has no proven role in the treatment of DLE.

XII-19. **The answer is C.** *(Chap. 205)* Lesions of cutaneous leishmaniasis progress from papules to plaques to atrophic scars with central necrosis and ulceration. Multiple primary lesions, regional adenopathy, and secondary bacterial infection are variably present. *Leishmania* parasites are transmitted by the bite of the female phlebotomine sandfly. While probing for a blood meal, sandflies regurgitate the parasite's flagellated promastigote stage into the host's skin, which eventually get phagocytized by macrophages. The larvae of *Trichinella spiralis* are found in undercooked pork and game meat and cause the syndrome of trichonosis. Inhalation of the spores of *Bacillus anthracis* causes the pulmonary form of anthrax infection. The tsetse fly is the vector for the trypanosome parasite, which can cause sleeping sickness. Mosquito bites transmit a number of infections, most notably malaria and a variety of viral infections such as viral encephalitis.

XII-20. **The answer is B.** *(Chap. 53)* Oral antifungal agents are required for effective treatment of dermaphytosis of the hair or nails. Treatment requires prolonged courses of drug (e.g., 2–18 months) and exposes the patient to an increased risk of adverse reaction to the drug. All of the oral agents carry a risk of hepatotoxicity. They should not be used in women who are pregnant or breast-feeding. Griseofulvin is approved for dermatophyte infections of the skin, hair, or nails. Itraconazole and terbinafine are approved for onychomycosis. With terbinafine therapy, there is also a risk of drug-drug interaction with drugs that require the P450 enzyme for metabolism. Most treatment courses require serial monitoring of liver enzymes to avoid drug-induced hepatitis or liver failure.

REFERENCES

Adrogué HJ, Madias NE: Management of life-threatening acid–base disorders. *N Engl J Med* 338:26–34, 1998

Baker DG, Schumacher HR, Jr: Acute monoarthritis. *N Engl J Med* 329:1013–1020, 1993

Bennett CL: Thrombotic thrombocytopenic purpura associated with clopidogrel. *J Am Coll Cardiol* 50:1138, 2007

Beral V et al: Breast cancer and breastfeeding. *Lancet* 360: 187–195, 2002

Brickner ME, Hillis LD, Lange RA: Congenital heart disease in adults. *N Engl J Med* 342:256–263, 2000

Camm AJ, Garratt CJ: Adenosine and supraventricular tachycardia. *N Engl J Med* 325:1621–1629, 1991

Collaborative Group on Hormonal Factors in Breast Cancer: Breast cancer and breast feeding: Collaborative reanalysis of individual data from 47 epidemiologic studies in 30 countries, including 50302 women with breast cancer and 96973 women without the disease. *Lancet* 360: 187–195, 2002

Crapo R et al: Arterial blood gas reference values for sea level and an altitude of 1400 meters. *Am J Respir Crit Care Med* 160:1525–1531, 1999

Dezee KJ et al: Treatment of excessive anticoagulation with phytonadione (Vitamin K): A meta-analysis. *Arch Intern Med* 166:391–397, 2006

Duggan C et al: Inherited and acquired risk factors for venous thromboembolic disease among women taking tamoxifen to prevent breast cancer. *J Clin Oncol* 21: 3588–3593, 2003

Eagle KA et al: ACC/AHA guideline update for perioperative cardiovascular evaluation for noncardiac surgery—executive summary. *J Am Coll Cardiol* 39:542, 2002

Frank MM: Complement in the pathophysiology of human disease. *N Engl J Med* 316:1523–1530, 1987

Hahn AF: The challenge of respiratory dysfunction in Guillain-Barré syndrome. *Arch Neurol* 58(6):871–872, 2001

Ifudu O: Care of patients undergoing hemodialysis. *N Engl J Med* 339:1054–1062, 1998

Laffey JG et al: Ventilation with lower tidal volumes as compared with traditional tidal volumes for acute lung injury. *N Engl J Med* 343:812–814, 2000

Lawn ND et al: Anticipating mechanical ventilation in Guillain-Barré syndrome. *Arch Neurol* 58:893–898, 2001

Lee TH et al: Derivation and prospective validation of a simple index for prediction of cardiac risk of major noncardiac surgery. *Circulation* 100:1043, 1999

Loftus EV: Microscopic colitis: Epidemiology and treatment. *Am J Gastroenterol* 98(12 Suppl):S31–S36, 2003

The Matisse Investigators: Subcutaneous fondaparinux versus intravenous unfractionated heparin in the initial treatment of pulmonary embolism. *N Engl J Med* 349:1695–1702, 2003

Morris TA et al: No difference in risk for thrombocytopenia during treatment of pulmonary embolism and deep venous thrombosis with either low-molecular-weight heparin or unfractionated heparin: A metaanalysis. *Chest* 132:1131, 2007

Ost D, Fein AM, Feinsilver SH: The solitary pulmonary nodule. *N Engl J Med* 348:2535–2542, 2003

Ridker PM, et al: Mutation in the gene coding for coagulation factor V and the risk of myocardial infarction, stroke, and venous thrombosis in apparently healthy men. *N Engl J Med* 332:912, 1995

Rubin HR et al: Patient ratings of dialysis care with peritoneal dialysis versus hemodialysis. *JAMA* 291:321–333, 2002

Shen J et al: Polymorphic makers of the glycogen debranching enzyme gene allowing linkage analysis in families with glycogen storage disease type III. *J Med Genet* 34:34–38, 1997

Smith RA et al: American Cancer Society Guidelines for the early detection of cancer, 2004. *CA Cancer J Clin* 54:41–52, 2004

Smitt PS et al: Paraneoplastic cerebellar ataxia due to autoantibodies against a glutamate receptor. *N Engl J Med* 342:21–27, 2000

Wilt TJ et al: Saw palmetto extracts for treatment of benign prostatic hyperplasia: A systematic review. *JAMA* 280: 1604–1609, 1998

NOTES

NOTES

NOTES

NOTES

NOTES

NOTES

COLOR ATLAS

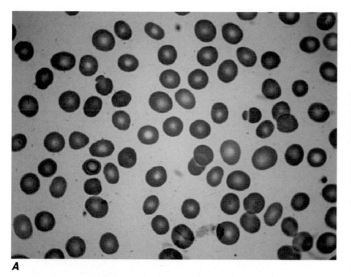

A

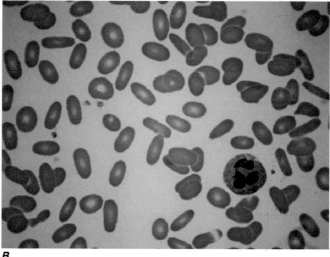

B

Figure III-21

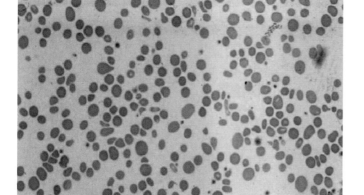

C

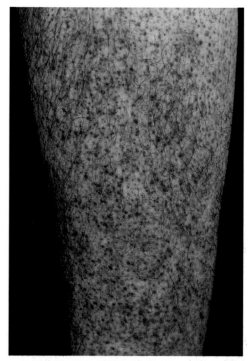

Figure II-3

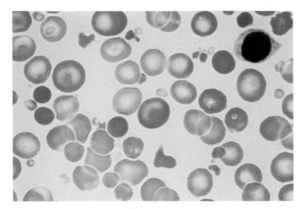

Figure III-6

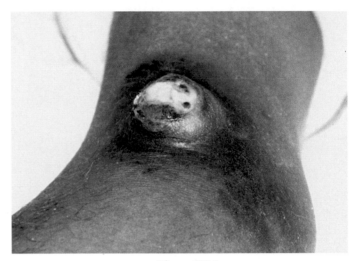

Figure IV-2

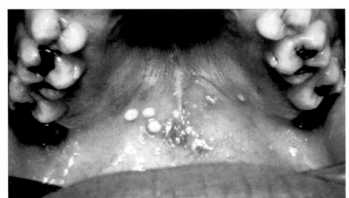

Figure IV-57

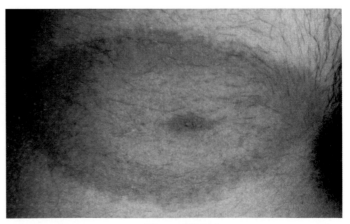

Figure IV-121

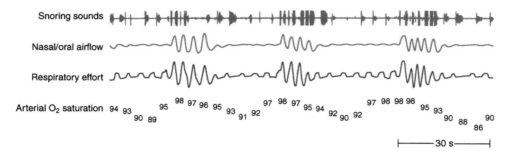

Figure VI-32

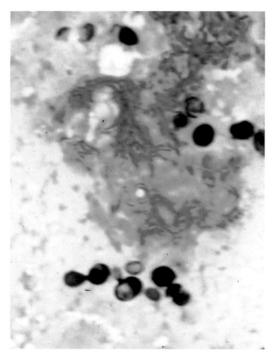

Figure VI-30

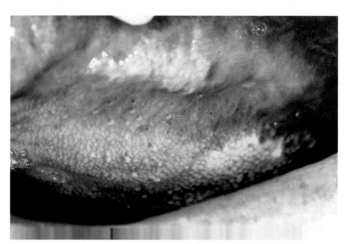

Figure IV-158

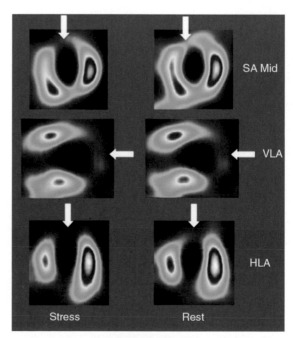

Figure V-115

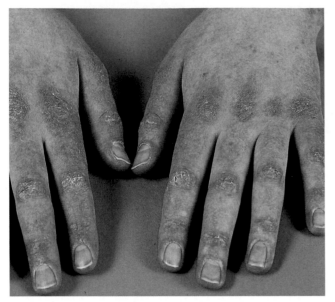

Figure XI-62

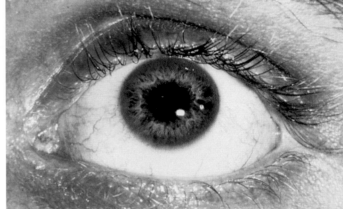

Figure X-14

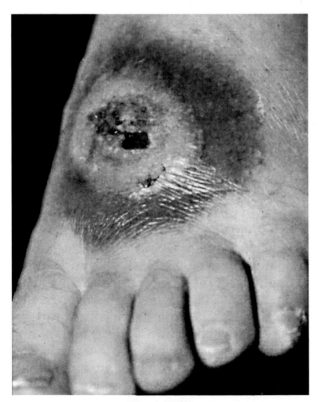

Figure XII-3

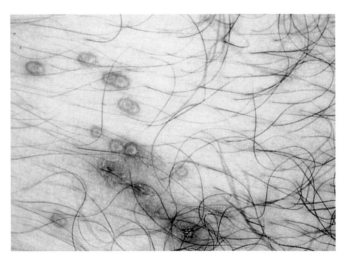

Figure XII-6

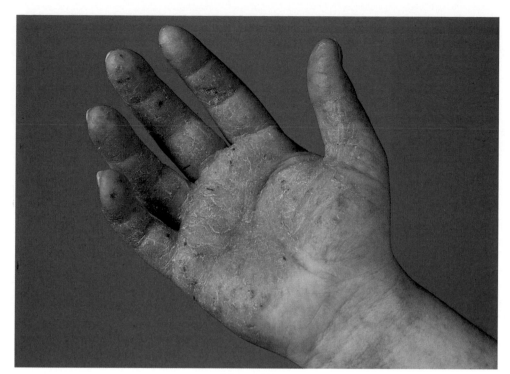

Figure XII-8

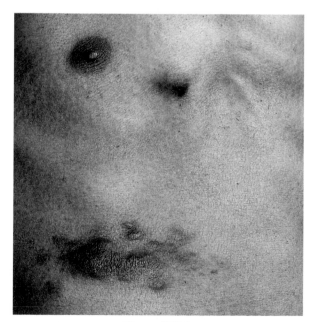

Figure XII-9

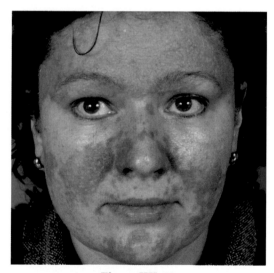

Figure XII-11

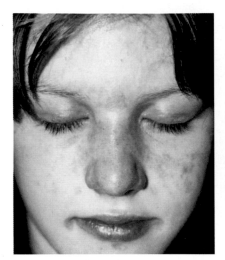

Figure XII-13

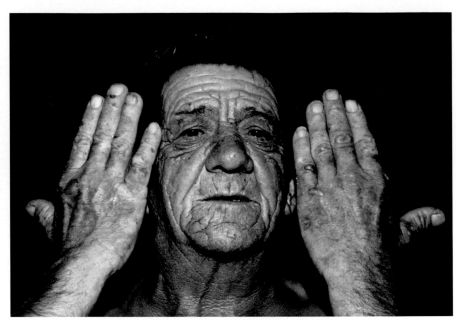

Figure XII-12

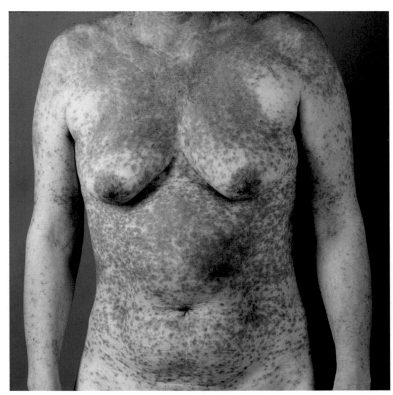

Figure XII-15

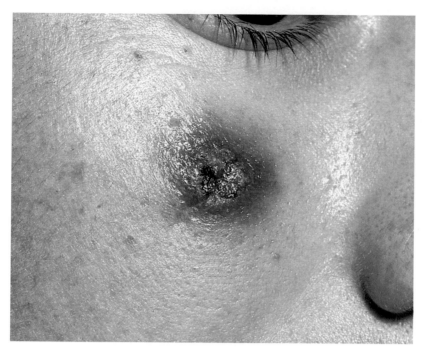

Figure XII-19

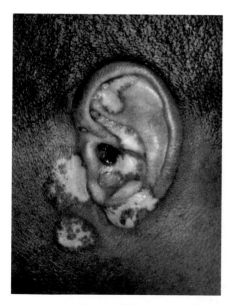

Figure XII-18

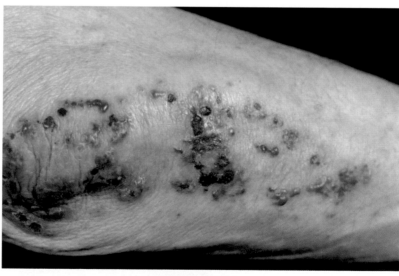

Figure XII-16

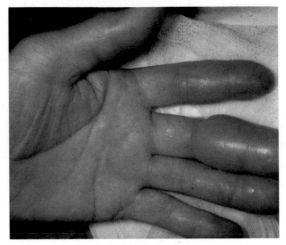

Figure I-36

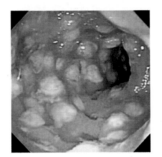

Figure VIII-76

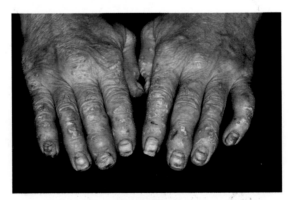

Figure IX-49